Contents

CHAPTER 3
Neuromuscular Physical Therapy 53

CHAPTER 4
Cardiac, Vascular and Lymphatic Physical Therapy 95

CHAPTER 5
Pulmonary Physical Therapy ...127

CHAPTER 9
Geriatric Physical Therapy 223

CHAPTER 10
Therapeutic Exercise Foundations 251

CHAPTER 11
Therapeutic Modalities 269

CHAPTER 12
Gait, Functional Training, Equipment and Devices 295

CHAPTER 13
Teaching & Learning 327

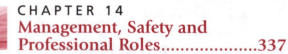

CHAPTER 14
Management, Safety and
Professional Roles....................337

CHAPTER 15
Research and Evidence-Based
Practice.....................................365

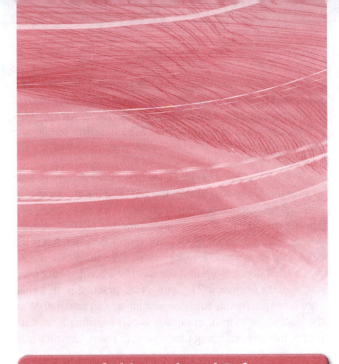

Introduction

RAYMOND P. SIEGELMAN

KAREN E. RYAN

Purpose of This Book and Software

TherapyEd's PTA Exam Review & Study Guide, 3rd Edition, Karen Ryan, author is designed to help you, the physical therapist assistant (PTA) candidate focus your preparation for the National Physical Therapy Examination [NPTE] for Physical Therapist Assistants. Each chapter is presented in easy-to-read outline format. The chapters emphasize the major elements presented in the Content Outline of the NPTE. Specific chapters focus on pediatric, geriatric, cardiopulmonary, neurological, musculoskeletal and other aspects of physical therapy practice. It is vital for the PTA candidate to be able to incorporate knowledge of normal and pathological conditions, interventions and patient response to clinical situations. Additionally, Chapter 1 is dedicated to helping you structure your review process and prepare to take the licensure examination. It is hoped that the outlined contents presented will help organize and focus your review and do so in an efficient and effective manner. This text will provide a basic review. You may elect to pursue a more in-depth review of topics, terms or procedures that may require additional study by referring to recommended references.

The software containing simulated examinations should enable you to determine whether you have sufficient mastery of a particular content area and are able to apply it correctly to the clinical situation described in the question. The practice examination format tries to mimic the actual NPTE format. There is a question counter and running clock at the top of the computer screen. You have the ability to mark and retrieve questions you would like to view again. The computer programming will analyze your results and will provide feedback to help you focus on deficient areas and need for additional study. The computer-based questions with the correct answer in bold type and rationales are provided in the back of this text. The exercise of reading and interpreting these practice questions should also help prepare you for the various forms and appearances of the actual NPTE multiple-choice questions.

What is the Procedure for Obtaining and Retaining a License to Practice as a PTA?

Regulation (licensure, registration, certification) of health care practitioners by the states and other jurisdictions of the United States is a means by which the public is protected from incompetent or immoral practitioners. In the United States, nearly all jurisdictions require PTAs to be regulated in some manner to practice. Regulation is a function of the state or territorial governments, not the federal government. The onus is on the candidate for regulation to demonstrate competency.

All jurisdictions which regulate PTAs require the candidate to successfully complete the National Physical Therapy Examination for Physical Therapist Assistants. What can be confusing is that each state may have different requirements to fulfill in order to become eligible to take the NPTE. These requirements may differ from state to state or within the same state depending upon whether or not the candidate graduated from a PTA program accredited by the Commission on Accreditation in Physical Therapy (CAPTE). Each state has sovereignty over PTA regulation.

Contact the individual regulatory board in the state or jurisdiction in which you are seeking regulation to obtain applications and information about requirements and procedures. Complete the application materials and submit them to the regulatory authority in which you seek regulation along with required payment. On receiving and approving your application, the regulatory authority will approve your application and then notify the Federation of State Boards of Physical Therapy (FSBPT) of your eligibility to sit for the NPTE. If you are not ready to begin full time studying, do not forward all of the necessary monies or documentation to the state. When the FSBPT receives notification of your eligibility to sit for the examination, you will be sent an authorization-to-test letter. You will have 60 days from the date on this letter in which to schedule and take the NPTE. You may schedule your examination at a Prometric testing center by phone or online using the information provided in your authorization letter. You will be required to pay a computer usage fee upon scheduling your examination. Within the 60-day time frame you may cancel and/or reschedule your appointment; however, there may be a charge associated with this. On completion, the examination will be scored by the FSBPT and results reported to the regulatory authority in the jurisdiction in which you applied for regulation. The regulatory authority will notify you of the results. Results may be available in as little as 2 days; it may take as long as 7 to 10 days.

Candidates with documented disabilities may receive special accommodation during the examination. Special seating, extra time, a reader or other considerations are possible. Any special accommodation must be requested through and preapproved by the regulatory board. Candidates are encouraged to contact the FSBPT as well as review the *NPTE Candidate Handbook* for further information.

Some additional factors candidates may encounter are as follows:

JURISPRUDENCE EXAMINATION: some states require candidates to pass an examination concerning the rules, regulations and laws governing practice of physical therapy in that state. This written examination is in addition to the NPTE. PTAs who are already licensed and wish to obtain another license when moving to a different state may have to successfully complete a jurisprudence examination if required by that state.

FEES: all states require a fee to apply for and renew a license. There are separate fees to sit for the NPTE, which are paid to the FSBPT. Computer usage fees must also be paid to Prometric upon scheduling your examination. Fees vary widely and can change yearly.

TESTS OF ENGLISH LANGUAGE PROFICIENCY: various tests of spoken, written or comprehended English may be required if English is not a first language. Standards and requirements differ from state to state. Personal interviews may also be required.

AIDS AWARENESS TRAINING: a requirement for licensure in some states.

FINGERPRINTING, FBI CHECK, VACCINATION, MALPRACTICE INSURANCE: one or more may be required by some jurisdictions.

CREDENTIALS EVALUATION: may be required by PTAs who graduated from programs that are outside the United States or from programs not accredited by the CAPTE. This process may be required to establish eligibility to take the NPTE.

TEMPORARY LICENSE: some states grant a temporary license to a candidate eligible to take the NPTE. This allows the individual to practice under supervision prior to taking and passing the NPTE. If a candidate fails the NPTE, the temporary license may be revoked or it may be extended if the candidate immediately reapplies to take the exam again. Again, this depends upon the state. If a state does not offer a temporary license, a PTA may NOT practice in that state until all requirements for licensure have been satisfied. With the implementation of computer-based examinations, temporary licenses are being phased out in many jurisdictions.

TRANSFER OF SCORES TO OTHER JURISDICTIONS: all jurisdictions use the criterion-referenced grading method which standardizes exam scoring and allows transfer of passing scores without a problem. The FSBPT is responsible for score transfer. Contact the Score Transfer Service at http://www.fsbpt.net/pt. You may transfer your scores online or download the Score Transfer Request Form and mail the completed form to the Federation. There is a fee for this service. If you maintain regulation, you should not have to retake the NPTE if you move to a different state. However, if you are not licensed or regulated, let your regulation lapse or never took the examination, you will probably have to take it when seeking a license in jurisdictions that require PTA regulation.

RETAKING THE NPTE: some states limit the number of times one may take the NPTE. Three times per 12-month period is the limit for sitting for the examination. Some states only allow three opportunities to take the NPTE in total. If you fail, the state may impose a stipulation that you show evidence of some form of remedial work or study before retaking the NPTE. The state has an obligation to protect the public from practitioners who do not demonstrate competency.

LICENSE/REGULATION RENEWAL: after one, two or three years regulation must be renewed to continue practicing. The state or jurisdiction typically sends out a renewal notice. Sometimes renewal is an easy procedure. You just pay the fee and return the form. In some states, verification of continuing education units may be required to renew. The regulation may lapse if there is a failure to notify the state of a change of address and, thereby, not receive a renewal notice, or if there is a failure to respond to a renewal notice in a timely fashion, or if other requirements are not met. It is illegal to practice without valid regulation. The state may require a number of conditions be met in order to reinstate lapsed regulation. One condition might include retaking the

NPTE even if you had previously passed. Inform the regulatory board of any change of address. Do not let your regulation lapse!

CONTINUING EDUCATION: many states require the PTA to acquire a specific number of continuing education units (CEUs) in order to renew regulation. Documentation, approval and reporting of CEUs vary from state to state. The state may also require evidence of continuing active practice in order to renew. Continuing education requirements change from time to time; the regulation holder is responsible to know and meet any current requirements. Be sure to track the regulatory body's requirements on a regular basis. Currently, the American Physical Therapy Association and the Federation of State Boards are exploring alternative means for continued competency measurement or monitoring.

ENDORSEMENT: with valid regulation in one jurisdiction, a PTA may apply to another state for a "license by endorsement." All criteria established by the new state must be met. This can include taking a jurisprudence exam for that state, interviews, letters of recommendation, AIDS awareness, CEUs and so on. Contact the regulatory board in the state where license by endorsement is sought to get information and applications. Start the process early—it can take months!

How Is the Examination Developed?

The FSBPT is the organization that helps the various regulatory boards to coordinate the regulation of physical therapy practice. It is the FSBPT that owns the National Physical Therapy Examinations for both PTAs and physical therapists.

A large number of practitioners, educators and others contribute questions to the FSBPT. These items are designed to test knowledge and problem solving that reflects entry-level competency and the current practice expectations for PTAs. The exam covers knowledge of both entry-level academic and clinical training.

Various committees and psychometricians of the Federation help develop the "blueprint" for NPTE content, construct and fine-tune the questions. From a large pool of items, a group selects those that will be used on each examination.

Currently, the Federation does not publish the number of forms that exist for the exam; however, they do identify that a test taker can take the exam three times and not get the same items or same exam. Each examination adheres to the content blueprint in order to comprehensively and fairly assess a candidate's competency to practice. There is a degree of stability, consistency and continuity from examination to examination in terms of what is being assessed. Yet, each examination is a unique document with its own make-up and mix of old, new or revised questions. Questions are not derived from one specific textbook or narrow point of view. A list of texts commonly used in PTA programs can be found on the FSBPT website. Terminology is consistent with that used in the *Guide to Physical Therapist Practice* and other commonly used texts. There is usually a retooling of the examination questions every year; however, the Content Outline does not change and the basic examination format and content remain the same. When the Content Outline changes (and it does from time to time!) the examination reflects those changes. The FSBPT is moving to a format in which there are not specific versions of the exam, but a test bank from which exam questions are drawn. In this case, each exam taken would be different, but each would still meet the current blueprint. Items in the test bank will still go through the entire process used by the FSBPT to validate the question and determine its criterion referenced score prior to its use in scoring an exam.

Each candidate who sits for the NPTE must accept the NPTE Security Agreement. In part, this agreement states that it is illegal and unethical to recall (memorize) and share questions that are on the NPTE or to solicit questions that are on the NPTE from candidates who have taken the exam. The FSBPT has and will continue to actively prosecute individuals who violate the Security Agreement. This Security Agreement is necessary since questions may be reused on subsequent examinations.

The American Physical Therapy Association does not develop, oversee or administer the examination.

What Areas Does the Examination Cover?

There is a great emphasis on applying knowledge to the management of patient/client clinical situations and problems to safely and effectively treat patients consistent with the principles of best practice. However, the examination also deals with topics peripheral to direct patient care. These topics can include the PTA's role in safety, knowledge of professional roles, ethical decision making, teaching and learning and evidence-based practice.

The examination is very comprehensive. Ensure that your preparation reflects the composition of the current examination. Naturally, not every item or sub-item listed below will be covered on each examination. The examination consists of 200 questions. Of those, only 150 questions will count toward your score. The test is delivered in 4 blocks of 50 questions at a time. The test taker can go back and forth between the questions within one block, but once that block of questions is submitted, it is not available for further review. The additional 50 questions are used by the Federation to check their validity for future use. This content outline is based on the 150 questions that are scored.

Content Outline for the NPTE for the PTA

Effective March 2008 the 150 questions that count toward the test takers' score will be based on the NPTE Content Outline 2008 as developed by the FSBPT. The information that follows has been adapted from the NPTE Content Outline 2008, copyright 2007. The exam content is divided into three large groups of questions with the largest portion of the examination content, approximately 73%, falling into the actual delivery of physical therapy interventions to patients throughout the life span and affecting different body systems. Understanding and use of equipment and devices and the application of therapeutic modalities will make up 14.67% of the exam. The next category makes up 12.67% of the questions; Safety & Professional Roles, Teaching/Learning and Evidence-Based Practice.

The following categories and division designations identify content areas covered in the NPTE. In addition, they will be used to report your score on the practice exams included on the CD in this text. This will allow you to continue to assess your areas of strength and areas that require improvement as your studies proceed.

Category A

Clinical Application of Physical Therapy Principles and Foundational Sciences (A)

To correctly answer questions in this category, the test taker will need to apply knowledge of the scientific principles of pathology, diseases and conditions affecting the body systems to effectively treat patients across their life span. There will be a total of 59 items in this category, or 39.33% of the NPTE. This category includes:

1. Anatomy and physiology of the systems
2. Pathologies/conditions of the systems
3. Diseases or conditions of the systems to provide effective treatments
4. Medical management of the systems such as medical tests, medications, surgical procedures
5. Physiological response to environmental factors and characteristics; for example, air and water temperature, humidity, water depth and buoyancy, altitude
6. Effects of activity and exercise on the systems (including the physiological response to various types of tests/measures and interventions)
7. Joint structure, mobility and function

Number of Questions by System

Cardiovascular & Pulmonary (I A) = 10 questions
Musculoskeletal (II A) = 15 questions
Neuromuscular & Nervous
   Systems (III A) = 14 questions
Integumentary (IV A) = 4 questions
Other Systems—Metabolic & Endocrine,
   Gastrointestinal, Multisystem (V A) = 16 questions

Category B

Data Collection (B)

To correctly answer questions in this category, the test taker will need to understand the reaction of body systems to the various tests and measures and make correct clinical judgments related to results for patients across their life span. There will be a total of 23 items in this category, or 15.33% of the NPTE. This category includes:

1. Appropriate types of tests/measures and their applications
2. Movement analysis of the various systems
3. Physiological response of the systems
4. Kinesiology/kinematics

Number of Questions by System

Cardiovascular & Pulmonary (I B) = 4 questions
Musculoskeletal (II B) = 9 questions
Neuromuscular & Nervous
   Systems (III B) = 7 questions
Integumentary (IV B) = 2 questions
Other Systems—Metabolic &
   Endocrine (V B) = 1 question

Category C

Intervention (C)

In this section, the test taker will answer questions related to the impact of the application of interventions on the systems across the life span. There will be a total of 27 items in this category, or 18.00% of the NPTE. This category includes:

1. Application of interventions to the systems
2. Appropriate types of interventions
3. Physiological response to interventions
4. Secondary effects or complications from intervention to the systems
5. Effects or secondary effects on systems from interventions applied to other body systems
6. Motor control and motor learning related to the neuromuscular system
7. Wound management techniques
8. Cognition, affect, memory, arousal

Number of Questions by System

Cardiovascular & Pulmonary (I C)	= 5 questions
Musculoskeletal (II C)	= 8 questions
Neuromuscular & Nervous Systems (III C)	= 9 questions
Integumentary (IV C)	= 3 questions
Other Systems—Metabolic & Endocrine (V C)	= 2 questions

Category D

Equipment & Devices (D); and Therapeutic Modalities (D)

To correctly answer questions in this category, the test taker will need to apply knowledge of the implementation and use of equipment and devices and the application of therapeutic modalities. One will need to incorporate an understanding of context and other factors influencing the use of equipment, devices and therapeutic modalities. These situations will be applied to patient and client treatment across their life span. There will be a total of 22 items in this category, or 14.67% of the NPTE. This category includes:

Equipment & Devices (D)

1. Assistive and adaptive devices
2. Prosthetic and orthotic devices
3. Protective and supportive devices
4. Gravity-assisted devices
5. Bariatric equipment and devices

Therapeutic Modalities (D)

1. Indications, contraindications and precautions for the implementation of modalities
2. Physical agents such as athermal agents, heat and cold therapeutic agents, hydrotherapy, light agents, sound agents
3. Mechanical modalities, including compression therapies, mechanical motion devices and traction
4. Electrotherapeutic medication delivery—iontophoresis
5. Electrical stimulation including functional electrical stimulation (FES), high-volt pulsed galvanic stimulation (HVPC), neuromuscular electrical stimulation (MNES) and transcutaneous electrical nerve stimulation (TENS).

Category E

Safety & Professional Roles (E); Teaching/Learning (E); Evidence-Based Practice (E)

To correctly answer questions in this category, the test taker will need to understand and apply principles of safety and patient protection into scenarios to ensure the healthcare worker makes decisions to protect patient safety and security in a trustworthy environment. The test taker will need to incorporate theories of teaching and learning into clinical environments to effectively communicate with patients and clients. Also included in this category are questions related to basic research methodology and data collection techniques that are necessary for interpretation of information and research to support evidence-based practice. There will be a total of 19 items in this category, or 12.67% of the NPTE. This category includes:

Safety & Professional Roles (E)

1. Risk factors for falls and use of restraints and equipment
2. Preparedness for emergency situations and performance of CPR
3. Proper body mechanics (use of, observation of, instruction in)
4. Injury prevention
5. Implement infection control measures (standard and universal precautions)
6. Legal obligations for reporting abuse and neglect
7. Patient and client rights related to legislation
8. Human resource and legal issues
9. Standards of documentation for patient care
10. Risk guidelines (documentation, policies and procedures and incident reports)
11. Roles and responsibilities of all healthcare providers and support staff

Teaching & Learning (E)

1. Teaching and learning theories, techniques and strategies that include cognitive, motor impairments and abilities
2. Communication skills encompassing different styles and modes (verbal, nonverbal)

Evidence-Based Practice (e)

1. Suitability and application of outcomes measures
2. Data collection techniques, including surveys and direct observation
3. Basic research concepts and interpretation, such as validity and reliability

Levels of Question Difficulty

The NPTE for PTAs attempts to ascertain how a candidate deals with a variety of different situations in order to determine how the assistant will function in a clinical setting.

Many of the questions require problem solving at the middle to upper levels of cognitive functioning, those written at the comprehension and application levels. PTA candidates should be well prepared to answer questions written at the comprehension and application level.

KNOWLEDGE: questions require recall of specific bits of information whether it is medical terminology, the name of something, a classification, a category or a specific sequence of events. This is the information that forms the basis of physical therapy practice. Without a sound knowledge foundation, higher level problem solving becomes difficult or nearly impossible. Knowledge is obtained by memorization, repetition, use of acronyms such as RICE, flash cards and so on. Questions on the NPTE assume competency in this knowledge base. There should not be any questions at this low cognitive level on the examination.

COMPREHENSION: questions at this level expect one to understand the significance of the facts, terminology or knowledge. What are the implications of the information? Why is this information relevant? For example, why does a second-degree ankle sprain result in edema formation?

Debating, sharing and exchanging information with a colleague, supervisor or in small groups can help to promote comprehension of information. Expect there to be many questions written at this level on the examination.

APPLICATION: questions are based on the relevance, implications or significance one can attach to familiar or unfamiliar clinical or administrative scenarios. These types of questions can also require, for example, the application of procedures, rules, theories and guidelines to clinical situations. The comprehended knowledge has to be manipulated, altered or used to fit a particular case. For example, given a particular patient or established therapeutic goals, how can one apply the principles of exercising under water to facilitate movement, decrease or increase weight bearing, in-

crease the speed of movement and so on? Another example might involve appropriate application of APTA's *Guide for Conduct of the Physical Therapist Assistant* to a clinical or ethical situation.

To help prepare, try to relate new situations to what is already familiar. Apply different approaches or outlooks to a variety of patient care problems or administrative dilemmas. Working in small peer groups might be helpful. There will likely be a fair number of application questions on the NPTE and they can challenge your problem-solving abilities.

ANALYSIS: questions require the interpretation of a variety of factors and an understanding of the differences, similarities and interrelationships among those concepts. These types of questions require analysis of anatomical, physiological, pathological, psychological, administrative and other factors. Each factor has to be quickly examined in light of the situation presented in the question. The meaning of the factors is determined. Critical thinking is then used to reach conclusions. Analysis might be required when reacting to life-threatening situations; communicating with patients, families, caregivers, healthcare workers or students; making ethical decisions; modifying an intervention based on a patient's reaction and so on. Often, a list of reasonable possibilities is presented and the best or most likely possibility has to be selected by the test taker. Given a particular scenario, sometimes the least likely goal or intervention is requested. Use of sound clinical judgment is essential. This type of decision making, or "thinking on one's feet" is done frequently by clinicians. Use the practice questions on the software-simulated examinations as a means of self-assessment and then follow up in areas of weakness. Expect some analysis questions.

LEVELS OF EXAM QUESTIONS

QUESTION LEVEL AND DESCRIPTION	RELEVANCE TO NPTE	NPTE EXAM PREPARATION STRATEGY
Knowledge Recall of basic information and facts. For example, spinal cord levels, muscle attachments, diagnoses, wheelchair measurements.	A solid knowledge foundation of entry-level information is required to answer clinical scenario questions that will be posed on the NPTE. It is very unlikely that you will find a question written at this level on the exam.	A strong commitment to studying specific facts and information acquired during your PTA education is needed. This text provides extensive information in an outline format to ease your review. Memorization of specific facts and information you will need to apply to solving clinical problem posed in the questions is highly suggested.
Comprehension Understanding of information to determine significance, consequences, or implications. For example, the impact of spasticity on function.	The NPTE is not a "matching" type of test. You will not be able to simply recall information to be successful in answering a question. You must be able to apply facts and knowledge to multiple clinical scenarios. You can expect to find many questions written at this level on the examination.	When studying the text to review basic content and foundational knowledge, ask yourself how and why this fundamental information is important, how you will use the information to administer and modify interventions to persons across the lifespan. Studying with a peer or a group can provide you with additional insights about the relevance, significance, consequences, and implications of the information.
Application Use of information and application of rules, procedures, or theories to new situations. For example, the modification of a treatment for a patient who has a recent hip replacement in addition to an acute CVA.	The NPTE requires you to use your knowledge and comprehension as described above, along with the competencies you developed during your clinical experiences, in a manner that best fits the specific scenario identified in the exam item. You can expect to find many questions written at this level on the examination.	Continue to actively apply information that you review in the text book to new and novel clinical situations. Consider how the information you are processing can be used for patients with different diagnoses, of different ages, and with differing levels of health and wellness. The exam items included on the CD in this text are constructed such that you must use these comprehension and application skills to correctly answer the items. Review the analysis of your performance after you have completed the exam to help identify how well you are applying your knowledge.

continued		
QUESTION LEVEL AND DESCRIPTION	RELEVANCE TO NPTE	NPTE EXAM PREPARATION STRATEGY
Analysis Recognition of interrelationships between principles and interpretation or evaluation of data presented. For example, the most appropriate focus for discharge planning for a parent with a traumatic brain injury.	It is unlikely the NPTE for the physical therapist assistant will contain items that are written at the analysis level.	Critically review the rationales provided in the text of the correct and incorrect responses to the exam questions. Review the content area(s) you did not get correct. Reflect with a peer or study group can be beneficial in helping to determine your gaps in analysis of exam items.

Methods of Reading Multiple-Choice Questions

Carefully read the stem of each question. What is the focus of the question? Try to think about the information using what you know and your judgment. Then read each choice carefully. Begin the process of eliminating one option at a time. Every time you are able to rationalize the elimination of an option, the odds of answering the question correctly go up dramatically. Be careful, sometimes options have some correct information, but it is not correct or germane for the question asked!

If the stem of the question is long or involved, you might wish to read the options first. In this way, when you read the stem of the question, you may be able to better focus on the relevance of the information presented.

As the exam progresses, your reading skills will tend to deteriorate. You may have to rest your eyes for a minute or stand up and walk away from the computer screen for a short time. If your mind is no longer processing information properly, you may answer questions incorrectly that you should normally get right. Stop what you are doing and rest for a few moments. It is fruitless to continue until you can clearly refocus on the contents before you on the computer screen. You might have to take a longer break after you complete a section.

There are specific strategies that may be helpful in answering multiple-choice questions. These include:

1. Look for opposites in the list of options. These are the extremes of a concept such as positive/negative, inversion/eversion, hypoglycemia/hyperglycemia, spasticity/flaccidity and so on. Examine opposites first. If you cannot eliminate both of them immediately, there is a good chance that one is the correct answer. If you can eliminate both opposites right away, the chances drop to 50/50 for selecting the correct response from the remaining two choices.

2. Identify choices that are so similar that it is difficult to choose between them. These may be choices which say exactly the same thing in slightly different ways. If you cannot discriminate between them, it is possible that both are incorrect. For example, if one option in a question is the primary muscle of inspiration, and another option in the same question is the diaphragm, they both say the same thing and need to be eliminated. Sometimes a choice that is unique or different, but not far-fetched, merits greater consideration than others.

3. Identify clues in the stem which may be helpful in focusing your thoughts. For example, the examiners present a recently discharged patient who can transfer independently but cannot ambulate independently for more than 20 feet. Your judgment should lead you to conclude that the patient is probably homebound. Therefore, if you were asked to choose among exercises or activities, the one best suited for home use might be most appropriate.

4. Look for key words or phrases in the stem. If you see *best, most important, first, primary* and so forth, it means you have to set priorities. All of the options could correctly answer the question; however, you must go through the process of rank ordering and elimination to select the best option. Try to eliminate any obviously unrealistic choices first and work backward toward what you consider the top priority.

5. Look for overlapping facts in the options. If you ascertain that a fact or statement in a choice is incorrect and you see the same fact or statement in another option, both choices can be eliminated. For example, given a patient problem, two options in the question are:
   (1) Pallor and diaphoresis
   (2) Tachycardia and diaphoresis
   If you determine that diaphoresis is never a sign of this problem in (1), then you must automatically eliminate choice (2) as well.

6. Identify options that are crucial for the survival or safety of the patient. These always receive high priority. Give less credibility to those responses that provide false reassurance to the patient, are overly optimistic, or do not address the patient's or family's feelings. Give more credibility to empathetic responses. Don't always choose a response which gives away responsibility to someone else. There may be certain situations where the examiners want the PTA to assume responsibility unless it is outside the scope of practice or skill level of the PTA.

7. Look for negative words or phrases in the stem. Phrases such as *except for, all but, least important* and so on denote that you must search for an answer that is false, unacceptable, low priority or contraindicated. The negative word or words are in bold type. The most common way of handling these negative questions is to label each

choice either TRUE or FALSE relative to the scenario presented. You should wind up with three TRUES and one FALSE. The FALSE choice would be the correct answer if you categorized everything appropriately.

8. Don't look for a particular pattern of answers that would cause you to alter a choice you believe to be correct. For example, do not eliminate a correct choice because you chose that same letter or number option in the preceding item or series of items. Questions are selected and placed randomly in the exam. Don't look for or think about answer patterns.

9. Don't overanalyze a question. Read the question at face value. Don't go outside of the gist of the information in the stem of the question to try and reach a conclusion. Sufficient information should be available. Adding your own hypothetical conditions to the situation presented could easily lead you astray.

How Can the Examination Review Be Structured?

Once you have completed your entry-level PTA education, you bring all of your academic and clinical experience to the table in preparation for the NPTE. Four to 6 weeks of independent structured review should be adequate. More time might be necessary for candidates for whom English is a second language or who were not educated through a CAPTE accredited PTA program. Candidates with learning disabilities may also need additional preparation time as the processing of information might take more time. The 1-day Licensure Examination Preparatory Course, such as the type offered since 1989 by TherapyEd, can be quite helpful. Extensive student feedback has indicated that this preparation course is effective in providing up-to-date information on examination expectation and trends. Study hints and additional means of self-assessment provide even more focus and direction for exam preparation.

Please show respect for the examination process. Procrastination, skimpy review and a lack of under-standing about the nature of the NPTE could lead to disappointing results. The expenses incurred to retake the examination and the potential loss of income because of failure to obtain regulation could be significant. If not successful, your self-esteem will take a mighty blow. **See Chapter 1 for further details on testing success.**

Analysis of Strengths and Weaknesses

A shotgun approach to exam preparation is not the best way to utilize your time. Systematically, try to form a composite picture of your PTA education and experiences. **See Chapter 1 for further direction and assistance with assessing areas of strength and weakness.**

ACADEMIC PROGRAM: even accredited PTA programs can vary widely in terms of the quantity and quality of the content covered. Many programs are superb. Other programs may have curricular or faculty shortcomings. There could be a lack of emphasis on content that might be important for the NPTE. Try to recollect which content areas were presented in a comprehensive manner and which areas left something to be desired. Were there any gaps in your basic preparation that may be emphasized on the NPTE? Were academic standards poorly enforced? Will this require you to spend more time gathering or reviewing information in these areas? These factors can play a role when confronting the NPTE which conforms to a standard that is outside of the academic setting.

CLASSROOM PERFORMANCE: generally speaking, strong classroom performers should fare well on the NPTE as long as they take the time to properly prepare.

Students who performed marginally in their program; whose basic PTA program lacked rigor or whose English skills are not well developed may have more difficulty with the NPTE and require additional study and focus.

CLINICAL EXPERIENCES/AFFILIATIONS: if the range of clinical experiences was limited in terms of settings, patient populations, types of interventions or degree of responsibility, exam candidates may have difficulty in their ability to answer questions requiring application of clinical knowledge or judgment. An exam candidate with no clinical exposure in such areas as prosthetics, cardiac rehabilitation, wound or burn care, pediatrics and so on might have more difficulty in reaching conclusions requiring the proper or best intervention in these areas. Many NPTE questions require an amalgam of clinical experience as well as academic knowledge to solve problems. Selected use of the *Guide to Physical Therapist Practice* may prove useful in areas of deficient clinical preparation. Specific practice patterns interventions and outcomes may be delineated.

ANALYSIS OF SAMPLE QUESTION RESULTS: at appropriate times, attempt to answer the practice questions in the simulated examinations in the accompanying software. The computer scoring will assist you in identifying content areas and domains in which your performance was good as well as those areas that need more work. This analysis can serve as a basis for structuring further review and study. After taking the examinations, be sure to read the rationale for the simulated examination questions in this *Review & Study Guide*.

Based on your personal analysis, write down areas of weakness and try to rank order them in terms of which areas might require the most remedial work. Set priorities based on the Content Outline emphasis and expectations of the examination. Recall that the NPTE for PTAs is based primarily on entry-level knowledge and judgment.

Discipline

About a month or two prior to your scheduled examination, establish a routine to spend 6 days a week reviewing material. Set up realistic and potentially achievable short-term goals as to what you wish to accomplish each day. Take 1 day off per week to pursue other interests. Give yourself a break! However, when you are reviewing, allot about 2 to 3 hours of concentrated and uninterrupted time each day. Study in a quiet and well-lit space. Do not study when you are ill or overly tired. If you work during the week, perhaps weekends will afford you more flexibility or time for the review. If you break your routine, add compensatory time. Answer the computer-based sample questions as a means of diagnosing strengths and weaknesses. Trying to memorize sample questions and rationales is not a satisfactory means of preparation. Practice questions serve as templates for a multitude of item possibilities and primarily as diagnostic tools. You must review basic physical therapy knowledge and be able to apply that knowledge to a variety of problems, settings, circumstances and situations. Some people may benefit from small peer group study sessions.

Even though the review is for the purpose of passing the NPTE, we have received feedback through the years that this retrospective overview of one's PTA education has helped to sharpen and focus many aspects of clinical practice as well.

The Role of Critical Reasoning in Licensure Examination Performance

What is Critical Reasoning?

Critical reasoning is the process of drawing conclusions - a process we each go through many times in a day. We utilize our knowledge, skills, experiences, and logic to make conclusions about everyday situations. In order to successfully draw conclusions, we must make a concerted effort to embark on this decision-making process with purpose, clarity, accuracy, and thoroughness.

How does this relate to the NPTE, and why should you spend time focusing your attention on this process? Some individuals erroneously believe that the NPTE only tests your ability to recall facts that are readily found in textbooks. Although factual knowledge is an important foundation for the exam, the questions on the NPTE are designed to compel you to test your ability to reason out clinical scenarios and to make prudent decisions about the situation described in each question. Each question on the NPTE will be an opportunity for you to draw on your knowledge, skills, and clinical experiences to arrive at a justifiable, reasonable conclusion to the situation proposed in

the question. You arrive at a correct conclusion primarily by use of clinical reasoning.

Five subtypes

There are five main subtypes, each one of these is important to understand, as the circumstances surrounding a situation will determine the critical strategy we employ to the critical reasoning process. This is based on expert consensus of many critical thinking experts and reported by Peter and Noreen Facione (1990a, 1990b, 2006). Each one of these is important to understand as the circumstances surrounding a situation will determine the critical reasoning strategy we employ. These subtypes are: inductive reasoning, deductive reasoning, analysis, inference and evaluation.

INDUCTIVE REASONING: Inductive reasoning requires clinical judgment and ongoing expansion of our knowledge base. It begins with observations and reasoning in specific situations and progresses to the ability to draw conclusions from more generalized situations with a larger set of circumstances. It is important since it provides insight into understanding populations and not just individuals.

Regarding the physical therapist assistant's role, inductive reasoning is critical for effective treatment planning in order to meet the goals set in the plan of care established by the PT. It allows the PTA to weigh all the viable treatment options, rather than just one, and select the most appropriate choice given the entire set of circumstances.

Example: when working with a patient with back pain, TENS was able to decrease the pain for this specific patient when nothing else would work. We may initially assume that all back pain, therefore, will respond positively to TENS. While this thinking is flawed, it may lead us to further explore the use of TENS for pain management of areas other than the low back or may encourage us to consider the use of other modalities for addressing back pain in different individuals.

DEDUCTIVE REASONING: Deductive reasoning is the opposite of inductive reasoning: we begin with a larger set of circumstances and theories that we then apply to the specific situation we are addressing. It involves drawing conclusions based on facts, laws, rules or accepted principles. Research both requires deductive reasoning skills as well as provides essential information toward making clinical decisions based on its findings.

Deductive reasoning is important to the PTA as it provides the reasons for the decisions we make. It is also helpful in providing a starting point as well as a structured process from which to work in our clinical decision making. The clinician must have a good background knowledge of the information prior to making decisions in this fashion, as utilizing incorrect procedures or flawed knowledge will result in unsound conclusions.

Example: we have a standard protocol for the use of transcutaneous electrical neural stimulation (TENS) for pain control based on data gathered over the course of its use on multiple individuals and, therefore, we are able to utilize this protocol on a variety of individuals with various types of pain rather than starting from the beginning each time.

ANALYSIS: Analysis is the process of "making sense out of pieces": interpreting the meaning of information, determining relationships within the information presented, and then making assumptions or judgments about that information.

This type of reasoning is important to the PTA as it allows the individual to draw conclusions based on observations, a frequent occurrence in the implementation of the treatment plan. The PTA must continually determine what is relevant and irrelevant information in order to effectively analyze the situation.

Example: the PTA examines ROM readings taken over the past week and makes a determination if the patient is progressing as expected based on the diagnosis and outlined plan of care.

INFERENCE: Inference involves making logical judgments based on concepts, beliefs, assumptions, and evidence rather than direct observations. This process often relies on the assistant's prior clinical experiences in making predictions about future occurrences.

This is a skill the PTA utilizes to make assumptions as to what he or she can expect from a certain clinical situation. It is often employed to answer patient questions about their future: length of stay, possible recovery, or ongoing disabilities that may be expected.

Example: the PTA reviews the chart of a patient prior to seeing him/her the first time. The patient's diagnosis is right anterior cerebral artery CVA. Immediately, the PTA begins to make predictions about what to expect when meeting the patient the first time, including possible personality changes, greater LE involvement than UE, and urinary incontinence.

EVALUATION: Evaluation involves relying on guiding principles to determine a course of action as well as validating the decisions we do make. It involves the "gut instinct" we utilize in decision making, often forcing us to rely on ethical principles to find solutions where there are no easy answers. It can be difficult for concrete thinkers, as there is often not a black or white answer.

The PTA often utilizes evaluation when determining if a referral back to the PT for further evaluation is indicated. This process becomes easier as the individual has more experience in practice and clinical decision making.

Example: when working with a patient with a history of recent MI to complete shoulder exercises, the patient begins to sweat profusely and complain of nausea and lightheadedness. The PTA must weigh what is happening and determine whether or not the symptoms he/she is observing are related to the shoulder exercises or symptomatic of a new heart problem.

Improving critical reasoning

In order to be successful on the national examination, each of the above reasoning skills must be utilized. Critical reasoning is not learned and improved in a quick lesson or by simply reading the definition of each subtype. It requires practice with items that test these skill areas and provide feedback on your performance. The good news is that you already have this information contained in this study guide! Each practice question in the book has an accompanying rationale for the correct and incorrect choices. Additionally, each question has an explanation for the subtype of critical reasoning and the knowledge or skill required to arrive at a correct conclusion. Paying attention to these areas will help you to build your knowledge and experiences with critical reasoning skills and prepare you for the NPTE.

Individuals will often say, "I'm not a good test taker", "They are trying to trick me", "I don't know what the question is asking", or "They ask questions that have no right answers". The truth is, you have demonstrated some level of competence in test-taking and critical reasoning as evidenced by your success at reaching this point in your education. If you are still having the above feelings, however, this is likely an indicator of a failure in one of the subtypes of critical reasoning.

Often individuals believe the inability to answer test questions is related to a lack of content knowledge. While this is one plausible explanation for lack of success, the bigger problem for students is possessing the knowledge but having the inability to utilize the information.

As part of the preparation process to take the examination, you should identify your aptitude for critical reasoning in each of the subtypes. After the areas of weakness are identified, various strategies can be utilized to help improve critical reasoning with the hope of improving performance on the examination. Each of the simulated examination in this text are labeled with the type of critical reasoning utilized. The following five symbols have been assigned to help you identify these:

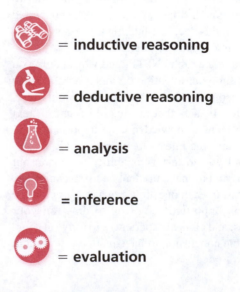

= **inductive reasoning**

= **deductive reasoning**

= **analysis**

= **inference**

= **evaluation**

After you receive the analysis of the practice test results from the CD, refer back to your incorrect responses and see if there is a pattern to the types of questions you are answering incorrectly related to a subtype of critical reasoning. Do you notice that you have difficulty with certain types of questions, such as ones that encourage evaluative or inferential reasoning? This will help you to identify a potential area for improvement and guide your future studies. If you notice that you have a weakness in a certain area of reasoning, do not despair. Being aware of the issue is a good first step.

Once you have identified a weakness in critical reasoning, take some time to reflect on why this is so. Ask yourself the following questions and determine how they may be true of your situation.

- Do I have difficulty taking specific information and applying it to larger populations? This could indicate challenges in inductive reasoning.
- Do I prefer to follow my instincts rather than what a protocol may provide? This could indicate challenges in deductive reasoning.
- Do I tend to misjudge what is presented in the form of pictures, graphs, and chart? This could indicate challenges in analytical reasoning.
- Do I have difficulty thinking about how situations may evolve over time or making assumptions about a situation? This could indicate challenges in inferential reasoning.
- Do I rely on protocols and guidelines more than gut instinct? Do I feel anxious when I have questions I cannot find answers to in a textbook ? This could indicate challenges in evaluative reasoning.

Other Courses of Action

This study guide helps you to identify potential weak areas so that you are the most prepared for succeeding on the NPTE. More detailed information about critical reasoning is beyond the scope and focus of this book. However, if you find that you want additional information about critical reasoning and practice with questions that test critical thinking and reasoning skills, the following resources are recommended to help you practice honing these skill areas:

- **Insight Assessment, Inc.** http://www.insightassessment.com/. Offers periodic free mini-tests with rationales for correct and incorrect answers. Also offers resources that discuss the various types of reasoning.
- **Coping.org.** http://www.coping.org/write/percept/critical.htm. Offers information about the various types of reasoning and challenges with the reasoning process.
- **Nosich, G. M.** (2001). *Learning to Think Things Through: A Guide to Critical Thinking in the Curriculum*, 2nd ed. Prentice Hall.A handy guide written to help students engage in critical thinking.
- **Richard Bowles.** http://richardbowles.tripod.com/gmat/critreas/critreas.htm. Richard Bowles offers a practice

critical reasoning test to improve critical reasoning skills at his personal website.
- **San Jose State University.** http://www.sjsu.edu/depts/itl/7/part2/indded.html. Offers free practice tests for inductive and deductive reasoning and explanations of the difference between the two types of reasoning.

Specific Reasoning References

Facione, P. (2006). *Critical Thinking: What It Is and Why It Counts*. Millbrae, CA: The California Academic Press.

Facione, P. (1990a). *Critical Thinking: A Statement of Expert Consensus for Purposes of Educational Assessment and Instruction: Research Findings and Recommendations*. Newark, DE: The American Psychological Association. ERIC Document Reproduction Service. No. ED 315423.

Facione, P. (1990b). *Critical Thinking: A Statement of Expert Consensus for Purposes of Educational Assessment and Instruction ("Executive Summary: The Delphi Report")*. Millbrae, CA: The California Academic Press.

Facione, N. C., &Facione, P. A. (2006).*The Health Sciences Reasoning Test HSRT: Test Manual 2006 Edition*. Millbrae, CA: The California Academic Press.

Final Review

A review consisting of JUST answering or memorizing sample questions is often unsatisfactory. The sample questions in the accompanying computer software are not actual NPTE questions. These questions are to be used for diagnostic or learning purposes. It is possible that on the NPTE you may see some questions that cover content similar to some practice questions. However, the NPTE questions may be phrased differently and have entirely different answers. You, most likely, will encounter questions with an entirely new or different focus than the simulated examinations.

A final review should refocus on those areas that are emphasized on the examination and that you have identified as areas of personal weakness. You may wish to retake the simulated examinations if time permits.

Preplanning for the Day of the Examination

SCHEDULING: schedule your examination for a time of day when you work and think your best. If you are an "early bird" and are more alert in the morning, schedule a morning test time. If you are the "night owl type" and don't function well until noon, schedule your examination for the afternoon.

TRAVEL: make travel and lodging arrangements in advance if it is necessary to travel to the testing site. Bring a map and directions with you. Directions are available at www.2test.com

or www.prometric.com. Drive to the examination site the night before so you know the route the next day; be sure to plan for such factors as traffic flow during rush hour, work day versus weekend and so on. Plan to arrive at the examination site early. Remember you must arrive at least 30 minutes prior to your scheduled exam to complete required documentation, fingerprinting and photographing. Bring some money to cover any parking fees.

BRING: prior to your scheduled exam, be sure to gather important documentation and items you will need to have with you. You will need (1) authorization-to-test letter; (2) identification (being sure you have at least one form of currently valid government-issued photo ID such as your driver's license or passport, and one other form of ID that has your name preprinted on it and your signature on it; a Social Security card is not acceptable); (3) be sure you have glasses or contacts with you if you need them. Be aware that your first and last name on both forms of identification must exactly match the first and last name as it appears on your authorization to test letter.

PRIOR TO THE EXAM: eat a good meal prior to taking the examination; avoid energy draining carbohydrate-loaded foods. Be sure you are hydrated. It would be best to avoid beverages filled with stimulants such as caffeine. Avoid use of medications such as antihistamines or muscle relaxants, alcohol or the use of other substances that may affect your alertness. Dress comfortably and wear layers to help accommodate for any variations in temperature at the test site. You may want to use the restroom prior to entering the testing room.

ARRIVAL TIME: arrive 30 minutes prior to the start of your examination.

UPON ARRIVAL: your thumbprint and photograph will be taken at the Prometric Center. You will need to sign appropriate paperwork.

DURING THE EXAM: you will be videotaped and visually monitored during the examination. Each time you leave your testing station be sure you sign off of your computer and ensure a "scheduled break" or "unscheduled break" screen is showing; failure to do so can result in an invalid exam. Each time you reenter the testing room you will be required to submit another thumbprint.

What Should You Do or Expect Just Before the Examination?

The day prior to the examination make sure you have gathered, in one spot, all necessary documents, materials, identifications, medications, eyeglasses and items of a personal nature. Do not rush around the day of your scheduled NPTE searching for these things. It will heighten your anxiety. Do not cram or stay up until late hours reviewing material. Do not go to a party the night before the exam (after it's over, OK!). Try and get a good night's sleep.

Expect to be a little nervous. Prometric personnel are used to anxious individuals. They will try and put you at ease and explain testing procedures. If you are overly anxious, your ability to process the questions and retrieve information might be impaired. Anxiety can lead you to dwell more on the consequences of the examination, such as possible failure, rather than focusing on the content of the questions presented. Practice whatever relaxation strategies you find helpful— pursed lip breathing, visualization, progressive relaxation, etc. If you have disciplined yourself to review material in a thorough and methodical way, your self-confidence will increase as does the likelihood of a positive outcome.

During the Examination

Expect the whole examination procedure to last up to 4.5 hours or so. You may use the restroom during the examination; however, the clock on the computer screen keeps ticking away while you are gone. There are one scheduled break and two unscheduled breaks allowed during the examination. The scheduled break occurs after the second block of questions has been completed and submitted; the clock will stop during this break. You are allowed up to 15 minutes for this break. We suggest you take advantage of the scheduled break to stretch your legs and get up and move around a bit. The two unscheduled breaks may be used between question blocks; time on the clock continues to elapse during these breaks. You must "sign-off" of the computer correctly during these breaks to avoid an invalid exam. Food or drink is not allowed at the computer cubicle during the examination. Books, purses, digital watches, cell phones, digital devices, etc, are not allowed in the testing room. There may be lockers available at the test center for these items during the exam. Test centers have rules regarding the type of clothing, watches or digital devices and your actions during the examination. Be sure to ask about them prior to beginning the exam. Keep money, medications, tissues, reading glasses or other valuables in a pocket. At some centers, you may be allowed to go to the reception area to move about or get a drink of water during a break. At other centers, your movement might be limited.

Prometric personnel will orient you regarding the examination procedures. A preexam computer tutorial should familiarize you with the keyboard commands and other functions. We urge you to take the tutorial and ask for clarification of any detail prior to the start of the examination. If you are dissatisfied with the lighting, seating, ability to read the computer screen, noise levels or other factors, request a change to another computer cubicle before the exam starts.

Consider using earplugs to block out any distracting noise. Other test takers may be coming or going or receiving an orientation during your examination. Prometric personnel can supply headphones while taking the exam to help dampen noise. You may not be permitted to wear earplugs. You will be allowed to use scratch paper in the form of a white board and dry erase marker during the examination to make any notes to yourself. Prometric testing centers will provide this. It will be collected at the conclusion of the examination.

There are 200 multiple-choice questions on the exam. Each question has four possible choices. Select the one best choice that answers each item. Four hours are allocated for the actual examination. The examination is divided into sections of 50 questions each. The sections are balanced in terms of content covered. During the examination, you may electronically mark questions you have skipped or wish to review at the end of that section. We do not recommend skipping questions; answer each question to the best of your ability. Use educated guesses if you must. You are not penalized for guessing. Once a section has been completed, you can review marked or any questions, and change answers as often as you would like; however, once you submit the questions in that section, they are not available for review at a later time. Do remember that this review time is still using time within your allotted 4 hours. Sections are not individually timed. You may take as much or as little time as you wish for each section. There is a scheduled break after the second section, question 100, for 15 minutes' duration that does not count against your 4-hour total allotted time. There is a running clock on the computer screen identifying time remaining to complete the examination. If you complete the examination prior to the allocated time, you may leave early.

Once the examination has commenced, communicate only with Prometric personnel. An innocent remark to a nearby test taker or glancing at another computer screen might be mistaken for an attempt to cheat. Candidates attempting to cheat, by whatever means, can face serious consequences. Trying to obtain regulation to practice as a PTA by fraudulent means is a crime. Don't even think about doing it.

What Are Some Strategies that Might Help When Taking the Actual Examination?

Time management is crucial. There are 200 items to answer in 4 hours. This amounts to an allotment of a little over 1 minute per question. Do not skip or fail to answer a question. Unanswered questions are automatically wrong. You must complete an average of 50 questions per hour to finish all of the examination questions. When you have completed the first 50 questions, check the running clock on the computer screen. Have you completed them in an hour or less? If not, you must increase your pace or it will be unlikely you will get to all of the questions. Some people prefer to check the computer clock at the end of the first hour and then note the number of questions answered. Either way, pace yourself properly. Remember, in the third hour of the exam your reading skills will tend to deteriorate and it may take longer to process each question. If English is your second language, you must think in English. Failure to think in English will make it very difficult for you to finish the exam on time as well as be a source of examination interpretation errors.

What should you do if there are only 2 minutes left and you have not had a chance to read or answer all of the questions? Do not leave anything blank. Quickly, choose answers for each question even if you have not had a chance to read the question. There are no penalties for guessing or entering an incorrect answer. Perhaps you will be lucky and get a few correct! If you finish early, you may leave or spend the remaining time going over questions you marked and wish to review. Do not change answers unless you have a very good reason for doing so. More often than not, people change correct answers to incorrect ones.

How are the NPTE for the PTA Graded and the Scores Reported?

All jurisdictions now employ the criterion-referenced performance standard. Using this system, a test score is interpreted in terms of an individual's mastery of a specified content domain. A passing criterion or standard is established by the FSBPT for each examination. A candidate must reach or exceed the designated cut score of competency to pass the examination. The cut score represents the minimal acceptable level of exam performance consistent with the safe and effective practice expected of the PTA. A panel of content experts establishes the passing score after screening questions for performance characteristics and bias. The examinee's performance is not compared with the performance of others who took the same examination. There are different forms of the examination which are used when taking the exam by computer. Each form of the NPTE has its own criterion-referenced passing grade. Thus, when taking the computer-based examination, your examination might differ from another individual's and have a different passing grade. Grading on the curve, use of a fixed percentage and the number of questions answered correctly are methods no longer in use for determining passing scores.

Reporting the grades to candidates can be confusing. Because versions of the examination might differ as to level of difficulty, scaled scores rather than the absolute number of questions answered correctly (raw score) are reported to candidates. The scaled scoring range is from 200 to 800, with 600 always reflecting the cut score. Thus, if the passing raw score was determined to be 105 out of 150 questions for a particular version of the NPTE, the 105 would equal a scaled score of 600. If a candidate achieved a score of 600 or better, the state licensing board would notify the candidate of their success and issue a license providing that all other conditions were satisfied.

Some states still convert the scaled passing score to another system based on the number 70 or 75. Thus, your score could be reported as being above or below the number 70 or 75. This does not necessarily mean that you scored above or below 70% or 75% or correctly or incorrectly answered 70 or 75 questions. It is merely an arbitrary numbering system used to denote a pass/fail line.

What Happens If You Have to Retake the NPTE?

Remember, most candidates are successful the first time! If you receive bad news about your NPTE results, life goes on but gets a bit more complicated. You might lose your temporary license if the state or jurisdiction has granted you one. If you are working as a PTA, you might lose your job or be downgraded to another position. If you have accepted a future position and fail to get a license, your employer might opt not to save the position for you.

Undoubtedly, you will experience various emotions which could include anger, frustration, depression, low self-esteem and embarrassment.

What can be done? You can go online and download the Performance Feedback Request Form from the FSBPT. This report compares your test performance, in various categories, with other candidates who sat for the same examination. It gives the number of questions in a category, your percentage score and the average percentage score of others in that category. The current cost is $75 plus a $3 credit card fee for this service. No personal checks accepted. For examination security reasons, no one has access to or can revisit their actual examination. You may contact http://www.fsbpt.org or call 1-703-739-9420.

Our advice is not to dwell on past failures. Carefully evaluate your performance. Think about areas on the previous examination(s) with which you had some difficulty. Were there any gaps in your academic or clinical knowledge? Did you find it difficult to answer questions requiring judgment or application of knowledge?

Focus on the next examination. Reinstitute a program of disciplined self-study. Consider taking a preparation course if you had not previously attended one. Do not retake the NPTE too quickly. We have found that candidates who retake the examination without adjusting their behaviors or correcting deficiencies wind up with the same disappointing results. There is no magic potion that helps you pass the examination. The onus is on you to demonstrate competency to practice. Take a positive and determined outlook. Approach the next examination with self-confidence and a minimum of anxiety.

Useful Web Links and E-mail Addresses

http://www.fsbpt.org
The Federation of State Boards of Physical Therapy
Information on licensure, addresses and links to state physical therapy boards, information about the NPTE and the role of the Federation.
http://www.fsbpt.net/pt
Website regarding transfer of exam scores and other related information.
http://www.2test.com
Locations of Prometric Testing and Assessment Centers
http://www.apta.org
The American Physical Therapy Association
Information about the profession, policies regarding the role of the physical therapist assistant, resources in selected areas of practice, etc.
http://www.TherapyEd.com
TherapyEd (previously known as International Educational Resources)
Information about examination preparatory courses and materials for physical and occupational therapists, PTAs and occupational therapy assistants

chapter 1

Testing Success

KAREN E. RYAN

Educational Preparation

You are likely now in the process of completing, or have just completed, your college education to become a physical therapist assistant (PTA). Good for you! Following graduation you are getting ready to embark on an amazing career—once you get past this one little (clearly we say this facetiously) hurdle of passing this one little licensure exam.

While you were in school you successfully figured out how to answer your instructors' exam questions. If your instructors had you answer questions that were written at the comprehension and application level, you are well on your way to being ready to study for the licensure examination.

Now you need to review facts from 2–3 years of college-level preparation to ensure your readiness to take and pass the licensure exam.

Purpose and Structure of the Licensure Examination

Purpose of the Licensure Examination

1. Protection of the public is the number one reason clinicians need to get a license in a state to practice.
2. Answer exam questions with that reason in mind—SAFETY.
   a. Is this safe to perform on this patient (think about diagnosis, condition, stage of healing, etc)?
   b. Am I as a PTA legally allowed to make this decision?
   c. Are there contraindications to performing the intervention?
   d. Is this patient presenting with signs and symptoms of intolerance, poor response to treatment?
3. This examination does not ask you to apply specific licensure laws from your state.
   a. Be sure to check with the licensing authority in the state or jurisdiction where you are seeking a license. You may have to take a "jurisprudence" examination.
      (1) An examination given by state (or jurisdiction) in which licensure is being sought.
      (2) Tests applicant's knowledge of rules, regulations and laws governing the practice of physical therapy in that state or jurisdiction.

4. This examination will apply the principles of appropriate care and delegation as identified by overseeing bodies such as the American Physical Therapy Association and the Centers for Medicare and Medicaid Services.

How Is the Exam Developed?

1. The examination is developed by the Federation of State Boards of Physical Therapy (FSBPT).

2. The examination is based on a "blueprint," or matrix, the FSBPT develops based on a survey of physical therapy practice. This survey of practice occurs approximately once every 5 years.
   a. Physical therapists (PTs) and PTAs across the country are surveyed and asked what entry level (a PTA graduate on day 1 of the job) PTAs do, and at what frequency.
   b. This survey and return information is reviewed by a panel of experts (PTs and PTAs) and the blueprint is developed.

Number and Delivery of Questions

1. You will answer 200 questions. Only 150 will count toward your actual score.
   a. The other 50 questions are "trial" questions being tested for validity and reliability.
   b. You will not know which questions are "trial" questions so you must answer each as if it were being scored. Do not leave any answers blank.
      (1) Trial questions will appear in just the same manner as the scored items. They will appear in any/all of the blocks of questions.

2. Breaks during the examination.
   a. You will have 4 hours to complete the exam.
   b. You are allowed one scheduled break and two unscheduled breaks during the examination.
      (1) The scheduled break occurs upon completion and submission of question #100 (the second block of questions).
         (a) You are allowed up to 15 minutes for this break.
         (b) You can stop the break at any time within the allotted 15 minutes.
         (c) This break does not count against your 4-hour allotted testing time; the time clock stops during this break.
      (2) You may take the two unscheduled breaks at the end of any block of questions.
         (a) The time clock continues to count down during each of these breaks.

c. You will have an opportunity prior to beginning the exam to participate in a practice session which will familiarize you with the exam delivery.
   (1) This does not count against your 4 hours. We suggest you take advantage of this opportunity.

3. The examination will be delivered in "blocks" of 50 questions. We suggest you plan on 60 minutes per 50-question block.
   a. You will have access to fifty (50) questions (one block) at a time.
      (1) You can spend as much or as little time as you need on each block. There is no time within the blocks, just the 4-hour maximum time.
      (2) You can go back and forth through questions in each block as many times as you choose.
      (3) We recommend one time through to answer questions and identify ("mark") those you want to come back to and review.
   b. Spend approximately 1 minute per question (50 minutes) to allow 10 minutes for review.
   c. After the last question in each block, you will be given the opportunity to review items in the block.
      (1) You can select "Review all Questions" (every question in that block) or "Review Marked Questions" (just the questions you want to go back and review).
         (a) Use the "mark" option carefully. If you choose to "mark" most of the questions in the block, you will have a difficult time getting through them all thoroughly.
         (b) If you choose to "mark" items sparingly you can take time and review those critical questions for which you need more time.
   d. **Red Flag:** Be cautious when changing answers during your review.
      (1) **Red Flag:** Do not be tempted to change your answer without good reason!
         (a) Change only if you recall specific evidence to do so.
         (b) Change if you accidentally chose a different answer than you intended.
         (c) Change if you misread the question.
   e. At the end of the block you will be prompted to "Submit" your questions. Once you choose this option, this block of questions is gone and you will automatically start the next block.
   f. Make sure you answer every question even if you are giving it your "best guess." Remember if an answer is blank, it is automatically wrong.

4. At the conclusion of the exam, you will be given an opportunity to complete a survey of the exam and exam process.
   a. This survey is delivered on the computer following your examination.

Question Format

1. **Each question is a multiple-choice item.**
   a. Questions do not relate to prior or upcoming questions. Consider each question separately on its own merits and information.

2. **Each question will have four specific choices.**
   a. The choices do not link to each other.
   b. Each question is its own entity and does not link to any other question.

3. **Red Flag: You will be expected to answer with the "best answer" from the choices provided.**
   a. **Red Flag:** That does not mean it is the only correct answer there might be in physical therapy—it means those are your only choices.

4. **Use the methods of answering multiple-choice questions discussed in the Introduction Section in the *PTA Examination Review & Study Guide* to select the best choice.**

5. **You are not "penalized" for getting an answer wrong.**
   a. Never leave a question blank; always answer it.
   b. If you have to use an educated guess, you will have at least a 25% chance of getting it correct; a blank answer is 100% wrong all of the time.

Question (Item) Difficulty

1. **The bulk of the examination will have questions that are written at the Comprehension and Application levels. (See *PTA Examination Review & Study Guide*, Introduction).**
   a. This means each question will present a problem, situation or condition for which you must make a correct decision.
   b. You will need to apply knowledge from multiple "chapters" and "classes" from school to solve the problem presented.
      (1) Simply having information memorized is not sufficient for this level of test question.

2. **The examination covers persons from young to old. You must be able to apply information across the life span.**

3. **You must be able to apply interventions and concepts to persons who have multiple system involvement. You must be able to correctly problem-solve situations.**

4. **Remember the questions are not meant to "trick" you. They are meant to make you tie relevant pieces of information together to solve problems presented.**

Structuring Your Exam Review

Determine What You Need to Do to Prepare

1. **Do you need to review content?**
   a. It is likely you will need to review some content—2 years of schooling covers a lot of information. Remember, information has to be reviewed with the premise of "How will I use this to provide safe intervention to patients across their life span? Is this intervention or assessment appropriate and indicated for the specific patient condition? What effect will this intervention have on the patient as a whole?"
      (1) **Red Flag:** Studies show that the act of applying concepts to situations and the act of using concepts and knowledge to answer specific questions is more effective than simply studying—for example, reading and reviewing information.
   b. You will know you need to review content if you are unable to verbalize viable correct options to a test item without seeing the four choices you are given.

   c. It is critical to recognize that simply reviewing information with the intent of "memorizing" it for later use will likely result in failing results.

2. **Do you need to practice test-taking strategies?**
   a. You likely need some practice answering exam questions if you are unable to use multiple-choice test-taking strategies to help manage test items in a timely, scientific and efficient manner.
   b. It is critical that you realize that just taking multiple examinations is not a content review.

3. **Do you have anxiety about taking the exam?**
   a. Most of us have anxiety related to an examination situation. Clearly this exam can be one of the major challenges presented to us in our lifetimes. Remember that anxiety is not always a bad thing—it can heighten our senses, increase our level of alertness and increase our adrenaline level. When these responses are controlled, they will not interfere with your taking and passing the exam.

⚑(1) **Red Flag:** When you are anxious about taking the exam, it is a normal response.

    (a) Use stress management techniques to gain control of your anxiety.

      • Deep breathing.

      • Progressive relaxation.

      • Visualization techniques.

(2) When anxiety is not under control, it can negatively affect your performance on the exam.

⚑b. **Red Flag:** Recognize that undue anxiety is likely the result of poor preparation for exam day. Only you are in control of this situation. Take your review process seriously and approach it with an organized plan and you will be better prepared to take and pass your licensure examination.

Establish Control Over the Study and Review Process

1. **Begin the review process 4–6 weeks prior to the date you plan to take the exam. If English is your second language, or if you struggled as a student, you may need up to 8 weeks of review and exam preparation.**

    a. Remember, once you have applied, paid for, and submitted all of the required paperwork you will receive a letter from the FSBPT that gives you 6 weeks in which you must schedule and take your examination.

      (1) This time frame can be extended, but additional fees will be required.

2. **Set a regular study schedule and follow it.**

    a. Plan between 2–3 hours at a time, 6 days a week. Take a day off from your studying to enjoy those things you enjoy and that will energize you.

      (1) Be sure to schedule physical activity, and time with friends/family/significant others.

      (2) Involve those close to you in helping increase your success rate. Have them help with daily responsibilities; have them help with flash cards if you need to memorize facts, etc.

      (3) Limit internal stimuli like hunger, extraneous thoughts and fatigue. Get enough rest and include physical activity (even if it is light activity like walking) to help keep you fresh.

      (4) Limit external stimuli from television, telephones, laundry, pets, children, etc.

      (5) Capture spare minutes for studying by carrying note cards or sheets of notes with you.

Assess Areas of Strength and Weakness

1. **Take one of the practice examinations. After the examination you will be provided with feedback identifying the areas in which you had incorrect responses.**

    a. For example, did you get incorrect responses in the musculoskeletal or lymphatic areas? Did you get incorrect responses related to clinical application of physical therapy principles, intervention, data collection, etc?

    b. Make note of those areas.

2. **Use the FSBPT Exam Blueprint to clarify specific information the exam will cover.**

    a. For example, if you tested weak in the area of clinical application for the cardiovascular system, review the bullet points for this category of the examination and base your studies on these content areas.

3. **Read the rationale for each answer you had incorrect and write notes to yourself identifying information you want/need to go back and review.**

    a. Be specific. For example: "Review the blood supply of the brain and explain potential effects and responses to occlusion or hemorrhage"; "Explore the effects of environment on persons with multiple sclerosis"; "Explain the physiology of the metabolic system and how it may affect interventions I apply to the patient/client."

4. **Now you are ready to begin an organized and purposeful review process.**

Structuring a Purposeful Review Process

1. **Choose one of the areas identified in the steps listed above. Identify what resources (notes, texts) you will need to do an in-depth review of that subject area.**

2. **Gather those resources and use one 2- to 3-hour study session to review this subject area. Determine how many subject areas you can review in this study session based on how extensive the review process needs to be.**

    a. TherapyEd's **PTA Examination Review & Study Guide** is designed to give you a complete review of content in one resource. You may want to use the table of contents to identify multiple chapters within the text where you can find review content.

    b. The PTA **Course Manual**, only available to students taking our courses, is a "one-stop-shopping center" for ready reference lists, tables, with additional information, tables and explanations.

    c. Your course texts and notes will provide additional detail when you are unable to draw complete conclusions for the information provided in our resources.

3. **Summarize and utilize what you have read.**

    a. Read and review the material you have gathered with purpose.

      (1) Upon reading a section in whatever source you use, stop and summarize by writing down "how" you

will use this information. For example, explain how this information affects interventions you will provide, or how it affects performing data collection on a patient/client who is an infant, young child, adolescent, adult, young adult, older adult.

b. Try Mind Mapping—this is great if you are a visual or kinesthetic learner! (Figure 1-1).

   (1) In the center of a page write down the concept you are trying to learn or use.

   (2) From there diagram curving branches coming off of the center concept. These branches identify streams of information related to the central topic.

   (3) Write them with different colored ink or highlight with contrasting colors. It has been shown in studies that concepts can be better understood and recalled with the use of colors.

4. **Continue this process until you have reviewed all necessary areas of concern.**

Reassess Your Areas of Strength and Weakness

1. Take another of the review examinations provided on the CD in the *National PTA Examination Review & Study Guide*.

2. Continue as identified in Section C above.

The 6-Week Training Program for Exam Preparation (Table 1-1)

1. **Take TherapyEd's Examination Preparation course.**
   a. If you are unable to attend a course, take one of the simulated examinations on the CD included in this text.
   b. Analyze your areas of strength and weakness.
   c. Develop your focused review program.
   d. Follow through with focused review for 2–3 weeks.

2. **Take the next simulated examination from the CD enclosed.**
   a. Reassess your areas of strength and weakness.
   b. Develop your focused review program. Follow through with focused review for 2–3 weeks.

3. **Take the second simulated examination from the CD enclosed.**
   a. Reassess your areas of strength and weakness.

b. Develop your focused review program. Follow through with focused review for 5–10 days.

4. **Take 2–3 days off from studying and let your mind rest.**

5. **Avoid last-minute studying or reviewing the night before. This can just lead to anxiety and be detrimental to your testing performance.**

6. **Take the NPTE.**

Table 1-1 ➤ 6-WEEK TRAINING PROGRAM FOR EXAM PREPARATION

TherapyEd
Evanston, Illinois
United States of America

**6 Week Training Program
for Exam Preparation**

Class Ends
Focused study
2 weeks

⬇

**1ˢᵗ Practice Test
Reassess Areas for Improvement**

Focused study
2 weeks

⬇

**2ⁿᵈ Practice Test
Reassess Areas for Improvement**

Focused study
2 weeks

⬇

**3ʳᵈ Practice Test
Reassess Areas for Improvement**

Focused study
5-10 days

⬇

Take a day or two off

⬇

Licensure exam

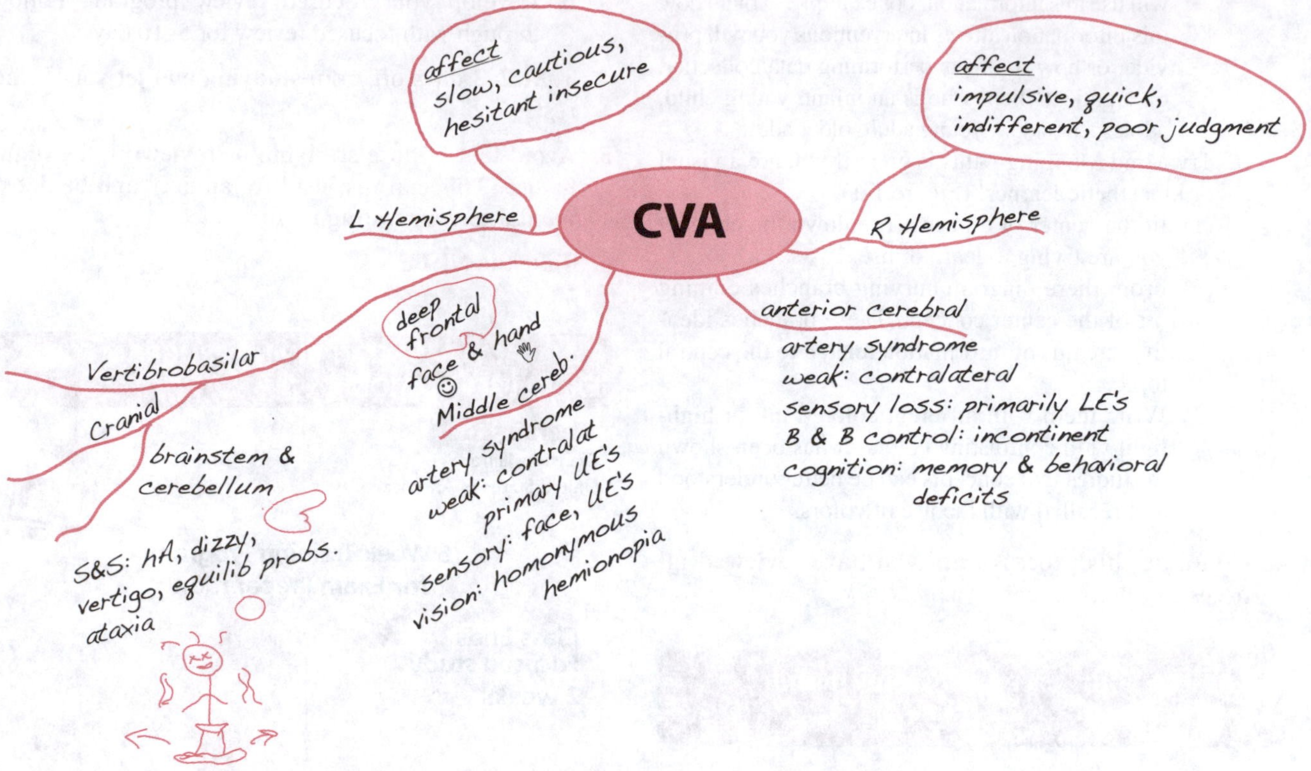

Figure 1-1 • Mind Map: Presentation of a Patient Following Cardiovascular Accident

---

Application Concepts

Making the Most of Your Study Time

- Use practice exams as a mechanism to determine your areas of strength and areas of weakness.
- Begin your study on the areas in which you tested weak.
- Establish a good study plan based on areas of identified strength and weakness.
- Use the NPTE content outline as a syllabus to structure study areas and content. This information can be found in the Introduction of this text.
- Use TherapyEd's *Review and Study*, as well as the *Course Manual*, to access information quickly.
- Structure your study so that you are applying clinical concepts of anatomy, pathology, physiology and medical management in providing intervention and performing data collection with patients and clients.
- Apply concepts to patients and clients of all ages.

chapter *2*

Musculoskeletal System

ROBERT ROWE

Focus Areas for Content Review:

- Anatomy and physiology of the musculoskeletal system.
- Pathologies and injuries of the musculoskeletal system commonly seen in physical therapy.
- Physical therapy interventions; indications and contraindications, appropriate responses, PTA response to adverse reaction, effects of interventions on the musculoskeletal system.

- Musculoskeletal tests and measures indicating patient ability to participate in and/or indication to discontinue intervention as well as to document the patient's progress toward the established goals.
- Principles of progression of intervention activities as related to musculoskeletal conditions commonly encountered in physical therapy.

Clinical Application—Soft and Bony Tissues

Tissue Structure and Function

1. **Collagen types I and II.**
   a. Type I: tightly woven fibers collected into bundles; thick, rugged and stiff.
      (1) Demonstrate very little extensibility when placed under stress.
      (2) Found in ligaments.
      (3) Found in tendons.
      (4) Found in joint capsule.
   b. Type II: more loosely woven fibers collected into a network; more flexible than type I.
      (1) Fiber network helps maintain shape and provide internal strength in tissues.
      (2) Found in hyaline cartilage.

2. **Elastin fibers.**
   a. Formed into an interwoven network within tissues.
   b. Resists tensile (stretching) forces.
   c. Elastin in tissues allows it to withstand a stretch and return readily to previous shape.
      (1) Found in cartilage.
      (2) Found in spinal ligaments.

3. **Dense irregular connective tissue.**
   a. Contains a high density of collagen type I fibers.
   b. Has a high degree of tensile strength and low degree of extensibility.
   c. Has multidirectional fiber orientation, contributing to its ability to withstand multidirectional forces.
   d. Found in:
      (1) Joint capsule.
      (2) Periosteum.
      (3) Aponeurosis.
      (4) Dermis.
   e. Contributes to joint stability.
   f. Low vascularity and low water content contribute to slower healing time frame.
      (1) The tension placed on these tissues during joint motion retrains undesirable motion.

4. **Dense regular connective tissue.**
   a. Contains a high density of collagen fibers that contribute to high tensile strength.
   b. Has the most tensile strength and is the least extensible (stretchy) of connective tissue types.
   c. Fiber orientation is unidirectional (parallel), contributing to its ability to withstand unidirectional forces.
   d. Found in:
      (1) Ligaments.
      (2) Tendons.
   e. Low vascularity and low water content contribute to slower healing time frame.

5. **Loose irregular connective tissue.**
   a. Contains lower density collagen fibers that exhibit multidirectional fiber organization.
   b. Tissues are more pliable and extensible than dense regular or dense irregular connective tissues.
   c. Found in:
      (1) Superficial fascial sheaths.
      (2) Muscle and nerve sheaths.
   d. Relatively higher vasculature and water content contribute to faster healing times.
      (1) Tissue is easiest tissue to mobilize following trauma or period of immobilization.

6. **Articular cartilage.**
   a. Found on joint surfaces.
      (1) Matrix at bottom layers firmly anchors it to the ends of bones.
      (2) Fibers arranged in a scaffold-type arrangement; contributes to its significant strength.
      (3) Responds well to compressive forces by dispersing stresses.
      (4) Reduces friction between joint surfaces.
   b. Is a type of hyaline cartilage; however, it is unable to nourish itself.
      (1) Receives its nourishment from synovial fluid through the "milking" action that occurs when cartilage is deformed during joint loading.
   c. Is avascular and aneural.

7. **Fibrocartilage.**
   a. Shares properties of dense irregular connective tissue and articular cartilage.
   b. Demonstrates significant ability to absorb and disperse multidirectional loads.
   c. Found in:
      (1) Intervertebral disc.
      (2) Labrum.
      (3) Meniscus.
   d. Nourishment obtained through "milking" action occurring through joint loading forces.
      (1) In synovial joint, nutrients are diffused through synovial fluid.
      (2) In joints such as the intervertebral disc and pubis symphysis, nutrients are diffused across fluid contained in surrounding trabecular bone.
   e. Healing.
      (1) Some tissue repair may occur where vascularized structures attach near it; e.g., ligaments of the spine, joint capsule in the knee.
      (2) Portions that do not attach near a blood supply demonstrate poor healing ability: e.g., innermost portions of the meniscus.

8. **Bone.**
   a. Provides rigid support system for body.
   b. Joints allow for a system of levers contributing to movement.
   c. Comprised of two basic layers:

(1) A strong, dense outer layer (compact bone) contributes to its strength.
   (a) Contains the haversian system which contributes to maintenance and repair of bone.
(2) A softer, mesh inner layer (cancellous bone) serves to store marrow.
   d. Covered with periosteum, a fibrous connective tissue, which serves to provide blood supply to the bone as well as an attachment site for tendons and ligaments.
   e. Is continuously remodeling and reshaping.
      (1) A balance between osteoblast (bond formation) and osteoclast (bone remodeling or absorbing) activity maintains this homeostatic state.

9. **Muscle.**
   a. Consists of light and dark bands of contractile fibers that respond to a stimulus to contract.
      (1) Actin and myosin filaments interlink and become closer together during muscle contraction and slide farther apart during muscle relaxation.
   b. Demonstrates elasticity.
   c. Strength of muscle.
      (1) Dependent on its cross-sectional area; greater cross-sectional area = greater strength and visa versa.
      (2) Is most weak at the end ranges of complete relaxation and complete contraction.
      (3) Is most strong at the mid ranges of its available ROM.

Effects of Aging on Structure and Function

1. **Mechanical properties.**
   a. The ability to withstand forces diminishes with age.
   b. Amount of deterioration highly variable between individuals.
   c. Accumulated microtrauma through normal "wear and tear" can contribute to structural failure.
   d. Tissues diminish in their ability to rehydrate, thus decreasing the ability to withstand forces placed upon them.
      (1) Contributes to decreasing ability of tissue to distribute forces between bony surfaces.
   e. With stress, bundles of fibers in connective tissues lose their ability align themselves.
      (1) Results in decreased ability to withstand more rapidly applied forces.

2. **Effects of aging can be somewhat modified.**
   a. Good nutrition contributes to improved overall function as well as tissue function.
   b. Proper hydration is important for all body systems to function normally.
   c. Appropriate strengthening and aerobic activities can contribute to overall function and good health.

Effects of Immobilization

1. **Histology and normal mechanics of tissues are changed with immobilization.**

2. **Fibrosis and adhesions occur in tissues.**
   (a) Water content of tissues decreases and contributes to cross-linking of collagen fibers.
   (b) Collagen being laid down to repair tissue is laid down in a "haphazard" fashion (commonly called *cross-linking*) which further limits tissue mobility.

3. **Decreased tensile forces placed on the structures contribute to a decline in strength of tissues.**
   (a) Studies demonstrate that ligaments that have been subjected to immobilization and subsequent rehabilitation, do not regain the same tensile strength they had to begin with.

4. **Bone and cartilage will lose mass, volume and strength.**

5. **This decrease in strength can begin within days of immobilization.**

Clinical Application
- Tissues are designed to withstand a myriad of forces placed upon them.
- Articular and fibrocartilage rely on the "milking" action of joint movement and muscle contraction/relaxation to maintain nourishment.
- Bone is continuously remodeling and relies on compressive forces to maintain its health: e.g. those achieved by weight bearing and muscle contraction and relaxation.
- Immobilization alters the immediate and ultimate strength of soft tissues.

Response to Stress

1. **Soft tissue.**
   a. Connective tissues are designed to respond to stresses placed upon them at rest and at work (during activity).
   b. Ability of the tissue to withstand stress, without tissue failure, is dependent upon:
      (1) The health of the tissue prior to the load.
      (2) The force applied to the tissue.
      (3) The rate at which the force is applied.
      (4) The viscoelastic qualities of the tissue.
      (5) This action is depicted through the stress-strain curve (Figure 2-1).
   c. When an external force is applied correctly, within the limits of the connective tissue's ability to withstand the force, an elastic change occurs.
      (1) Maintenance of range of motion (ROM) of the tissue.

   d. When an external force is applied correctly, to the limits of the connective tissue's ability to withstand the force, a plastic change occurs.
      (1) Increased ROM of the tissue.
   e. When the force applied exceeds the tissue's ability to withstand the force, a tear (strain or sprain) occurs: e.g., "twisting" an ankle, hyperextending a shoulder.
      (1) The extent of the injury to a muscle or tendon is identified at the "degree" of strain or sprain (Table 2-1).

2. **Scar tissue formation in soft tissues.**
   a. Occurs in four phases.
   b. Each phase responds differently to mobilization forces.
   c. Phases of scar tissue formation:
      (1) Phase 1: inflammatory phase.
         (a) Occurs immediately.
         (b) Lasts from 24–36 hours.
         (c) Predominated by migration of fluids and macrophages to the damaged site; facilitates the healing response.
         (d) Generally immobilization or limited use is important to limit tissue damage and allow initial healing to occur without increasing inflammatory response.
      (2) Phase 2: granulation phase.
         (a) Relative increase in vascularity.
         (b) Granulation tissue forming.
         (c) Timing of phase dependent on specific tissues; generally more vascular tissues heal more quickly.
         (d) Muscle and epithelial tissue heals faster.
         (e) Tendon and ligament heal more slowly.
         (f) Some movement is generally allowed; highly dependent on tissue injured.
      (3) Phase 3: scar tissue formation.
         (a) Characterized by increasing fibroblasts and collagen production.
            - Collagen is laid down in an unorganized fashion and begins binding to damaged areas.

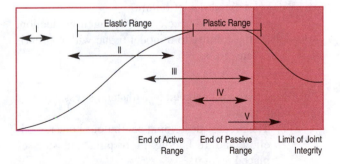

STRESS-STRAIN CURVE & RANGE OF JOINT PLAY

Figure 2-1 • Grades of movement.
(Adapted from Grieve GP. *Mobilization of the Spine. A Primary Handbook of Clinical Method.* 5th ed. Churchill Livingstone, New York, 1991.)

Table 2-1 ➤ DEGREE OF MUSCLE STRAIN, TENDON INJURY AND LIGAMENT SPRAIN

	1° STRAIN	2° STRAIN	3° STRAIN	1° SPRAIN	2° SPRAIN	3° SPRAIN	TENDINITIS
Definition	A few fibers of muscle torn	Approximately ½ muscle fibers torn	All muscle fibers torn (rupture)	A few fibers of ligament torn	Approximately ½ ligament fibers torn	All ligament fibers torn	Inflammation of tendon, tendon degeneration
Mechanism of Injury	Excessive load or stretch	Excessive load or stretch, crush injury	Excessive load or stretch	Excessive load or stretch	Excessive load or stretch	Excessive load or stretch	Overuse, excessive load or stretch; also aging
Weakness	Minor	Moderate, potentially > due to pain	Moderate to significant	Minor	Minor to significant	Minor to significant	Minor to significant
Muscle Spasm	Minor	Moderate to significant	Moderate	Minor	Minor	Minor	Minor
Swelling	Minor	Moderate to significant	Moderate to significant	Minor	Moderate	Moderate to significant	Minor to significant, potential thickening
Disability, Loss of Function	Minor	Moderate to significant	Significant, reflex inhibition and pain	Minor	Moderate to significant	Moderate to significant, joint instability	Minor to significant
Pain with Isometric Contraction	Minor	Moderate to significant	Minor to no pain	No	No	No	Minor to significant
Pain with Stretch	Yes	Yes	No, unless other tissues also damaged	Yes	Yes	No, unless other tissues also damaged	Yes
ROM	Decreased	Decreased	May increase or decrease, dependent on swelling	Decreased	Decreased	Decreased	May increase or decrease, dependent on swelling Dislocation of subluxation possible
Joint Play	Normal	Normal	Normal	Normal	Normal	Normal to excessive	Normal

(b) Scar tissue at this time can be easily remodeled with appropriate stresses applied.

(c) Lasts from 3–8 weeks depending on original tissue makeup (vascularity).

(4) Phase 4: maturation.

(a) Scar tissue matures during this phase; solidifies and shrinks.

(b) Maximal stresses can be placed on tissue without risk of failure.

(c) Continued accelerated collagen production, thus ability to remodel tissue with appropriate stress.

3. Bone tissue.

a. Bone tissue is designed to withstand stress.

b. Wolf's law.

(1) The process describing continuous bone remodeling and reshaping in response to stresses placed upon it.

(2) Muscle contraction and relaxation, such as that occurring during resisted exercise, places sufficient stress on bone to stimulate this remodeling and reshaping process.

(3) Weight-bearing activities are particularly effective in stimulating remodeling and reshaping of bone.

c. Excessive stress placed on bone results in fracture.

d. Fracture types:

(1) Complete: bone is fractured all the way through, may be nondisplaced or displaced.

(a) Will require immobilization.

(b) Displaced will require relocation of the bone ends; may occur with local pain killers or under anesthesia.

(c) May require open reduction internal fixation (ORIF); through surgical intervention the fracture is reduced and pins, screw and/or plates are used to secure bone ends.

(2) Incomplete: bone demonstrates a disruption in its integrity; the disruption does not completely separate and fragments are still somewhat connected.

(a) Will require immobilization. Type used dependent upon location of fracture and whether it is a weight-bearing area or not.

(3) Stress fracture: fine, hairline fracture occurring with little to no soft tissue damage.

(a) Can be difficult to diagnose; often best seen on x-ray 3–4 weeks following incident.

(b) Often seen with runners, dancers, participants in aerobics or track.

(4) Open fracture: one in which the bone protrudes out of the skin.
    (a) Will require open reduction (surgical) and potentially internal fixation (placement of pins, screws, plates to secure bone segments).
(5) Greenstick: the bone is partially bent and partially broken (resembling what occurs when a green stick is bent); occurs in children (as their bones are more flexible than a teen's or adult's).

Principles of Kinesiology and Biomechanics

Selected Kinematics

1. **Arthrokinematics (accessory motion).**
   a. Defined as the movement between joint surfaces.
   b. There are three motions that describe movement of one joint surface on another:
   (1) *Roll* consists of one joint surface rolling on another such as a tire rolling on the road. An example of this would be movement between the femoral and tibial articular surfaces of the knee.
   (2) *Glide/slide* consists of a pure translatory motion of one surface gliding on another, as when a braked wheel skids. An example of this type of motion in human body would be movement of joint surface of proximal phalanx at head of a metacarpal bone of hand.
       (a) Joint mobilization techniques use this motion to restore accessory motion and restore joint play.
   (3) *Spin* consists of a rotation of the movable component of the joint. An example of this type of motion is movement between joint surfaces of radial head with humerus.
   (4) Combinations of all three motions can occur at joints. An example is movement between joint surfaces of humerus and scapula of shoulder.

2. **Osteokinematics (physiological motion).**
   a. Defined as movement between two bones; e.g., flexion, abduction.

3. **Convex-concave rule describes relationship between arthrokinematics and osteokinematics. See application box below.**
   a. When the concave joint surface is moving, gliding occurs in the same direction of bone movement.
   b. When the convex joint surface is moving, gliding occurs in the opposite direction of bone movement.

Response to Mobilization

1. **Effects of tissue mobilization techniques.**
   (a) Cross-linking is diminished and new collagen is laid down in a more orderly fashion.
   (b) Tissues become rehydrated and demonstrate improved viscosity.
   (c) Adhesions are partially ruptured facilitating tissue elongation.

Application Concepts—Convex/Concave Rule

The convex/concave rule describes the relationship between the angular motion of a joint (physiological motion) and the linear motion that occurs at the joint surface (accessory motion).

Concave Rule:

If the shape of the distal bone at the joint is concave, gliding (linear motion) occurs in the same direction as the angular movement. For example, the tibia is concave at the tibiofemoral joint. As the tibia moves anteriorly during knee extension, the joint surface glides anteriorly. If knee extension is limited, a grade III or IV anterior glide can help with regaining motion.

Convex Rule:

If the shape of the distal bone at the joint is convex, gliding occurs in the opposite direction of the angular movement. For example, the head of the humerus is convex at the glenohumeral joint. As the shaft of the humerus moves anteriorly during shoulder flexion, the joint surface of the humerus is gliding posteriorly. If shoulder flexion is limited, a grade III or IV posterior glide can help with regaining motion.

Joint Capsule

1. **Capsular positions.**
   a. Resting or loose-packed position (Table 2-2).
   (1) Joint position where capsule and other soft tissues are in most relaxed position.
   (2) Minimal joint surface contact.
   (3) **Red Flag:** May perform joint play and mobilization techniques in this position.
   b. Close-packed position (Table 2-2).
   (1) Joint position where capsule and other soft tissues are maximally tensed.

Table 2-2 ➤ RESTING AND CLOSE-PACKED POSITIONS

JOINT	CONVEX/CONCAVE RULE	CLOSE-PACKED POSITION	RESTING/LOOSE-PACKED POSITION
Glenohumeral	Convex	Full ABD (abduction) & full ER (external/lateral rotation)	55-70 ABD, 30 horizontal adduction, 0 rotation
Humeroulnar	Concave	Full extension & full supination	70 flexion, 10 supination
Humeroradial	Concave	90 flexion, 5 supination	Full extension & supination
Proximal radioulnar	Convex	5 supination, full extension	70 flexion, 35 supination
Distal radioulnar	Concave	5 supination	10 supination
Radiocarpal	Convex	Full extension & radial deviation	Neutral, with slight ulnar deviation
1st carpometacarpal	Concave coronal plane Convex sagittal plane	Full opposition	Halfway between end range flexion/extension and abduction/adduction
1st metacarpophalangeal	Concave	Full extension	Slight flexion
2nd-5th metacarpophalangeal	Concave	Full flexion	Slight flexion
Proximal & distal interphalangeal	Concave	Full extension	Slight flexion
Hip	Convex	Ligamentous: full extension, ABD & internal/medial rotation Bony: 90 flexion, slight ABD & ER	30 flexion, 30 ABD & slight ER
Patellofemoral	Concave	Full knee flexion	Full knee extension
Tibiofemoral	Concave	Full extension & ER	25 flexion
Talocrural	Concave	Full dorsiflexion	10 plantarflexion
Metatarsophalangeal	Concave	Full extension	neutral

(2) Maximal contact between joint surfaces.

➤ (3) **Red Flag:** Joint play and mobilization techniques cannot be properly performed in this position.

c. Characteristic "pattern" or restriction of proportional limitation or restriction in ROM secondary to capsular contraction (Table 2-3).

   (1) Each joint has its own characteristic "pattern" of proportional limitation.

2. End-feels.

   a. Normal physiological end-feel.

   (1) Soft: occurs with soft tissue approximation.

   (2) Firm: capsular and ligamentous stretching.

   (3) Hard: when bone and/or cartilage meet.

   b. Pathological end-feel.

   (1) Boggy: edema, joint swelling.

   (2) Firm with decreased elasticity: fibrosis of soft tissues.

   (3) Rubbery: muscle spasm.

   (4) Empty: loose then very hard; associated with muscle guarding or patient protecting from going into painful part of range.

   (5) Hypermobility: end-feel at a later time than opposite side.

3. Grading of accessory joint movement.

   a. Accessory joint movement or joint play is graded to assess arthrokinematic motion of the joint and/or when it is impractical or impossible to measure joint motion with a goniometer (Table 2-4).

Table 2-3 ➤ CAPSULAR PATTERNS

JOINT(S)	PROPORTIONAL LIMITATIONS
Glenohumeral	Greater limitation of external rotation, followed by abduction, and internal rotation
Humeroulnar	Loss of flexion > extension
Humeroradial	Loss of flexion > extension
Forearm	Equally restricted in pronation and supination in presence of elbow restriction
Wrist	Limitation: flexion = extension
Hip	Limited flexion/internal rotation > loss of extension > flexion
Tibiofemoral (knee)	Flexion grossly limited; slight limitation of extension
Talocrural (ankle)	Loss of plantarflexion > dorsiflexion
Talocalcaneal (subtalar)	Increasing limitations of varus; joint fixed in valgus (inversion > eversion)

Table 2-4 ➤ MANUAL GRADING OF ACCESSORY JOINT MOTION

GRADE	JOINT STATUS
0	Ankylosed
1	Considerable hypomobility
2	Slight hypomobility
3	Normal
4	Slight hypermobility
5	Considerable hypermobility
6	Unstable

From: Grieve GP. *Mobilization of the Spine; A Primary Handbook of Clinical Method*, 5th ed, Churchill Livingstone, New York, 1991, with permission.

b. Although interrater reliability is poor, intrarater reliability has been found to be acceptable.

c. Data gleaned provides clinicians with more specific data to help guide treatment approach.

Muscle Substitutions

1. **Occur as result of muscles that have become shortened/lengthened, have become weakened, have lost endurance, have developed impaired coordination or have become paralyzed.**

2. **Stronger muscles compensate for loss of motion.**

3. Common muscle substitutions:
   (a) Use of scapular stabilizers to initiate shoulder motion when shoulder abductors are weakened.
   (b) Use of lateral trunk muscles or tensor fascia latae (TFL) when abductors are weak.
   (c) Use of passive finger flexion by contraction of wrist extensors when finger flexors are weak (tenodesis).
   (d) Use of long head of biceps, coracobrachialis and anterior deltoid when pectoralis major is weak.
   (e) Use of lower back extensors, adductor magnus and quadratus lumborum when hip extensors are weak.
   (f) Use of lower abdominal, lower obliques, hip adductors and latissimus dorsi when hip flexors are weak.

Clinical Application – Soft Tissue Techniques Including Mobilization

Connective Tissue Mobilization for Tissue Tension

1. Transverse friction techniques:
   a. Press finger tip(s) perpendicular to tendon.
   b. Press down through superficial tissues; move superficial tissues on tendon.
      (1) Deeper tissues can most easily be accessed by placing the muscle on slack.
      (2) Slight tension on a tendon allows effective transverse friction.
   c. Use pressure in one direction on the tendon; e.g., always pull toward you or push away from you during each treatment session.
   d. Apply for 5–6 minutes per tendon or tendon area.
   e. Follow cross friction techniques with manual or active stretching of associated muscle.

2. Muscle techniques:
   a. Apply a longitudinal stroke, using finger tips or thumbs, along the muscle fibers.
      (1) This technique is designed to facilitate separating muscle bundles from each other.
   b. Muscle tissue is best reached with the muscle on slack.

3. Transverse muscle techniques:
   a. Apply a transverse force to a muscle bundle along any portion of the muscle that demonstrates decreased mobility.
   b. This technique helps mobilize the muscle fiber from its sheath.
   c. This technique can improve ROM and active strength of the muscle.

4. Fascia techniques:
   a. Use longitudinal strokes along fascial areas near bony surfaces that demonstrate limited mobility.
      (1) For example, anterior-lateral border along the tibia in shin splints, iliotibial band (ITB) anterior to the lateral knee, junction between ITB and biceps femoris.

Connective Tissue Mobilization for Lengthening

1. **Tissues must be stretched beyond their elastic limit and into their plastic range (see Figure 2-1).**

2. **Speed.**
   (a) The stretching force must be applied slowly enough to avoid tissue damage, as well as to avoid stimulating contractile tissue in muscle.
   (b) Gradually release the stretch.

3. **Duration.**
   a. The stretching force must be applied long enough to allow for remodeling (rearranging of collagen fiber bonds) of collagen fibers and redistribution of water to surrounding tissues.
   b. Long-duration stretches are typically recommended.
   c. Terms typically used to describe long-duration stretching techniques include.
      (1) Static.
      (2) Sustained.
      (3) Prolonged.
   d. Terms typically used to describe short-duration stretching techniques include.
      (1) Cyclic.

(2) Intermittent.

(3) Ballistic.

e. Evidence.

(1) It is generally accepted that stretches applied for 30–60 seconds (whether it be one to two 30-second stretches or six 10-minute stretches) are effective to gain ROM.

(2) Low-load and long-duration stretches yield the most significant elastic deformation and long-term plastic tissue responses.

4. Intensity.

a. Stretching force should be a low-magnitude force that is applied over time.

b. Low-intensity stretching has been shown to elongate dense connective tissues more effectively, with less tissue damage and post exercise soreness, than high-intensity stretch.

5. Frequency.

a. There is little evidence to support a specified frequency of stretching.

b. Consider:

(1) Acuity or chronicity of condition.

(2) Cause of/for the condition.

(3) Stage of tissue healing.

(4) Severity of loss of ROM.

6. Mode of stretch. See Chapter 10 for details.

Joint Mobilization

1. Indications and contraindications (Table 2-5).

2. Systems of "dosages" of joint mobilization techniques.

a. Maitland (oscillatory techniques) (See Figure 2-1).

(1) Grade I = small-amplitude oscillation at the beginning of the range.

(2) Grade II = large-amplitude oscillation before the point of tissue resistance.

(3) Grade III = large-amplitude oscillation that pushes into tissue resistance.

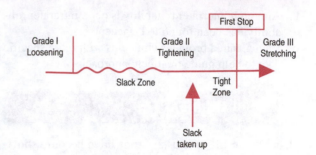
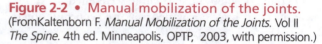

Figure 2-2 • Manual mobilization of the joints. (FromKaltenborn F. *Manual Mobilization of the Joints.* Vol II *The Spine.* 4th ed. Minneapolis, OPTP, 2003, with permission.)

(4) Grade IV = small-amplitude oscillation near the end of passive range.

(5) Grade V = small-amplitude, high-velocity manipulation past the end of passive range.

b. Uses of Maitland "doses."

(1) Grades I and II: primarily used to limit pain.

(a) Joint oscillations stimulate mechanoreceptors that block nociceptive pathways at the brain or spinal cord level and inhibit the perception of pain.

(2) Grades III and IV: primarily used to stretch maneuvers.

(3) Either physiological or joint play motions are used in mobilization techniques.

c. Kaltenborn (sustained translation) (See Figure 2-2).

(1) Grade I = small-amplitude translation with no tension applied to the joint capsule.

(2) Grade II = translation that stops just short of applying tension to the joint capsule.

(3) Grade III = translation that stretches/places tension on the joint capsule.

d. Uses of Kaltenborn "doses."

(1) Grade I: a distraction force used with all gliding motions; also used for pain relief.

(2) Grade II: distraction applied to asses joint reaction; this reaction either indicated increased or decreased distraction.

(a) Gentle grade II distraction is used intermittently to inhibit pain; used to maintain joint play when ROM is not allowed.

(3) Grade III: distractions and glides are used to stretch the joint structures to increase joint play.

Table 2-5 ➤ INDICATIONS AND CONTRAINDICATIONS TO JOINT MOBILIZATION

INDICATIONS	CONTRAINDICATIONS/PRECAUTIONS
Pain	Joint hypermobility
Muscle spasm and guarding	Joint effusion
	Inflammation
Joint hypomobility	Precautions
Functional limitation in joint ROM	Malignancy
	Unhealed fracture
	Bone disease
	Hypermobility in adjacent joints
	Systemic connective tissue diseases (rheumatoid arthritis)
	Individual is on blood-thinning medications

Application Concept

Physical therapist assistant students should be prepared to answer questions about joint kinematics and kinesiology as they relate to the clinical application of physical therapy concepts and interventions to patients/clients on the licensure examination. This may include the application of, effects of and responses to joint mobility techniques.

3. **Assessment of pain.**
   a. Pain before limit in tissue ROM: indicates injury is still in the inflammatory or early granulation phase of tissue healing.
      (1) Only small-amplitude rhythmic oscillation and/or distraction techniques are indicated.
   b. Pain occurs concurrently with reaching the tissue limitation: indicates the tissues are in the granulation phase and still healing.
      (1) Small-amplitude and large-amplitude rhythmic oscillation techniques "within" the tissue ROM are indicated; helps maintain joint nutrition and begins to assist with remodeling disorganized (haphazardly organized) scar tissues.
   c. Pain occurs after tissue limitation is met: indicates tissues are likely in the remodeling or maturation phase and can tolerate more aggressive stretching techniques.
      (1) Small-and large-amplitude rhythmic oscillations into tissue resistance are indicated to stretch tissues.

4. **Application considerations;**
   a. Position the joint so is it is freely available and the muscles are relaxed.
      (1) Position the joint capsule in the open packed position.
      (2) May need to reposition the joint so that it is in the least painful position.
   b. Examine joint play.
   c. Initiate mobilization techniques.

   (1) Begin with grades I and II.
   (2) Progress to higher grades as indicated per outcome goals.

5. **Force and direction of movements.**
   a. Treatment force is applied close to the opposing joint surface.
      (1) Position hand, fingers, thumb and mobilization belt so the greatest surface area is in contact with the patient's tissues for increased comfort.
   b. The entire bone is moved to accomplish the motion; do not use the bone as a lever so that the joint surface rolls.
   c. The plane of the concave bone is used to determine direction of the force applied.
   d. The treatment plane is perpendicular to a line running from the axis of rotation to the middle of the concave articular surface.
   e. Distraction techniques are applied perpendicular to the treatment plane.
   f. Gliding techniques are applied parallel to the treatment plane.
      (1) Apply the concave-convex rule.
         (a) If the moving surface is convex, the treatment glide should be opposite the direction in which the moving bone swings.
         (b) If the moving surface is concave, the treatment glide should be in the same direction the bone swings.
   g. Joint mobilization techniques should be used as a part of a comprehensive treatment program to improve joint mobility and joint range of motion.

Diagnostic Testing

Imaging

1. **Plain film radiograph (x-ray).**
   a. Used to demonstrate integrity of bony tissues. X-ray beams pass through the tissues resulting in varying shades of gray on the film depending on the density of the tissue they pass through. The more dense the structure (bone), the more white the structure will appear.
   b. A negative to this exam is that it exposes the patient to radiation.

2. **Computed tomography (CT scan).**
   a. Uses plain film x-ray slices that are enhanced by a computer to improve resolution. It is multiplanar so can be viewed from multiple directions.
   b. Typically used to assess complex fractures as well as facet dysfunction, disc disease or stenosis of the spinal canal or intervertebral foramen.
   c. CT does have the ability to demonstrate soft tissues, although not as well as magnetic resonance imaging (MRI).

3. **Discography.**
   a. Radiopaque dye is injected into the disc to identify abnormalities within the disc (annulus or nucleus). The needle is inserted into the disc with the assistance of radiography (fluoroscopy).

4. **MRI.**
   a. Uses magnetic fields rather than radiation.
   b. Offers excellent visualization of tissue anatomy. Utilizes two types of imaging known as T1 and T2. T1 demonstrates fat within the tissues and is

typically used to assess bony anatomy; T2 suppresses fat and demonstrates tissues with high water content. T2 is used to assess soft tissue structures.

5. **Arthrography.**
   a. Invasive technique injects water-soluble dye into area and is observed with a radiograph. Dye is observed as it surrounds tissues, demonstrating the anatomy by where fluid moves within the joint.
   b. Typically used to identify abnormalities with joints such as tendon ruptures.

6. **Bone scan (osteoscintigraphy).**
   a. Chemicals laced with radioactive tracers are injected.
   b. Isotope settles in areas where there is a high metabolic activity of bone.
   c. Radiograph is taken; demonstrates any "hot spots" of increased metabolic activity.
   d. Patients with dysfunctions, such as rheumatoid arthritis, possible stress fracture, bone cancer, infection within the bone, will often received a bone scan since these dysfunctions are known to have an increase in metabolic activity of bone in affected area.

7. **Diagnostic ultrasound.**
   a. Utilizes transmission of high-frequency sound waves, similar to therapeutic ultrasound.
   b. Provides real-time dynamic images and able to assess soft tissue dysfunctions.
   c. No known harmful effects are known at this time.

8. **Myelography.**
   a. Invasive technique using water-soluble dye. Dye is visualized as it passes through vertebral canal to observe anatomy within region.
   b. Seldom used because of many side effects.

Laboratory Tests

1. There is a potential for laboratory tests to help with diagnostic decision making.

2. The following are potential categories of tests:
   a. Blood tests.
   b. Serum chemistries.
   c. Immunological tests.
   d. Pulmonary function tests.
   e. Arterial blood gases.
   f. Fluid analysis.

Electrodiagnostic testing

1. Electroneuromyography (ENMG) and nerve conduction velocity (NCV) tests are commonly used to assess and/or monitor musculoskeletal conditions.

Clinical Application—Treatment of Musculoskeletal Conditions

Arthritic Conditions

1. **Degenerative joint disease (DJD; degenerative osteoarthritis/osteoarthrosis [OA]) (Table 2-6).**
   a. A degenerative process of varied etiology which includes mechanical changes, diseases and/or joint trauma.
   b. Characterized by degeneration of articular cartilage with hypertrophy of subchondral bone and joint capsule of weight-bearing joints.
   c. Many different medications are used to control pain, including corticosteroids and nonsteroidal anti-inflammatory drugs (NSAIDs). Glucocorticoids injected into joints that are inflamed and not responsive to NSAIDs. For mild pain without inflammation, acetaminophen may be used.
   d. Diagnostic tests utilized: plain film imaging demonstrates characteristic findings of OA (diminished joint space, decreased height of articular cartilage, presence of osteophytes) and lab tests help to rule out other disorders such as rheumatoid arthritis (RA).
   e. Clinical examination will assist in confirming diagnosis.
   f. Physical therapy goals, outcomes and interventions:
      (1) Joint protection strategies.
      (2) Maintain/improve joint mechanics and connective tissue functions.
      (3) Implementation of aerobic capacity/endurance conditioning or reconditioning such as aquatic programs.

2. **Rheumatoid conditions.**
   a. Ankylosing spondylitis (Marie-Strümpell, Bechterew's, rheumatoid spondylitis).
      (1) Progressive inflammatory disorder of unknown etiology that initially affects axial skeleton.
      (2) Initial onset (usually mid and low back pain for 3 months or more) before fourth decade of life.
      (3) First symptoms include mid and low back pain, morning stiffness and sacroiliitis.

Table 2-6 ➤ SUMMARY OF SYMPTOMS OBSERVED IN COMMON AND UNCOMMON DYSFUNCTIONS

DYSFUNCTION	SYMPTOMS OBSERVED
Degenerative Joint Disease/ Osteoarthritis	Pain and stiffness upon rising
	Pain eases through the morning (4 – 5 hours)
	Pain increases with repetitive bending activities
	Constant awareness of discomfort with episodes of exacerbation
	Describes pain as more soreness and nagging
Facet Joint Dysfunction	Stiff upon rising. Pain eases within an hour
	Loss of motion accompanied by pain
	Patient will describe pain as sharp with certain movements
	Movement in pain-free range usually reduces symptoms
	Stationary positions increase symptoms
Discal with Nerve Root Compromise	No pain in reclined or semireclined position
	Pain increases with increasing weight-bearing activities
	Describes pain as shooting, burning or stabbing
	Patient may describe altered strength or ability to perform activities of daily living
Spinal Stenosis	Pain is related to position
	Flexed positions decrease pain, and extended positions increase pain
	Describes symptoms as a numbness, tightness or cramping
	Walking for any distance brings on symptoms
	Pain may persist for hours after assuming a resting position
Vascular Claudication	Pain is consistent in all spinal positions
	Pain is brought on by physical exertion
	Pain is relieved promptly with rest (1 – 5 minutes)
	Pain is described as a numbness
	Patient usually has decreased or absent pulses
Neoplastic Disease	Patient will describe pain as gnawing, intense or penetrating
	Pain is not resolved by changes in position, time of day or activity level
	Pain will wake the patient

(4) Results in kyphotic deformity of the cervical and thoracic spine and a decrease in lumbar lordosis.

(5) Degeneration of peripheral and costovertebral joints may be observed in advanced stages.

(6) Affects men three times more often than women.

(7) Medications: NSAIDs such as aspirin are used to reduce inflammation and pain associated with condition. Corticosteroid therapy or medications to suppress immune system may be used to control various symptoms. Cytotoxic drugs (drugs that block cell growth) may be used in people who do not respond well to corticosteroids or who are dependent on high doses of corticos-

teroids. Tumor necrosis factor (TNF) inhibitors have been shown to improve some symptoms of ankylosing spondylitis.

(8) Diagnostic tests utilized: HLA-B27 antigen may be helpful, but not diagnostic by itself.

(9) Clinical examination will assist in confirming diagnosis.

(10) Physical therapy goals, outcomes and interventions:

(a) Implementation of flexibility exercises for trunk to maintain/improve normal joint motion and length of muscles in all directions, especially extension.

(b) Implementation of aerobic capacity/endurance conditioning or reconditioning such as aquatic programs.

(c) Implementation of relaxation activities to maintain/improve respiratory function.

• Breathing strategies to maintain/improve vital capacity.

b. Gout.

(1) Genetic disorder of purine metabolism characterized by elevated serum uric acid (hyperuricemia). Uric acid changes into crystals and deposits into peripheral joints and other tissues (e.g., kidneys).

(2) Most frequently observed at knee and great toe of foot.

(3) Medications: NSAIDS (specifically indomethacin), COX-2 inhibitors (cardiac side effects may limit use), colchicine, corticosteroids, adrenocorticotropic hormone (ACTH), allopurinol, probenecid and sulfinpyrazone.

(4) Diagnostic tests utilized: lab tests identify monosodium urate crystals in synovial fluid and/or connective tissue samples.

(5) Clinical examination will assist in confirming diagnosis.

(6) Physical therapy goals, outcomes and interventions.

(a) Patient/client education for injury prevention and reduction of involved joint(s).

(b) Early identification of condition with fast implementation of intervention is very important.

c. Psoriatic arthritis.

(1) Chronic, erosive inflammatory disorder of unknown etiology associated with psoriasis.

(2) Erosive degeneration usually occurs in joints of digits as well as axial skeleton.

(3) Both sexes are affected equally.

(4) Medications: acetaminophen for pain, NSAIDs, corticosteroids, disease-modifying antirheumatic drugs (DMARDs) can slow the progression of psoriatic arthritis, and biological response modifiers (BRMs) such as Enbrel (etanercept) are a

newly developed class of medicines. See Table 9-2 for a review of medications.

(5) Diagnostic tests utilized: lab tests are not useful except to rule out rheumatoid arthritis.

(6) Clinical examination will assist in confirming diagnosis.

(7) Physical therapy goals, outcomes and interventions:

   (a) Joint protection strategies.

   (b) Maintain/improve joint mechanics and connective tissue functions.

   (c) Implementation of aerobic capacity/endurance conditioning or reconditioning such as aquatic programs.

d. Rheumatoid arthritis (RA).

Also see Chapter 9.

(1) Chronic systemic disorder of unknown etiology that usually involves a symmetrical pattern of dysfunction in synovial tissues and articular cartilage of joints of hands, wrists, elbows, shoulders, knees, ankles and feet.

(2) Metacarpophalangeal (MCP) and proximal interphalangeal (PIP) joints are usually affected with characteristic pannus formation (inflammatory granulation tissue that covers joint surface), ulnar drift and volar subluxation of MCP joints; ulnar drift observed at PIPs in severe forms. Distal interphalangeal (DIP) joints are usually spared. Other deformities include swan neck and boutonniere deformities and Bouchard's nodes (excessive bone formation on dorsal aspect of PIP joints).

(3) Women have two to three times greater incidence than men.

(4) Juvenile rheumatoid arthritis (JRA) onset prior to age 16 with complete remission in 75% of children.

(5) Pharmacological management varies with disease progression and may include gold compounds and antirheumatic drugs (DMARDs) (e.g., hydroxychloroquine and methotrexate) early. NSAIDs (e.g., ibuprofen), immunosuppressive agents (e.g., cyclosporine, azathioprine and mycophenolate) or corticosteroids are commonly prescribed for long-term management.

(6) Diagnostic tests utilized: plain film imaging demonstrating symmetrical involvement within joints as well as laboratory testing. Positive test findings include an increased white blood cell count and erythrocyte sedimentation rate. Hemoglobin and hematocrit tests will show anemia and rheumatoid factor will be elevated.

(7) Clinical examination will assist in confirming diagnosis.

(8) Physical therapy goals, outcomes and interventions:

   (a) Joint protection strategies.

   (b) Maintain/improve joint mechanics and connective tissue functions.

   (c) Implementation of aerobic capacity/endurance conditioning or reconditioning such as aquatic programs.

Skeletal and Soft Tissue Conditions

1. **Osteoporosis. See Chapter 9.**

2. **Osteomalacia.**

  a. Characterized by decalcification of bones as result of a vitamin D deficiency.

  b. Symptoms include: severe pain, fractures, weakness and deformities.

  c. Medications: calcium, vitamin D and vitamin D injection in the form of calciferol (vitamin D2).

  d. Diagnostic tests utilized: plain films, lab tests (urinalysis and blood work), bone scan and potentially a bone biopsy.

  e. PT clinical examination will assist in confirming diagnosis.

  f. Physical therapy goals, outcomes and interventions:

    (1) Joint/bone protection strategies.

    (2) Maintain/improve joint mechanics and connective tissue functions.

    (3) Implementation of aerobic capacity/endurance conditioning or reconditioning such as aquatic programs.

3. **Osteomyelitis.**

  a. An inflammatory response within bone caused by an infection.

  b. Usually caused by *Staphylococcus aureus*, but could be another organism.

  c. More common in children and immunosuppressed adults than healthy adults and more common in males than females.

  d. Medical treatment consists of antibiotics. Proper nutrition is important as well. Surgery may be indicated if infection spreads to joints.

  e. Diagnostic tests utilized: lab tests for infection and possibly a bone biopsy.

  f. Clinical examination will assist in confirming diagnosis.

  g. Physical therapy goals, outcomes and interventions:

    (1) Joint/bone protection strategies as well as cast care.

    (2) Maintain/improve joint mechanics and connective tissue functions.

4. **Arthrogryposis multiplex congenita. See Chapter 8.**

5. **Osteogenesis imperfecta. See Chapter 8.**

6. **Osteochondritis dissecans.**

  a. A separation of articular cartilage from underlying bone (osteochondral fracture), usually involving medial femoral condyle near intercondylar notch and observed less frequently at femoral head and talar dome. Also affects the humeral capitellum.

b. Surgical intervention is indicated if fracture is displaced.

c. Diagnostic tests utilized: plain film or CT scan imaging to identify defect.

d. Clinical examination will assist in confirming diagnosis.

e. Physical therapy goals, outcomes and interventions:
   (1) Joint/bone protection strategies.
   (2) Implementation of flexibility exercises to maintain/improve normal joint motion and length of muscles.
   (3) Implementation of aerobic capacity/endurance conditioning or reconditioning such as aquatic programs.
   (4) Implementation of strength, power and endurance exercises.

7. **Myofascial pain syndrome.**

a. Characterized by clinical entity known as a "trigger point" which is a focal point of irritability found within a muscle. Trigger point can be identified as a taut palpable band within the muscle.

b. Trigger points may be active or latent. Active trigger points are tender to palpation and have a characteristic referral pattern of pain when provoked. Latent trigger points are palpable taut bands that are not tender to palpation, but can be converted into an active trigger point.

c. Onset is hypothesized to sudden overload, overstretching and/or repetitive/sustained muscle activities.

d. Medical intervention may include dry needling and/or injection of analgesic, possibly combined with a corticosteroid.

e. Diagnosis is made by clinical assessment with no diagnostic tests available.

f. Clinical examination will assist in confirming diagnosis.

g. Physical therapy goals, outcomes and interventions:
   (1) Implementation of flexibility exercises to maintain/improve normal joint motion and length of muscles.
   (2) Implementation of manual therapy for maintenance of normal joint mechanics.
       (a) Soft tissue/massage techniques and joint oscillations to reduce pain and/or muscle guarding.
       (b) Biomechanical faults caused by joint restrictions should be corrected with joint mobilization to the specific restrictions identified during the examination.
       (c) Use of "spray and stretch" technique.
       (d) Cryotherapy, thermotherapy, hydrotherapy, sound agents and transcutaneous electrical nerve stimulation (TENS) for symptomatic relief of pain.
       (e) Desensitization of trigger point with manual pressure.
   (3) Implementation of strength, power and endurance exercises.
       (a) Active assistive, active and resistive exercises.
       (b) Task-specific performance training.

8. **Tendinitis.**

a. An inflammation of tendon as result of microtrauma from overuse, direct blows and/or excessive tensile forces.

b. Medications: acetaminophen, NSAIDs and/or steroid injection.

c. Diagnostic tests utilized: possibly MRI.

d. Clinical examination will assist in confirming diagnosis. Specific special tests are available to assist with making diagnosis within each region/joint.

e. Physical therapy goals, outcomes and interventions:
   (1) Implementation of flexibility exercises to maintain/improve normal joint motion and length of muscles.
   (2) Implementation of manual therapy for maintenance of normal joint mechanics.
       (a) Soft tissue/massage techniques and joint oscillations to reduce pain and/or muscle guarding.
       (b) Biomechanical faults caused by joint restrictions should be corrected with joint mobilization to the specific restrictions identified during the examination.
   (3) Implementation of aerobic capacity/endurance conditioning or reconditioning.
   (4) Application of thermal agents for pain reduction, edema reduction and muscle performance.
       (a) Cryotherapy, thermotherapy, hydrotherapy and sound agents.
   (5) Patient/client education and training/retraining for instrumental activities of daily living (IADL).
       (a) Household chores, yard work, shopping, caring for dependents and home maintenance.

9. **Tendonosis.**

a. Common chronic tendon dysfunction whose cause and pathogenesis are poorly understood. Often referred to as chronic tendinitis; however, there is no inflammatory response noted.

b. Common in many tendons throughout body (supraspinatus, common extensor tendon of elbow, patella, Achilles').

c. Histological characteristics include hypercellularity, hypervascularity, no indication of inflammatory infiltrates and poor organization and loosening of collagen fibrils.

d. Medications: acetaminophen, NSAIDs and/or steroid injection.
e. Diagnostic tests utilized: possibly MRI.
f. Clinical examination will assist in confirming diagnosis. Specific special tests are available to assist with making diagnosis within each region/joint.
g. Physical therapy goals, outcomes and interventions:
(1) Implementation of flexibility exercises to maintain/improve normal joint motion and length of muscles.
(2) Implementation of manual therapy for maintenance of normal joint mechanics.
(a) Soft tissue/massage techniques and joint oscillations to reduce pain and/or muscle guarding.
(b) Biomechanical faults caused by joint restrictions should be corrected with joint mobilization to the specific restrictions identified during the examination.
(3) Implementation of aerobic capacity/endurance conditioning or reconditioning.
(4) Application of thermal agents for pain reduction, edema reduction and muscle performance.
(a) Cryotherapy, thermotherapy, hydrotherapy and sound agents.
(5) Patient/client education and training/retraining for IADL.
(a) Household chores, yard work, shopping, caring for dependents and home maintenance.

10. Bursitis.
a. Bursitis is an inflammation of bursa secondary to overuse, trauma, gout or infection.
b. Signs and symptoms of bursitis.
(1) Pain with rest.
(2) Passive ROM (PROM) and active ROM (AROM) are limited due to pain but not in a capsular pattern.
c. Medications: acetaminophen, NSAIDs and/or steroid injection.
d. Clinical examination will assist in confirming diagnosis.
e. Physical therapy goals, outcomes and interventions:
(1) Implementation of flexibility exercises to maintain/improve normal joint motion and length of muscles.
(2) Implementation of manual therapy for maintenance of normal joint mechanics.
(a) Soft tissue/massage techniques and joint oscillations to reduce pain and/or muscle guarding.
(b) Biomechanical faults caused by joint restrictions should be corrected with joint mobilization to the specific restrictions identified during the examination.
(3) Implementation of aerobic capacity/endurance conditioning or reconditioning.

(4) Application of thermal agents for pain re-duction, edema reduction and muscle performance.
(a) Cryotherapy, thermotherapy, hydrotherapy and sound agents.
(5) Patient/client education and training/retraining for IADL.
(a) Household chores, yard work, shopping, caring for dependents and home maintenance.

11. Muscle strains.
a. Characterized by an inflammatory response within a muscle following a traumatic event that caused microtearing of the musculotendinous fibers.
b. Pain and tenderness within that muscle.
c. Seen within muscles throughout the body.
d. Medications: acetaminophen and/or NSAIDs.
e. Diagnostic tests utilized: MRI if necessary.
f. Clinical examination will assist in confirming diagnosis.
g. Physical therapy goals, outcomes and interventions.
(1) Implementation of flexibility exercises to maintain/improve normal joint motion and length of muscles.
(2) Implementation of manual therapy for maintenance of normal joint mechanics.
(a) Soft tissue/massage techniques and joint oscillations to reduce pain and/or muscle guarding.
(b) Biomechanical faults caused by joint restrictions should be corrected with joint mobilization to the specific restrictions identified during the examination.
(3) Implementation of aerobic capacity/endurance conditioning or reconditioning.
(4) Application of thermal agents for pain re-duction, edema reduction and muscle performance.
(a) Cryotherapy, thermotherapy, hydrotherapy and sound agents.
(5) Patient/client education and training/retraining for IADL.
(a) Household chores, yard work, shopping, caring for dependents and home maintenance.

12. Myositis ossificans.
a. Painful condition of abnormal calcification within a muscle belly.
b. Usually precipitated by direct trauma which results in hematoma and calcification of the muscle.
c. Can also be induced by early mobilization and stretching with aggressive physical therapy following trauma to muscle.
d. Most frequent locations are quadriceps, brachialis and biceps brachii muscles.
e. Medications: acetaminophen and/or NSAIDs.
f. Surgical care is warranted only in patients with nonhereditary myositis ossificans and only after maturation of the lesion (6–24 months). Surgery is

indicated when lesions mechanically interfere with joint movement or impinge on nerves.

g. Diagnostic tests utilized: imaging (plain films, CT scan and/or MRI).

h. Clinical examination will assist in confirming diagnosis.

i. Physical therapy goals, outcomes and interventions:

(1) Implementation of flexibility exercises to maintain/improve normal joint motion and length of muscles. Must avoid being overly aggressive with muscle flexibility exercises, which may worsen condition.

(2) Implementation of manual therapy for maintenance of normal joint mechanics.

(a) Soft tissue/massage techniques and joint oscillations to reduce pain and/or muscle guarding. Avoid aggressive soft tissue/massage techniques, which may worsen condition.

(b) Biomechanical faults caused by joint restrictions should be corrected with joint mobilization to the specific restrictions identified during the examination.

(3) Implementation of aerobic capacity/endurance conditioning or reconditioning such as aquatic programs.

> ⚑ **Red Flag: Heterotopic Ossification**
>
> Heterotopic ossification is formation of bone in a muscle, tendon, joint capsule or ligament. If it occurs in muscle tissue, it is often called *myositis ossificans*. While the cause is unknown, musculoskeletal trauma, spinal cord injury, traumatic brain injury, burns to the extremities and aggressive stretching after immobilization increase the risk for patients of developing this disorder. The most commonly involved muscles are the quadriceps and brachialis. Signs of muscle involvement include muscle firmness and pain with palpation, muscle stiffness and pain with muscle stretch or contraction. If suspected, the involved tissues should be rested until the bone is reabsorbed. Massage, stretching and strengthening of involved muscles are contraindicated. Joint mobilization is contraindicated if the joint is involved.

> ⚑ **Red Flag: Complex Regional Pain Syndrome (CRPS)**
>
> CRPS I (reflex sympathetic dystrophy) is a potential complication following musculoskeletal trauma. CRPS II (causalgia) is a potential complication following peripheral nerve injury. CPRS involves a localized malfunction of the sympathetic nervous system.

> Symptoms include intense pain that is out of proportion to the injury, distally located edema, warmth, redness and sweating. Early recognition is important because progression can lead to tissue changes such as osteoporosis, muscle atrophy and contractures. Treatment includes edema reduction, desensitization training and weight bearing and/or distraction of the involved joints. Early mobility exercises and edema reduction following injury can help to prevent this disorder. See Chapter 3 for details.

13. Complex regional pain syndrome (CRPS). See Chapter 3.

14. Paget's disease (osteitis deformans). See Chapter 9.

15. Idiopathic scoliosis.

a. Two types: structural and nonstructural, both of unknown etiology.

b. Structural scoliosis is an irreversible lateral curvature of spine with a rotational component.

c. Nonstructural scoliosis is a reversible lateral curvature of spine without a rotational component and straightening as individual flexes spine.

d. Intervention for structural scoliosis includes bracing and possible surgery with placement of Harrington rod instrumentation. Rule of thumb is <25 degrees, do conservative physical therapy (see below); between 25 and 45 degrees use spinal orthoses. Surgery is generally performed for curves >45 degrees.

e. Diagnostic tests utilized: plain film imaging using full-length Cobb's method. CT scan and/or MRI may be used to rule out associated conditions.

f. Clinical examination will assist in confirming diagnosis.

g. Physical therapy goals, outcomes and interventions:

(1) Implementation of flexibility exercises to maintain/improve normal joint motion and length of muscles throughout trunk and pelvis.

(2) Implementation of strength, power and endurance exercises.

(3) Electrical stimulation to improve muscle performance.

(4) Application and patient education regarding spinal orthoses.

16. Torticollis.

a. Spasm and/or tightness of sternocleidomastoid (SCM) muscle with varied etiology.

b. Dysfunction observed is side-bending toward and rotation away from the affected SCM.

c. Medications: acetaminophen, muscle relaxants and/or NSAIDs.

d. Diagnostic tests utilized: none.

e. Physical therapy goals, outcomes and interventions:
(1) Implementation of flexibility exercises to maintain/improve normal joint motion and length of muscles.
(2) Implementation of manual therapy for maintenance of normal joint mechanics.
(a) Soft tissue/massage techniques and joint oscillations to reduce pain and/or muscle guarding.
(b) Biomechanical faults caused by joint restrictions should be corrected with joint mobilization to the specific restrictions identified during the examination.

Upper Extremity Disorders

1. **Shoulder conditions.**
a. Glenohumeral subluxation and dislocation.
(1) Most dislocations (95%) occur in anteriorinferior direction.
(2) Anterior-inferior dislocation occurs when abducted upper extremity is forcefully externally rotated causing tearing of inferior glenohumeral ligament, anterior capsule and occasionally glenoid labrum.
(3) Posterior dislocations are rare and occur with multidirectional laxity of glenohumeral joint.
(4) Posterior dislocation occurs with horizontal adduction and internal rotation of glenohumeral joint.
(5) Complications may include compression fracture of posterior humeral head (Hill-Sachs lesion), tearing of superior glenoid labrum from posterior to anterior (SLAP lesion), an avulsion of anteroinferior capsule and ligaments associated with glenoid rim (Bankart's lesion) and bruising of axillary nerve.
(6) Following surgical repair for dislocation/chronic subluxation, patients should avoid apprehension position (flexion to 90 degrees or greater, horizontal abduction to 90 degrees or greater and external rotation to 80 degrees).
(7) Diagnostic tests utilized: plain film imaging, CT scan and/or MRI.
(8) PT clinical examination. Apprehension tests will be positive.
(9) Medications.
(a) Acetaminophen for pain.
(b) NSAIDs for pain and/or inflammation.
(10) Physical therapy goals, outcomes and interventions:
(a) Physical therapy intervention is varied dependent upon the specific patient problems and whether surgery is performed.
(b) Biomechanical faults caused by joint restrictions should be corrected with joint mobi-

lization to the specific restrictions identified during the examination.
(c) Restoration of normal shoulder mechanics via strengthening/endurance/coordination exercises that focus on regaining dynamic scapulothoracic and glenohumeral stabilization and muscular reeducation.
b. Instability.
(1) Divided into two categories: traumatic (common in young throwing athletes) and atraumatic (individuals with congenitally loose connective tissue around the shoulder).
(2) Characterized by popping/clicking and repeated dislocation/subluxation of the glenohumeral joint.
(3) Unstable injuries will require surgery to reattach the labrum to the glenoid. Bankart's lesions will require surgery.
(4) Diagnosis made by clinical examination by comparing results of patient history with the AROM, PROM, resistive tests and palpation. MRI arthrograms are very effective in identifying labral tears.
(5) Medications.
(a) Acetaminophen for pain.
(b) NSAIDS for pain and/or inflammation.
(6) Physical therapy goals, outcomes and interventions.
(a) Physical therapy intervention emphasizes return of function without pain.
(b) Functional training and restoration of muscle imbalances using exercise to normalize strength, endurance, coordination and flexibility.
(c) Biomechanical faults caused by joint restrictions should be corrected with joint mobilization to the specific restrictions identified during the examination.
(d) For patients requiring surgery, the shoulder will usually be kept in a sling for 3 or 4 weeks. After 6 weeks, more sport-specific training can be done, although full fitness may take 3 or 4 months.
c. Labral tears.
(1) Glenoid labrum injuries are classified as either superior (toward the top of the glenoid socket) or inferior toward the bottom of the glenoid socket. A superior injury is known as a SLAP lesion (superior labrum, anterior [front] to posterior [back]) and is a tear of the rim above the middle of the socket that may also involve the biceps tendon. A tear of the rim below the middle of the glenoid socket is called a Bankart lesion and also involves the inferior glenohumeral ligament. Tears of the glenoid labrum may often occur with other shoulder injuries, such as a dislocated shoulder.

(2) Characterized by the following signs and symptoms:
- (a) Shoulder pain which cannot be localized to a specific point.
- (b) Pain is made worse by overhead activities or when the arm is held behind the back.
- (c) Weakness.
- (d) Instability in the shoulder.
- (e) Pain on resisted flexion of the biceps (bending the elbow against resistance).
- (f) Tenderness over the front of the shoulder.

(3) Unstable injuries will require surgery to reattach the labrum to the glenoid. Bankart's lesions will require surgery.

(4) Diagnosis made by clinical examination by comparing results of AROM, PROM, resistive tests and palpation. MRI arthrograms are very effective in identifying labral tears. The "gold" standard for identifying a labral tear is through arthroscopic surgery of the shoulder.

(5) Medications:
- (a) Acetaminophen for pain.
- (b) NSAIDs for pain and/or inflammation.

(6) Physical therapy goals, outcomes and interventions:
- (a) Physical therapy intervention emphasizes return of function without pain.
- (b) Functional training and restoration of muscle imbalances using exercise to normalize strength, endurance, coordination and flexibility.
- (c) Any underlying causes which contributed to the injury such as shoulder instability should be addressed.
- (d) Biomechanical faults caused by joint restrictions should be corrected with joint mobilization to the specific restrictions identified during the examination.
- (e) Following surgery, the shoulder will usually be kept in a sling for 3 or 4 weeks. After 6 weeks, more sport-specific training can be done, although full fitness may take 3 or 4 months.

d. Thoracic outlet syndrome (TOS).
(1) Compression of neurovascular bundle (brachial plexus, subclavian artery and vein, vagus and phrenic nerves and the sympathetic trunk) in thoracic outlet between bony and soft tissue structures.

(2) Compression occurs when size or shape of thoracic outlet is altered.

(3) Common areas of compression are:
- (a) Superior thoracic outlet.
- (b) Scalene triangle.
- (c) Between clavicle and 1st rib.
- (d) Between pectoralis minor and thoracic wall.

(4) Surgery may be performed to remove a cervical rib or a release of anterior and/or middle scalene muscle.

(5) Diagnostic tests utilized: plain film imaging to identify abnormal bony anatomy and MRI to identify abnormal soft tissue anatomy. Electrodiagnostic test to assess nerve dysfunction.

(6) PT clinical examination may include the following special tests:
- (a) Adson's test.
- (b) Roos' test.
- (c) Wright's test.
- (d) Costoclavicular test.

(7) Medications.
- (a) Acetaminophen for pain.
- (b) NSAIDs for pain and/or inflammation.

(8) Physical therapy goals, outcomes and interventions:
- (a) Physical therapy intervention will vary depending on the exact cause.
- (b) Includes postural reeducation.
- (c) Functional training and restoration of muscle imbalances using exercise to normalize strength, endurance, coordination and flexibility.
- (d) Biomechanical faults caused by joint restrictions should be corrected with joint mobilization to the specific restrictions identified during the examination.
- (e) Manipulations (typically 1st rib articulation) to diminish pain and soft tissue guarding.

e. Acromioclavicular and sternoclavicular joint disorders.
(1) Mechanism of injury is a fall onto shoulder with upper extremity adducted or a collision with another individual during a sporting event.

(2) Traditionally, degree of injury is graded from first to third degree.

(3) Upper extremity is positioned in neutral with use of sling in acute phase. Avoid shoulder elevation during the acute phase of healing.

(4) Diagnostic tests utilized: plain film imaging.

(5) PT clinical examination may include the shear test.

(6) Surgical repair is rare due to tendency of acromioclavicular joint degeneration following the repair.

(7) Medications:
- (a) Acetaminophen for pain.
- (b) NSAIDs for pain and/or inflammation.

(8) Physical therapy goals, outcomes and interventions:
- (a) Emphasize return of function without pain.
- (b) Functional training and restoration of muscle imbalances using exercise to normalize strength, endurance, coordination and flexibility.

(c) Manual therapy techniques to AC and SC joints and surrounding connective tissues such as soft tissue/massage, joint oscillations and mobilizations to normalize soft tissue and joint biomechanics.

f. Subacromial/subdeltoid bursitis.
  (1) Subacromial and subdeltoid bursae (which may be continuous) have a close relationship to rotator cuff tendons which makes them susceptible to overuse.
  (2) They can also become impinged beneath the acromial arch.
  (3) Diagnosis made by PT clinical examination. Differentiate from contractile condition by comparing results of AROM, PROM and resistive tests.
  (4) Medications:
    (a) Acetaminophen for pain.
    (b) NSAIDs for pain and/or inflammation.
  (5) Physical therapy goals, outcomes and interventions:
    (a) Refer to intervention for general bursitis/tendinitis/tendonosis (See section V.B.10).

g. Rotator cuff tendinitis.
  (1) Tendons of rotator cuff are susceptible to tendinitis due to relatively poor blood supply near insertion of muscles.
  (2) Results from mechanical impingement of the distal attachment of the rotator cuff on the anterior acromion and/or coracoacromial ligament with repetitive overhead activities.
  (3) Diagnostic tests utilized: MRI may be used, but sometimes not sensitive enough for accurate assessment.
  (4) PT clinical examination including the following special tests will be useful to make diagnosis.
    (a) Supraspinatus test.
    (b) Neer's impingement test.
  (5) Medications:
    (a) Acetaminophen for pain.
    (b) NSAIDs for pain and/or inflammation.
  (6) Physical therapy goals, outcomes and interventions.
    (a) Refer to intervention for general bursitis/tendinitis/tendonosis (See section V.B.8).

h. Impingement syndrome:
  (1) Characterized by soft tissue inflammation of the shoulder from impingement against the acromion with repetitive overhead AROM.
  (2) Diagnostic tests utilized: arthrogram or MRI may be used.
  (3) PT clinical examination including the following special tests will be useful to make diagnosis.
    (a) Neer's impingement test.
    (b) Supraspinatus test.
    (c) Drop arm test.

(4) Surgical repair of shoulder impingement. The patient should avoid shoulder elevation >90 degrees.
(5) Medications:
  (a) Acetaminophen for pain.
  (b) NSAIDs for pain and/or inflammation.
(6) Physical therapy goals, outcomes and interventions:
  (a) Restoration of posture.
  (b) Correction of muscle imbalances and biomechanical faults using strengthening, endurance, coordination and flexibility exercises to gain restoration of normal function.
  (c) Biomechanical faults caused by joint restrictions should be corrected with joint mobilization to the specific restrictions identified during the examination.

i. Internal (posterior) impingement.
  (1) Characterized by an irritation between the rotator cuff and greater tuberosity or posterior glenoid and labrum.
  (2) Often seen in athletes performing overhead activities. Pain commonly noted in posterior shoulder.
  (3) Diagnostic tests utilized: None.
  (4) PT clinical examination including posterior internal impingement test helps to identify this condition.
  (5) Medications:
    (a) Acetaminophen for pain.
    (b) NSAIDs for pain and/or inflammation.
  (6) Physical therapy goals, outcomes and interventions.
    (a) Correction of muscle imbalances and biomechanical faults using strengthening, endurance, coordination and flexibility exercises to gain restoration of normal function.
    (b) Biomechanical faults caused by joint restrictions should be corrected with joint mobilization to the specific restrictions identified during the examination.

j. Bicipital tendinitis.
  (1) Most commonly an inflammation of the long head of the biceps.
  (2) Results from mechanical impingement of the proximal tendon between the anterior acromion and the bicipital groove of the humerus.
  (3) Diagnostic tests utilized: MRI may be used, but sometimes not sensitive enough for accurate assessment.
  (4) PT clinical examination including the following special test will be useful to make diagnosis.
    (a) Speed's test.
  (5) Medications:
    (a) Acetaminophen for pain.
    (b) NSAIDs for pain and/or inflammation.

(6) Physical therapy goals, outcomes and interventions:

(a) Refer to intervention for general bursitis/tendinitis/tendonosis (See section V.B.8).

k. Proximal humeral fractures.

(1) Humeral neck fractures frequently occur with a fall onto an outstretched upper extremity among older osteoporotic women. Generally does not require immobilization or surgical repair since it is a fairly stable fracture.

(2) Greater tuberosity fractures are more common in middle-aged and elder adults. This is also usually related to a fall onto the shoulder and does not require immobilization for healing.

(3) Diagnostic tests utilized: plain film imaging.

(4) Medications:

(a) Acetaminophen for pain.

(b) NSAIDs for pain and/or inflammation.

(5) Physical therapy goals, outcomes and interventions:

(a) Physical therapy intervention emphasizes return of function without pain.

(b) Functional training and restoration of muscle imbalances using exercise to normalize strength, endurance, coordination and flexibility.

(c) Biomechanical faults caused by joint restrictions should be corrected with joint mobilization to the specific restrictions identified during the examination.

(d) Early PROM is important in preventing capsular adhesions.

l. Adhesive capsulitis (frozen shoulder).

(1) Characterized by a restriction in shoulder motion as a result of inflammation and fibrosis of the shoulder capsule, usually due to disuse following injury or repetitive microtrauma.

(2) Restriction follows a capsular pattern of limitation:

(a) Greatest limitation in external rotation, followed by abduction and flexion, and least restricted in internal rotation.

(3) Commonly seen in association with diabetes mellitus.

(4) Diagnosis made by clinical examination by comparing results of AROM, PROM, resistive tests and palpation.

(5) Medications:

(a) Acetaminophen for pain.

(b) NSAIDs for pain and/or inflammation.

(6) Physical therapy goals, outcomes and interventions:

(a) Physical therapy intervention emphasizes return of function without pain.

(b) Functional training and restoration of muscle imbalances using exercise to normalize strength, endurance, coordination and flexibility.

(c) Biomechanical faults caused by joint restrictions should be corrected with joint mobilization to the specific restrictions identified during the examination.

2. **Elbow conditions.**

a. Elbow contractures.

(1) Loss of motion in capsular pattern (loss of flexion greater than extension).

(2) Loss of motion in noncapsular pattern as the result of a loose body in the joint, ligamentous sprain and/or complex regional pain syndrome.

(3) Diagnosis made by clinical examination by comparing results of AROM, PROM, resistive tests and palpation.

(4) Medications:

(a) Acetaminophen for pain.

(b) NSAIDs for pain and/or inflammation.

(5) Physical therapy goals, outcomes and interventions:

(a) Biomechanical faults caused by joint restrictions should be corrected with joint mobilization to the specific restrictions identified during the examination.

(b) Soft tissue/massage techniques, modalities, flexibility exercises and functional exercises including strengthening, endurance and coordination.

(c) Splinting may be an effective adjunct to physical therapy management in regaining loss of motion for capsular restrictions.

b. Lateral epicondylitis ("tennis elbow").

(1) Most often a chronic inflammation of the extensor carpi radialis brevis (ECRB) tendon at its proximal attachment to the lateral epicondyle of the humerus.

(2) Onset is gradual, usually the result of sports activities or occupations that require repetitive wrist extension or strong grip with the wrist extended, resulting in overloading the ECRB.

(3) PT clinical examination includes:

(a) Tests to rule out involvement or relationship to cervical spine condition.

(b) Lateral epicondylitis tests to clearly identify condition.

(4) Medications:

(a) Acetaminophen for pain.

(b) NSAIDs for pain and/or inflammation.

(5) Physical therapy goals, outcomes and interventions:

(a) Correction of muscle imbalances and biomechanical faults using strengthening, endurance, coordination and flexibility exercises to gain restoration of normal function.

(b) Biomechanical faults caused by joint restrictions should be corrected with joint mobilization to the specific restrictions identified during the examination.

(c) Education regarding prevention.

(d) Cryotherapy, thermotherapy, hydrotherapy, sound agents and TENS for symptomatic relief of pain.

(e) Counterforce bracing is frequently used to reduce forces along the ECRB.

c. Medial epicondylitis (golfer's elbow).

(1) Usually an inflammation of the pronator teres and flexor carpi radialis tendons at their attachment to the medial epicondyle of the humerus.

(2) Occurs as the result of chronic overuse in sports such as baseball pitching, driving golf swings, swimming or occupations that require a strong hand grip and excessive pronation of the forearm.

(3) Diagnostic tests utilized: none.

(4) PT clinical examination including medial epicondylitis test helps to identify this condition.

(5) Physical therapy goals, outcomes and interventions:

(a) Intervention is similar to lateral epicondylitis.

d. Distal humeral fractures:

(1) Complications can include loss of motion, myositis ossificans, malalignment, neurovascular compromise, ligamentous injury, and CRPS.

(2) Supracondylar fractures must be examined quickly for neurovascular status due to high number of neurological (typically radial nerve involvement) and vascular structures that pass through this region (may lead to Volkmann's ischemia). In youth, it is important to assess growth plate as well. These fractures have high incidence of malunion.

(3) Lateral epicondyle fractures are fairly common in young people and typically require an open reduction internal fixation (ORIF) to ensure absolute alignment.

(4) Diagnostic tests utilized: plain film imaging.

(5) Medications:

(a) Acetaminophen for pain.

(b) NSAIDs for pain and/or inflammation.

(6) Physical therapy goals, outcomes and interventions:

(a) Physical therapy intervention includes pain reduction and limiting the inflammatory response following trauma and/or surgery.

(b) Improving flexibility of shortened structures, strengthening and training to restore functional use of upper extremity (UE).

e. Osteochondrosis of humeral capitellum.

(1) Osteochondritis dissecans affects central and/or lateral aspect of capitellum or radial head. An osteochondral bone fragment becomes detached from articular surface, forming a loose body in joint. Caused by repetitive compressive forces between radial head and humeral capitellum. Occurs in adolescents between 12 and 15 years of age.

(2) Panner's disease is a localized avascular necrosis of capitellum leading to loss of subchondral bone with fissuring and softening of articular surfaces of radiocapitellar joint. Etiology is unknown but occurs in children age 10 or younger.

(3) Diagnostic tests utilized: plain film imaging.

(4) Medications:

(a) Acetaminophen for pain.

(b) NSAIDs for pain and/or inflammation.

(5) Physical therapy goals, outcomes and interventions:

(a) Physical therapy intervention includes rest with avoidance of any throwing or UE loading activities (e.g., gymnastics).

(b) When patient is pain free, initiate flexibility and strengthening/endurance/coordination exercises.

(c) During late phases of rehabilitation, a program to slowly increase load on joint is initiated. If symptoms persist, surgical intervention is necessary.

(d) After surgery, initial focus of rehabilitation is to minimize pain and swelling using modalities. Flexibility exercises are begun immediately following surgery.

(e) Thereafter, a progressive strengthening program is initiated.

(f) Biomechanical faults caused by joint restrictions should be corrected with joint mobilization to the specific restrictions identified during the examination.

f. Ulnar collateral ligament injuries.

(1) Occur as result of repetitive valgus stresses to medial elbow with overhead throwing.

(2) Clinical signs include pain along medial elbow at distal insertion of ligament. In some cases, paresthesias are reported in ulnar nerve distribution with positive Tinel's sign.

(3) Diagnostic tests utilized: MRI.

(4) PT clinical examination including medial ligament instability test helps to identify this condition.

(5) Medications:

(a) Acetaminophen for pain.

(b) NSAIDs for pain and/or inflammation.

(6) Physical therapy goals, outcomes and interventions:

(a) Initial intervention includes rest and pain management.

(b) After resolution of pain and inflammation, strengthening exercises that focus on elbow flexors are initiated. Taping can also be used for protection during return to activities.

g. Nerve entrapments.
  (1) Ulnar nerve entrapment.
    (a) Various causes which include direct trauma at the cubital tunnel, traction due to laxity at medial aspect of elbow, compression due to a thickened retinaculum or hypertrophy of flexor carpi ulnaris muscle, recurrent subluxation or dislocation and DJD that affects the cubital tunnel.
    (b) Clinical findings include medial elbow pain and paresthesias in ulnar distribution, and a positive Tinel's sign.
  (2) Median nerve entrapment.
    (a) Occurs within pronator teres muscle and under superficial head of flexor digitorum superficialis with repetitive gripping activities required in occupations (e.g., electricians) and with leisure time activities (e.g., tennis).
    (b) Clinical signs include an aching pain with weakness of forearm muscles and positive Tinel's sign with paresthesias in median nerve distribution.
  (3) Radial nerve entrapment.
    (a) Entrapment of distal branches (posterior interosseous nerve) occurs within radial tunnel (radial tunnel syndrome) as result of overhead activities and throwing.
    (b) Clinical signs include lateral elbow pain that can be confused with lateral epicondylitis, pain over supinator muscle, and paresthesias in a radial nerve distribution. Tinel's sign may be positive.
  (4) Diagnostic tests utilized: electrodiagnostic tests.
  (5) Clinical examination helps to identify this condition.
  (6) Medications:
    (a) Acetaminophen for pain.
    (b) NSAIDs for pain and/or inflammation.
    (c) Neurontin for neuropathic pain.
  (7) Physical therapy goals, outcomes and interventions:
    (a) Early intervention includes rest, avoiding exacerbating activities, use of NSAIDs, modalities and soft tissue/massage techniques to reduce inflammation and pain.
    (b) Protective padding and night splints to maintain slackened position of involved nerves.
    (c) Nerve gliding to improve neurodynamics.
    (d) With reduction in pain and paresthesias, rehabilitation program should focus on strengthening/endurance/coordination exercise of involved muscles to achieve muscle balance between agonists and antagonists, normal flexibility of shortened structures and normalization of strength/endurance/coordination.
    (e) Intervention should also include functional training, patient education and self-management techniques.

Neurodynamic Exercises

Nerve entrapment by edema, scar tissue or other tissue constrictions limits the nervous system's ability to dissipate tensile forces during movement. Excessive tensile force (traction) on the nervous system can lead to pain, paresthesia and muscle weakness. Neurodynamic exercises are designed to maintain or regain lost nervous system mobility. Tension in a peripheral nerve is related to specific positions of the limbs and spine, much like tension in a muscle during a stretching exercise. A "nerve glide" exercise involves alternating tension between the distal and proximal portions of the nerve to achieve a gliding movement of the nerve.

h. Elbow dislocations.
  (1) Posterior dislocations account for most dislocations occurring at elbow.
    (a) Posterior dislocations are defined by position of olecranon relative to the humerus.
    (b) Posterolateral dislocations are most common and occur as the result of elbow hyperextension from a fall on the outstretched upper extremity.
    (c) Posterior dislocations frequently cause avulsion fractures of medial epicondyle secondary to traction pull of medial collateral ligament.
  (2) Anterior and radial head dislocations account for only 1%–2% of all elbow dislocations.
  (3) With a complete dislocation, ulnar collateral ligament will rupture with possible rupture of anterior capsule, lateral collateral ligament, brachialis muscle and/or wrist flexor and extensor muscles.
  (4) Clinical signs include rapid swelling, severe pain at the elbow and a deformity with olecranon pushed posteriorly.
  (5) Diagnostic tests utilized: plain film imaging.
  (6) Medications:
    (a) Acetaminophen for pain.
    (b) NSAIDs for pain and/or inflammation.
  (7) Physical therapy goals, outcomes and interventions:
    (a) Initial intervention includes reduction of the dislocation.
    (b) If elbow is stable, there is an initial phase of immobilization followed by rehabilitation focusing on regaining flexibility within limits of stability and strengthening.
    (c) If elbow is not stable, surgery is indicated.

3. Wrist and hand conditions.
  a. Carpal tunnel syndrome (repetitive stress syndrome).
    (1) Compression of the median nerve at the carpal tunnel of the wrist as the result of inflammation of the flexor tendons and/or median nerve.
    (2) Commonly occurs as result of repetitive wrist motions or gripping, with pregnancy, diabetes and rheumatoid arthritis.
    (3) Must rule out potential of cervical spine dysfunction, thoracic outlet syndrome or peripheral nerve entrapment that is mimicking this condition.
    (4) Diagnostic tests utilized: electrodiagnostic testing.
    (5) Common clinical findings include exacerbation of burning, tingling, pins and needles and numbness into median nerve distribution at night and a positive Tinel's sign and/or Phalen's test. Long-term compression causes atrophy and weakness of thenar muscles and lateral two lumbricals.
    (6) Medications:
      (a) Acetaminophen for pain.
      (b) NSAIDs for pain and/or inflammation.
    (7) Physical therapy goals, outcomes and interventions:
      (a) Biomechanical faults caused by joint restrictions should be corrected with joint mobilization to the specific restrictions identified during the examination.
      (b) Soft tissue/massage techniques, modalities, flexibility exercises and functional exercises including strengthening, endurance and coordination.
  b. DeQuervain's tenosynovitis.
    (1) Inflammation of extensor pollicis brevis and abductor pollicis longus tendons at first dorsal compartment.
    (2) Results from repetitive microtrauma or as a complication of swelling during pregnancy.
    (3) Diagnostic tests utilized: MRI, but usually not necessary to make diagnosis.
    (4) Clinical signs include: pain at anatomical snuffbox, swelling, decreased grip and pinch strength, positive Finkelstein's test (which places tendons on a stretch).
    (5) Medications:
      (a) Acetaminophen for pain.
      (b) NSAIDs for pain and/or inflammation.
    (6) Physical therapy goals, outcomes and interventions.
      (a) Biomechanical faults caused by joint restrictions should be corrected with joint mobilization to the specific restrictions identified during the examination.
      (b) Soft tissue/massage techniques, modalities, flexibility exercises and functional exercises

including strengthening, endurance and coordination.
  c. Colles' fracture.
    (1) Most common wrist fracture resulting from a fall onto an outstretched UE. These fractures are immobilized between 5 and 8 weeks. Complication of median nerve compression can occur with excessive edema.
    (2) Characteristic "dinner fork" deformity of wrist and hand results from dorsal or posterior displacement of distal fragment of radius with a radial shift of wrist and hand.
    (3) Diagnostic tests utilized: plain film imaging.
    (4) Complications may include loss of motion, decreased grip strength, CRPS and carpal tunnel syndrome.
    (5) Medications:
      (a) Acetaminophen for pain.
      (b) NSAIDs for pain and/or inflammation.
    (6) Physical therapy goals, outcomes and interventions:
      (a) Early physical therapy intervention that focuses on normalizing flexibility is paramount to functional recovery of wrist and hand.
      (b) Biomechanical faults caused by joint restrictions should be corrected with joint mobilization to the specific restrictions identified during the examination.
      (c) Soft tissue/massage techniques, modalities, flexibility exercises and functional exercises including strengthening, endurance and coordination.
  d. Smith's fracture.
    (1) Similar to Colles' fracture except distal fragment of radius dislocates in a volar direction causing a characteristic "garden spade deformity."
    (2) Diagnostic tests utilized: plain film imaging.
    (3) Medications:
      (a) Acetaminophen for pain.
      (b) NSAIDs for pain and/or inflammation.
    (4) Physical therapy goals, outcomes and interventions:
      (a) Intervention is similar to Colles' fracture.
  e. Scaphoid fracture:
    (1) Results from a fall onto outstretched UE in a younger person. Most commonly fractured carpal.
    (2) Diagnostic tests utilized: plain film imaging.
    (3) Complications include a high incidence of avascular necrosis of the proximal fragment of the scaphoid secondary to poor vascular supply. Carpals are immobilized between 4 and 8 weeks.
    (4) Medications:
      (a) Acetaminophen for pain.
      (b) NSAIDs for pain and/or inflammation.
    (5) Physical therapy goals, outcomes and interventions:

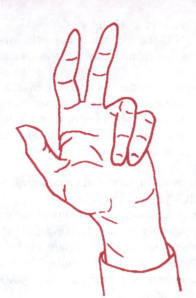

Figure 2-3 • Dupuytren's contracture.
(Adapted from Magee DJ. *Orthopedic Physical Assessment.* 2nd ed. Philadelphia, Saunders, 1992.)

(a) Early intervention includes maintenance of flexibility of distal and proximal joints while UE is casted. Later intervention emphasizes strengthening, stretching and joint and soft tissue mobilizations to regain full functional use of wrist and hand.

f. Dupuytren's contracture (Figure 2-3).
 (1) Observed as banding on palm and digit flexion contractures resulting from contracture of palmar fascia which adheres to skin.
 (2) Affects men more often than women.
 (3) Contracture usually affects the metacarpophalangeal (MCP) and proximal interphalangeal (PIP) joints of fourth and fifth digits in nondiabetic individuals and affects third and fourth digits most often in individuals with diabetes.
 (4) Medications:
  (a) Acetaminophen for pain.
  (b) NSAIDs for pain and/or inflammation.
 (5) Physical therapy goals, outcomes and interventions:
  (a) Physical therapy intervention includes flexibility exercise to prevent further contracture and splint fabrication/application.
  (b) Once contracture is under control, promote restoration of normal hand function through functional exercises.
  (c) Physical therapy intervention following surgery includes wound management, edema control and progression of functional exercise.

g. Boutonnière deformity (Figure 2-4).
 (1) Results from rupture of central tendinous slip of extensor hood.

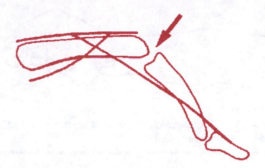

Figure 2-4 • Boutonnière deformity.
(From Magee DJ. *Orthopedic Physical Assessment.* 2nd ed. Philadelphia, Saunders, 1992.)

 (2) Observed deformity is extension of MCP and distal interphalangeal (DIP) with flexion of PIP.
 (3) Commonly occurs following trauma or in rheumatoid arthritis with degeneration of the central extensor tendon.
 (4) Medications:
  (a) Acetaminophen for pain.
  (b) NSAIDs for pain and/or inflammation.
 (5) Physical therapy goals, outcomes and interventions:
  (a) Physical therapy intervention includes edema management, flexibility exercises of involved and uninvolved joints, splinting or taping and functional strengthening/endurance/coordination exercises.

h. Swan neck deformity (Figure 2-5).
 (1) Results from contracture of intrinsic muscles with dorsal subluxation of lateral extensor tendons.
 (2) Observed deformity is flexion of MCP and DIP with extension of PIP.
 (3) Commonly occurs following trauma or with rheumatoid arthritis following degeneration of lateral extensor tendons.
 (4) Diagnostic tests utilized: plain film imaging, but may not be necessary.
 (5) Medications:
  (a) Acetaminophen for pain.
  (b) NSAIDs for pain and/or inflammation.

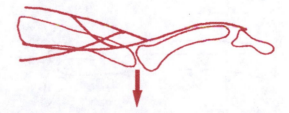

Figure 2-5 • Swan neck deformity.
(From Magee DJ. *Orthopedic Physical Assessment.* 2nd ed. Philadelphia, Saunders, 1992.)

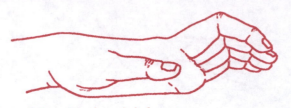

Figure 2-6 • Ape hand deformity.
(From Magee DJ. *Orthopedic Physical Assessment.* 2nd ed. Philadelphia, Saunders, 1992.)

    (6) Physical therapy goals, outcomes and interventions:
        (a) Physical therapy intervention includes edema management, flexibility exercises of involved and uninvolved joints, splinting or taping and functional strengthening/endurance/coordination exercises.

  i. Ape hand deformity (Figure 2-6).
    (1) Observed as thenar muscle wasting with first digit moving dorsally until it is in line with second digit.
    (2) Results from median nerve dysfunction.
    (3) Diagnostic tests utilized: electrodiagnostic testing.
    (4) Medications:
        (a) Acetaminophen for pain.
        (b) NSAIDs for pain and/or inflammation.
    (5) Physical therapy goals, outcomes and interventions:
        (a) Physical therapy intervention includes edema management, flexibility exercises of involved and uninvolved joints, splinting or taping and functional strengthening/endurance/coordination exercises.

  j. Mallet finger (Figure 2-7).
    (1) Rupture or avulsion of extensor tendon at its insertion into distal phalanx of digit.
    (2) Observed deformity is flexion of DIP joint.
    (3) Usually occurs from trauma forcing distal phalanx into a flexed position.
    (4) Diagnostic tests utilized: possibly MRI.
    (5) Medications:

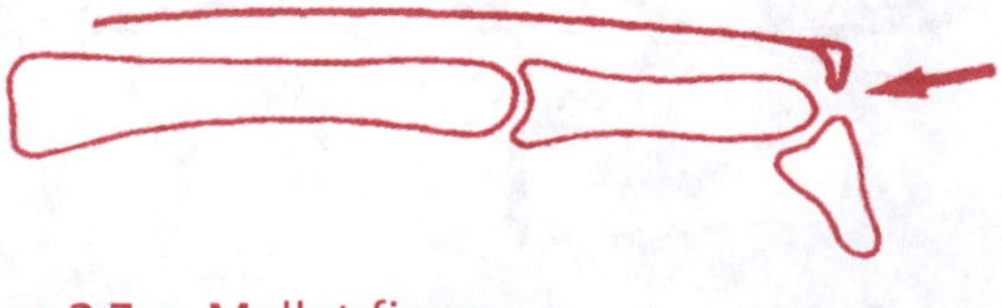

Figure 2-7 • Mallet finger.
(From Magee DJ. *Orthopedic Physical Assessment.* 2nd ed. Philadelphia, Saunders, 1992.)

        (a) Acetaminophen for pain.
        (b) NSAIDs for pain and/or inflammation.
    (6) Physical therapy goals, outcomes and interventions:
        (a) Physical therapy intervention includes edema management, flexibility exercises of involved and uninvolved joints, splinting or taping and functional strengthening/endurance/coordination exercises.

  k. Gamekeeper's thumb.
    (1) A sprain/rupture of ulnar collateral ligament of MCP joint of first digit.
    (2) Results in medial instability of thumb.
    (3) Frequently occurs during a fall while skiing when increasing forces are placed on thumb through ski pole. Immobilized for 6 weeks.
    (4) Diagnostic tests utilized: possibly MRI.
    (5) Medications:
        (a) Acetaminophen for pain.
        (b) NSAIDs for pain and/or inflammation.
    (6) Physical therapy goals, outcomes and interventions.
        (a) Physical therapy intervention includes edema management, flexibility exercises of involved and uninvolved joints, splinting or taping and functional strengthening/endurance/coordination exercises.

  l. Boxer's fracture.
    (1) Fracture of neck of 5th metacarpal.
    (2) Frequently sustained during a fight or from punching a wall in anger or frustration.
    (3) Casted for 2–4 weeks.
    (4) Diagnostic tests utilized: plain film imaging.
    (5) Medications:
        (a) Acetaminophen for pain.
        (b) NSAIDs for pain and/or inflammation.
    (6) Physical therapy goals, outcomes and interventions:
        (a) Physical therapy intervention includes edema management, flexibility exercise initially at uninvolved joints followed by involved joints after sufficient healing has occurred.
        (b) Initiation of functional strengthening/endurance/coordination occurs when flexibility is restored.

Lower Extremity Conditions

1. **Hip conditions.**
  a. Avascular necrosis (AVN) of the hip (osteonecrosis).
    (1) Multiple etiologies resulting in an impaired blood supply to the femoral head.
    (2) Hip ROM is decreased in flexion, internal rotation and abduction.
    (3) Diagnostic tests utilized: plain film imaging, bone scans, CT and/or MRI may be utilized.

CHAPTER 2

(4) Symptoms include pain in the groin and/or thigh and tenderness with palpation at the hip joint.

(5) Coxalgic gait.

(6) Medications:

(a) Acetaminophen for pain.

(b) NSAIDs for pain and/or inflammation.

(c) Corticosteroids contraindicated since they may be causative factor. Patient taking steroids for some other condition should have dose decreased.

(7) Physical therapy goals, outcomes and interventions:

(a) Joint/bone protection strategies.

(b) Maintain/improve joint mechanics and connective tissue functions.

(c) Implementation of aerobic capacity, endurance conditioning or reconditioning such as aquatic programs.

(d) Postsurgical intervention includes regaining functional flexibility, improving strength/endurance/coordination and gait training.

b. Legg-Calvé-Perthe's disease (osteochondrosis). See Chapter 8.

c. Slipped capital femoral epiphysis. See Chapter 8.

d. Femoral anteversion and antetorsion.

(1) Excessive femoral anteversion or antetorsion (30 degrees or greater) leads to squinting patellae and toeing in.

(2) With an angle less than 0 degree (retroversion), femoral neck is rotated backward in relation to femoral condyles.

(3) Diagnostic tests utilized: plain film imaging.

(4) Clinical examination including Craig's test helps to identify this condition.

(5) Physical therapy goals, outcomes and interventions.

(a) Maintain/improve joint mechanics and connective tissue functions.

e. Coxa vara and coxa valga.

(1) Angle of femoral neck with shaft of femur is <120 degrees; coxa vara results.

(2) Angle of femoral neck with shaft of femur is >135 degrees; coxa valga results.

(3) Coxa vara usually results from a defect in ossification of head of femur. Coxa vara and coxa valga may result from necrosis of femoral head occurring with septic arthritis.

(4) Diagnostic tests utilized: plain film imaging.

(5) Physical therapy goals, outcomes and interventions.

(a) Maintain/improve joint mechanics and connective tissue functions.

f. Trochanteric bursitis.

(1) An inflammation of deep trochanteric bursa from a direct blow, irritation by iliotibial band (ITB) and biomechanical/gait abnormalities causing repetitive microtrauma.

(2) This condition is common in patients with rheumatoid arthritis.

(3) Diagnostic tests utilized: none.

(4) Diagnosis made by clinical examination. Differentiate from contractile condition by comparing results of AROM, PROM and resistive tests.

(5) Medications.

(a) Acetaminophen for pain.

(b) NSAIDs for pain and/or inflammation.

(6) Physical therapy goals, outcomes and interventions.

(a) Refer to intervention for general bursitis/tendinitis/tendonosis (See section V.B.10).

g. ITB tightness/friction disorder.

(1) Etiology: tight ITB, abnormal gait patterns.

(2) Results in inflammation of trochanteric bursa.

(3) Noble compression test is positive when friction is introduced over the lateral femoral condyle during knee extension. Ober's test will also demonstrate tightness in ITB.

(4) Medications:

(a) Acetaminophen for pain.

(b) NSAIDs for pain and/or inflammation.

(5) Physical therapy goals, outcomes and interventions:

(a) Reduction of pain and inflammation utilizing modalities, soft tissue techniques and manual therapy techniques such as soft tissue/massage and joint oscillations.

(b) Correction of muscle imbalances and biomechanical faults using strengthening, endurance, coordination and flexibility (ITB, hamstrings, quadriceps and hip flexors) exercises to gain restoration of normal function.

(c) Biomechanical faults caused by joint restrictions should be corrected with joint mobilization to the specific restrictions identified during the examination.

(d) Gait training and patient education regarding the selection of running shoes and running surfaces. Orthoses may be fabricated.

h. Piriformis syndrome.

(1) Piriformis muscle is an external rotator of hip and can become overworked with excessive pronation of foot, which causes abnormal femoral internal rotation. Considered a tonic muscle which is active with motion of sacroiliac joint, particularly sacrum.

(2) Tightness or spasm of piriformis muscle can result in compression of sciatic nerve and/or sacroiliac dysfunction.

(3) Diagnostic tests utilized: possibly electrodiagnostic tests for sciatic nerve.

(4) Signs and symptoms include:

(a) Restriction in internal rotation.

(b) Pain with palpation of piriformis muscle.

(c) Referral of pain to posterior thigh.

(d) Weakness in external rotation, positive piriformis test.

(e) Uneven sacral base.

(5) Perform lower extremity biomechanical examination to determine if abnormal biomechanics are the cause. Must rule out involvement of lumbar spine and/or sacroiliac joint.

(6) Medications:

(a) Acetaminophen for pain.

(b) NSAIDs for pain and/or inflammation.

(c) Neurontin for neuropathic pain.

(7) Physical therapy goals, outcomes and interventions.

(a) Reduction of pain utilizing modalities and manual therapy techniques such as soft tissue/massage to piriformis muscle.

(b) Joint oscillations to hip or pelvis to inhibit pain.

(c) Correction of muscle imbalances and biomechanical faults using strengthening, endurance, coordination and flexibility exercises to gain restoration of normal function.

(d) Restore muscle balance and patient education regarding protection of the sacroiliac joint (e.g., instruction not to step off a curb onto the dysfunctional lower extremity).

(e) Correction of biomechanical faults may include orthoses or orthotic devices for feet.

2. Knee conditions:

a. Ligament sprains.

(1) Four major ligaments may be involved with knee sprains (anterior cruciate, posterior cruciate, medial collateral and lateral collateral).

(2) Injury to the ligaments may result in a single plane or rotary instability.

(a) Anterior cruciate ligament (ACL) laxity may result in single plane anterior instability.

(b) Posterior cruciate ligament (PCL) laxity may result in single plane posterior instability.

(c) ACL and medial collateral ligament (MCL) laxity may result in anteromedial rotary instability.

(d) ACL and LCL laxity may result in anterolateral rotary instability.

(e) PCL and MCL laxity may result in posteromedial rotary instability.

(f) PCL and LCL laxity may result in posterolateral rotary instability.

(3) Classification of injury:

(a) First degree, resulting in little or no instability.

(b) Second degree, resulting in minimal to moderate instability.

(c) Third degree, resulting in extreme instability.

(4) "Unhappy triad" includes injury to the MCL, ACL and the medial meniscus resulting from a combination of valgum, flexion and external rotation forces applied to knee when the foot is planted.

(5) Diagnostic tests utilized: MRI. Difficult to visualize complete ACL on MRI, so often read incorrectly as partially torn even if normal.

(6) Refer to knee special tests that help to identify ligamentous instabilities of knee joint.

(7) Reconstruction frequently involves a combination of intra-articular and extra-articular procedures.

(8) Medications:

(a) Acetaminophen for pain.

(b) NSAIDs for pain and/or inflammation.

(9) Physical therapy goals, outcomes and interventions:

(a) Physical therapy intervention is varied depending on whether the patient undergoes a surgical procedure as well as type of surgery that is performed.

(b) Reduction of pain and inflammation utilizing modalities, soft tissue techniques and manual therapy techniques such as oscillations.

(c) Postoperatively, continuous passive motion (CPM) devices may be used to maintain/promote flexibility of the joint.

(d) Correction of muscle imbalances and biomechanical faults using strengthening, endurance, coordination and flexibility exercises to gain restoration of normal function.

(e) Biomechanical faults caused by joint restrictions should be corrected with joint mobilization to the specific restrictions identified during the examination.

(f) Progression to functional training based on patient's occupation and/or recreational goals.

b. Meniscal injuries.

(1) Result from a combination of forces to include tibiofemoral joint flexion, compression, and rotation which places abnormal shear stresses on the meniscus.

(2) Symptoms include lateral and/or medial joint pain, effusion, joint popping, knee giving way during walking, limitation in flexibility of knee joint and joint locking.

(3) Diagnostic tests utilized: MRI typically done, but not always sensitive enough to confirm tear.

(4) PT clinical examination including the following special tests will be useful to make diagnosis.

(a) McMurray's test.

(b) Apley's test.

(5) Medications:

(a) Acetaminophen for pain.

(b) NSAIDs for pain and/or inflammation.

(6) Physical therapy goals, outcomes and interventions.

(a) Reduction of pain and inflammation utilizing modalities, soft tissue/massage techniques to surrounding muscles and manual therapy techniques such as joint oscillations to inhibit pain.

(b) Correction of muscle imbalances and biomechanical faults using strengthening, endurance, coordination and flexibility exercises to gain restoration of normal function.

(c) Biomechanical faults caused by joint restrictions should be corrected with joint mobilization to the specific restrictions identified during the examination.

(d) Progression to functional training based on patient's occupation and/or recreational goals.

c. Patellofemoral conditions:

(1) Abnormal patella positions:

(a) Patella alta.
- Malalignment in which patella tracks superiorly in femoral intercondylar notch.
- May result in chronic patellar subluxation.
- Positive camel back sign (two bumps over anterior knee region instead of typical one. Two bumps, since patella is riding high within femoral condyles so there is a superior bump; tibial tuberosity forms second bump inferiorly).

(b) Patella baja.
- Malalignment in which patella tracks inferiorly in femoral intercondylar notch.
- Results in restricted knee extension with abnormal cartilaginous wearing resulting in DJD.

(c) Lateral patellar tracking.
- Could result if there is an increase in "Q angle" with a tendency for lateral subluxation or dislocation.

(d) Diagnostic tests utilized: plain film imaging including "sunrise" view.

(e) Physical therapy goals, outcomes and interventions:
- Regaining functional strength of structures surrounding knee, particularly vastus medialis oblique (VMO) muscle; regaining normal flexibility of ITB and hamstrings orthoses (if appropriate) and patellar bracing/taping.

(2) Patellofemoral pain syndrome (PFPS).

(a) Common dysfunction that may occur on its own or in conjunction with other entities. May have been caused by trauma or by congenital/developmental dysfunction.

(b) May be interrelated with chondromalacia patellae and/or patella tendinitis.

(c) Common result is an abnormal patellofemoral tracking that leads to abnormal patellofemoral stress.

(d) Occasionally surgery is indicated.

(e) Diagnostic tests utilized: possibly MRI to rule out other dysfunctions.

(f) Medications:
- Acetaminophen for pain.
- NSAIDs for pain and/or inflammation.

(g) Physical therapy goals, outcomes and interventions:
- Patellofemoral (McConnell) taping is helpful to inhibit pain during rehabilitation.
- Patella mobilization indicated with restrictions of patella glides: e.g., if patella is in a lateral glide position and has decreased medial glide, perform a medial glide joint mobilization to the patella.
- Correction of muscle imbalances and biomechanical faults using strengthening, endurance, coordination and flexibility exercises to gain restoration of normal function.

(3) Patellar tendinitis.

(a) May be related to overload and/or jumping-related activities/sports.

(b) May also be interrelated to patellofemoral dysfunction.

(c) Diagnosis made by clinical examination.

(d) Medications:
- Acetaminophen for pain.
- NSAIDs for pain and/or inflammation.
- Corticosteroid injection or by mouth.

(e) Physical therapy goals, outcomes and interventions:
- Refer to intervention for general bursitis/tendinitis/tendonosis (See section V.B.8).

d. Pes anserine bursitis.

(1) Typically caused by overuse or a contusion.

(2) Must be differentiated from tendinitis.

(3) Diagnosis made by PT clinical examination. Differentiate from contractile condition by comparing results of AROM, PROM and resistive tests.

(4) Medications:

(a) Acetaminophen for pain.

(b) NSAIDs for pain and/or inflammation.

(c) Corticosteroid injection or by mouth.

(5) Physical therapy goals, outcomes and interventions:

(a) Refer to intervention for general bursitis/tendinitis/tendonosis (See section V.B.10).

e. Osgood-Schlatter (jumper's knee).

(1) Mechanical dysfunction resulting in traction apophysitis of the tibial tubercle at the patellar tendon insertion.

(2) Diagnostic tests utilized: plain film findings demonstrate irregularities of the epiphyseal line.

(3) Occasionally surgery is indicated.

(4) Diagnosis made by clinical examination.

(5) Medications:

   (a) Acetaminophen for pain.

   (b) NSAIDs for pain and/or inflammation.

(6) Physical therapy goals, outcomes and interventions.

   (a) Modify activities to prevent excessive stress to irritated site.

f. Genu varum and valgum.

   (1) Normal tibiofemoral shaft angle is 6 degrees of valgum.

   (2) Genu varum is an excessive medial tibial torsion commonly referred to as "bowlegs."

   (3) Genu varum results in excessive medial patellar positioning and the pigeon-toed orientation of the feet.

   (4) Genu valgum is an excessive lateral tibial torsion commonly referred to as "knock-knees."

   (5) Genu valgum results in excessive lateral patellar positioning.

   (6) Diagnostic tests utilized: plain film imaging.

   (7) Diagnosis made by clinical examination.

   (8) Physical therapy goals, outcomes and interventions:

      (a) Intervention includes decreased loading of knee while maintaining strength and endurance.

g. Fractures involving knee joint.

   (1) Femoral condyle.

      (a) Medial femoral most often involved due to its anatomical design.

      (b) Numerous etiological factors include trauma, shearing, impacting and avulsion forces.

      (c) Common mechanism of injury is a fall with knee subjected to a shearing force.

   (2) Tibial plateau.

      (a) Common mechanism of injury is a combination of valgum and compression forces to knee when knee is in a flexed position.

      (b) Often occurs in conjunction with a medial collateral ligamentous injury.

   (3) Epiphyseal plate.

      (a) Mechanism of injury is frequently a weight-bearing torsional stress.

      (b) Presents more frequently in adolescents where an ACL injury would occur in an adult.

   (4) Patella.

      (a) Most common mechanism of injury is a direct blow to patella as result of a fall.

   (5) Diagnostic tests utilized: plain film imaging most likely, unless complex fracture, which would benefit from CT.

   (6) Medications:

(a) Acetaminophen for pain.

(b) NSAIDs for pain and/or inflammation.

(7) Physical therapy goals, outcomes and interventions:

   (a) Physical therapy intervention emphasizes return of function without pain.

   (b) Early flexibility is important in preventing capsular adhesions.

3. **Conditions of the lower leg.**

   a. Anterior compartment syndrome (ACS).

   (1) Increased compartmental pressure resulting in a local ischemic condition.

   (2) Multiple etiologies; direct trauma, fracture, overuse and/or muscle hypertrophy.

   (3) Symptoms of chronic or exertional compartment syndrome are produced by exercise or exertion and described as a deep cramping feeling.

   (4) Symptoms of acute ACS are produced by sudden trauma causing swelling within the compartment.

   (5) Diagnosis made by PT clinical examination.

   (6) Acute ACS is considered a medical emergency and requires immediate surgical intervention with fasciotomy.

> **Red Flag: Compartment Syndrome**
>
> Compartment syndrome involves swelling within a fascial compartment that compresses the muscles, nerves, blood vessels and lymph vessels within the compartment. It usually occurs in the compartments of the forearm or lower leg. Symptoms include swelling with paresthesia and severe pain. Acute compartment syndrome requires immediate medical intervention to prevent tissue death and permanent disability.

   b. Anterior tibial periostitis (shin splints).

   (1) Musculotendinous overuse condition.

   (2) Three common etiologies include:

      (a) Abnormal biomechanical alignment.

      (b) Poor conditioning.

      (c) Improper training methods.

   (3) Muscles involved include anterior tibialis and extensor hallucis longus.

   (4) Pain elicited with palpation of lateral tibia and anterior compartment.

   (5) Diagnosis made by PT clinical examination.

   (6) Medications:

      (a) Acetaminophen for pain.

      (b) NSAIDs for pain and/or inflammation.

   (7) Physical therapy goals, outcomes and interventions.

      (a) Correction of muscle imbalances and biomechanical faults using strengthening, endurance and coordination exercises.

(b) Flexibility exercises for anterior compartment muscles as well as the triceps surae to gain restoration of normal function.

c. Medial tibial stress syndrome.
  (1) Overuse injury of the posterior tibialis and/or the medial soleus resulting in periosteal inflammation at the muscular attachments.
  (2) Etiology is thought to be excessive pronation.
  (3) Pain elicited with palpation of the distal posteromedial border of the tibia.
  (4) Diagnosis made by PT clinical examination.
  (5) Medications:
    (a) Acetaminophen for pain.
    (b) NSAIDs for pain and/or inflammation.
  (6) Physical therapy goals, outcomes and interventions:
    (a) Correction of muscle imbalances and biomechanical faults using strengthening, endurance and coordination exercises.
    (b) Flexibility exercises for anterior compartment muscles as well as the triceps surae to gain restoration of normal function.

d. Stress fractures:
  (1) Overuse injury resulting most often in microfracture of the tibia or fibula.
  (2) 49% of all stress fractures involve the tibia, and 10% involve the fibula.
  (3) Three common etiologies: abnormal biomechanical alignment, poor conditioning and improper training methods.
  (4) Diagnostic tests utilized: plain film imaging and bone scan.
  (5) Medications:
    (a) Acetaminophen for pain.
    (b) NSAIDs for pain and/or inflammation.
  (6) Physical therapy goals, outcomes and interventions:
    (a) Correction of muscle imbalances and biomechanical faults using strengthening, endurance and coordination exercises.
    (b) Flexibility exercises for anterior compartment muscles as well as the triceps surae to gain restoration of normal function.

4. Foot and ankle conditions.
a. Ligament sprains.
  (1) 95% of all ankle sprains involve lateral ligaments.
  (2) With lateral sprains, foot is plantar flexed and inverted at time of injury.
  (3) The most common grading system is as follows:
    (a) Grade I: no loss of function with minimal tearing of the anterior talofibular ligament.
    (b) Grade II: some loss of function with partial disruption of the anterior talofibular and calcaneofibular ligaments.
    (c) Grade III: complete loss of function with complete tearing of the anterior talofibular and calcaneofibular ligaments with partial tear of the posterior talofibular ligament.
  (4) Diagnostic tests utilized: MRI if necessary.
  (5) Instability is evaluated using anterior drawer and talar tilt special tests.
  (6) Medications:
    (a) Acetaminophen for pain.
    (b) NSAIDs for pain and/or inflammation.
  (7) Physical therapy goals, outcomes and interventions:
    (a) Physical therapy intervention is varied depending on whether the patient undergoes a surgical procedure as well as type of surgery that is performed.
    (b) Reduction of pain and inflammation utilizing modalities, soft tissue techniques and manual therapy techniques such as oscillations.
    (c) Correction of muscle imbalances and biomechanical faults using strengthening, endurance, coordination and flexibility exercises to gain restoration of normal function.
    (d) Biomechanical faults caused by joint restrictions should be corrected with joint mobilization to the specific restrictions identified during the examination.
    (e) Progression to functional training based on patient's occupation and/or recreational goals.

b. Achilles' tendinitis/tendonosis.
  (1) Differentiate whether an inflammatory tendinitis or a chronic tendonosis.
  (2) PT clinical examination including Thompson's test helps to identify this condition.
  (3) Medications:
    (a) Acetaminophen for pain.
    (b) NSAIDs for pain and/or inflammation.
    (c) Corticosteroid injection or by mouth.
  (4) Physical therapy goals, outcomes and interventions:
    (a) Refer to intervention for general bursitis/tendinitis/tendonosis (See section V.B.8 and 9).

c. Fractures of foot and ankle.
  (1) Unimalleolar involves the medial or lateral malleolus.
  (2) Bimalleolar involves the medial and lateral malleoli.
  (3) Trimalleolar involves the medial and lateral malleoli and the posterior tubercle of the distal tibia.
  (4) Diagnostic tests utilized: plain film imaging.
  (5) Medications:
    (a) Acetaminophen for pain.
    (b) NSAIDs for pain and/or inflammation.
  (6) Physical therapy goals, outcomes and interventions:

(a) Physical therapy intervention emphasizes return of function without pain.

(b) Functional training and restoration of muscle imbalances using exercise to normalize strength, endurance, coordination and flexibility.

(c) Early PROM is important in preventing capsular adhesions.

d. Tarsal tunnel syndrome:

(1) Entrapment of the posterior tibial nerve or one of its branches within the tarsal tunnel.

(2) Over/excessive pronation, overuse problems resulting in tendinitis of the long flexor and posterior tibialis tendon and trauma may compromise space in the tarsal tunnel.

(3) Symptoms include; pain, numbness and paresthesias along the medial ankle to the plantar surface of the foot.

(4) Diagnostic tests utilized: electrodiagnostic tests.

(5) Positive Tinel's sign at the tarsal tunnel.

(6) Medications:

(a) Acetaminophen for pain.

(b) NSAIDs for pain and/or inflammation.

(c) Neurontin for neuropathic pain.

(7) Physical therapy goals, outcomes and interventions:

(a) Intervention includes the use of orthoses to maintain neutral alignment of the foot.

e. Flexor hallucis tendonopathy.

(1) Identified as a tendinitis in the acute stage or can present as a chronic tendonosis. Commonly seen in ballet performers.

(2) Medications:

(a) Acetaminophen for pain.

(b) NSAIDs for pain and/or inflammation.

(c) Corticosteroid injection or by mouth.

(3) Physical therapy goals, outcomes and interventions:

(a) Refer to intervention for general bursitis/tendinitis/tendonosis (See section V.B.8 and 9).

f. Pes cavus (hollow foot).

(1) Numerous etiologies to include genetic predisposition, neurological disorders resulting in muscle imbalances and contracture of soft tissues.

(2) Deformity observed includes an increased height of longitudinal arches, dropping of anterior arch, metatarsal heads lower than hindfoot, plantar flexion and splaying of forefoot and claw toes.

(3) Function is limited owing to altered arthrokinematics resulting in limited ability to absorb forces through foot.

(4) Diagnosis made by clinical examination including thorough biomechanical lower quarter exam.

(5) Physical therapy goals, outcomes and interventions.

(a) Intervention includes patient education emphasizing limitation of high impact sports (i.e., long-distance running and ballet), use of proper footwear and fitting for orthoses.

g. Pes planus (flat foot).

(1) Etiologies include genetic predisposition, muscle weakness, ligamentous laxity, paralysis, excessive pronation, trauma or disease (e.g., rheumatoid arthritis).

(2) Normal in infant and toddler feet.

(3) Deformity observed may include a reduction in height of medial longitudinal arch.

(4) Decreased ability of foot to provide a rigid lever for push off during gait as result of altered arthrokinematics.

(5) Diagnosis made by clinical examination including thorough biomechanical lower quarter exam.

(6) Physical therapy goals, outcomes and interventions:

(a) Intervention emphasizes patient education, use of proper footwear and orthotic fitting.

h. Talipes equinovarus (clubfoot).

(1) Two types: postural and talipes equinovarus.

(2) Etiology.

(a) Postural, which results from intrauterine malposition.

(b) Talipes equinovarus, which is an abnormal development of the head and neck of the talus as the result of heredity or neuromuscular disorders: e.g., myelomeningocele.

(3) Deformity observed:

(a) Plantar flexed, adducted and inverted foot (postural).

(b) Talipes equinovarus has three components: plantar flexion at talocrural joint, inversion at subtalar, talocalcaneal, talonavicular and calcaneocuboid joints. Supination is observed at midtarsal joints.

(4) Diagnosis made by PT clinical examination including thorough biomechanical lower quarter exam.

(5) Physical therapy goals, outcomes and interventions.

(a) Manipulation followed by casting or splinting for postural condition.

(b) Talipes equinovarus requires surgical intervention to correct deformity followed by casting or splinting.

i. Equinus.

(1) Etiology can include congenital bone deformity, neurological disorders such as cerebral palsy, contracture of gastrocnemius and/or soleus muscles, trauma or inflammatory disease.

(2) Deformity observed: plantar flexed foot.

(3) Compensation secondary to limited dorsiflexion includes subtalar or midtarsal pronation.

(4) Diagnosis made by PT clinical examination including thorough biomechanical lower quarter exam.

(5) Physical therapy goals, outcomes and interventions.

(a) Physical therapy intervention includes flexibility exercises of shortened structures within foot, joint mobilization to joint restrictions identified in examination, strengthening to intrinsic and extrinsic foot muscles and orthotic management.

j. Hallux valgus.

(1) Etiology is varied to include biomechanical malalignment (excessive pronation), ligamentous laxity, heredity, weak muscles and footwear that is too tight.

(2) Deformity observed: a medial deviation of head of first metatarsal from midline of body; metatarsal and base of proximal first phalanx moves medially, distal phalanx then moves laterally.

(3) Normal metatarsophalangeal angle is 8–20 degrees.

(4) Diagnosis made by clinical examination including thorough biomechanical lower quarter exam.

(5) Physical therapy goals, outcomes and interventions.

(a) Early orthotic fitting and patient education.

(b) Later management requires surgery followed by flexibility exercises to restore normal function, strengthening exercises, and possible joint mobilization to identified restrictions.

k. Metatarsalgia.

(1) Etiologies

(a) Mechanical: tight triceps surae group and/or Achilles' tendon, collapse of transverse arch, short first ray, pronation of forefoot.

(b) Structural changes in transverse arch possibly leading to vascular and/or neural compromise in tissues of forefoot.

(c) Changes in footwear.

(2) Complaint frequently heard is pain at first and second metatarsal heads after long periods of weight bearing.

(3) Diagnosis made by PT clinical examination including thorough biomechanical lower quarter exam.

(4) Medications:

(a) Acetaminophen for pain.

(b) NSAIDs for pain and/or inflammation.

(c) Neurontin for neuropathic pain.

(5) Physical therapy goals, outcomes and interventions:

(a) Intervention includes correction of biomechanical abnormality (improving flexibility of triceps surae), modalities to decrease pain.

(b) Prescription and/or creation of orthoses.

(c) Patient education regarding selection of footwear.

l. Metatarsus adductus.

(1) Etiology: congenital, muscle imbalance or neuromuscular diseases such as polio.

(2) Two types: rigid and flexible.

(3) Deformity observed.

(a) Rigid results in a medial subluxation of tarsometatarsal joints. Hindfoot is slightly in valgus with navicular lateral to head of talus.

(b) Flexible is observed as adduction of all five metatarsals at the tarsometatarsal joints.

(4) Diagnosis made by PT clinical examination including thorough biomechanical lower quarter exam.

(5) Physical therapy goals, outcomes and interventions.

(a) Intervention includes strengthening and regaining proper alignment of foot (i.e., through use of orthoses).

m. Charcot-Marie-Tooth disease.

(1) Peroneal muscular atrophy that affects motor and sensory nerves.

(2) May begin in childhood or adulthood.

(3) Initially affects muscles in lower leg and foot, but eventually progresses to muscles of hands and forearm.

(4) Slowly progressive disorder that has varying degrees of involvement depending on degree of genetic dominance.

(5) Diagnostic tests utilized: electrodiagnostic tests.

(6) Diagnosis made by PT clinical examination including thorough biomechanical lower quarter exam.

(7) Medications:

(a) Acetaminophen for pain.

(b) NSAIDs for pain and/or inflammation.

(c) Neurontin for neuropathic pain.

(8) Physical therapy goals, outcomes and interventions:

(a) No specific treatment to prevent since it is an inherited disorder.

(b) Physical therapy intervention centers on preventing contractures/skin breakdown and maximizing patient's functional capacity to perform activities.

(c) Patient education and training regarding braces and ambulatory assistive devices.

n. Plantar fasciitis.

(1) Etiology usually mechanical.

(a) Chronic irritation of plantar fascia from excessive pronation.

(b) Limited ROM of first metatarsophalangeal (MTP) and talocrural joint.

(c) Tight triceps surae.

(d) Acute injury from excessive loading of foot.

(e) Rigid cavus foot.

(2) Results in microtears at attachment of plantar fascia.

(3) Diagnostic tests utilized: none.

(4) Diagnosis made by PT clinical examination including thorough biomechanical lower quarter exam. Differentiated from tarsal tunnel syndrome by a negative Tinel's sign.

(5) Medications:

(a) Acetaminophen for pain.

(b) NSAIDs for pain and/or inflammation.

(c) Corticosteroid injection or by mouth.

(6) Physical therapy goals, outcomes and interventions:

(a) Physical therapy intervention includes regaining proper mechanical alignment.

(b) Modalities to reduce pain and inflammation.

(c) Flexibility of the plantar fascia for the pes cavus foot.

(d) Careful flexibility exercises for triceps surae.

(e) Joint mobilization to identified restrictions.

(f) Night splints.

(g) Strengthening of invertors of foot.

(h) Patient education regarding selection of footwear and orthotic fitting.

o. Forefoot/rearfoot deformities.

(1) Rearfoot varus (subtalar varus, calcaneal varus).

(a) Etiology: abnormal mechanical alignment of tibia, shortened rearfoot soft tissues or malunion of calcaneus.

(b) Deformity observed: rigid inversion of calcaneus when subtalar joint is in neutral position.

(c) Diagnosis made by PT clinical examination including thorough biomechanical lower quarter exam.

(d) Physical therapy goals, outcomes and interventions:

- Regaining proper mechanical alignment.
- Improving flexibility of shortened soft tissues.
- Orthotic fitting and patient education regarding selection of footwear.

(2) Rearfoot valgus.

(a) Etiology: abnormal mechanical alignment of the knee (genu valgum) or tibial valgus.

(b) Deformity observed: eversion of calcaneus with a neutral subtalar joint.

(c) Owing to increased mobility of hindfoot, fewer musculoskeletal problems develop from this deformity than occurs with rearfoot varus.

(d) Diagnosis made by PT clinical examination including thorough biomechanical lower quarter exam.

(e) Physical therapy goals, outcomes and interventions.

- Regaining proper mechanical alignment.
- Improving flexibility of shortened soft tissues.
- Orthotic fitting and patient education regarding selection of footwear.

(3) Forefoot varus.

(a) Etiology: congenital abnormal deviation of head and neck of talus.

(b) Deformity observed: inversion of forefoot when subtalar joint is in neutral.

(c) Diagnosis made by PT clinical examination including thorough biomechanical lower quarter exam.

(d) Physical therapy goals, outcomes and interventions.

- Regaining proper mechanical alignment.
- Improving flexibility of shortened soft tissues.
- Orthotic fitting and patient education regarding selection of footwear.

(4) Forefoot valgus.

(a) Etiology: congenital abnormal development of head and neck of talus.

(b) Deformity observed: eversion of forefoot when the subtalar joint is in neutral.

(c) Diagnosis made by PT clinical examination including thorough biomechanical lower quarter exam.

(d) Physical therapy goals, outcomes and interventions.

- Regaining proper mechanical alignment.
- Improving flexibility of shortened soft tissues.
- Orthotic fitting and patient education regarding selection of footwear.

Spinal Conditions

1. Muscle strain.

a. May be related to sudden trauma, chronic or sustained overload or abnormal muscle biomechanics secondary to faulty function (abnormal joint or muscle biomechanics).

b. Commonly will resolve without intervention, but if trauma is too great or if related to chronic etiology, will benefit from intervention.

c. Diagnosis made by PT clinical examination by comparing results of flexibility (AROM/PROM), resistive tests and palpation.

d. Medications:

(1) Acetaminophen for pain.

(2) NSAIDs for pain and/or inflammation.

(3) Corticosteroid injection or by mouth.

(4) Muscle relaxants; e.g., Flexeril (cyclobenza-prine) or Valium (diazepam).

(5) Trigger point injections.

e. Physical therapy goals, outcomes and interventions:

(1) Biomechanical faults caused by joint restrictions should be corrected with joint mobilization.

(2) Patient education regarding the elimination of harmful positions and postural reeducation.

(3) Spinal manipulation for pain inhibition is generally indicated for this condition.

2. **Spondylolysis/spondylolisthesis.**

a. Etiology: thought to be congenitally defective pars interarticularis.

b. Spondylolysis is a fracture of the pars interarticularis with positive "Scotty dog" sign on oblique radiographic view of spine.

c. Spondylolisthesis is the actual anterior or posterior slippage of one vertebra on another following bilateral fracture of pars interarticularis.

d. Spondylolisthesis can be graded according to amount of slippage from 1 (25% slippage) to 4 (100% slippage).

e. Diagnostic tests utilized: plain film (oblique to see fracture and lateral views to see slippage).

f. PT clinical examination including stork test helps to identify this condition.

g. Medications:

(1) Acetaminophen for pain.

(2) NSAIDs for pain and/or inflammation.

(3) Corticosteroid injection or by mouth.

(4) Muscle relaxants.

(5) Trigger point injections.

h. Physical therapy goals, outcomes and interventions:

(1) Biomechanical faults caused by joint restrictions should be corrected with joint mobilization to the specific restrictions identified during the examination.

(2) Exercise should focus on dynamic stabilization of trunk with particular emphasis on abdominals and trunk extension with multifidus muscle working from a fully flexed position of trunk up to neutral, but not into trunk extension.

(3) Avoid extension and/or other positions that add stress to defect (i.e., extension, ipsilateral sidebending and contralateral rotation).

(4) Patient should be educated regarding the elimination of positions of extension and should be reeducated on posture.

(5) Braces such as Boston brace and TLSO (thoracolumbosacral orthosis) have traditionally been used, but frequency is decreasing.

(6) Spinal manipulation may be contraindicated for this condition, particularly at the level of defect.

3. **Spinal or intervertebral stenosis.**

a. Etiology: congenital narrow spinal canal or intervertebral foramen coupled with hypertrophy of the spinal lamina and ligamentum flavum or facets as the result of age-related degenerative processes or disease.

b. Results in vascular and/or neural compromise.

c. Signs and symptoms (see Table 2-6).

(1) Bilateral pain and paresthesia in back, buttocks, thighs, calves and feet.

(2) Pain is decreased in spinal flexion, increased in extension.

(3) Pain increases with walking.

(4) Pain relieved with prolonged rest.

d. Diagnostic tests utilized: imaging including plain films, MRI and/or CT scan. Occasionally, myelography is helpful.

e. PT clinical examination including bicycle (van Gelderen's) test helps to identify this condition and differentiate it from intermittent claudication.

f. Medications:

(1) Acetaminophen for pain.

(2) NSAIDs for pain and/or inflammation.

(3) Corticosteroid injection or by mouth.

(4) Muscle relaxants.

(5) Trigger point injections.

g. Physical therapy goals, outcomes and interventions.

(1) Biomechanical faults caused by joint restrictions should be corrected with joint mobilization to the specific restrictions identified during the examination.

(2) Perform flexion biased exercise and exercises that promotes dynamic stability throughout the trunk and pelvis.

(3) Avoid extension and/or other positions that narrow the spinal canal or intervertebral foramen (i.e., extension, ipsilateral side bending and ipsilateral rotation).

(4) Manual and/or mechanical traction.

(a) Traction.

• Cervical spine positioning is at 15 degrees of flexion to provide the optimum intervertebral foraminal opening.

• Contraindications include joint hypermobility, pregnancy, rheumatoid arthritis, Down's syndrome or any other systemic disease which affects ligamentous integrity.

4. **Disc conditions:**

a. Internal disc disruption.

(1) Internal structure of disc annulus is disrupted; however, external structures remain normal. Most common in lumbar region.

(2) Symptoms include constant deep achy pain, increased pain with movement, no objective neurological findings, although patient may have referred pain into lower extremity.

(3) Regular CT or myelogram will not demonstrate any abnormal findings. Can be diagnosed by CT discogram or an MRI.

(4) Clinical examination helps to identify this condition.

(5) Medications:

(a) Acetaminophen for pain.

(b) NSAIDs for pain and/or inflammation.

(c) Muscle relaxants.

(d) Trigger point injections.

(e) Corticosteroid injection or by mouth.

(6) Physical therapy goals, outcomes and interventions:

(a) Biomechanical faults caused by joint restrictions should be corrected with joint mobilization to the specific restrictions identified during the examination.

(b) Spinal manipulation may be contraindicated for this condition.

(c) Patient education regarding proper body mechanics, positions to avoid, limiting repetitive bending and twisting movements, limiting upper extremity overhead and sitting activities and carrying heavy loads.

b. Posterolateral bulge/herniation.

(1) Most commonly observed disc disorder of lumbar spine due to three structural deficiencies:

(a) Posterior disc is narrower in height than anterior disc.

(b) Posterior longitudinal ligament is not as strong and only centrally located in lumbar spine.

(c) Posterior lamellae of annulus are thinner.

(2) Etiology: overstretching and/or tearing of annular rings, vertebral endplate and/or ligamentous structures from high compressive forces or repetitive microtrauma.

(3) Results in loss of strength, radicular pain, paresthesia and inability to perform activities of daily living.

(4) Diagnostic tests utilized: MRI.

(5) PT Clinical examination helps to identify this condition.

(6) Medications:

(a) Acetaminophen for pain.

(b) NSAIDs for pain and/or inflammation.

(c) Muscle relaxants.

(d) Trigger point injections.

(e) Corticosteroid injection or by mouth.

(7) Physical therapy goals, outcomes and interventions:

(a) Exercise program to promote dynamic stability throughout trunk and pelvis as well as to provide optimal stimulus for regeneration of disc.

(b) Positional gapping for 10 minutes to increase space within region of space occupying lesion: e.g., if left posterolateral lumbar herniation present.

• Have patient lying on right side with pillow under right trunk (accentuating trunk side bending right).

• Flex both hips and knees.

• Rotate trunk to left (or pelvis to right).

• Patient can be taught to perform this at home.

(c) Spinal manipulation may be contraindicated for this condition, particularly at the level of the herniation.

(d) Patient education regarding proper body mechanics, positions to avoid, limiting repetitive bending and twisting movements, limiting upper extremity overhead and sitting activities and carrying heavy loads.

(e) Manual and/or mechanical traction.

• Traction: cervical spine positioning is at 15 degrees of flexion to provide the optimum intervertebral foraminal opening.

• Contraindications include joint hypermobility, pregnancy, rheumatoid arthritis, Down's syndrome or any other systemic disease which affects ligamentous integrity.

• Efficacy of traction for intervention of disc conditions is currently under scrutiny.

c. Central posterior bulge/herniation.

(1) More commonly observed in the cervical spine but can be seen in the lumbar spine.

(2) Etiology: overstretching and/or tearing of annular rings, vertebral endplate and/or ligamentous structures (posterior longitudinal ligament) from high compressive forces and/or long-term postural malalignment.

(3) Results in loss of strength, radicular pain, paresthesia, inability to perform activities of daily living and possible compression of the spinal cord with central nervous system symptoms; e.g., hyperreflexia and a positive Babinski's reflex (Table 2-7).

(4) Diagnostic tests utilized: MRI.

(5) Clinical examination helps to identify this condition.

(6) Medications:

(a) Acetaminophen for pain.

(b) NSAIDs for pain and/or inflammation.

(c) Muscle relaxants.

(d) Trigger point injections.

(e) Corticosteroid injection or by mouth.

(7) Physical therapy goals, outcomes and interventions:

• Refer to posterolateral intervention (section 4.b) above.

d. Anterior bulge/herniation is very rare due to structural integrity of anterior intervertebral disc.

Table 2-7 ➤ TRUNK AND RIBCAGE MUSCULAR AND NEUROLOGICAL LEVELS

ACTION TO BE TESTED	MUSCLES	CORD SEGMENT	NERVES
Inspiration	Diaphragm levator costarum, external intercostals, anterior internal intercostals	C3-C5 T1-T12	Phrenic Intercostal
Forced expiration	Internal obliques, transverse abdominis, external obliques, posterior internal intercostals, rectus abdominis	T7-L1 T7-T12 T1-T12 T7-T12	Intercostal Intercostal Intercostal Intercostal
Spine extension	Erector spinae, transversospinalis, interspinales, rotatores intertransversarii	T1-T12, L1-L5, S1-S3	
Spine flexion	Rectus abdominis/external obliques, internal obliques, psoas minor	T7-T12 T7-L1 L1	Intercostal Intercostal Lumbar plexus
Spine lateral flexion (hip hiking in reverse)	Quadratus lumborum	T12-L3	Lumbar plexus
Spine rotation	Rotators, internal/external obliques, intertransversarii, transversospinalis	as above	

Adapted from Chusid JG. *Correlative Neuroanatomy and Functional Neurology*, Lange Medical Publications, Los Altos, CA, 1970; and Kendall FP; McCreary EK, Provance PG. *Muscles Testing and Function*, 4th ed, Baltimore, Williams & Wilkins, 1993.

5. **Facet joint conditions:**
   a. DJD.
      (1) Etiology: DJD is part of normal aging process because of weight-bearing properties of facets and intervertebral joints.
      (2) Results in bone hypertrophy, capsular fibrosis, hypermobility or hypomobility of joint and proliferation of synovium.
      (3) Symptoms include reduction in mobility of the spine, pain and possible impingement of associated nerve root resulting in loss of strength and paresthesias (see Table 1-8).
      (4) Diagnostic tests utilized: plain film imaging.
      (5) Clinical examination including lumbar quadrant test helps to identify this condition.
      (6) Medications:
         (a) Acetaminophen for pain.
         (b) NSAIDs for pain and/or inflammation.
         (c) Muscle relaxants.
         (d) Trigger point injections.
         (e) Corticosteroid injection or by mouth.
      (7) Physical therapy goals, outcomes and interventions:
         (a) Exercise program to promote dynamic stability throughout trunk and pelvis as well as to provide optimal stimulus for regeneration of facet cartilage and/or capsule.
         (b) Biomechanical faults caused by joint restrictions should be corrected with joint mobilization to the specific restrictions identified during the examination.
         (c) Spinal manipulation may be useful for this condition.
   b. Facet extrapment (acute locked back).
      (1) Caused by abnormal movement of fibroadipose meniscoid in facet during extension (from

flexion). Meniscoid does not properly reenter joint cavity and bunches up, becoming a space-occupying lesion, which distends capsule, causing pain.
      (2) Flexion is most comfortable for patient and extension increases pain.
      (3) Medications:
         (a) Acetaminophen for pain.
         (b) NSAIDs for pain and/or inflammation.
         (c) Muscle relaxants.
         (d) Trigger point injections.
         (e) Corticosteroid injection or by mouth.
      (4) Physical therapy goals, outcomes and interventions.
         (a) Positional facet joint gapping and/or manipulation are appropriate treatments.

6. **Acceleration/deceleration injuries of cervical spine.**
   a. Formerly known as "whiplash."
   b. Occurs when excess shear and tensile forces are exerted on cervical structures.
   c. Structures injured may include facets/articular processes, facet joint capsules, ligaments, disc, anterior/posterior muscles, fracture to odontoid process and spinous processes, temporomandibular joint (TMJ), sympathetic chain ganglia, spinal and cranial nerves.
   d. Signs and symptoms:
      (1) Early include headaches, neck pain, limited flexibility, reversal of lower cervical lordosis and decrease in upper cervical kyphosis, vertigo, change in vision and hearing, irritability to noise and light, dysesthesias of face and bilateral upper extremities, nausea, difficulty swallowing and emotional lability.
      (2) Late include chronic head and neck pain, limitation in flexibility, TMJ dysfunction, limited

tolerance to ADL, disequilibrium, anxiety and depression.

e. Common clinical findings include postural changes, excessive muscle guarding with soft tissue fibrosis, segmental hypermobility and gradual development of restricted segmental motion cranial and caudal to the injury (segmental hypomobility).

f. Diagnostic tests utilized: plain film imaging, CT and/or MRI.

g. Medications:
    (1) Acetaminophen for pain.
    (2) NSAIDs for pain and/or inflammation.
    (3) Muscle relaxants.
    (4) Trigger point injections.
    (5) Corticosteroid injection or by mouth.

h. Physical therapy goals, outcomes and interventions.
    (1) Spinal manipulation is generally indicated for this condition.
    (2) Correction of muscle imbalances and biomechanical faults using strengthening, endurance, coordination and flexibility exercises to gain restoration of normal function.
    (3) Biomechanical faults caused by joint restrictions should be corrected with joint mobilization to the specific restrictions identified during the examination.
    (4) Progression to functional training based on patient's occupation and/or recreational goals.
    (5) Patient education regarding the elimination of harmful positions and postural reeducation.
    (6) Manual and/or mechanical traction.
        (a) Traction.
            • Cervical spine positioning is at 15° of flexion to provide the optimum intervertebral foraminal opening.
            • Contraindications include joint hypermobility, pregnancy, rheumatoid arthritis, Down syndrome or any other systemic disease which affects ligamentous integrity.

7. **Hypermobile spinal segments.**
    a. An abnormal increase in ROM at a joint due to insufficient soft tissue control (i.e., ligamentous, discal, muscle or a combination of all three).
    b. Diagnostic tests utilized: plain film imaging, particularly dynamic flexion/extension views.
    c. Medications:
        (1) Acetaminophen for pain.
        (2) NSAIDs for pain and/or inflammation.
        (3) Muscle relaxants.
        (4) Trigger point injections.
        (5) Sclerosing injections.
        (6) Corticosteroid injection or by mouth.
    d. Physical therapy goals, outcomes and interventions:
        (1) Pain reduction modalities to reduce irritability of structures.
        (2) Passive ROM within a normal range of movement.

(3) Passive stabilization with corsets, splints, casts, tape and collars.

(4) Increase strength/endurance/coordination especially in the multifidus, abdominals, extensors and gluteals, which control posture.

(5) Regain muscle balance.

(6) Patient education regarding postural reeducation, limiting excessive overloading, limiting sustained activities and limiting end-range postures.

8. **Sacroiliac joint (SIJ) conditions.**
    a. Cause and specific pathology is unknown. Since this is a joint, it is assumed that it can become inflamed, develop degenerative changes or abnormal movement patterns.
    b. Anatomically and functionally SIJ is closely related to lumbar spine, so a thorough examination of both regions is indicated if a patient presents with pain in either.
    c. Diagnostic tests utilized: plain film imaging and possibly MRI. Occasionally double-blind injections may be used to assist in making the diagnosis (first injection is provocative in nature and second injection is analgesic. If increased "same" pain with first injection and decreased pain following second injection, joint is determined to be pathological).
    d. Clinical examination including the following special tests will be useful to make diagnosis:
        (1) Gillet's test.
        (2) Ipsilateral anterior rotation test.
        (3) Gaenslen's test.
        (4) Long-sitting (supine to sit) test.
        (5) Goldthwait's test.
    e. Medications:
        (1) Acetaminophen for pain.
        (2) NSAIDs for pain and/or inflammation.
        (3) Muscle relaxants.
        (4) Trigger point injections.
        (5) Corticosteroid injection or by mouth.
    f. Physical therapy goals, outcomes and interventions.
        (1) Spinal manipulation such as SIJ gapping is generally indicated for this condition to inhibit pain, reduce muscle guarding and restore normal joint motion.
        (2) Correction of muscle imbalances throughout pelvis using strengthening, endurance, coordination and flexibility exercises to gain restoration of normal function.
        (3) Biomechanical faults caused by joint restrictions should be corrected with joint mobilization to the specific restrictions identified during the examination.
        (4) Patient should be educated regarding the elimination of harmful positions and reeducated on posture.
        (5) Sacroiliac belts may be useful in some patients.

9. Repetitive/cumulative trauma to back.

a. Disorders of the nerves, soft tissues and bones precipitated or aggravated by repeated exertions or movements of the back, occurring most often in the workplace.

b. Repetitive trauma disorders account for 48% of all reported occupational diseases.

c. Diagnosis is difficult with up to 85% of back pain nondiagnosed.

d. Typically causes one of the conditions previously listed above: muscle, disc and/or joint impairment.

e. Vocational factors which contribute to back pain include physically heavy static work postures, lifting, frequent bending and twisting, and repetitive work and vibration.

f. Chronic disability may be reduced by enrollment in a work-conditioning program which includes patient education, aerobic exercises, general strengthening and functional stability exercises that promote endurance for work-related activities.

g. Intervention should be focused on prevention, consisting of education. If this phenomenon leads to a condition listed above, follow the specific intervention associated with that condition.

10. Other conditions affecting the spine (see Table 2-6):

a. Bone tumors.

  (1) May be primary or metastatic.

    (a) Primary tumors include multiple myeloma (which is most common primary tumor of bone), Ewing's sarcoma, malignant lymphoma, chondrosarcoma, osteosarcoma and chondromas.

    (b) Metastatic bone cancer has primary sites in lung, prostate, breast, kidney and thyroid.

    (c) Patient history should always include questions about a prior episode of cancer.

    (d) Signs and symptoms include pain which is unvarying and progressive, is not relieved with rest or analgesics and is more pronounced at night (Figure 2-8).

    (e) Diagnostic tests utilized: plain film imaging, CT and/or MRI as well as laboratory tests.

b. Visceral tumors.

  (1) Esophageal cancer symptomatology may include pain radiating to the back, pain with swallowing, dysphagia and weight loss.

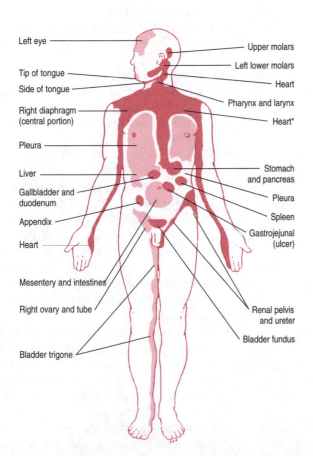
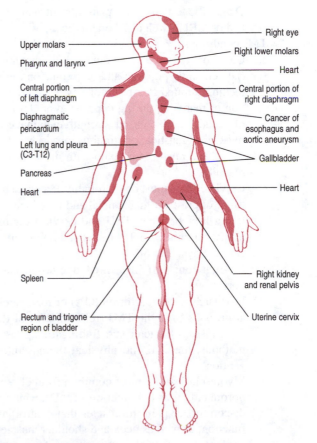

*The pain of coronary insufficiency can involve any aspect of the anterior chest but is more common in the substernal region.

Figure 2-8 • Pain referred from viscera.
(From Rothstein J et al. *The Rehabilitation Specialists' Handbook*. 3rd ed. Philadelphia, Davis, 1998:484–485.)

(2) Pancreatic cancer symptomatology includes a deep gnawing pain that may radiate from the chest to the back.

(3) Diagnostic tests utilized: plain film imaging, CT and/or MRI as well as laboratory tests.

c. Gastrointestinal conditions:

(1) Acute pancreatitis may manifest itself as midepigastric pain which radiates through to back.

(2) Cholecystitis may present with abrupt severe abdominal pain and right upper quadrant tenderness, nausea, vomiting and fever.

(3) Diagnostic tests utilized: plain film imaging, CT and/or MRI as well as laboratory tests.

d. Cardiovascular and pulmonary conditions.

(1) Heart and lung disorders can refer pain to chest, back, neck, jaw and upper extremity.

(2) Abdominal aortic aneurysm (AAA) usually appears as nonspecific lumbar pain.

(3) Diagnostic tests utilized: plain film imaging, CT and/or MRI as well as laboratory tests.

(4) Will be identified as pain during examination of abdominal region.

e. Urological and gynecological conditions:

(1) Kidney, bladder, ovarian and uterine disorders can refer pain to the trunk, pelvis and thighs.

(2) Diagnostic tests utilized: plain film imaging, CT and/or MRI as well as laboratory tests.

f. TMJ conditions.

a. Common signs and symptoms include joint noise (i.e., clicking, popping and/or crepitation), joint locking, limited flexibility of jaw, lateral deviation of mandible during depression or elevation of mandible, decreased strength/endurance of muscles of mastication, tinnitus, headaches, forward head posture and pain with movement of mandible.

b. Cervical spine must be thoroughly examined because of close biomechanical and functional relationships between TMJ and cervical region. Many patients with TMJ have a component of cervical dysfunction.

c. Dysfunctions fall into three diagnostic categories:

(1) DJD such as osteoarthritis (OA) or rheumatoid arthritis (RA) in the TMJ (refer to OA and RA for causes, characteristic findings, diagnostic methods, medical and physical therapy intervention).

(2) Myofascial pain is most common form of temporomandibular dysfunction (TMD), which is discomfort or pain in muscles that control jaw function, as well as neck and shoulder muscles. (Refer to myofascial pain syndrome for causes, characteristic findings, diagnostic methods, medical and physical therapy intervention.)

(3) Internal derangement of joint, meaning a dislocated jaw, displaced articular disc or injury to condyle.

(a) Loss of functional mobility may result from increased activity in muscles of mastication as result of stress and anxiety.

(b) Causes:
- Trauma, leading to joint edema, capsulitis, hypomobility/hypermobility or abnormal function of ligaments, capsule and/or muscles.
- Congenital anatomical anomalies: change in shape of palate.
- Abnormal function such as repeatedly chewing ice or hard candy, paranormal breathing (mouth breather), forward head posture.

(c) Diagnostic tests utilized: plain film imaging and/or MRI if necessary.

(d) Clinical examination helps to identify this condition.

(e) Medications:
- Acetaminophen for pain.
- NSAIDs for pain and/or inflammation.
- Muscle relaxants.
- Trigger point injections.
- Corticosteroid injection or by mouth.

(f) Physical therapy goals, outcomes and interventions.
- Postural reeducation regarding re-gaining the normal anterior-posterior curves and left-right symmetry of the spine.
- Modalities for reduction of pain and inflammation.
- Biofeedback to minimize effects of stress and/or anxiety.
- Joint mobilization if restriction in TMJ is present. Primary glide is inferior, which gaps joint, stretches the capsule and allows relocation of anteriorly displaced disc.
- Flexibility and muscle-strengthening exercises (e.g., Rocobado's jaw opening while maintaining the tongue in contact with the palate and isometric mandibular exercises).
- Patient education (e.g., foods to avoid and maintaining proper postural alignment).
- Night splints may be prescribed by the dentist to maintain resting jaw position.
- Educate patient regarding resting position of tongue on hard palate.
- It is critical to normalize the cervical spine posture prior to the patient receiving any permanent dental procedures and/or appliances.

Orthopaedic Surgical Repairs

1. **Surgical repairs of upper extremity.**
   a. Rotator cuff tears.
      (1) Usually degenerative and occur over time with impingement of supraspinatus tendon between greater tuberosity and acromion.
      (2) Signs and symptoms include:
         (a) Significant reduction of AROM into abduction.
         (b) No reduction of PROM.
         (c) Drop arm test is positive.
         (d) Poor scapulothoracic and glenohumeral rhythm.
      (3) Diagnostic tests utilized: arthrogram traditionally had been the "gold standard" test. MRI may be done, but may not be as sensitive.
      (4) Physical therapy goals, outcomes and interventions.
         (a) Rehabilitation is initiated following a period of immobilization with surgical intervention.
         (b) Physical therapy intervention emphasizes **return** of normal strength/endurance/coordination of muscles, joint mechanics, flexibility (AROM/PROM), and scapulothoracic and glenohumeral rhythm with overhead function.
   b. Tendon injuries and repairs of the hand.
      (1) Flexor tendon repairs.
         (a) First 3–4 weeks, distal extremity is immobilized with a protective splint with wrist and digits flexed. Rubber band traction is applied to maintain interphalangeal joints in 30–50 degrees of passive flexion.
         (b) Physical therapy goals, outcomes and interventions.
            • Patient can perform resisted extension and passive flexion within constraints of splint. AROM to tolerance is initiated at 4 weeks.
            • Goal is to manage all soft tissues through wound-healing phases by providing collagen remodeling which preserves free tendon gliding.
            • Early intervention consists of wound management, edema control and passive exercises.
            • Active extension exercises are initiated first followed by flexion.
            • Resistive and functional exercises are introduced when full AROM is achieved.
      (2) Extensor tendon repairs.
         (a) Distal repairs are immobilized such that the distal interphalangeal joints are in neutral for 6–8 weeks.
         (b) Physical therapy goals, outcomes and interventions.
            • AROM is initiated at 6 weeks with proximal interphalangeal joints in neutral.
            • Goal is to manage all soft tissues through wound-healing phases by providing collagen remodeling which preserves free tendon gliding.
            • Early intervention consists of wound management, edema control and passive exercises.
            • Active extension exercises are initiated first, followed by flexion.
            • Resistive and functional exercises are introduced when full AROM is achieved.
         (c) Proximal repairs are immobilized with the wrist and digital joints in extension for 4 weeks.
         (d) Physical therapy goals, outcomes and interventions.
            • Early AROM/PROM in flexion with metacarpophalangeal joint in extension. At 6 weeks, full AROM is initiated into flexion and extension.

2. **Surgical repairs of lower extremity.**
   a. Total hip replacement/arthroplasty (THR).
      (1) This information may vary depending on surgical procedure and/or MD preference/protocol. Must be familiar with postoperative protocol for each patient relative to procedure and/or MD.
      (2) Cemented versus noncemented.
         (a) Cemented hips can tolerate full weight-bearing immediately following surgery.
         (b) Cement may crack with aging causing a loosening of prosthesis. Noncemented technique is more stressful on bones during the surgical procedure.
         (c) Noncemented procedures are typically used with younger and/or more active individuals. Cemented technique may be better for individuals with fragile bones or for those who will benefit from immediate ability to weight bear: e.g., those with dementia or significant debilitation.
      (3) Bed positioning with a wedge to prevent adduction.
      (4) Patient should avoid the position of hip flexion >90 degrees with adduction and internal rotation. Partial weight-bearing to tolerance is initiated on the second postsurgery day using crutches or a walker with typical surgical procedures.
      (5) Physical therapy goals, outcomes and interventions:
         (a) Physical therapy intervention focus on bed mobility, transitional movements, ambulation and return to premorbid ADL.

b. Open reduction internal fixation (ORIF) following femoral fracture.
  (1) Patient will typically be non weight-bearing for 1–2 weeks using crutches or a walker. Thereafter, the patient will be partial weight-bearing as tolerated.
  (2) Physical therapy goals, outcomes and interventions:
    (a) Physical therapy intervention focus on bed mobility, transitional movements, ambulation and return to premorbid ADL.
c. Total knee replacements/arthroplasty (TKR).
  (1) TKR surgery is typically performed as a result of severe DJD of the knee joint which has led to pain and impaired function.
  (2) Physical therapy goals, outcomes and interventions:
    (a) Goals of early rehabilitation (1–3 weeks) include muscle reeducation, soft tissue mobilization, lymphedema reduction, initiation of PROM (e.g., a continuous passive motion [CPM] machine is used in the hospital following surgery), AROM and reduction of postsurgical swelling.
    (b) Goals of the second phase of rehabilitation include regaining endurance, coordination and strength of the muscles surrounding the knee. Also functional activities to include progressive ambulation stair climbing and transitional training based on healing and the type of prosthesis used.
    (c) Goals and outcomes of the last phase of rehabilitation include returning the patient to premorbid ADL. Functional and endurance training and proprioceptive exercises are introduced during this phase.
    (d) The weight-bearing status of patients with a cemented prosthesis is at the level of the patient's tolerance. Patients with cementless prostheses are progressed according to the time frame for fracture healing. Weight bearing 1–7 weeks is 25%, 50% by week 8, 75% by week 10 and 100% weight-bearing without an assistive device by week 12.
    (e) Avoidance of forceful mobilization and PROM into flexion >9 degrees is important because of the mechanical restraints of the prosthesis.
    (f) Biomechanical faults caused by joint restrictions should be corrected with joint mobilization to the specific restrictions identified during the examination.
d. Ligamentous repairs of knee.
  (1) Six phases of rehabilitation are followed with ACL and PCL reconstructive surgery.
  (2) ACL reconstruction (Table 2-8).

Table 2-8 ➤ HAMSTRING VERSUS PATELLA TENDON GRAFT FOR ACL RECONSTRUCTION

PROS/ CONS	HAMSTRING GRAFTS	PATELLA TENDON GRAFTS
Pros	1. Typically fewer symptoms. postoperatively 2. Greater return to pre-injury level of activity. 3. Typically allows earlier rehabilitation.	1. Better at maintaining graft tension postoperatively 2. Typically less expensive. 3. Faster healing time.
Cons	1. Typically more expensive. 2. Believed to be more technically difficult procedure. 3. Rehabilitation can be more difficult (i.e., slower).	1. Increased potential for anterior knee pain and later patellofemoral osteoarthrosis. 2. Increased potential for knee extension deficit. 3. Potential delay in rehabilitation secondary to more atrophy of quadriceps.

    (a) Immediately following surgery, a continuous passive motion unit (CPM) is utilized with PROM from 0–70 degrees of flexion.
    (b) Motion is increased to 0–120 degrees by the sixth week.
    (c) Reconstruction is usually protected with a hinged brace set at 20–70 degrees of flexion initially.
    (d) Patient is non–weight-bearing for approximately 1 week.
    (e) Weight-bearing progresses as tolerated to full weight-bearing.
    (f) Patient is weaned from brace between the second and fourth weeks.
  (3) Posterior cruciate ligament reconstruction.
    (a) Generally similar to ACL repair except patient is often initially in hinged brace at 0 degree during ambulation.
  (4) Physical therapy goals, outcomes and interventions following ACL and PCL surgical repairs:
    (a) Six phases of rehabilitation are as follows: preoperative, maximum protection, controlled motion, moderate protection, minimum protection and return to activity.
    (b) Specific interventions:
      • Soft tissue/massage techniques to quadriceps and hamstring muscles to reduce muscle guarding.
      • Joint oscillations to inhibit joint pain and muscle guarding.
      • Correction of muscle imbalances and biomechanical faults using strengthening, endurance, coordination and flexibility exercises to gain restoration of normal function.
      • Biomechanical faults caused by joint restrictions should be corrected with joint

mobilization to the specific restrictions identified during the examination.
- Progression to functional training based on patient's occupation and/or recreational goals.

e. Lateral retinacular release:

(1) Typically performed as a result of patellofemoral pain syndrome (PFPS). Purpose of procedure is to restore normal tracking of the patella during contraction of the quadriceps muscle.

(2) Physical therapy goals, outcomes and interventions.

(a) Intervention should emphasize closed kinetic chain exercises to streng then quadriceps muscles and regain dynamic balance of all structures (contractile and noncontractile) surrounding knee.

(b) Normalizing the flexibility of the hamstrings, triceps surae and ITB will help restore mechanical alignment.

(c) Mobilization of patella is important to maintain nutrition and decrease the likelihood of adhesions.

f Meniscal arthroscopy.

(1) Partial meniscectomy.

(a) Partial weight-bearing as tolerated when full knee extension is obtained.

(b) Physical therapy goals, outcomes and interventions:

- Initial goals focus on edema/effusion control.
- AROM is urged post surgical day 1.
- Isotonic and isokinetic strengthening by day 3.
- Jogging on the ball of the foot or toes is recommended to decrease the loading of the knee joint.

(2) Repairs.

(a) Patient will be non–weight-bearing for 3–6 weeks.

(b) Rehabilitation of the joint begins within 7–10 days of procedure.

(c) Physical therapy goals, outcomes and interventions:

- Soft tissue/massage techniques to quadriceps and hamstring muscles to reduce muscle guarding.
- Joint oscillations to inhibit joint pain and muscle guarding.
- Correction of muscle imbalances and biomechanical faults using strengthening, endurance, coordination and flexibility exercises to gain restoration of normal function.
- Biomechanical faults caused by joint restrictions should be corrected with joint

mobilization to the specific restrictions identified during the examination.
- Progression to functional training based on patient's occupation and/or recreational goals.

3. **Surgical repairs of spine.**

a. Rehabilitation varies according to the type of surgery performed.

b. A back protection program and early mobilization exercises should be initiated prior to surgery.

c. Patients should avoid prolonged sitting, heavy lifting and long car trips for approximately 3 months.

d. Repetitive bending with twisting should always be avoided.

e. With microdiscectomies, rehabilitation time is decreased because the fibers of the annulus fibrosus are not damaged.

f. With laminectomy/discectomy, early movement and activation of paraspinal musculature (especially multifidus) is necessary.

g. Multilevel vertebra fusion:

(1) Typically requires 6 weeks of trunk immobility with bracing.

(2) Once brace is removed and movement is allowed, important to regain as much normal/functional movement as possible while restoring functional activation of muscles.

(3) With combined anterior/posterior surgical approach, bracing is seldom used.

h. With Harrington rod placement for idiopathic scoliosis, rehabilitation goals focus on early mobilization in bed and effective coughing.

(1) The patient can begin ambulation between the fourth and seventh postoperative days.

(2) The patient should avoid heavy lifting and excessive twisting and bending.

i. Physical therapy goals, outcomes and interventions following surgical interventions.

(1) Soft tissue/massage techniques to paraspinal muscles to reduce muscle guarding.

(2) Joint oscillations to inhibit joint pain and muscle guarding.

(3) Correction of muscle imbalances using strengthening, endurance, coordination and flexibility exercises to gain restoration of normal function. Make sure that multifidus function is restored.

(4) Must develop dynamic stabilization for muscles of trunk and pelvis during all functional activities.

(5) Biomechanical faults caused by joint restrictions should be corrected with joint mobilization to the specific restrictions identified during the examination.

(6) Progression to functional training based on patient's occupation and/or recreational goals.

Interventions for Patients/Clients with Musculoskeletal Conditions

Interventions for Patients/Clients with Acute Conditions

1. **Acute phase:**
   a. Immobilization with limited (1–2 days) bed rest. Use of braces, slings, corsets, cervical collars, assistive devices and taping.
   b. Control inflammatory response (rest, ice, compression, elevation [RICE]).
      (1) Physical agents: ice and electric stimulation.
      (2) Compression and elevation to reduce and prevent effusion and swelling.
      (3) NSAIDs.
      (4) Rest/relaxation to reduce pain.
      (5) Soft tissue/massage techniques.
   c. Assisted movement of injured tissues.
   d. Joint oscillations (grades I and II) for pain relief.
   e. Therapeutic exercise:
      (1) Dose of 40%–60% of one repetition maximum (i.e., high repetition with low resistance) to stimulate regeneration of tissue and revascularization.
      (2) Exercise should be nontraumatic, meaning no pain and/or increased edema as a result of the exercise.
   f. Educate patient/client on joint protection strategies.

2. **Subacute phase:**
   a. Avoidance of continued irritation and repetitive trauma.
      (1) Modify activities at home/work/recreation.
      (2) Modify use of equipment or type of equipment at home/work/recreation.
      (3) Correct biomechanical faults such as leg length discrepancy, abnormal foot biomechanics, abnormal throwing motion.
   b. Joint mobilization.
   c. Continued therapeutic exercise including flexibility/endurance/coordination exercise.
   d. Postural reeducation.
   e. Biomechanical education.

3. **Functional restoration phase.**
   a. Maintain or return to optimum level of patient function.
   b. Normalize flexibility of joints and related soft tissues.
   c. Restore loading capacity of connective tissues to normal strength.
   d. Functional strengthening exercises.
   e. Functional stabilization of the involved joint/region.

Phases of Treatment for a Muscle/Tendon Injury

Acute Phase (Inflammatory Phase of Healing)

Patients in this phase often have pain at rest due to inflammation.

Treatment should consist of PRICE: Protection, rest, ice, compression and elevation.

Edema should be controlled because excessive edema can lead to reduced circulation, increased pain and increased fibrosis, which restricts movement.

Stretching the involved tissue is contraindicated due to the weakness of the newly formed tissue.

Pain-free AROM or gentle isometrics in a midrange position can help with circulation and prevent the negative effects of immobilization.

Massage can also help with circulation and prevent adhesions.

Subacute Phase (Repair Phase of Healing)

Patients in this phase should only have pain with activities that overstress the healing tissues.

Stretching to regain flexibility is most effective during this phase of treatment.

Progressive strengthening should be carefully monitored to prevent damage to the healing tissues.

Return-to-Function Phase (Remodeling Phase of Healing)

Patients should have no pain by this phase and should gradually return to previous activities.

Interventions for Patients/Clients with a Chronic Condition

1. **Determine possible causative factors.**
   a. Abnormal remodeling of injured tissues.
   b. Chronic low-grade inflammation due to repetitive stresses of tissues.

2. **Reduce stresses to tissues:**
   a. Identify/eliminate the magnitude of loading.
   b. Identify/eliminate direction of forces.
   c. Identify and eliminate any biomechanical barriers that are preventing healing: e.g., a leg length discrepancy.
   d. Educate patient regarding protection of joints and associated soft tissues.

3. **Regain structural integrity.**
   a. Improving flexibility.
   b. Postural reeducation.

c. Increasing tissue's capacity to tolerate loading.
d. Functional strengthening/endurance/coordination exercises.

4. **Resume optimal patient function and prevention of reoccurrence.**
   a. Patient education regarding causative factors in dysfunction.
   b. Work conditioning.

Specific Interventions

1. **Soft tissue/myofascial techniques.**
   a. These techniques aid in reduction of metabolites from muscle, reactivating a muscle which has not been functioning secondary to guarding and ischemia, revascularization of muscle and decrease guarding in a muscle.
   b. Autonomic: stimulation of skin and superficial fascia to facilitate a decrease in muscle tension.
   c. Mechanical: movement of skin, fascia and muscle causes histological and mechanical changes to occur in soft tissues to produce improved mobility and function. Examples include acupressure and osteopathic mechanical stretching techniques.
   d. Goals: decrease pain, edema and muscle spasm, increase metabolism and cutaneous temperature, stretch tight muscles and other soft tissues, improve circulation, strengthen weak muscles and mobilize joint restrictions.
   e. Indications: patients with soft tissue and joint restriction that results in pain and limits ADL.
   f. Contraindications:
      (1) Absolute: soft tissue breakdown, infection, cellulitis, inflammation and/or neo-plasm.
      (2) Relative: hypermobility and sensitivity.
   g. Traditional massage techniques such as effleurage and petrissage.
   h. Functional massage:
      (1) Three techniques used to assist in reactivation of a debilitated muscle and/or to increase vascularity to a muscle.
      (a) Soft tissue without motion.
         • Traditional technique; however, hands do not slide over skin. Instead they stay in contact with skin while hands and skin move together over the muscle.
         • Direction of force is parallel to muscle fibers and total stroke time should be 5–7 seconds.
      (b) Soft tissue with passive pumping.
         • Place muscle in shortened position and with one hand place tension on muscle parallel to muscle fibers.
         • Other hand passively lengthens muscle and simultaneously gradually releases tension of hand in contact with muscle.
      (c) Soft tissue with active pumping.
         • Place muscle in lengthened position and with one hand place tension on muscle perpendicular to muscle fibers.
         • Other hand guides limb as patient actively shortens muscle. Simultaneously as muscle shortens, gradually release tension of hand in contact with muscle.
   i. Transverse friction massage.
      (1) Used to initiate an acute inflammatory response for a tissue that is in metabolic stasis such as a tendonosis.
      (2) Involved tendon is briskly massaged in a transverse fashion (perpendicular to the direction of the fibers).
      (3) Performed for 5–10 minutes and tends to be very uncomfortable for the patient.
   j. Movement approaches require the patient to actively participate in treatment. Examples include:
      (1) Feldenkrais:
         (a) Facilitates development of normal movement patterns.
         (b) The practitioner uses skillful, supportive, gentle hands to create a sense of safety, maintain supportive contact, while introducing new movement possibilities in small, easily available increments.
      (2) Muscle energy techniques.
         (a) Include voluntary contraction in a precisely controlled direction, at varying levels of intensity, against an applied counterforce from the clinician.
         (b) Purpose is to gain motion that is limited by restrictions of the neuromuscular system.
         (c) Modification of proprioceptive neuromuscular facilitation (PNF) technique.
      (3) PNF hold-relax-contract technique.
         (a) Antagonist of the shortened muscle is contracted to achieve reciprocal inhibition and increased range.
         (b) Refer to Chapter 3.

2. **Articulatory techniques.**
   a. Joint oscillation.
      (1) Inhibits pain and/or muscle guarding.
      (2) Lubricates joint surfaces.
      (3) Provides nutrition to the joint structures.
      (4) It is suggested by Maitland that grades III and IV oscillations are beneficial to stretch tight connective tissues.
      (5) Grades of movement as described by Maitland (see Figure 2-1).
         (a) Five grades of joint play in neutral:
            • Grade I oscillations are small amplitude at the beginning of the range of joint play.
            • Grade II oscillations are large amplitude at the midrange of joint play.

- Grade III oscillations are large amplitude at the end range of joint play.
- Grade IV oscillations are small amplitude at the end range of joint play.
- Grade V is a manipulation of high velocity and low amplitude to the anatomical endpoint of a joint. Technically this is not an oscillation since it is a single movement rather than a repetitive movement.

(b) Indications for use of oscillation grades per Maitland:
- Grades I and II used to improve joint lubrication/nutrition as well as decrease pain and muscle guarding.
- Grades III and IV used to stretch tight muscles, capsules and ligaments.
- Grade V used to regain normal joint mechanics as well as decrease pain and muscle guarding.

(6) Contraindications:
(a) Absolute: joint ankylosis, malignancy involving bone, diseases that affect the integrity of ligaments (RA and Down syndrome), arterial insufficiency and active inflammatory and/or infective process.
(b) Relative: arthrosis (DJD), metabolic bone disease (osteoporosis, Paget's disease and tuberculosis), hypermobility, total joint replacement, pregnancy, spondylolisthesis, use of steroids and radicular symptoms.

b. Joint mobilization.
(1) To stretch/lengthen/deform collagen to normalize arthrokinematic glide of joint structures.
(2) Grades of translatoric glide as described by Kaltenborn (see Figure 2-2).
(a) Grade I:
- "Loosening" translatoric glide.
- Movement is a very small amplitude traction force.
- Used to relieve pain and/or decompress a joint during joint glides performed within examination or intervention.
(b) Grade II:
- "Tightening" translatoric glide.
- Movement takes up slack in tissues surrounding joint.
- Used to alleviate pain, assess joint play and/or reduce muscle guarding.
(c) Grade III:
- "Stretching" translatoric glide.
- Movement stretches the tissues crossing joint.
- Used to assess end feel or to increase movement (stretch tissue).
(3) Traction: manual, mechanical and self-or auto-traction.
(a) Vertebral bodies separating.
(b) Distraction and gliding of facet joints.

(c) Tensing of the ligamentous structures of the spinal segment.
(d) Intervertebral foramen widening.
(e) Spinal muscles stretching.
(4) Contraindications:
(a) Absolute: joint ankylosis, malignancy involving bone, diseases that affect the integrity of ligaments (RA and Down's syndrome), arterial insufficiency and active inflammatory and/or infective process.
(b) Relative: arthrosis (DJD), metabolic bone disease (osteoporosis, Paget's disease and tuberculosis), hypermobility, total joint replacement, pregnancy, spondylolisthesis, use of steroids and radicular symptoms.

c. Manipulation.
(1) Inhibit pain and/or muscle guarding.
(2) Improve translatoric glide in cases of joint dysfunction due to restriction.
(3) Healthcare practitioners who commonly perform manipulative thrusts include physical therapists, osteopaths, chiropractors, and medical doctors.
(4) Types of manipulations:
(a) Generalized.
- Fairly forceful long-lever techniques that are intended to include as many vertebral segments as possible.
- More commonly performed by chiropractic practitioners.
(b) Specific.
- Aimed at having an effect on either a specific segment or only a few vertebral segments.
- Uses minimal force with short-lever arms.
- Often includes "locking" techniques based on biomechanics to ensure that a specific vertebral segment receives the manipulative thrust.
- More commonly performed by physical therapists.
(c) Midrange.
- Very gentle, short-lever arm techniques.
- Barrier is created in midrange by specific positioning of patient as well as creating tautness in surrounding soft tissues.
- More commonly performed by osteopathic practitioners.
(5) Contraindications:
(a) Absolute: joint ankylosis, malignancy involving bone, diseases that affect the integrity of ligaments (RA and Down's syndrome), arterial insufficiency and active inflammatory and/or infective process.
(b) Relative: arthrosis (DJD), metabolic bone disease (osteoporosis, Paget's disease and tuberculosis), hypermobility, total joint replacement, pregnancy, spondylolisthesis, use of steroids and radicular symptoms.

3. **Neural tissue mobilization.**
   a. Movement of neural structures to regain normal mobility.
   b. Tension tests for upper and lower extremities (i.e., dural stretch test).
      (1) Movement of soft tissues that may be restricting neural structures (e.g., crossfriction massage for adhesions of the radial nerve to the humerus at a fracture site).
      (2) Indications: used for patients who have some type of restriction in neural mobility anywhere along the course of the nerve.
      (3) Postural reeducation: to open up the intervertebral foramen and decrease tension to tissues.
      (4) Contraindications: extreme pain and/or increase in abnormal neurological signs.

4. **Therapeutic exercise for musculoskeletal conditions.**
   a. Therapeutic exercise is indicated for the following reasons.
      (1) Decrease muscle guarding.
      (2) Decrease pain.
      (3) Increase vascularity of tissue.
      (4) Promote regeneration and/or speed up recovery of connective tissues such as cartilage, tendons, ligaments, capsules, intervertebral discs.
      (5) Mobilize restricted tissue to increase flexibility.
      (6) Increase endurance of muscle.
      (7) Increase coordination of muscle.
      (8) Increase strength of muscle.
      (9) Sensitize muscles to minimize joints going into excessive range in cases of hypermobility.
      (10) Develop dynamic stability and functional movement patterns allowing for optimal function within the environment.
   b. Home exercise program for patients/clients with musculoskeletal conditions.
      (1) Patient's home program will consist of exercises to reinforce clinical program.
      (2) Necessary to perform enough repetitions to have the desired physiological effect on appropriate tissues as well as develop coordination and endurance to promote dynamic stability within functional patterns.
   c. Refer to Chapter 10 for more details.

Manual Therapy Approaches in Rehabilitation

1. **All approaches provide a philosophical basis, subjective evaluation, objective examination, a diagnosis and a plan of care.**

2. **Approaches can be divided into two categories:**
   a. Physician-generated.
      (1) Mennell, who believed the joint is the dysfunctional unit.
      (2) Osteopaths suggest any component of the somatic system is responsible for dysfunction.
      (3) Cyriax, who contends that dysfunction is due to interplay between contractile and noncontractile tissues.
   b. Physical therapist-generated.
      (1) McKenzie, who feels that postural factors precipitate discal dysfunction. Treatment emphasizes the use of extension exercises.
      (2) Maitland, who proposes that the subjective evaluation should be integrated with objective measures in determining the dysfunctional area.
      (3) Kaltenborn, who believes that abnormal joint mobility and soft tissue changes account for dysfunction.
   c. Chiropractic-generated.
      (1) Focus is to restore normal joint function through soft tissue and joint manipulation. Chiropractors believe that restoration of normal biomechanical function affects other systems of the body as well, thus improving the patient's state of health in many ways.

Relevant Pharmacology

1. **NSAIDs.**
   a. Most commonly prescribed medication for pain relief for musculoskeletal dysfunction.
   b. Examples include: ibuprofen (Motrin), naproxen sodium (Aleve), salsalate (Discalced) and indomethacin (Indocin).
   c. Provide analgesic, anti-inflammatory and antipyretic capabilities.
   d. Adverse side effects could include gastrointestinal irritation, fluid retention, renal or liver problems and prolonged bleeding.
   e. COX-2 inhibitors have decreased gastrointestinal irritation, but rofecoxib (Vioxx) was withdrawn from the market secondary to its relationship with heart-related conditions. Other COX-2 inhibitors such as colecoxib (Celebrex) and valdecoxib (Bextra) are being evaluated for their safety and possible association with heart-related conditions.

2. **Muscle relaxants.**
   a. Commonly prescribed for skeletal muscle spasm.
   b. Examples include: cyclobenzaprine HCl (Flexeril), methocarbamol (Robaxin) and carisoprodol (Soma).
   c. Act on the central nervous system to reduce skeletal muscle tone by depressing the internuncial neurons of the brain stem and spinal cord.
   d. Adverse side effects could include drowsiness, lethargy, ataxia and decreased alertness.

3. **Nonnarcotic analgesics.**
   a. Prescribed when NSAIDs are contraindicated.
   b. Examples include acetaminophen (Tylenol).

c. Act on the central nervous system to alter response to pain and have antipyretic capabilities.

d. Adverse side effects are negligible when taken in recommended doses. Excessive amounts of acetaminophen may lead to liver disease or acute liver shutdown.

Psychosocial Considerations

1. **Malingering (symptom magnification syndrome).**
   a. Defined as a behavioral response where displays of symptoms control the life of the patient, leading to functional disability.
   b. There may be psychological advantages to illness:
      (1) The patient may feel protected from the threatening world.
      (2) Uncertainty or fear about the future.
      (3) Social gain.
      (4) Reduces stressors.
   c. Therapist needs to recognize symptoms and respond to the patient.
      (1) Tests to evaluate malingering back pain may include the Hoover's and Burn's tests and Waddell's signs.

(a) Hoover's test involves the therapist's evaluation of the amount of pressure the patient's heels place on the therapist's hands when the patient is asked to raise one lower extremity while in a supine position.

(b) Burn's test requires the patient to kneel and bend over a chair to touch the floor.

(c) Waddell's signs evaluate tenderness, simulation tests, distraction tests, regional disturbances and overreaction. Waddell's scores can be predictive of functional outcome.

(2) Functional capacity evaluations are used to evaluate psychosocial as well as physical components of disability.

(3) Emphasize regaining functional outcomes, not pain reduction.

2. **Secondary gain.**
   a. Usually some type of financial gain for staying ill.
      (1) Worker's compensation.
      (2) Larger settlement for injury claims.
   b. Frequently seen in clinics that manage industrial injuries.
   c. May not want to return to work for various reasons associated with the work environment; e.g., stress, dislike of coworkers.

3

Neuromuscular Physical Therapy

TIFFANY BOHM

Focus Areas for Content Review:

- Anatomy and physiology of the neuromuscular system.
- Pathologies and injuries of the neuromuscular system commonly seen in physical therapy.
- Physical therapy interventions; indications and contraindications, appropriate responses, PTA response to adverse reaction, effects of interventions on the musculoskeletal system.

- Tests and measures indicating patient ability to participate in and/or indication to discontinue intervention as well as to document the patient's progress toward the established goals.
- Principals of progression of intervention activities as related to neuromuscular conditions commonly encountered in physical therapy.

Anatomy and Physiology of the Neuromuscular System

Organization of the Nervous System

1. **Central nervous system (CNS).**
   a. Brain.
   b. Spinal cord.

2. **Peripheral nervous system (PNS).**
   a. Afferent system: conveys information from sensory receptors to the CNS.
   b. Efferent system: conveys information from the CNS to muscles and glands.
      (1) Somatic nervous system: conveys information to skeletal muscles.
      (2) Autonomic nervous system (ANS): conveys information to smooth muscle, cardiac muscle, and glands.

3. **Sympathetic division.**
   a. Stress responses.
   b. Prepares body for "fight or flight" and emergency responses.
      (1) Raises heart rate and blood pressure.
      (2) Constricts peripheral blood vessels and redistributes blood to organs.
      (3) Inhibits peristalsis.

4. **Parasympathetic division.**
   a. Relaxation responses.

   b. Conserves and restores homeostasis.
      (1) Slows heart rate and reduces blood pressure.
      (2) Increases peristalsis and glandular activity.

Structural Components

1. **Neuron.**
   a. Individual nerve cell that is responsible for conduction of impulses.
   b. Parts.
      (1) Soma (cell body).
      (2) Dendrites: provide large surface area to receive information.
      (3) Axons: conduct impulses away from the cell body, sometimes long distances.

2. **Neuroglia.**
   a. Support and protect neurons but do not transmit signals.
   b. Includes astrocytes, oligodendrocytes, Schwann's cells, microglia.

Grouping of Neural Tissue

1. **Nerve: grouping of neurons outside the CNS.**

2. **Tract: grouping of neurons inside the CNS.**

3. Ganglia: grouping of neuron cell bodies outside the CNS.

4. White matter: myelinated axons from many neurons.

5. Gray matter: cell bodies and dendrites and/or unmyelinated axons.

6. Upper motor neuron: brain and spinal cord.

7. Lower motor neuron: peripheral nerve.

Physiology

1. Terminology.
   a. Resting potential: difference in electrical potential across the cell membrane when information is not being transmitted.
      (1) Positive ion charge outside the membrane and negative ion charge inside the membrane that is maintained by sodiumpotassium pumps.
   b. Depolarization: potential becomes less negative than the resting potential via potassium rushing into the cell.
      (1) Generates an action potential or nerve impulse that travels along the neuron.
   c. Saltatory conduction.
      (1) Nerve impulse jumps between spaces in the myelin sheath known as nodes of Ranvier.
      (2) Increases speed of impulse conduction.
   d. Synapse.
      (1) Location of signal transmission between the presynaptic cell axon and postsynaptic cell dendrite or effector organ.
      (2) Determines which chemical or electrical signals are released and transferred.
   e. Neurotransmitters.
      (1) Chemical messengers released by the presynaptic membrane.
      (2) Bind to receptors on the postsynaptic membrane to cause excitation or inhibition of the postsynaptic membrane.
   f. Neuromodulators.
      (1) Alter neural function by activating membrane channels or genes within the cell.
      (2) Effect occurs within seconds and can last from minutes to days.
   g. All-or-none principle.
      (1) If a stimulus is strong enough, it generates an action potential.
      (2) If it is not, an action potential will not occur.
      (3) No matter how strong the stimulus, the action potential is always the same as long as it is threshold level.
   h. Refractory periods.
      (1) Absolute refractory period: when the membrane is depolarized and it is not possible to create another action potential.
      (2) Relative refractory period: hyperpolarization period when a stronger than normal stimulus would be required to produce another action potential.
   i. Repolarization: restoration of the membrane to resting potential when potassium is pushed out of the cell.

2. Types of sensory axons.
   a. Ia and Ib.
      (1) Large and myelinated for fast conduction speed.
      (2) Carry proprioceptive information (muscle, tendon or ligament stretch).
   b. II and A-beta.
      (1) Medium size and myelinated for medium speed of conduction.
      (2) Carry fine touch information.
   c. A-delta and C.
      (1) Small with little or no myelination, therefore they transmit slowly.
      (2) Free nerve endings carrying temperature, coarse touch and nociception.

Brain

1. Brainstem.
   a. Midbrain.
      (1) Connects pons to diencephalon.
      (2) Contains ascending and descending tracts.
      (3) Contains oculomotor and trochlear cranial nerve nuclei.
      (4) Contains relay stations for visual and auditory reflexes.
      (5) Substantia nigra.
         (a) Large motor nucleus connecting with the basal ganglia and cortex.
         (b) Important in motor control and muscle tone.
   b. Pons.
      (1) Connects the medulla oblongata to the midbrain.
      (2) Allows passage of ascending and descending tracts.
      (3) Contains nuclei for trigeminal, abducens, facial and vestibulocochlear cranial nerves and nuclei for regulation of respiration.
   c. Medulla oblongata.
      (1) Connects spinal cord with the pons.
      (2) Contains all ascending and descending tracks.
      (3) Contains glossopharyngeal, vagus, spinal accessory and hypoglossal cranial nerve nuclei.
      (4) Contains important centers for vital sign functioning: cardiac, respiratory, vasomotor centers and reticular formation (maintenance of consciousness and arousal).

---

*Substantia nigra and subthalamic nuclei function closely with basal ganglia and are often considered part of the basal ganglia.
*Regulation of posture and muscle tone.

2. **Diencephalon.**
   a. Thalamus.
      (1) Group of nuclei deep within the cerebrum.
      (2) Receives all sensory stimuli except olfactory.
      (3) Interprets crude sensory information.
   b. Hypothalamus.
      (1) Primary role is homeostasis.
      (2) Regulates body temperature, sugar and fat metabolism and water balance.
      (3) Primitive drives for eating, sexual behavior, rage, aggression, emotion, thirst, hunger and sleep/wake cycles.

3. **Cerebrum.**
   a. General information.
      (1) Constitutes the bulk of the brain.
      (2) Convolutions of gray matter:
         (a) Composed of unmyelinated axons with gyri and sulci.
         (b) Separates lobes.
            • Lateral central fissure: separates temporal lobe from frontal and parietal lobes.
            • Longitudinal cerebral fissure: separates the two hemispheres.
            • Central sulcus: separates frontal lobe from the parietal lobe.
      (3) White matter: myelinated axons.
         (a) Fibers connect the hemispheres and regions of the brain, allow for communication between the structures.
      (4) Deeper structures.
         (a) Basal ganglia: caudate, putamen and globus pallidus.
         (b) Portions of limbic system.
            • Housed within cerebrum and diencephalon.
            • Associated with feeding, aggression, emotions and endocrine aspects of sexual response.
   b. Lobes (Table 3-1).
      (1) Primary cortices: receive incoming messages.
      (2) Association areas: link various parts of the cortex and integrate and interpret information.

4. **Cerebellum.**
   a. Located behind the pons and medulla in the posterior fossa.
   b. Functions.
      (1) Equilibrium.
      (2) Regulation of muscle tone.
      (3) Maintenance of posture and voluntary movement control.
      (4) Coordinates smooth voluntary movements.
      (5) Motor learning.
      (6) Sequencing of movements.

5. **Cranial nerves (Table 3-2).**

Table 3-1 ➤ LOBES OF CEREBRUM

LOBE	PRIMARY FUNCTIONS
Frontal	• Primary motor cortex (precentral gyrus): responsible for voluntary movements on contralateral side of the body • Broca's area: motor components of speech • Cognition, judgment, attention, abstract thinking and emotional control
Parietal	• Primary sensory cortex (postcentral gyrus): integrates sensation from contralateral side of body • Short-term memory • Perception of touch, proprioception, pain and temperature sensations
Temporal	• Primary auditory cortex: receives auditory information • Associative auditory cortex: processing of auditory information • Wernicke's area: comprehension of spoken word • Long-term memory • Visual perception
Occipital	• Primary visual cortex: receives visual information • Visual association cortex: processes visual information and applies meaning

Table 3-2 ➤ CRANIAL NERVES

NUMBER	NAME	SENSORY/MOTOR	FUNCTION
I	Olfactory	Sensory	Smell
II	Optic	Sensory	Visual acuity
III	Oculomotor	Motor	Turns eye up, down and in
IV	Trochlear	Motor	Turns adducted eye down
V	Trigeminal	Sensory	Facial sensation
		Motor	Muscles of mastication (temporalis and masseter)
VI	Abducens	Motor	Turns eye out
VII	Facial	Sensory	Taste on anterior two/thirds of tongue
		Motor	Facial expressions
VIII	Vestibulocochlear	Sensory	Vestibular: vestibular ocular reflex (VOR); balance
			Cochlear: hearing acuity
IX	Glossopharyngeal	Sensory	Taste on posterior one-third of tongue
		Motor	Gag reflex; pharynx control: soft palate rising with "ah" sound
X	Vagus	Sensory	Autonomic nervous system functions
		Motor	Gag reflex; pharynx control: soft palate rising with "ah" sound
XI	Spinal Accessory	Motor	Trapezius muscle: elevation of shoulders Sternocleidomastoid muscle: turning head to side
XII	Hypoglossal	Motor	Tongue movements

6. Blood supply.

a. Anterior system.

(1) Supplies the frontal, parietal and parts of temporal lobe.

(2) Aortic arch common carotid artery bifurcates to form internal and external carotid arteries; internal carotid enters cranium, bifurcates to form anterior and middle cerebral arteries.

b. Posterior system.

(1) Supplies brainstem, cerebellum, medial temporal lobe and occipital lobes.

(2) Subclavian artery vertebral arteries unite to form basilar artery, bifurcates to form posterior cerebral arteries.

c. Circle of Willis: anterior and posterior systems connect at the base of the brain to ensure adequate circulation to the brain.

7. Support structures.

a. Skull: rigid, bony chamber with an opening (foramen magnum) at its base.

b. Meninges: three membranes surrounding the brain.

(1) Dura mater: dense and fibrous outermost layer.

(2) Arachnoid layer: delicate, vascular middle layer.

(3) Pia mater: thin, vascular inner membrane covering the brain surface.

c. Cerebrospinal fluid.

(1) Protects the brain and aids in the exchange of nutrients and waste products.

(2) Produced in the choroid plexuses in the ventricles.

(3) Circulates within the subarachnoid space, ventricles and central canal of the spinal cord.

d. Blood-brain barrier: protective structure that selects what can and cannot enter the CNS.

Application Concepts

- Medulla oblongata: contains centers for vital sign functioning of the cardiac, respiratory and vasomotor centers. It is responsible for the maintenance of consciousness and arousal.
- Hypothalamus: critical for maintaining homeostasis. Controls primitive drives including those related to rage, aggression, emotion, thirst and hunger, as well as the sleep/wake cycle.
- Basal ganglia: regulates posture and muscle tone.
- Cerebellum: regulates maintenance of posture and voluntary movement control.

Spinal Cord

1. Begins as continuation of medulla oblongata and extends from foramen magnum to inferior border of L1 in conus medullaris to convey information to/from the brain and periphery.

2. Protection and coverings.

a. Vertebral canal: bony structure formed by the vertebral foramina that houses the spinal cord and cauda equina.

b. Meninges: continuous with the meninges of the brain.

3. Spinal cord cross-section.

a. Gray matter and white matter.

b. Divided into regions.

(1) Anterior/ventral regions carry motor information.

(2) Posterior/dorsal regions carry sensory information.

4. Spinal nerves.

a. Divided into 30 segments:

(1) Eight cervical, 12 thoracic, 5 lumbar, 5 sacral and a few coccygeal segments.

(2) Cauda equina: nerves arising from the distal tip of the spinal cord.

(3) Refer to musculoskeletal chapter 10 for myotome and dermatome distributions.

b. Dorsal and ventral roots branch off spinal cord and combine to form spinal nerve.

(1) Dorsal roots carry sensory information.

(2) Ventral roots carry motor information.

c. Spinal nerve splits into dorsal (posterior) and ventral (anterior) rami.

(1) Dorsal rami innervate the deep muscles and skin of the back.

(2) Ventral rami innervate the superficial back, lateral and anterior trunk and extremity muscles.

d. Plexuses.

(1) Network of adjoining nerves formed by ventral rami in the cervical and lumbosacral region.

(2) Brachial plexus (C5-T1) innervates the upper extremity and some cervical muscles.

(3) Lumbosacral plexus (T12-S2) innervates the lower extremity muscles.

5. Spinal reflexes.

a. Involuntary responses to stimuli.

b. Monosynaptic or stretch reflex.

(1) Stimulus: muscle stretch.

(2) Reflex arc: afferent Ia from muscle spindle to alpha motoneuron and back to muscle of origin.

(3) Aids with maintenance of muscle tone.

(a) Autogenic facilitation: contraction of the agonist.

(b) Reciprocal inhibition: inhibition of antagonist muscle.

c. Polysynaptic or inverse stretch reflex.

(1) Stimulus: muscle contraction.

(2) Reflex arc: afferent Ib from Golgi's tendon organ via inhibitory interneuron to muscle of origin.

(3) Functions for agonist inhibition and stretch-protection reflex.

Application Concepts

- Many neurological medications act as agonists or antagonists to either mimic or block the action of neurotransmitters and neuromodulators.
- Since the ability to maintain a stable internal environment (homeostasis) is controlled by the hypothalamus, damage to this area may cause problems with temperature, water and behavioral regulation.
- While no two insults are identical, each area of the brain has a specific function and, therefore, a patient with damage to a given area will likely follow the general guidelines of predicted dysfunction and ensuing functional return that can be expected.
- Cranial nerve nuclei are located in the brainstem. Subsequently, damage to the brainstem can lead to a variety of cranial nerve dysfunctions.

Physical Therapy Examination and Data Collection

Physical Therapist Assistant's Role and Responsibilities

1. Demonstrate competence in performing specific data collection techniques as delegated by the supervising PT.

2. Perform a thorough review of the patient's medical record after the patient history and systems review have been performed by the PT.

3. Use information from the data collection process to progress patient interventions within the plan of care established by the PT.

4. Differentiate appropriate and adverse changes that need to be reported to the physical therapist and other members of the health care team.

Application Concept

- Failure to review the medical chart for daily updates or identify subtle changes in the patient's current status can potentially lead to the PTA treating a patient with newly developed contraindications.

Patient History and Medical Record Review

1. The PT is responsible for the history and medical review; performed at initial evaluation.

2. Present symptoms, past medical history and psychosocial history, including current living situation and family/social support.

3. Diagnostic procedures completed.
   a. Cerebral angiography: shows areas of increased and decreased vascularity.
   b. Computed tomography (CT): shows presence of abnormal changes in tissue density.
   c. Magnetic resonance imaging (MRI): identifies tumors, demyelination and vascular abnormalities.
   d. Electroencephalography (EEG): records ongoing electrical activity of the brain, commonly used when assessing seizures.

Resting Posture

1. Performed at initial evaluation by PT, ongoing by PT and PTA to determine progress.

2. Observe in all functional positions.

3. Observe for typical patterns of spasticity following CNS insult (Table 3-3).

Level of Consciousness

1. Performed at initial evaluation by PT, ongoing by PT and PTA to determine progress.

2. Orientation to person, place and time (oriented ×3).

3. Response to stimuli.
   a. Purposeful, nonpurposeful, no response.
   b. Verbal, tactile, painful stimuli, simple commands.

4. Level of arousal.
   a. Alert: responds fully and appropriately to stimuli and examiner.
   b. Lethargic: appears drowsy; can respond to questions but falls asleep easily.
   c. Obtunded: responds slowly and is confused; decreased interest in environment.
   d. Stupor: only aroused from sleep with painful stimuli; minimal awareness of self and environment.
   e. Coma: cannot be aroused and no response to external stimuli or environment.

Table 3-3 ➤ TYPICAL PATTERNS OF SPASTICITY IN UPPER MOTOR NEURON SYNDROME

UPPER LIMBS	ACTIONS	MUSCLES AFFECTED
Scapula	Retraction, downward rotation	Rhomboids
Shoulder	Adduction and internal rotation, depression	Pectoralis major, latissimus dorsi, teres major, subscapularis
Elbow	Flexion	Biceps, Brachialis, Brachioradialis
Forearm	Pronation	Pronator teres, Pronator quadratus
Wrist	Flexion, adduction	F. carpi radialis
Hand	Finger flexion, clenched fist	F. dig. profundus/sublimis, Add. pollicis brevis, F. pollicis brevis
	Thumb adducted in palm	

LOWER LIMBS	ACTIONS	MUSCLES AFFECTED
Pelvis	Retraction (hip hiking)	Quadratus lumborum
Hip	Adduction (scissoring)	Add. longus/brevis
	Internal rotation	Add. magnus, gracilis
	Extension	Gluteus maximus
Knee	Extension	Quadriceps
Foot & ankle	Plantar flexion	Gastrocsoleus
	Inversion	Tibialis posterior
	Equinovarus	
	Toes claw	
	(MP ext., PIP flex, DIP ext.)	Long toe flexors
	Toes curl	Ext. hallucis longus
	(PIP, DIP flex)	Peroneus longus
Hip & knee	Flexion	Iliopsoas
(prolonged sitting posture)		Rectus femoris, pectineus
	Sacral sitting	Hamstrings
Trunk	Lateral flexion with concavity rotation	Rotators
		Internal/external obliques
COG forward	Excessive forward flexion	Rectus abdominis, external obliques
(prolonged sitting posture)	Forward head	Psoas minor

The form and intensity of spasticity may vary greatly, depending upon the CNS lesion site and extent of damage. The degree of spasticity can fluctuate within each individual (i.e., due to body position, level of excitation, sensory stimulation, and voluntary effort). Spasticity predominates in antigravity muscles (i.e., the flexors of the upper extremity and the extensors of the lower extremity). If left untreated, spasticity can result in movement deficiencies, subsequent contractures, degenerative joint changes, and deformity.
Adapted from Mayer NH, Esquenazi A, Childers MK. Common patterns of clinical motor dysfunction. Muscle and Nerve 6:S21, 1997.

5. Glasgow Coma Scale.
   a. Consciousness is related to degree of eye opening, motor response and verbal response.
   b. Score ranges from 3 to 15.
      (1) Mild brain injury = score of 13 to 15.
      (2) Moderate brain injury = score of 9 to 12.
      (3) Severe brain injury (coma) = score ≤8.

Arousal, Mentation and Cognition

1. Information used by PTA to correctly modify educational approach used during intervention.

2. Attention.
   a. Length of attention span.
   b. Sustained attention: ability to attend to task without redirection.
   c. Divided attention: ability to shift attention from one task to another.
   d. Focused attention: ability to stay on task in the presence of detractors.
   e. Ability to follow single and multistep commands.

3. Memory.
   a. Immediate recall: recall of items after a brief interval (5 minutes).
   b. Short-term recall: recall of recent events. (What did you have for breakfast?).
   c. Long-term recall: remote recall of past events. (Where were you born?).

4. Emotional responses/behaviors.
   a. Safety, judgment: impulsivity and lack of inhibition.
   b. Affect, mood: irritability, agitation, depression and withdrawal.

   c. Egocentricity.

   d. Insight into disability.

   e. Ability to follow rules of social conduct.

   ⚑ Red Flag

     • A patient with impulsivity, lack of behavioral inhibition and/or poor insight into his/her disability can be a safety concern to those around him/her as well as him/ herself.

5. Higher level cognitive abilities.

   a. Judgment, problem solving.

   b. Abstract reasoning.

   c. Ability to learn new information and generalize learning to new situations.

   d. Ability to order components of cognitive or functional task.

6. Mini-mental status examination (MMSE).

   a. Brief screening test for cognitive dysfunction.

   b. Maximum score of 30.

     (1) Mild cognitive impairment: 21–24.

     (2) Moderate cognitive impairment: 16–20.

     (3) Severe mental impairment: ≤15.

Aerobic Capacity and Endurance

1. Performed by PT and PTA prior to, during and immediately following intervention.

2. Vital signs at rest, during and after activity: HR, RR, BP.

⚑ Red Flag

   • Failure to assess vital signs for an accurate baseline can lead to an emergency situation with patients demonstrating unstable cardiopulmonary functioning.

3. Autonomic nervous system responses indicating stress.

   a. Wide pupillary reactions.

   b. Hyper alertness.

   c. Increases in heart rate, pulse rate and/or respiratory rate.

   d. Nausea.

   e. Diaphoresis.

   f. Perceived exertion, dyspnea or angina. See RPE scale Chapter 4, Box 4–1.

4. Observe for signs of postural hypotension/ orthostatic hypotension.

   a. Blood pressure drops with change from supine to sitting position.

   b. Decrease of systolic blood pressure >20 mm Hg or diastolic blood pressure >10 mm Hg.

   c. Lightheadedness, syncope, mental confusion, weakness.

   ⚑ Red Flag

     • Orthostatic hypotension must be identified immediately and the patient carefully monitored as he/she is at an increased risk of syncope and falls.

Sensory Testing (Table 3-4)

1. Performed at initial evaluation by PT, ongoing by PT and PTA to determine progress.

2. Testing considerations.

   a. Ensure patient comprehends instructions and can communicate responses.

   b. Occlude vision.

   c. Apply stimulus in random, unpredictable order to avoid summation.

   d. Always pose a choice. (Hot or cold?).

   e. Check for objective manifestations: withdrawal, blinking or wincing.

   f. Document location of deficits by utilizing dermatome chart (Figure 3-1).

3. Exteroceptive (superficial) sensations.

   a. Sharp/dull discrimination.

   b. Temperature.

   c. Light touch.

4. Proprioceptive (deep) sensations.

   a. Movement sense (kinesthesia).

   b. Joint position sense.

   c. Vibration sense.

5. Combined (cortical) sensations.

   a. Stereognosis.

   b. Two-point discrimination.

   c. Texture recognition.

   d. Tactile localization.

   e. Graphesthesia.

   f. Barognosis.

Perceptual Dysfunction

1. Information used by PTA to correctly modify educational approach used during intervention.

2. Basic information.

   a. Suspect perceptual dysfunction if patient has difficulty with functional mobility skills or activities of daily living for reasons that cannot be accounted for by specific sensory, motor or comprehension deficits.

   b. Language impairments, hearing loss or visual disturbance can be masked as perceptual dysfunction.

3. Homonymous hemianopsia.

   a. Loss of contralateral $1/2$ of the visual field in each eye.

   b. Results from a lesion in the optic tract.

   ⚑ Red Flag

     • The presence of homonymous hemianopsia is a safety concern for ambulatory patients as they are unable to fully visualize the environment and avoid potential dangers.

Table 3-4 ➤ SENSORY TESTING

Exteroceptive (superficial) sensations

TEST	TEST	NORMAL RESPONSE
Sharp/dull discrimination	• Alternate between sharp and dull points applied on the tested location.	• Identify touch as either sharp or dull.
Temperature	• Patient is given test tubes with either hot or cold water.	• Correctly identify the test tube as having hot or cold water.
Light touch	• Lightly touch the patient in the tested location with a cotton ball.	• Verbalize when the touch is felt.

Proprioceptive (deep) sensations

TEST	TEST	NORMAL RESPONSE
Kinesthesia	• Therapist moves the patient's limb in various directions.	• Identifies the direction of motion (up/down, bent/straight, etc)
Proprioception	• Therapist places the joint/limb in a position.	• Able to mimic or verbalize the position of the joint.
Vibration	• A tuning fork is applied to a bony prominence, vibrating or not.	• Identifies whether the tuning fork is vibrating or not.

Combined (cortical) sensations

TEST	TEST	NORMAL RESPONSE
Stereognosis	• Object is placed in the patient's hand	• Able to identify the object by touch only.
Two-point discrimination	• Using calipers, test whether patient feels one or two points.	• Given normal ranges, accurately identifies 1 or 2 points.
Texture recognition	• Patient is given objects with similar shape/size but of different textures.	• Able to identify the various textures (soft, hard, rough, etc)
Tactile localization	• Touch the patient in the tested location with a cotton ball or finger.	• Identifies when and where the touch occurs.
Graphesthesia	• Draw a letter in palm of patient's hand.	• Able to identify the letter.
Barognosis	• Place similar objects with varying weights in the patient's hand.	• Able to identify differences in weight.

4. **Body scheme/body image disorders.**
   a. Body scheme disorder (somatognosia): inability to identify body parts or their relationship to each other.
   b. Visual spatial neglect (unilateral neglect): ignores one side of the body and stimuli coming from that side.
   c. Right/left discrimination disorder: unable to identify right and left sides of the body.
   d. Anosognosia: severe denial, neglect or lack of awareness of dysfunction.
   ➤ **Red Flag**
   • Anosognosia presents a safety risk for the patient and those around him/her as he/she may not recognize the dangers and engage in activities unsafe for his/her functioning level.

5. **Spatial relations disorders.**
   a. Figure-ground discrimination disorder: inability to pick out an object from the background on which it rests.
   b. Form constancy disorder: inability to pick out an object from an array of similarly shaped objects.
   c. Spatial relations deficit: inability to properly place objects in relationship to one another.
   d. Position in space deficit: inability to determine up/down, in/out, under/over.

   e. Topographical disorientation: inability to navigate a familiar route on own.
   f. Depth/distance perception disorder: unable to accurately judge depth or distance.
   g. Vertical disorientation: unable to accurately determine what is upright.
   ➤ **Red Flag**
   • The presence of spatial relations disorders makes independent ambulation a safety concern without extensive practice and development of compensatory strategies.

6. **Agnosia.**
   a. Inability to recognize familiar objects with one sensory modality.
   b. Retains the ability to recognize the same object with other sensory modalities.

7. **Apraxia.**
   a. Inability to perform purposeful movements when there is no loss of sensation, strength, coordination or comprehension.
   b. Breakdown in ability to conceptualize and/or perform motor components of a task.
   c. Ideomotor apraxia: cannot perform the task on command but can do the task when left on own.

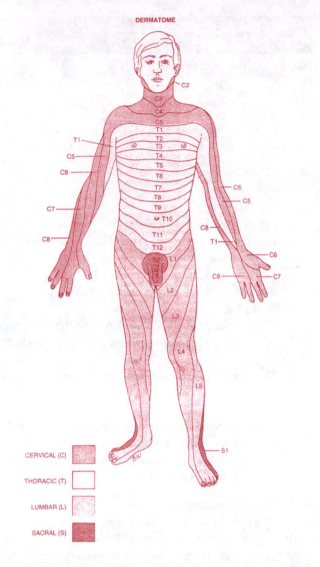

DERMATOME

CERVICAL (C)

THORACIC (T)

LUMBAR (L)

SACRAL (S)

Figure 3-1 • from IER's National PTA Examination Review & Study Guide 2008 edition by Karen E. Ryan

d. Ideational apraxia: cannot perform the task at all either on command or on own.

Motor Function

1. **Performed at initial evaluation by PT, ongoing by PT and PTA to determine progress.**

2. **Muscle tone.**
   a. Normal tone is necessary for skilled, coordinated, selective movement.
   b. Types of abnormalities (Table 3-5).
   c. Quantification of tone.
      (1) Modified Ashworth's scale for spasticity (Table 3-6).
         (a) No change in resistance with normal tone.
         (b) Faster movements will increase resistance if spasticity is present.

Table 3-5 ➤ MUSCLE TONE ABNORMALITIES

HYPERTONIA	
Spasticity	• Always an Upper Motor Neuron (UMN) lesion
Decorticate rigidity	• Always an UMN lesion • Sustained flexor posturing in the upper extremities • Sustained extensor posturing in the lower extremities • Diencephalon lesion • Sign of severe impairment
Decerebrate rigidity	• Always an UMN lesion • Sustained extensor posturing in the upper and lower extremities • Brainstem lesion • Sign of severe impairment
Rigidity	• Always an UMN lesion • Resistance to passive stretch in agonist and antagonist • Basal ganglia lesion
Cogwheel rigidity	• Ratchet-like response to quick passive movement; catches/releases/catches
Leadpipe rigidity	• Constant rigidity
HYPOTONIA	
Flaccidity	• LMN lesion • Cerebellar lesion • Following spinal or cerebral shock–resolves or changes to spasticity

(2) Assess reflex integrity.
   (a) Deep tendon reflexes (DTRs).
   (b) Superficial cutaneous.
   (c) Developmental reflexes.
d. Signs of hypertonia.
   (1) Increased resistance to passive range of motion.
      (a) Limb feels stiff, resistive to movement.
      (b) Increases further with increased velocity of quick stretch.
   (2) Clonus.
      (a) Maintained stretch stimulus or quick stimulus produces a cyclical, spasmodic contraction.
      (b) Common in plantarflexors, wrist flexors and jaw.
   (3) Hyperactive reflexes.
e. Signs of hypotonia.
   (1) Decreased or no resistance to passive range of motion.

Table 3-6 ➤ MODIFIED ASHWORTH SCALE

GRADE	DESCRIPTION
0	• No increased tone
1 or 1+	• Slight increase in tone
2	• Moderate increase in tone
3	• PROM is difficult
4	• Affected joints are non-moveable (ankylosed)

Table 3-7 ➤ DEEP TENDON REFLEXES COMMONLY TESTED

SITE	NERVE ROOT LEVEL
Biceps	C5-C6
Triceps	C7-C8
Brachioradialis	C5-C6
Hamstrings	L5-S3
Quadriceps	L2-L4
Achilles	S1-S2

Table 3-8 ➤ GRADING SCALE FOR MUSCLE STRETCH REFLEXES

GRADE	DESCRIPTION
0	Absent
1+	Hyporeflexia
2+	Normal
3+	Hyperreflexia
4+ and 5+	Increasingly abnormal hyperreflexia

(2) Hypoactive reflexes.
f. Influences on tone.
  (1) Increased patient effort.
  (2) Stress and anxiety.
  (3) Position of patient and influence of tonic reflexes.
  (4) Fever/infection increases tone.

3. **Reflex integrity. PT most likely to evaluate, PTA may or may not perform; however should understand impact on intervention.**
  a. Deep tendon reflexes (DTR) (Table 3-7).
    (1) Also called stretch reflex or monosynaptic stretch reflex.
    (2) Testing.
      (a) Position muscle in mid range.
      (b) Tap tendon with reflex hammer or tips of fingers.
      (c) Jendrassik's maneuver: patient hooks fingers together and isometrically attempts to pull them apart to increase sensitivity of DTR in lower extremities.
    (3) Grading (Table 3-8).

  b. Babinski.
    (1) Superficial cutaneous reflex.
    (2) Test: quick stroke to lateral border of the sole of the foot.
    (3) Normal response: flexion of 1st toe.
    (4) Abnormal response: extension of 1st toe.
  ⮑ **Red Flag**
    • Presence of a Babinski's reflex after 2 years of age is a sign of upper motor neuron dysfunction.
  c. Developmental reflexes and reactions: refer to Pediatrics chapter.
  ⮑ **Red Flag**
    • Persistent, absent or asymmetric reflexes usually indicate early brain damage and affect normal development and rehabilitation at any age (refer to Table 8-1 for normals).

4. **Muscle performance.**
  a. Strength, power and endurance.
  b. Upper motor neuron lesion (Table 3-9).
    (1) Results from damage to the brain or spinal cord.

Table 3-9 ➤ DIFFERENTIAL DIAGNOSIS: COMPARISON OF UPPER MOTOR NEURON (UMN) AND LOWER MOTOR NEURON (LMN) SYNDROMES

	UMN LESION	LMN LESION
Location of lesion	Central nervous system	Cranial nerve nuclei/nerves
Structures involved	Cortex, brainstem, corticospinal tracts, spinal cord	SC: anterior horn cell, spinal roots, peripheral nerve
Disorders	Stroke, traumatic brain injury, spinal cord injury	Polio, Guillain-Barré, PNI, peripheral neuropathy, radiculopathy
Tone	Increased: hypertonia	Decreased or absent: hypotonia, flaccidity
	Velocity dependent	Not velocity dependent
Reflexes	Increased: hyperreflexia, clonus	Decreased or absent: hyporeflexia
	Exaggerated cutaneous and autonomic reflexes: + Babinski	Cutaneous reflexes decreased or absent
Involuntary Movements	Muscle spasms: flexor or extensor	With denervation: fasciculations
Strength	Weakness or paralysis: ipsilateral (stroke) or bilateral (SCI)	Limited distribution: segmental or focal pattern
	Corticospinal: contralateral if above decussation in medulla;	Root-innervated pattern
	Ipsilateral if below	
	Distribution: never focal	
Muscles bulk	Variable, disuse atrophy	Neurogenic atrophy; rapid, focal, severe wasting
Voluntary Movements	Impaired or absent: dyssynergic patterns, obligatory synergies	Weak or absent if nerve interrupted

(2) Weakness.
  (a) May be present but masked by hypertonicity.
  (b) May be due to opposition from a spastic antagonist.
  (c) Resulting from disuse atrophy.
c. Lower motor neuron lesion (see Table 3-9).
  (1) Weakness and decreased muscle tone will be present in the involved muscles.
  (2) May develop disuse atrophy in the involved and uninvolved muscles.
d. Testing protocols.
  (1) Manual muscle testing.
    (a) Utilize traditional manual muscle testing when possible.
    (b) Make notations regarding alterations in test position/patient response.
  (2) Handheld dynamometry.
  (3) Isokinetic dynamometry.
  (4) Timed tests for power and endurance.

5. **Voluntary movement patterns.**
a. Coordinated movement requirements control of speed, distance, direction, rhythm, varying levels of muscle tension and trunk/proximal joint stability.
b. Common considerations associated with coordination impairments.
  (1) Abnormal synergy patterns (Table 3-10).
  (2) Associated reactions.
    (a) Ramiste's phenomenon: resisted hip abduction/adduction of uninvolved extremity causes the same reaction in the involved extremity.
    (b) Homolateral limb synkinesis: flexing involved UE causes flexion of involved LE.

  (3) Substitution patterns due to pain or muscle weakness.
  (4) Assess for signs of cerebellar dysfunction (Table 3-11).
  (5) Assess for signs of basal ganglia dysfunction (Table 3-12).
  ⌦ Red Flag
    • Presence of basal ganglia or cerebellar lesions can lead to decreased patient safety with balance activities and ambulation.
c. Specific testing guidelines.
  (1) Describe head, trunk and limb movement.
  (2) Movement control.
    (a) Are movements precise?

Table 3-10 ➤ ABNORMAL SYNERGIES

Synergy Patterns

	FLEXION SYNERGY	EXTENSION SYNERGY
Upper Extremity		
Scapula	Retraction & elevation	Protraction (pec minor)
Shoulder	Abduction & ER	Adduction & IR (subscapularis)
Elbow	Flexion	Extension
Forearm	Supination	Pronation
Wrist & finger	Flexion	Flexion
Lower Extremity		
Hip	Flexion, abduction & ER	Extension and adduction
Knee	Flexion	Extension
Ankle	DF & inversion	PF & inversion
Toe	DF	PF

Table 3-11 ➤ CEREBELLAR DYSFUNCTION SIGNS AND TESTS

TERM	DESCRIPTION	COMMON TEST
Ataxia	• General term used to describe uncoordinated movement, includes dysmetria, intention tremor	
Dysmetria	• Inability to accurately judge the distance to reach a goal or target • Hypermetria or hypometria	• Pointing, past pointing • Heel on shin
Hypotonia	• Low tone	• Passive movement • Deep tendon reflex testing
Dysdiadochokinesia	• Difficulty performing rapid alternating movements (RAM)	• Pronation/supination • Finger to nose • Knee flexion/extension
Movement decomposition	• Movements are performed in distinct segments instead of fluid motions	• AROM
Intention tremor	• Involuntary, oscillatory movement • Appears with voluntary movement, decreases/absent at rest	• Observation with movement
Postural tremor	• Appears while attempting to hold limb still or while holding trunk still during sitting or standing	• Observation with movement
Dysarthria	• Slurring of speech due to impaired motor control of speech structure	• Examined by the speech therapist

Table 3-12 ➤ BASAL GANGLIA DYSFUNCTION SIGNS

TERM	DESCRIPTION	COMMON TEST
Bradykinesia	• Poverty of movement	• Observation of functional tasks
Akinesia	• Without movement • Unable to initiate movement	• Observation of attempts at functional tasks
Rigidity	• Cogwheel • Leadpipe • Present at rest	• Passive movement
Resting tremor	• Disappears with voluntary movement	• Observation at rest
Chorea	• Involuntary, relatively quick twitches or "dancing" movements	• Observation at rest
Athetosis	• Involuntary, slow irregular, twisting, sinuous movements • Occur more in upper extremities	• Observation at rest

    (b) Can the patient make continuous and appropriate motor adjustments if speed and direction of movement are changed?

    (c) Does occluding vision alter performance?

  (3) Speed/rate control: does increasing the speed of performance affect quality of motor performance?

  (4) Steadiness: can a position be maintained without swaying, tremors or extra movements?

  (5) Fatigue: does the patient fatigue rapidly, and does the quality of movement change with onset of fatigue?

  (6) Reaction time: does movement occur in a reasonable amount of time?

   ⚑ **Red Flag**
     • Decreased reaction time should be identified and compensatory strategies outlined to prevent potential safety issues.

 d. Specific tests.

  (1) Active ROM testing for examining abnormal synergy patterns.

  (2) Nonequilibrium tests of coordination (Table 3-13).

  (3) Equilibrium tests of coordination (Table 3-14).

  (4) Scoring.

    (a) 0 (unable).

    (b) 1 (severe impairment).

    (c) 2 (moderate impairment).

    (d) 3 (minimal impairment).

    (e) 4 (normal performance).

Gait and Locomotion

1. Performed at initial evaluation by PT, ongoing by PT and PTA to determine progress.

2. Observation for normal/abnormal patterns, timing, speed of ambulation and wheelchair mobility.

 a. Indoor/outdoor surfaces.

 b. Level/uneven terrain.

 c. During functional activities such as opening/closing doors and on/off elevators.

⚑ **Red Flag**
  • Failure to assess and practice ambulation on a variety of surfaces and in all of the environments the patient will encounter does not adequately prepare the patient for safe ambulation upon discharge.

3. Common gait deviations associated with CNS insult.

 a. Cerebellar impairment.

  (1) Wide base of support.

  (2) Arms at high guard (raised and away from body).

  (3) Slow initiation of swing with forceful termination.

 b. Basal ganglia impairment.

  (1) Narrow base of support, decreased step length, shuffling gait.

  (2) Decreased arm swing and trunk rotation.

  (3) Festination: increased velocity propulsion.

  (4) Akinesia or dyskinesia: difficulty starting and stopping gait.

Balance

1. Performed at initial evaluation by PT, ongoing by PT and PTA to determine progress.

2. The control of relative position of body parts by skeletal muscles with respect to gravity and each other.

 a. Center of mass (COM): in anatomical position, it is located just anterior to S2.

 b. Base of support (BOS): body surface area in contact with the environmental surface.

 c. Limits of stability (LOS): perimeter of the base of support.

3. Systems contributing to balance.

 a. Visual system: visual acuity, depth perception and visual field deficits.

 b. Somatosensory: proprioception and cutaneous sensation (touch, pressure) of lower extremities and trunk, especially feet and ankles.

Table 3-13 ➤ NONEQUILIBRIUM COORDINATION TESTS

1. Finger to nose	The shoulder is abducted to 90 degrees with the elbow extended. The patient is asked to bring the tip of the index finger to the tip of the nose. Alterations may be made in the initial starting position to assess performance from different planes of motion.
2. Finger to assistant's finger	The patient and PTA sit opposite each other. The PTA's index finger is held in front of the patient. The patient is asked to touch the tip of their index finger to the PTA's index finger. The position of the PTA's finger may be altered during testing to assess ability to change distance, direction and force of movement.
3. Finger to finger	Both shoulders are abducted to 90 degrees with the elbows extended. The patient is asked to bring both hands toward the midline and approximate the index fingers from opposing hands.
4. Alternate nose to finger	The patient alternately touches the tip of the nose and the tip of the PTA's finger with the index finger. The position of the PTA's finger may be altered during testing to assess ability to change distance, direction and force of movement.
5. Finger opposition	The patient touches the tip of the thumb to the tip of each finger in sequence.
6. Mass grasp	An alternation is made between opening and closing fist (from finger flexion to full extension). Speed may be gradually increased.
7. Pronation/supination	With elbows flexed to 90 degrees and held close to body, the patient alternately turns the palms up and down. This test also may be performed with shoulders flexed to 90 degrees and elbows extended. The ability to reverse movements between opposing muscle groups can be assessed at many joints. Examples include active alternation between flexion and extension of the knee, ankle, elbow, fingers and so forth.
8. Tapping (hand)	With the elbow flexed and the forearm pronated, the patient is asked to "tap" his or her hand on the knee.
9. Tapping (foot)	The patient is asked to "tap" the ball of one foot on the floor without raising the knee; heel maintains contact with floor.
10. Pointing and past pointing	The patient and PTA are opposite each other, either sitting or standing. Both patient and PTA bring shoulders to a horizontal position of 90 degrees of flexion with elbows extended. Index fingers are touching or the patient's finger may rest lightly on the PTA's. The patient is asked to fully flex the shoulder (fingers will be pointing toward ceiling) and then return to the horizontal position such that index fingers will again approximate. Both arms should be tested, either separately or simultaneously. A normal response consists of an accurate return to the starting position. An abnormal response there is typically a "past pointing," or movement beyond the target. Several variations to this test include movements in other directions such as toward 90 degrees of shoulder abduction or toward 90 degrees of shoulder flexion (finger will point toward floor). Following each movement, the patient is asked to return to the initial horizontal starting position.
11. Alternate heel to knee; heel to toe	From a supine position, the patient is asked to touch the knee and big toe alternately with the heel of the opposite extremity.
12. Toe to examiner's finger	From a supine position, the patient is instructed to touch the great toe to the examiner's finger. The position of finger may be altered during testing to assess ability to change distance, direction and force of movement.
13. Heel on shin	From a supine position, the heel of one foot is slid up and down the shin of the opposite lower extremity.
14. Drawing a circle	The patient draws an imaginary circle in the air with either upper or lower extremity (a table or the floor also may be used). This also may be done using a figure-eight pattern. This test may be performed in the supine position for lower extremity assessment.
15. Fixation or position holding	Upper extremity: The patient holds arms horizontally in front (sitting or standing). Lower extremity: The patient is asked to hold the knee in an extended position (sitting).

Tests should be performed first with eyes open and then with eyes closed. Abnormal responses include a gradual deviation from the "holding" position and/or a diminished quality of response with vision occluded. Unless otherwise indicated, tests are performed with the patient in a sitting position. Vary speed from slow to fast, observe control.

From O'Sullivan S, Schmidt T: Physical Rehabilitation: Assessment and Treatment, 4th ed, F.A. Davis, 2001, pg 166, with permission.

c. Vestibular: motor responses to positional and movement changes.

d. Musculoskeletal: strength and range of motion of lower extremities and trunk.

➢ **Red Flag**
   • Since vision is a major component of balance, training of other systems must be incorporated in rehabilitation to assist patients with adapting to the visual changes that typically occur with age or are present with a number of neurological dysfunctions.

4. **Assessing balance and LOS.**
   a. Observe maximum sway in any direction.
   b. Check static balance.
      (1) Sitting tests: holding a steady position, with and without upper extremity support.
      (2) Standing tests: double limb and single limb support.
      (3) Romberg's test.
         (a) Stand with feet together.
         (b) First with eyes open, then with eyes closed for 30 seconds each.
      (4) Sharpened or tandem Romberg.
         (a) Stand in tandem heel to toe position.
         (b) First with eyes open, then with eyes closed for 30 seconds each.

Table 3-14 ➤ EQUILIBRIUM COORDINATION TESTS

1. Standing in a normal, comfortable posture.
2. Standing, feet together (narrow base of support).
3. Standing, with one foot directly in front of the other in tandem position (toe of one foot touching heel of opposite foot).
4. Standing on one foot.
5. Arm position may be altered in each of the above postures (i.e., arms at side, over head, hands on waist, and so forth).
6. Displace balance unexpectedly (while carefully guarding patient).
7. Standing, alternate between forward trunk flexion and return to neutral.
8. Standing, laterally flex trunk to each side.
9. Standing, eyes open (EO) to eyes closed (EC); ability to maintain an upright posture without visual input is referred to as a *positive Romberg sign*.
10. Standing in tandem position, eyes open (EO) to eyes closed (EC) (*Sharpened Romberg*).
11. Walking, placing the heel of one foot directly in front of the toe of the opposite foot (tandem walking).
12. Walking along a straight line drawn or taped to the floor, or place feet on floor markers while walking.
13. Walk sideways, backward, or cross-stepping.
14. March in place.
15. Alter speed of ambulatory activities; observe patient walking at normal speed, as fast as possible, and as slow as possible.
16. Stop and start abruptly while walking.
17. Walk and pivot (turn 90, 180 or 360 degrees).
18. Walk in a circle, alternate directions.
19. Walk on heels or toes.
20. Walk with horizontal and vertical head turns.
21. Step over or around obstacles.
22. Stairclimbing with and without using handrail; one step at-a-time versus step-over-step.
23. Agility activities (coordinated movement with upright balance); jumping jacks, alternate flexing and extending the knees while sitting on a Swiss ball.

From O'Sullivan S, Schmidt T: Physical Rehabilitation: Assessment and Treatment, 4th ed, F.A. Davis, 2001, pg 165, with permission.

➤ **Red Flag**
   - Many clinicians fail to examine and rehabilitate static balance, tending more toward the dynamic balance tasks associated with ambulation. Both are equally important and, given the importance of static balance in daily function as well as a preparatory activity for dynamic balance, assessment of one should not be neglected.

  c. Dynamic/functional balance.
   (1) Standing up, walking, turning and stopping.
   (2) With ambulation, navigate an obstacle course or complete multiple tasks simultaneously (i.e., walking while talking).
   (3) BOS challenges: sitting or standing on a moveable surface (Dynadisk, balance board, dense foam).

5. Functional balance tests (Table 3-15).
6. Functional balance grades (Table 3-16).

Environmental, Home, and Work (Job/School/Play) Barriers

1. Administer a structured questionnaire to identify barriers.
2. Ask routine interview questions to determine barriers.
3. Identify common and frequently occurring barriers in home and work environments.
   a. Curbs, steps with and without railings, uneven terrain, busy streets.
   b. Inaccessible travel routes to and within environments.
   c. Throw rugs, dense carpeting.
   d. Accessibility of safety call buttons or switches.
   e. Work station, computer monitor height.

➤ **Red Flag**
   - Barriers present in the patient's environment must be identified to provide a comprehensive rehabilitation program ensuring safety for the patient.

Assistive and Adaptive Devices

1. Assess patient's and caregiver's safe use of the device via subjective reports regarding care, function and benefit of device.
2. Assess alignment and fit of the device.
3. Assess proper working order of wheelchairs and ambulatory assistive devices.

➤ **Red Flag**
   - Assistive and adaptive devices are only useful if they are fit to the patient and in proper working order.

Orthotic, Protective and Supportive Devices

1. Assess skin changes after use of an orthosis for changes signifying normal or abnormal pressure points.
2. Ability of patient and/or family member to don/doff and care for an orthosis.
3. Subjective reports from patient and caregiver regarding care, function and benefit of orthosis.
4. Normal characteristics of function with use of orthosis.
5. Changes in function with use of orthosis.

Table 3-15 ➤ FUNCTIONAL BALANCE TESTS

TEST	DESCRIPTION	REFERENCE VALUES
Performance-Oriented Mobility Assessment (POMA, Tinetti)	Examines balance (balance subtest, nine items including sitting, sit-to-stand, standing, standing feet together, turn 360 degrees, sternal nudge, stand on one leg, tandem stand, reaching up, bending over, stand-to-sit, timed rising) and walking (gait subtest, eight items including gait initiation, path, turning timed walk, step over obstacles)	Maximum score is 28; patients who score <19 are at high risk for falls; patients who score 19–24 are at moderate risk
Berg Balance Scale	Examines functional balance (14 items) including sitting unsupported, sit-to-stand, stand-to-sit, transfers; in standing: EO to EC, feet together, forward reach, pick object off floor, head turns, turning 360 degrees, stepping up, tandem stand, stand on one leg	Maximum score is 56; patients who score <45 are at high risk for falls; with scores 54–46, a 1-point drop is associated with a 6%–8% increase in fall risk
Timed Up and Go (TUG)	Examines functional balance during rise from a chair, walk 3 m, turn, and return to chair. Performance on the Get Up & Go test (GUG) is untimed	Normal intact adults can perform the test in ≤10 seconds; 11–20 seconds is considered normal for frail elderly or disabled patients; patients who take >20 seconds are at increased risk for falls; patients who take >30 seconds are at high risk
Functional Reach (FR)	Examines maximal distance a person can reach forward beyond arm's length while maintaining a fixed position in standing (single item test)	Forward reach norms: above average >12.2 inches, below average <5.6 inches; a forward reach of <10 is indicative of increased fall risk
Multidirectional Reach Test (MDRT)	Examines maximal distance a person can reach forward, backward, and lateral to right and left	Backward: above average >7.6 inches, below average <1.6 inches; lateral: above average >9.4 inches, below average <3.8 inches
Short Physical Performance Battery (SPPB)	Includes repeated chair stands (sit-to-stand rises), semitandem, tandem, and side-by-side stands as well as a timed 8 ft (2.44 meter) walk	Tests are scored in terms of time to complete: 5 sit-to-stands, 10 sec in each of the standing conditions and 8 ft walk. An ordinal score is given for each section. Summary ordinal score: 0 (worst performance) to 12 (best performance)

Self-Care and Home-Management (Including Activities of Daily Living [ADL])

1. Administer standard questionnaire regarding patient's abilities with ADL.

2. Observe and report patient's use of basic adaptive skills in ADL.

3. Functional rating scales.
   a. The Functional Independence Measure (FIM).
      (1) Measures patient ability in six areas: self-care, sphincter control, transfers, locomotion, communication and social cognition.
      (2) Scale.
         (a) 7–complete independence without assistive device.
         (b) 6–complete independence with assistive device.
         (c) 5–supervision or assistance with set-up required.
         (d) 4–minimum assistance required.
         (e) 3– moderate assistance required.
         (f) 2–maximum assistance required.
         (g) 1– total assistance required.
   b. Katz's index of ADL: evaluates degree of assistance needed in bathing, dressing, toileting, transferring, continence and feeding.
   c. Outcome and assessment information set (OASIS): assesses ADL/IADL such as grooming, dressing, transferring, laundry and shopping.

Table 3-16 ➤ FUNCTIONAL BALANCE GRADES

GRADE	STATIC BALANCE	DYNAMIC BALANCE
Normal	Maintains balance without hand-hold support	Accepts maximal challenge and easily weight shifts in all directions throughout the full range
Good	Maintains balance without hand-hold support, demonstrating limited postural sway	Accepts moderate challenge (pick up item off floor without losing balance)
Fair	Maintains balance with hand-hold support and occasional minimal assistance	Accepts minimal challenge (maintain balance while turning head or body)
Poor	Requires hand-hold support and modmax assistance to maintain balance	Unable to accept challenge or move without loss of balance

Community and Work (Job/School/Play) Integration/Reintegration

1. Administer standard questionnaire to identify abilities.

2. Observe and report patient performance on IADL.

Application Concepts
- Any home exercise program utilized will likely be dependent on the mentation of a patient, thereby necessitating a thorough assessment of the individual's initial and continuing status of mental functioning.

- Feedback is used throughout therapeutic intervention. Decreased sensory functioning will limit the type of feedback that can be used. For example, an individual who is severely hard of hearing should not be given feedback solely in the form of verbal instruction but via visual and tactile cueing as well.
- Perceptual disorders can be severely limiting to a patient's rehabilitation potential and return to function.
- Synergies can be used to allow independent movement that otherwise would not be possible.
- Many neurological dysfunctions lead to decreased ambulation ability and safety concerns. Gait deviations must be identified early and remediated or compensated for prior to allowing the patient being recommended for discharge.

Intervention Strategies for Patients with Neurological Dysfunction

Roles and Responsibilities of PTA

1. Understand the plan of care for the patient directed to him/her.

2. Define the indications, contraindications and precautions of interventions delegated by the PT.

3. Use information from the data collection process to monitor patient status and progress patient toward short- and long-term goals.

4. Adjust or withhold intervention based on patient status as determined through observation and data collection.

5. Participate in patient status judgments by reporting changes to supervising PT and requesting reexamination or revision to plan of care.

6. Utilize data collection and communication to participate in determining a patient's progress toward specific outcomes as established in the plan of care by the PT.

7. Educate the patient and significant others.

8. Participate in the discharge planning process.
   ▷ Red Flag
   - The PTA must know the contraindications and precautions for each patient he/she is working with to know when it is safe to continue therapy within the plan of care and when to refer back to the physical therapist.

Application Concept
These approaches can be used on patients/clients who fall outside of the neuromuscular system as well: e.g., orthopedic, geriatric.

General Intervention Considerations

1. Monitor heart rate and blood pressure for any patient with cardiac complications.

2. Modify the intensity of the intervention if indicated by the cardiac response.

3. Use commands and instructions consistent with the cognitive and communication abilities of the patient.

4. Always begin with demonstration of the entire task, start to finish, at the appropriate speed, while identifying key components for successful task completion.

5. Examine influences of tone, the amount of resistance of muscles to passive elongation.
   a. If patient has high tone that increases during exercise, decrease the intensity of intervention, utilize inhibition techniques and/or increase the external support.
   b. If the patient has low tone, monitor for stability to prevent unwanted stress on the joints and utilize facilitation techniques.

6. When ready, the clinician should advance the difficulty of exercise/activity (Table 3-17).

Table 3-17 ➤ EXERCISE/ACTIVITY DIFFICULTY

TO ALTER DIFFICULTY LEVEL	ACTIVITY COMPONENT	EXAMPLE
To decrease	Widen/broaden the base of support	• Work in supine instead of sitting • Work in bilateral stance instead of unilateral stance
	Decrease the number of segments involved	• Work in prone on elbows instead of sitting and weightbearing on an extended upper extremity • Work in tall kneeling instead of standing
	Decrease the range of movement	• Roll between $^{\circ}/_{\checkmark}$ turn from prone and $^{\circ}/_{\checkmark}$ turn from supine • Reach in a narrow, unilateral range in sitting instead of full range, cross midline
	Increase the stability of the support surface	• Work on sitting on a mat table instead of an exercise ball • Work on ambulation over level, tile surface instead of gravel
	Decrease stage of motor control	• Use rhythmic initiation in sidelying instead of weight shifting in sitting • Work on stepping forward and back with unaffected extremity instead of walking
To increase	Narrow the base of support	• Work in standing instead of sitting • Work in heel to toe stance instead of bilateral stance
	Increase the number of segments involved	• Work in quadruped instead of sitting • Work in standing instead of sitting
	Increase the range of movement	• Roll from supine to prone and reverse • Reach across midline in sitting
	Decrease the stability of the support surface	• Work on sitting on an exercise ball instead of on a chair • Work on ambulation over foam mats instead of level tile

CHAPTER 3

⮫Red Flag

- The PTA should not attempt to follow any therapeutic intervention or treatment approach for which he/she does not possess a full knowledge of the concepts of treatment and how to safely and competently apply these concepts to a given patient situation.

Intervention Approaches

1. **Neurodevelopmental Treatment (NDT).**
   a. Developed by Karel Bobath, MD, and Berta Bobath, PT.
   b. Basic concepts.
      (1) Normal movement sequences and balance reactions are the focus of therapy so an accurate analysis of the patient's movement patterns is essential.
      (2) Motor learning of patterns of movement can be facilitated by repetition and experience in the environment.
      (3) Abnormal tone, primitive reflex patterns and mass synergies result in abnormal patterns of posture and movement and interfere with normal recovery and function.
      (4) Inhibition of unwanted activity precedes practice of normal motor patterns.
   c. Techniques.
      (1) Active movements are guided or assisted.

   (2) Low effort maximizes performance in the presence of tonal disorders, while high effort, maximal resistance results in unwanted activity and is avoided.
   (3) Avoid any substitution movements.
   (4) Minimize verbal instructions or feedback during movement.
   (5) Ensure movement success and avoid repeated failures.
   (6) Normalize postural tone.
   (7) Abnormal patterns of movements and reflexes are inhibited or prevented.
   (8) Normalize sensory/perceptual experiences.
   (9) Emphasize normal functional activities that are meaningful and goal oriented, utilizing both affected and intact body segments.

2. **Proprioceptive Neuromuscular Facilitation (PNF).**
   a. Developed by Herman Kabat, MD, and Margaret Knott, PT, and later modified by Dorothy Voss, PT.
   b. Basic concepts
      (1) Facilitation of total patterns of movement focuses on motor learning in synergistic muscle patterns.
      (2) Normal movements are spiral and diagonal in character.
      (3) Proprioceptive elements (e.g., maximal resistance and stretch) and irradiation from strong muscles can be used to strengthen weak muscles in a pattern.

Table 3-18 ➤ PNF TECHNIQUES FOR FACILITATION

NEW TERMINOLGY (OLD TERMINOLOGY)	DESCRIPTION	INDICATIONS
Combination of Isotonics (Agonist Reversals)	• Combination of concentric, isometric and eccentric contractions of one muscle	• Weak postural muscles • Poor eccentric control of body weight with movement transitions • Decreased AROM • Poor muscular control
Stabilizing Reversals (Alternating Isometrics)	• In an alternating pattern, agonist and antagonist muscle contract isometrically	• Decreased stability • Poor antigravity control • Weakness
Contract-Relax	• Isotonic movement in rotation followed by an isometric contraction of antagonist at point of limitation with voluntary relaxation and push into new range	• Limited ROM resulting from muscle tightness or spasticity
Hold-Relax	• Isometric contraction of antagonist followed by relaxation and PROM into new range	• Limited ROM resulting from muscle tightness, spasm or pain
Rhythmic Initiation	• Voluntary relaxation followed by passive movement through an increasing ROM then active assisted, active and finally resisted movements	• Inability to initiate movement • Poorly coordinated movements • Hypertonicity • Motor learning deficits • Communication disorders
Rhythmic Rotation	• Voluntary relaxation combined with slow, passive, rhythmic rotations	• Hypertonia • Limited ROM or function
Rhythmic Stabilization	• Simultaneous isometric contraction (cocontraction) [cocontraction as elsewhere] of agonist and antagonist muscles	• Decreased stability in weightbearing • Poor antigravity control • Limited ROM caused by muscle tightness
Dynamic Reversals (Slow Reversals)	• Slow isotonic contractions of agonist and then antagonist	• Decreased AROM • Weak antagonistic muscles • Poor reciprocal control • Muscular hypertonicity
Repeated Stretch (Repeated Contractions)	• Repeated isotonic contractions induced by quick stretch and enhanced with resistance at point of weakness in range	• Weakness • Fatigue • Decreased ability to perform fucntional movement

(4) Total patterns of movement and posture are important preparatory patterns for advanced functional skills (e.g., gait).

c. Techniques for facilitation (Table 3-18).

d. Diagonal patterns of movement (Table 3-19).

(1) Named for motions occurring at the proximal joint (shoulder or hip).

(2) Intermediate joint (elbow or knee) may be flexing or extending.

➢ **Red Flag**

• Continuing to work only in synergistic patterns as the patient regains isolated, voluntary movements can decrease the patient's rehabilitation potential.

Table 3-19 ➤ PNF DIAGONAL PATTERNS

Upper extremity

PATTERN	SHOULDER MOTIONS	VERBAL CUE
D1F	• Flexion-adduction-external rotation	• "Close your hand, turn, and pull your arm up across your face."
D1E	• Extension- abduction-internal rotation	• "Open your hand, turn, and push your arm down and out."
D2F	• Flexion-abduction-external rotation	• "Open your hand, turn, and lift your arm up and out."
D2E	• Extension-adduction-internal rotation	• "Close your hand, turn, and pull your arm down and across your body."

Lower extremity

PATTERN	HIP MOTIONS	VERBAL CUE
D1F	• Flexion-adduction-external rotation	• "Bring your foot up, turn, and pull your leg up and across your body."
D1E	• Extension- abduction-internal rotation	• "Push your foot down, turn, and push your leg down and out."
D2F	• Flexion-abduction-internal rotation	• "Lift your foot up, turn, and lift your leg up and out."
D2E	• Extension-adduction-external rotation	• "Push your foot down, turn, and pull your leg down and in."

3. **Movement therapy in hemiplegia.**
   a. Developed by Signe Brunnstrom, PT.
      (1) Some aspects of this approach are not consistent with current practice.
      (2) Classification of the stages of recovery based on Brunnstrom's work is helpful to understanding recovery and outcome.
   b. Basic concepts.
      (1) Sensorimotor recovery occurs in a sequential pattern that can vary between and within limbs while peaking at any stage.
      (2) Patients with very little recovery must first gain control of basic limb synergies.
      (3) Once initial control is achieved, out-of-synergy combinations are promoted.
   c. Techniques.
      (1) Facilitation of volitional control movement.
         (a) Reflexes: some aspects of concept regarded as inappropriate.
         (b) Proprioceptive inputs: resistance, weight bearing, stretching and tapping.
         (c) Exteroceptive inputs: rubbing, stroking.
         (d) Eye contact and appropriate verbal commands.
         (e) Use of unaffected side to facilitate affected side via transfer effects.
         (f) Progress control from small range to large range and isometric to isotonic contractions.
         (g) Fatigue, pain and heavy resistance are avoided, as these decrease control.
         (h) Positive reinforcement and repetition are keys to successful motor learning.
      (2) Patterns of movement.
         (a) Training activities focus on the out-of-synergy combinations needed for everyday function.
         ⚑ **Red Flag**
            • The patient must be able to produce out-of-synergy movements to utilize the movement therapy in hemiplegia approach.

4. **Sensory stimulation techniques.**
   a. Combines several of the treatment approaches and is based on the work of Rood.
   b. Basic concepts.
      (1) Indications.
         (a) Patients who demonstrate absent or disordered motor control and would benefit from the use of augmented feedback.
         (b) Most useful in the early stages of motor learning with limited movement potential.
      (2) Contraindications.
         (a) Patients who will not benefit from a hands-on approach.
         (b) Patients with sufficient motor control to perform and refine a motor skill based on intrinsic feedback mechanisms.

⚑ **Red Flag**
   • Extrinsic feedback should not be utilized with patients who have or can learn the ability to use intrinsic feedback so as not to facilitate dependence on the clinician.
      (3) Response to stimulation is dependent upon multiple factors including level of intactness of CNS, initial level of arousal and type and amount of stimulation.
      (4) Early use of sensory stimulation techniques should be phased out as soon as possible in favor of active control by the learner.
      (5) Multiple techniques or repeated application of the same technique may be necessary to produce the desired response in patients functioning at low levels.
   c. Techniques (Table 3-20).

5. **Compensatory training approach.**
   a. General concepts.
      (1) Indicated to offset or adapt to residual impairments and disabilities.
      (2) Focus is on early resumption of functional independence with reliance on uninvolved segments for function.
      (3) Changes are made in the patient's overall approach to tasks.
      (4) Patient is made aware of movement deficiencies and alternate ways to accomplish tasks, including substitution.
   ⚑ **Red Flag**
      • Compensatory strategies should not be taught until it becomes obvious the patient will not be able to rehabilitate a given skill. If used too early, compensatory mechanisms will become habit, and this can slow or even prevent development of the desired skill.
   b. Concerns with the compensation approach.
      (1) Focus on using uninvolved segments to accomplish daily tasks may suppress recovery and contribute to learned nonuse of the impaired segments.
      (2) Focus on task-specific learning may lead to the development of splinter skills that cannot be easily generalized to other tasks or environmental situations.
   c. May be the only approach possible if severe motor deficits are present or no additional recovery is anticipated.
   d. Strategies.
      (1) Simplify activities and adapt environment to facilitate relearning of skills and enhance performance.
      (2) Energy conservation and activity pacing are important to ensure completion of all daily movement requirements.

Table 3-20 ➤ PROPRIOCEPTIVE TECHNIQUES

INHIBITORY TECHNIQUES	RESPONSE
Prolonged, slowly applied stretch	Inhibits agonist muscle, decreases tone
Inhibitory pressure (firm pressure on long tendons)	Inhibits muscle, decreases tone
FACILITATION TECHNIQUES	**RESPONSE**
Quick stretch, tapping of muscle belly or tendon	Facilitates agonist muscle, inhibits antagonist
Resistance	Recruits motor units; facilitates, strengthens agonist contraction
Joint approximation	Enhances joint awareness, facilitates co contraction, action of postural extensors, stabilizing muscles
Joint traction	Enhances joint awareness, action of flexors; relieves muscle spasm
EXTEROCEPTIVE STIMULATION TECHNIQUES	
INHIBITORY TECHNIQUES	**RESPONSE**
Maintained touch (maintained pressure)	Produces calming effect, generalized inhibition
Slow stroking (continuous, slow stroking to spinal posterior primary rami)	Produces calming effect, generalized inhibition
Prolonged icing	Produces inhibition of muscle tone, spasm and pain
Neutral warmth	Produces generalized inhibition of tone, relaxation, calming effect, decreased pain
FACILITATION TECHNIQUES	**RESPONSE**
Light touch, quick icing facilitation	Initiates phasic, withdrawal reactions
VESTIBULAR STIMULATION TECHNIQUES	
INHIBITORY TECHNIQUES	**RESPONSE**
Slow, maintained vestibular stimulation (slow, repetitive rocking)	Produces generalized inhibition of tone, relaxation, calming effect
Inverted positioning (head down position) BP	Elicits generalized activation of postural extensors, calming effect, decreased HR and BP
FACILITATION TECHNIQUES	**RESPONSE**
Fast, irregular vestibular stimulation (spinning, fast rolling)	Produces generalized facilitation of tone, improved motor coordination, improved retinal image stability

(3) Establish a new functional pattern focusing on key task elements.

(4) Repeated practice working toward consistency and efficiency.

(5) Use orthoses to support/control afflicted segments.

Motor Control/Motor Learning

1. **Motor control.**
   a. Motor program.
      (1) A set of prestructured muscle commands that, when initiated, result in the production of a coordinated movement sequence.
      (2) A learned task that can be carried out largely uninfluenced by peripheral feedback.
   b. Motor plan.
      (1) An overall strategy for movement.
      (2) An action sequence requiring the coordination of a number of motor programs.
   c. Stages of motor control.
      (1) Mobility.
          (a) Movements in dependent postures that are poorly controlled.
          (b) Distal mobility.
      (2) Stability.
          (a) The ability to maintain an antigravity posture in a weight-bearing position.
          (b) Proximal stability.
      (3) Controlled mobility.
          (a) The ability to move within or between postures.
          (b) Distal stability with proximal mobility.
      (4) Skill.
          (a) Highly coordinated movements.
          (b) Proximal stability with distal mobility.
   d. Feedback.
      (1) Afferent information sent by various sensory receptors to control centers.
      (2) Feedback updates control centers about the correctness of movement while it progresses to shape ongoing movement.
      (3) Feedback allows motor responses to be adapted to the demands of the environment.
   e. Feedforward.

(1) Readies the system in advance of movement.
  (a) Anticipatory responses that adjust the system for incoming sensory feedback or for future movements.
f. Motor skill acquisition.
  (1) Behavior is organized to achieve a goal-directed task.
  (2) Active problem solving/processing is required for the development of a motor program, motor plan or to motor learn.
  (3) Adaptive to specific environmental demands.
    (a) Closed environment: static and controlled by the clinician.
    (b) Open environment: variable and changing with distracters presented.
  (4) CNS recovery/reorganization is dependent upon experience.

2. Motor learning.
a. General concepts.

(1) A change in the capability of a person to perform a skill.
(2) Result of practice or experience.
b. Stages of motor learning (Table 3-21).
c. Measures of motor learning.
  (1) Performance: level of automaticity, effort and speed of decision making.
  (2) Retention: ability to demonstrate the skill after a period of no practice.
  (3) Generalizability: capability to apply what has been learned to similar tasks.
  (4) Resistance to contextual change: capability to apply what has been learned to other environmental contexts.
d. Feedback.
  (1) Intrinsic feedback: sensory information normally acquired during performance of a task.
  (2) Augmented feedback: externally presented feedback, such as verbal cueing, that is added during normally acquired task performance.

CHAPTER 3

Table 3-21 ➤ STAGES OF MOTOR LEARNING AND TRAINING STRATEGIES	
COGNITIVE STAGE CHARACTERISTICS	**TRAINING STRATEGIES**
The learner • develops an understanding of task, *cognitive mapping* • assesses abilities, task demands • identifies stimuli, contacts memory • selects response, performs initial approximations of task • structures motor program • modifies initial responses ***"What to do"*** decision	Highlight purpose of task in functionally relevant terms. Demonstrate ideal performance of task to establish a *reference of correctness* Have patient verbalize task components and requirements. Point out similarities to other learned tasks Direct attention to critical task elements **Select appropriate feedback** • Emphasize intact sensory systems, intrinsic feedback systems • Carefully pair extrinsic feedback with intrinsic feedback • High dependence on vision: have patient watch movement • Provide **Knowledge of Performance (KP):** focus on errors as they become consistent; do not cue on large number of random errors • Provide **Knowledge of Results (KR):** focus on success of movement outcome Ask learner to evaluate performance, outcomes; identify problems, solutions Use reinforcements (praise) for correct performance and continuing motivation **Organize feedback schedule** • *Feedback* after every trial improves performance during early learning • *Variable feedback* (summed, fading, bandwidth designs) increases depth of cognitive processing, improves retention; may decrease performance initially **Organize initial practice** • Stress controlled movement to minimize errors • Provide adequate rest periods using *distributed practice* if task is complex, long, or energy costly or if learner fatigues easily, has short attention, or has poor concentration • Use manual guidance to assist as appropriate • Break complex tasks down into component parts, teach both parts and integrated whole • Use *bilateral transfer* as appropriate • Use *blocked (repeated) practice* of same task to improve performance • Use *variable practice* (serial or random practice order) of related skills to increase depth of cognitive processing and retention; may decrease performance initially • Use *mental practice* to improve performance and learning, reduce anxiety **Assess, modify arousal levels as appropriate** • High or low arousal impairs performance and learning • Avoid stressors, mental fatigue **Structure environment** • Reduce extraneous environmental stimuli, distractors to ensure attention, concentration • Emphasize closed skills initially gradually progressing to open skills

(Continued on following page)

Table 3-21 ➤ continued

ASSOCIATED STAGE CHARACTERISTICS	TRAINING STRATEGIES
The learner practices movements, refines motor program, spatial and temporal organization; decreases errors, extraneous movements Dependence on visual feedback decreases, increases for use of proprioceptive feedback; cognitive monitoring decreases ***"How to do"*** decision	**Select appropriate feedback** • Continue to provide KP; intervene when errors become consistent • Emphasize proprioceptive feedback, "feel of movement" to assist in establishing an internal reference of correctness • Continue to provide KR; stress relevance of functional outcomes • Assist learner to improve self-evaluation, decision-making skills • Facilitation techniques, guided movements are counterproductive during this stage of learning **Organize feedback schedule** • Continue to provide feedback for continuing motivation; encourage patient to self-assess achievements • Avoid excessive augmented feedback • Focus on use of variable feedback (summed, fading, bandwidth) designs to improve retention **Organize practice** • Encourage consistency of performance • Focus on variable practice order (serial or random) of related skills to improve retention **Structure environment** • Progress toward open, changing environment • Prepare the learner for home, community, work environments
AUTONOMOUS STAGE CHARACTERISTICS	**TRAINING STRATEGIES**
The learner practices movements; continues to refine motor responses, spatial and temporal highly organized; movements are largely error-free; minimal level of cognitive monitoring ***"How to succeed"*** decision	Assess need for conscious attention, automaticity of movements **Select appropriate feedback** • Learner demonstrates appropriate self-evaluation, decision-making skills • Provide occasional feedback (KP, KR) when errors evident **Organize practice** • Stress consistency of performance in variable environments, variations of tasks (open skills) • High levels of practice (massed practice) are appropriate **Structure environment** • Vary environments to challenge learner • Ready the learner for home, community, and work environments Focus on competitive aspects of skills as appropriate; e.g., wheelchair sports

From: O'Sullivan S, Schmitz T. Physical Rehabilitation. 5th ed, Philadelphia, FA Davis, 2007, with permission.

    (a) Knowledge of results (KR): augmented feedback about the outcome of a movement.

    (b) Knowledge of performance (KP): augmented feedback about the nature of the movement produced.

  (3) Feedback schedules.

    (a) Terminal: given after task completion to facilitate long-term retention.

    (b) Summed: given after a set of trials is completed.

    (c) Fading: given frequently at first and then progressively decreased.

    (d) Bandwidth: given only if performance falls outside a designated margin of error.

 e. Practice.

  (1) Blocked practice: practice of a single motor skill repeatedly (111 222 333).

  (2) Serial practice: practice of a group or class of motor skills in serial or predictable order (123 123 123).

  (3) Random practice: practice of a group or class of motor skills in random order (213 123 312 123).

  (4) Variable practice: practice with a variety of circumstances in order to increase generalizability and long-term retention.

  (5) Massed practice: relatively continuous practice with a small amount of rest time.

  (6) Distributed practice: rest time is greater than practice time.

  (7) Mental practice: cognitive rehearsal of a skill without physical performance.

 f. Transfer.

  (1) The effects, either positive or negative, of having previous practice of a skill or skills upon the learning of a new skill or upon performance in a new context.

  (2) Part-whole transfer: complex motor task is broken into its component parts for separate practice before practice of the integrated whole.

  (3) Bilateral transfer: improvement in movement skill performance with one limb results from practice with the opposite limb.

 g. Strategies for effective learning.

(1) Frequency: feedback given after every trial improves performance, while variable feedback improves learning and retention.

(2) Type of feedback: early training should focus on visual feedback, while later training should focus on proprioceptive feedback.

(3) Environment: reduce extraneous environmental stimuli (closed environment) early in learning, while later learning focuses on adaptation to environmental demands (open environment).

(4) Supportive feedback can be used to shape behavior, motivate patient.

(5) Assist learner in recognizing/pairing intrinsic feedback with movement responses.

(6) Provide appropriate augmented feedback.

(a) Knowledge of results: simply identifies success or failure of the end product.

(b) Knowledge of performance.
- Early in learning, focus feedback on correct aspects of performance.
- Later in learning, focus feedback on errors as they become consistent.
- Avoid feedback dependence.
  * Reduce augmented feedback as soon as possible.
  * Foster active introspection, decision making by learner.

(7) Establish practice schedule based on functional goal.

(a) Distributed practice is used when superior performance is desired, motivation is low or the learner has a short attention, poor concentration or fatigues easily.

(b) Massed practice is used when a task is new and the learner needs repetition to learn.

(c) Use random or serial practice order, rather than blocked practice, to improve learning and retention.

(d) Use mental practice when the task has a large cognitive component or to decrease fear and anxiety.

(8) Use part-whole transfer when a task is complex, has highly independent parts or the learner has limited memory, attention or difficulty with only a particular portion of a larger task.

(9) Until patient develops adaptability and generalizability, transfer of learning will be optimized when tasks are highly similar.

(10) With learners who have attention deficits or who mentally fatigue easily, focus on key task elements, give frequent rest periods and limit feedback.

(11) Involve learner in goal setting to make practice functionally relevant and desirable for the patient to learn.

Promote Ambulation Independence

1. **Preambulation mat activities, with progression.**

a. Rolling: log, segmental, counterrotation.

b. Prone on elbows: PNF holding activities, active head movements, weight shifting.

c. Prone on hands: PNF holding activities, active head movements, head movements with scapular depression, forward and lateral movements.

d. Hook-lying: static holding, PNF holding activities, movements out of midline.

e. Bridging: static hold, modify BOS (feet closer, arms closer, arms crossed on trunk), slow-reversal-hold pelvic activities, active to resisted hip abduction and adduction.

f. Quadruped: static hold, PNF holding activities, weight shifting, multidirectional rocking, lifting one extremity (usually begin with arm, then leg) and progress to arm and opposite leg together.

g. Sitting: with arm support, remove arm support, static hold, PNF holding activities, active head and arm movements, weight shifting within BOS, weight shifting outside BOS.

h. Kneeling: arm support on solid surface and progress to movable support, static hold, PNF holding activities, minisquats for eccentric hip control, weight shifting, balance activities, active arm activities, throw and catch ball, hip hiking.

i. Half-kneeling: static hold, PNF holding activities, weight-shifting activities, slow-reversal and slow-reversal-hold pelvis movements.

j. Modified plantigrade (standing with arm support): static hold, PNF holding activities to shoulders and pelvis, weight-shifting activities, unweighting one lower extremity.

k. Standing: tonic hold, PNF holding activities, active weight shifting with feet in parallel progressing to one forward of the other, active arm and head movements, balance activities (throw/ catch ball, reaching, etc), stepping activities.

2. **Preambulation parallel bar activities.**

a. Entire progression should be demonstrated and then each component reviewed prior to the patient performing the task.

b. Emphasize correct sit-to-stand procedure: scoot to edge of chair, push from the arms of the chair, and pull feet back under knees.

c. Consideration with parallel bar activities.

(1) Clinician should be positioned inside the parallel bars directly in front of the patient.

(2) Initial balance activities are modified depending on the patient's weight-bearing status and specific requirements for treatment.

(3) Monitor the patient's circulatory status closely and be aware if the patient is experiencing orthostatic hypotension.

(4) Assess the patient's limits of stability by determining how far the center of gravity can be displaced while still maintaining balance.

d. Anterior-posterior and lateral weight shifts, first with stable hand placement, then with alteration of hand placement.

e. Hip hiking: pelvic elevation by hiking one hip at a time. Resistance can be added as skill level improves.

f. Standing push-ups: hands placed on the bars just anterior to the thighs, and body weight is lifted by simultaneous elbow extension and shoulder depression.

g. Stepping forward and backward with manual resistance applied to the pelvis for increased difficulty.

h. Forward progression: patient should maintain a loose, open grip on the bars and push down rather than pull up on the bars to best mimic ambulation with use of an assistive device.

i. Turning: patient is instructed to turn toward the stronger side, stepping in a small circle, not pivoting on a single extremity.

⚑ **Red Flag**

- While most patients should be encouraged to turn toward the stronger side during turning, patients with an acute total hip replacement must follow the precautions outlined by the physician. This may necessitate turning toward or away from the affected side.

j. Return to seated position: cue patient to back up, release stronger hand from bar and then reach back for the wheelchair armrest.

k. Advanced parallel bar activities.
   a. Resisted forward ambulation: resistance can be applied manually to the pelvis or the shoulders.
   b. Backward ambulation: initially without resistance, then add manual resistance at the pelvis.

c. Sidestepping: turn sideways and holds onto the bar with bilateral UE, initially without resistance, then progress to manual contacts at the pelvis.

d. Braiding: crossed sidestep with one limb advancing alternately anteriorly and posteriorly across the other limb.

⚑ **Red Flag**

- Braiding should not be utilized with patients who have total hip precautions limiting adduction past midline.

Application Concepts

- A variety of intervention techniques are available to the clinician. Selection of the appropriate approach should be based upon the patient's goals and functional status as well as the clinician's ability to apply the concepts of the given approach.
- Due to the nature of neurological dysfunction, greater length of time and practice may be required to rehabilitate the patient.
- Motor control and motor learning are the basis upon which all rehabilitation is developed. It is essential to implement rehabilitation with an understanding of these concepts to ensure success and greatest possible return to independent function.
- The PTA must be aware of the influences that increase tone (heat, stress, etc.) for a given patient and attempt to avoid such triggers.
- Activities utilized with patients should mimic functional skills to the greatest degree possible in order to facilitate generalization and adaptation to the environments the patient will be functioning in following discharge from rehabilitation.

Conditions/Pathology/Diseases (CPD) with Intervention

Infectious Disorders

1. **Physical therapy management for all infectious disorders of the brain.**
   a. Symptomatic and supportive, including bed positioning, passive range of motion (PROM), skin care and safety measures if confusion is present.
   b. Clinician must know and follow standard precautions.

2. **Meningitis.**
   a. Basic information.
      (1) Inflammation of the meninges of the spinal cord or brain.

   (2) Etiology: bacterial or viral infection.
   (3) Patients with bacterial infection are usually sicker and experience a more rapid time course.

⚑ **Red Flag**

- If untreated, meningitis can result in seizures, coma and death.

   b. Medical management.
      (1) Bacterial: treat infective organism with antibacterial therapy.
      (2) Viral: treat symptoms.

3. **Encephalitis.**
   a. Basic information.
      (1) Severe inflammation of the brain.

(2) Etiology: viral (herpes simplex) or bacterial infection.

b. Clinical picture.
(1) Headache.
(2) Nausea and vomiting.
(3) Focal signs corresponding to area of brain involved.
(4) Seizures, coma and death.

c. Medical management.
(1) Bacterial: treat infected organism with antibacterial therapy.
(2) Viral: primarily symptomatic, but antiviral medication is available for herpes simplex virus.

4. Brain abscess.

a. Basic information.
(1) Localized infection in the brain.
(2) Etiology: encapsulated collection of pus accumulates in the brain.

b. Clinical picture.
(1) Signs of active infection: fever, chills and headache.
(2) Progression to focal neurological signs depending upon site of infection.

c. Medical management.
(1) Bacterial: treat infective organism with antibacterial therapy.
(2) Surgical drainage.

CNS Neoplasms

1. Classification.

a. Primary.
(1) Originate from cells found within the brain or spinal cord.
(2) Benign: may be operable or inoperable due to location.
(3) Malignant.

b. Secondary.
(1) Originate from cells outside the brain or spinal cord.
(2) Metastatic.

2. Clinical picture: dependent upon location of lesion.

a. Headache.
b. Mental and behavioral changes.
c. Motor, speech and/or language impairments.
d. Seizures.

3. Medical management: surgery, radiation therapy, chemotherapy and/or immunotherapy.

4. Physical therapy management.

a. Symptomatic and supportive.
b. Bed positioning, PROM, skin care, ambulation, assistive device assessment.

Degenerative Diseases of the CNS

1. Amyotrophic lateral sclerosis (ALS).

a. Basic information.
(1) Progressive upper and lower motor neuron disease.
(a) Amyotrophic: muscle fiber atrophy from peripheral nerve involvement.
(b) Degeneration and scarring of the motor neurons in the lateral aspect of the spinal cord, brainstem and cerebral cortex.
(2) Death usually results in 2–5 years due to respiratory compromise.

b. Clinical picture.
(1) Dependent upon upper and lower motor neuron and involvement.
(2) Eventually both upper motor neurons and lower motor neurons are involved.
(a) Lower motor neuron signs: asymmetrical, distal weakness with eventual progressive atrophy, facial weakness that results in difficulty with swallowing.
(b) Upper motor neuron signs: hyperactive tendon reflexes and spasticity.
(3) Cognition is not affected.
(4) Aerobic capacity and endurance progressively diminishes, with eventual respirator use required.
(5) Compromised cranial nerve integrity.
(6) Motor function progressively diminishes with eventual total dependency for mobility and ADL.

c. Medical management.
(1) There is no known cure.
(2) Medications to control symptoms, including drooling and spasticity.
(3) Aggressive respiratory management.

d. Physical therapy management.
(1) Symptomatic and supportive.
(2) Maintain ROM and prevent disuse atrophy.
(3) Teach energy conservation.
(4) Help patient maintain independence for as long as possible.
(5) Assess need for adaptive and assistive devices.
(6) Instruct the patient and caregiver in transfers, positioning and respiratory management (postural drainage, chest stretching).

↪ **Red Flag**
• Avoid overworking weakened, denervated muscles which can lead to more rapid breakdown of musculature and further limit the patient's function.

2. Multiple sclerosis (MS).

a. Basic information.
(1) Chronic, progressive demyelinating disease of the CNS with no known cure.

(2) Commonly affects young adults.

(3) Etiology is unknown, but most likely an autoimmune response to a virus.

(4) Demyelinating lesions (plaques) impair neural transmission and cause nerves to fatigue rapidly.

(5) Fluctuating periods.

(a) Relapse: worsening of symptoms.

(b) Remission: periods of decreased or no symptoms.

(c) May progress to permanent disability.

🏴 **Red Flag**

- During an acute relapse, exercise should be avoided. This is a direct contraindication to exercise.

(6) Categories.

(a) Relapsing-remitting MS.
- Cycles of exacerbation/remission with long periods of stability.
- May have minimal long-term impairment.

(b) Primary-progressive MS.
- Disease progresses from onset with no or occasional plateaus.
- May experience temporary, minor improvements.

(c) Secondary-progressive MS.
- Begins as relapsing-remitting MS.
- Turns into progressive course.

(d) Progressive-relapsing MS.
- Progressive course with acute relapses periodically.
- Loss of function and progressive worsening with each exacerbation.

b. Clinical picture.

(1) Dependent upon plaque sites.

(2) Early symptoms: paresthesias, diplopia and fatigue.

(3) Emotional dysregulation, mentation and cognition, including euphoria.

(4) Dysarthria and scanning speech.

(5) Sensory deficits: paresthesias, hyperpathia, dysesthesias, trigeminal neuralgia.

(6) Lhermitte's sign: electric shock–like sensation throughout the body produced by flexing the neck.

(7) Visual problems: diplopia, blurred vision, optic neuritis, scotoma (blind spot) and nystagmus.

🏴 **Red Flag**

- Ensure patient safety with functional skills given the prevalence of visual problems in patients with MS.

(8) Spasticity and hyperreflexia.

(9) Paresis.

(10) Impaired coordination: ataxia, intention tremors, dysmetria, dysdiadochokinesia.

(11) Vestibular dysfunction leading to impaired balance.

(12) Ataxia.

(13) Fatigue.

(a) Early afternoon fatigue and exhaustion common.

(b) High-energy periods in early morning.

(c) Some recovery in early evening.

(14) Impaired functional mobility skills.

c. Medical management.

(1) Corticosteroids shorten recovery during exacerbations.

(2) Avoid precipitating or exacerbating factors: infections, trauma, pregnancy and stress.

d. Physical therapy management.

(1) Minimize secondary complications.

(2) Maintain functional independence as much as possible.

(3) Manage fatigue/energy conservation.

(4) Patient and family education.

(5) Provide psychological and emotional support and encourage support group participation.

(6) Frenkel exercises.

(a) Coordination exercises performed in supine, sitting, standing and walking.

(b) Primarily for the LE but concepts can be applied to develop UE exercises.

(c) Progress from assisted independent and from unilateral to bilateral.

🏴 **Red Flag**

- Avoid factors that cause transient worsening of symptoms: heat, hyperventilation, dehydration, fatigue.

3. **Parkinson's disease (PD).**

a. Basic information.

(1) Chronic, progressive disease of the CNS.

(2) Basal ganglia disorder.

(a) Deficiency of dopamine and degeneration of the substantia nigra.

(b) Loss of inhibitory dopamine results in excessive excitatory output from cholinergic system of basal ganglia.

(3) Causes: commonly idiopathic but can also be infectious, atherosclerosis, toxic or drug induced.

b. Clinical picture.

(1) Slowly progressive with emergence of secondary impairments and permanent disability.

(2) Hoehn and Yahr classification system.

- I = Minimal or absent disability, unilateral symptoms.
- II = Minimal bilateral or midline involvement, no balance involvement.
- III = Impaired balance, some restrictions in activity.
- IV = All symptoms present and severe; stands and walks only with assistance.
- V = Confinement to bed or wheelchair.

(3) Common impairments: rigidity, bradykinesia, resting tremor, impaired postural reflexes.

(4) Mentation deficits: bradyphrenia (slowing of thought processes), depression and dementia in advanced stages.

(5) Communication.

  (a) Dysarthria.

  (b) Hypophonia (decreased speech volume) with mutism in advanced stages.

  (c) Masked face.

  (d) Micrographia: small writing.

(6) Musculoskeletal.

  (a) Contractures commonly present in flexors and adductors.

  (b) Persistent posturing in kyphosis with forward head.

  (c) Osteoporosis leading to high risk for fracture.

  ⚑ **Red Flag**

    • Since contracture development can lead to impaired posture, it is essential to include a stretching and positioning component in the rehabilitation program.

(7) Sensory impairments: abnormal cramp-like sensations that are poorly localized and perceptual deficits.

(8) Visual problems.

(9) Impaired skin integrity leading to decubitus ulcer development in later stages.

⚑ **Red Flag**

  • Ensure good patient and family education regarding positioning to avoid skin breakdown once the patient becomes wheelchair bound or bedridden.

(10) Impaired muscle tone/reflexes.

  (a) Rigidity (cogwheel or leadpipe).

  (b) Resting tremors that progress to intention tremors in later stages.

  (c) Pill-rolling tremor in hands.

(11) Impaired muscle strength associated with disuse and atrophy.

(12) Impaired motor control.

  (a) Bradykinesia: slowed movement.

  (b) Akinesia: absent movement/inability to initiate movement resulting in freezing episodes.

  (c) Slowed reaction time and movement time.

(13) Impaired balance and postural reactions.

(14) Festinating gait: shortened stride, decreased speed, increased cadence, decreased arm swing and trunk rotation.

(15) Impaired functional abilities.

(16) Decreased muscular and general body endurance.

 c. Medical management.

  (1) Levadopa/Sinemet (see Table 9–2).

  (2) Anticholinergic drugs for tremor control.

  (3) Surgery may be considered when medication does not control tremors and dyskinesia.

 d. Physical therapy management.

  (1) Prevent/minimize secondary complications.

  (2) Patient education on compensatory strategies.

  (3) Therapeutic exercise.

    (a) Improve rotational movements (PNF strategies).

    (b) Reduce rigidity.

    (c) Facilitate appropriate posture.

    (d) Flexibility exercises.

  (4) Functional mobility skills (i.e., rolling, supine to sit).

  (5) Relaxation strategies.

  (6) Improve balance, postural control and safety.

  (7) Improve cardiovascular endurance.

  (8) Energy conservation techniques.

  (9) Promote independence with ADL.

Cerebral Vascular Accident (CVA, Stroke)

1. **Basic information.**

 a. Sudden, focal neurological deficit resulting from ischemic or hemorrhagic lesions in the brain

 b. Etiologic categories.

  (1) Thrombus: formation or development of a blood clot within the cerebral arteries or their branches.

  (2) Embolus: traveling bits of matter (thrombi, tissue, fat, air, bacteria) that produce occlusion and infarction in the cerebral arteries.

  (3) Hemorrhage: abnormal bleeding as a result of rupture of a blood vessel.

    (a) Subarachnoid hemorrhage.

     • Blood between the arachnoid layer and the pia mater.

     • Most common causes: aneurysm and vascular malformations.

     • Symptoms depend upon location of the hemorrhage.

    (b) Subdural hemorrhage.

     • Blood between the dura mater and arachnoid layer.

     • Most often caused by trauma.

     • The body can reabsorb small volumes of blood but larger amounts must be surgically evacuated.

 c. Risk factors.

  (1) Atherosclerosis, hypercholesterolemia, hypertension and cardiac disease.

  (2) Diabetes.

  (3) Smoking, alcohol and drug abuse.

  (4) Transient ischemic attacks (TIAs).

    (a) Brief warning episodes of dysfunction lasting less than 24 hours.

(b) A precursor of major stroke in more than one-third of patients.

🏳 **Red Flag**

- Failure to educate patients on the risk factors associated with CVA could lead to an increased risk of additional insult.

d. Pathophysiology.
(1) Cerebral anoxia: lack of oxygen supply to the brain causing irreversible damage beginning 4–6 minutes after insult occurs.
(2) Cerebral infarction: irreversible cellular damage.
(3) Cerebral edema: accumulation of fluids within the brain; can result in elevated intracranial pressure and potential for herniation and death.

2. **Clinical picture.**
a. Syndromes (Table 3-22).
(1) Middle cerebral artery syndrome.
(2) Anterior cerebral artery syndrome.
(3) Posterior cerebral artery syndrome.
(4) Vertebrobasilar artery syndrome.
(5) Internal carotid artery syndrome.
b. Resting posture: initial tendency toward flaccidity, with progression to spasticity and abnormal resting postures.
c. Arousal, mentation and cognition.
(1) Impairments in orientation, attention, memory and ability to follow commands.
(2) Left versus right hemisphere lesions (Table 3-23).
(a) Patients with left hemisphere lesions (right hemiplegia) tend to be slow, cautious, insecure and hesitant.
(b) Patients with right hemisphere lesions (left hemiplegia) tend to be impulsive, quick, overestimate their ability and use poor judgment leading to safety concerns.

🏳 **Red Flag**

- Safety is a major concern with patients who have a right-sided CVA. Patients need to be taught safety awareness techniques, and family members should be educated in proper monitoring of the patient and environment for potential safety concerns.

(3) Emotional lability: tendency to cry or laugh easily and difficulty inhibiting same behavior.
d. Speech and communication impairments.
(1) Occur with damage to parieto-occipital cortex of the dominant hemisphere.
(2) Expressive dysfunction.
(a) Nonfluent aphasia (Broca's, expressive or motor aphasia).
- Occurs from damage to Broca's area.
- Results in speech that requires a great deal of effort to produce.
- When speech occurs, words are typically restricted, interrupted and awkward.

Table 3-22 ➤ CVA SYNDROMES

Anterior cerebral artery syndrome
Supplies medial part of the frontal and parietal lobe; basal ganglia and corpus callosum
- Contralateral sensory and motor loss with LE affected more than UE
- Mental impairment (confusion, amnesia, etc.)
- Urinary incontinence
- Apraxia (deficits in motor planning) affecting the ability to imitate movement and perform bimanual tasks
- Slow, delayed movement
- Lack of spontaneous movement
- Behavioral changes

Middle cerebral artery syndrome
Supplies lateral cerebral hemispheres, including frontal, temporal and parietal lobes
- Contralateral sensory motor loss, with face and UE affected more than LE
- Perceptual deficits
- Homonymous hemianopsia
- Broca's aphasia (expressive or motor aphasia)
- Wernicke's aphasia (receptive or sensory aphasia)
- Global aphasia

Posterior cerebral artery syndrome
Supplies occipital lobe, medial and inferior temporal lobe, thalamus and midbrain
- Contralateral sensory and motor loss
- Homonymous hemianopsia
- Visual agnosia, prosopagnosia and cortical blindness
- Oculomotor nerve palsy
- Involuntary movement
- Thalamic pain syndrome
- Pusher syndrome: pushing toward the paretic side in sitting, standing and when walking
- Involuntary movements (choreoathetosis, intention tremors and hemiballismus)

Vertebrobasilar artery syndrome
Supplies medulla, pons and cerebellum
- Wide variety of symptoms, both ipsilaterally and contralaterally
- Cranial nerve involvement (diplopia, dysphagia, dysarthria, deafness and vertigo)
- Ataxia
- Wallenberg's Syndrome (deficits in visual disturbances [nystagmus]; deficits in balance, gait coordination, temperature and pain sensation)
- Locked-in Syndrome (patient is awake and aware of their environment, however is unable to speak or control any muscles beyond the eyes; in complete locked-in syndrome the patient is unable to control eye movements)
- Complete basilar occlusion causes death as a result of ischemia to areas that control vital functions

Internal carotid artery syndrome
Supplies anterior cerebral artery and middle cerebral artery
- Complete occlusion results in extensive cerebral edema which causes coma and death
- Incomplete occlusion can cause a mixture of anterior and middle cerebral artery syndromes

(b) Verbal apraxia: impairment of voluntary articulation control.
(c) Dysarthria.
- Decreased ability to control movements of the jaw, tongue and respiratory structures needed for speech control.

Table 3-23 ➤ CVA SYNDROMES

Hemispheric Dysfunction

LEFT HEMISPHERE INJURY	STRATEGIES FOR THERAPEUTIC INTERVENTION
• Right side hemiplegia/paresis • Right side hemisensory loss • Speech-language impairments • Trouble planning/sequencing movement • Slow, cautious, anxious • Realistic in self-assessment • Communication is difficult • Can't do steps of task • Difficulty processing • Verbal cues are hard to process • Trouble expressing positive emotion	• Develop communication plan of words and gestures • Assess level of understanding • Give frequent feedback and support • Do not underestimate ability to learn

RIGHT HEMISPHERE INJURY	STRATEGIES FOR THERAPEUTIC INTERVENTION
• Left side hemiplegia/paresis • Left side hemisensory loss • Visual-perceptual deficits • Trouble sustaining movements • Quick and impulsive • Poor judgment; overestimates abilities • Safety is a concern • Can't put it all together • Abstract concepts are difficult • Visual cues are hard to process • Trouble perceiving emotions	• Use verbal cues; demonstrations or gestures may be confusing with presence of visual-perceptual deficits • Give frequent feedback • Focus on slowing down and controlling movements • Focus on safety • Avoid environmental clutter • Do not overestimate ability to learn

- Understand spoken language and use the correct words, but spoken words are difficult to understand.
  (3) Receptive dysfunction.
  (a) Fluent aphasia (Wernicke's or receptive aphasia).
    - Occurs from damage to Wernicke's area.
    - Spontaneous speech is preserved and fluent.
    - Auditory comprehension is severely impaired.
  (4) Global aphasia: combination of expressive and receptive aphasia resulting in major difficulty with both comprehension and production of language.
  e. Dysphagia: difficulty swallowing.
  ☞ **Red Flag**
    - Dysphagia can lead to aspiration, which places the patient at risk of respiratory distress or pneumonia. The clinician must be aware of specific diet restrictions the patient may have, including the thickness of liquids the patient is allowed to intake. Thin liquids increase risk.
  f. Sensory impairments.
  g. Perceptual dysfunction.
  h. Motor impairments.

(1) Muscle tone.
  (a) Flaccidity: transient decrease or lack of resistance to PROM occurring during a period of spinal shock immediately after injury.
  (b) Spasticity: increased resistance to PROM following spinal shock as function begins to return.
(2) Brunnstrom's Stages of Motor Recovery.
  (a) Stage 1: initial flaccidity, no voluntary movement.
  (b) Stage 2: emergence of spasticity, hyperreflexia, synergies (mass patterns of movement).
  (c) Stage 3: voluntary movement possible but only in synergies; spasticity at its peak.
  (d) Stage 4: voluntary control in isolated joint movements emerging, corresponding decline of spasticity and synergies.
  (e) Stage 5: increasing voluntary control out-of-synergy; coordination deficits present.
  (f) Stage 6: control and coordination near normal.
(3) Muscle performance impairments: decreased strength, power and endurance.
(4) Voluntary movement patterns.
  (a) Abnormal synergy patterns associated with cerebral stroke.
  (b) Ataxia and hypotonia associated with cerebellar stroke.
  (c) Extent of upper extremity and lower extremity involvement dependent upon extent of the infarct, etiology and vascular site.
i. Gait deficits (Table 3-24).
  (1) Trendelenburg's limp: lateral tilt to sound side resulting from weak hip abductors on the involved side.
  (2) Scissoring: results from spastic adductors.
  (3) Insufficient pelvic rotation during swing.
  (4) Equinus gait: heel does not touch down.
  (5) Varus foot: weight is borne on the lateral side of the foot.
  (6) Unequal step lengths.
  (7) Decreased cadence with uneven timing.

3. **Medical management.**
  a. Anticoagulation therapy for prevention: Coumadin, clot-busting medications.
  b. Surgical intervention: carotid endarterectomy.
  c. Tissue plasminogen activator (tPA).
    (1) Used to dissolve clots in the brain and restore blood flow.
    (2) Must be administered within 3 hours of insult to be effective; if administered via catheter into the brain, it can be used later.

4. **Physical therapy management.**
  a. Prevent or minimize secondary complications.
    (1) Positioning and PROM to prevent deformity and contracture development.

Table 3-24 ➤ COMMON GAIT DEVIATIONS SEEN IN PATIENTS WITH STROKE

HIP	
DEVIATION	**POSSIBLE CAUSES**
Retraction	Increased trunk and lower extremity muscle tone
Hiking	Inadequate hip and knee flexion, increased tone in the trunk and lower extremity
Circumduction	Increased extensor tone, inadequate hip and knee flexion, increased plantar flexion in the ankle or footdrop
Inadequate hip flexion	Increased extensor tone, flaccid lower extremity

KNEE	
DEVIATION	**POSSIBLE CAUSES**
Decreased knee flexion during swing	Increased lower extremity extensor tone, weak hip flexion
Excessive flexion during stance	Weakness or flaccidity in the lower extremity, increased flexor tone in the lower extremity
Hyperextension during stance	Hip retraction, increased extensor tone in the lower extremity, weakness in the gluteus maximus, hamstrings or quadriceps
Instability during stance	Increased lower extremity flexor tone, flaccidity, weakness of extensor muscles

ANKLE	
DEVIATION	**POSSIBLE CAUSES**
Footdrop	Increased extensor tone, flaccidity
Ankle inversion or eversion	Increased tone in specific muscle groups, flaccidity
Toe clawing	Increased flexor tone in the toe muscles

    (2) Maintain skin integrity.
    (3) Decrease shoulder pain.
       (a) Subluxation: caused by forces of gravity or traction and weakness of capsule and shoulder musculature.
       (b) Immobility can lead to adhesive capsulitis.
       (c) Poor dynamic stabilizers can lead to impingement syndrome.
       ➤ **Red Flag**
        • Poor handling techniques, such as pulling on the UE during transfers and PROM without scapular mobilization, can cause cumulative microtrauma that leads to increased shoulder pain.
  b. Promote awareness and use of hemiplegic side via tone-reducing activities (inhibition techniques) and facilitation of out-of-synergy, functional movements.
  c. Improve postural control and balance.
  d. Task-specific training utilizing goal-directed activities.
    (1) Focus on functional mobility skills: rolling, sitting, sit-to-stand, transfers, ambulation.
    (2) Develop practice schedules and utilize feedback to facilitate learning.

    (3) Focus on adapting movements to specific demands of the environment.
    (4) Utilize compensatory training when rehabilitation peaks.
  e. Promote independence with self-care and ADL.
  f. Improve respiratory and cardiovascular function.
    (1) Improve chest expansion and teach diaphragmatic breathing patterns.
    (2) Exercise training: cycle ergometry, walking.
  g. Muscle reeducation.
    (1) Biofeedback training.
       (a) Aids with increasing firing in paretic muscles and improving muscle control.
       (b) Helps to decrease firing in spastic muscles.
    (2) Functional electrical stimulation to stimulate muscle action and reduce spasticity.
  h. Constraint-induced movement therapy: "forced use" of the paretic extremity.
  ➤ **Red Flag**
    • Constraint-induced movement therapy should not be used until the subacute and chronic stages so as not to expand the area of injury.
  i. Provide emotional support to patient and family and encourage socialization.

Traumatic Brain Injury (TBI)

1. **Basic information.**
  a. Mechanism of injury is contact forces to skull and rotational acceleration forces causing varying degrees of injury to the brain.
  b. May be a focal lesion with a clinical presentation resembling hemiplegia or a diffuse lesion resulting in bilateral impairments.
  c. Types of head injury.
    (1) Open head injury: skull fracture and torn meninges with resultant brain exposure posing a risk of infection.
    (2) Closed head injury: no skull fracture or brain exposure but a risk of increased intracranial pressure exists.
    ➤ **Red Flag**
      • The clinician should be aware of the signs of increased intracranial pressure when working with a patient with a closed TBI. These include severe headache and rapid changes in level of consciousness.
  d. Pathophysiology.
    (1) Primary brain damage: due to forces on the brain at the time of impact.
      (a) Local brain damage: cerebral contusion, lacerations, swelling and herniation.
      (b) Coup-contracoup injury: injury occurring at point of impact and opposite point of impact with a high-velocity impact.

(c) Diffuse axonal injury.
- Disruption and tearing of axons and small blood vessels from shear-strain of angular acceleration.
- Results in neuronal death and petechial hemorrhages.
- Common causes: high-velocity impact and shaken baby syndrome.

(2) Secondary brain damage: changes due to the brain's reaction to trauma.

(a) Hypoxic-ischemic injury: results from systemic problems (cardiovascular and respiratory) that compromise cerebral circulation.

(b) Swelling/edema: can result in increased intracranial pressure and brain herniation (central, uncal or tonsilar).

(3) Concussion.

(a) Loss of consciousness, either temporary or permanent, resulting from head injury.

(b) Potential changes occur in HR, RR and BP.

(c) Extent of injury.

- Mild concussion: momentary loss of consciousness; retrograde amnesia.
- Classic concussion: transient loss of consciousness; mostly reversible in 24 hours; retrograde and posttraumatic amnesia.
- Severe concussion: loss of consciousness more than 24 hours; diffuse axonal injury and coma are present.

2. **Clinical picture.**

a. Arousal, mentation, cognition.

(1) Glasgow coma scale (GCS).

(2) Rancho Los Amigos level of cognitive functioning (LOCF) (Table 3-25).

(a) Outlines predictable sequence of cognitive and behavioral recovery.

(b) Eight levels of behavior.

(3) I = no response.

(4) II and III = decreased response levels.

(5) IV, V and VI = confused levels.

(6) VII and VIII = appropriate levels.

Table 3-25 ► LEVELS OF COGNITIVE FUNCTIONING (LOCF) RANCHOS LOS AMIGO	
LEVEL	**BEHAVIORS TYPICALLY DEMONSTRATED**
I	No responses. Patient appears to be in a deep sleep and is completely unresponsive to any stimuli.
II	Generalized response. Patient reacts inconsistently and nonpurposefully to stimuli in a nonspecific manner. Responses are limited and often the same regardless of stimulus presented. Responses may be physiologic changes, gross body movements, and/or vocalization.
III	Localized response. Patient reacts specifically but inconsistently to stimuli. Responses are directly related to the type of stimulus presented. May follow simple commands in an inconsistent, delayed manner, such as closing eyes or squeezing hand.
IV	Confused-agitated. Patient is in heightened state of activity. Behavior is bizarre and nonpurposeful relative to immediate environment. Does not discriminate among persons or objects; is unable to cooperate directly with treatment efforts. Verbalizations frequently are incoherent and/or inappropriate to the environment; confabulation may be present. Gross attention to environment is very brief; selective attentions often nonexistent. Patient lacks short-term and long-term recall.
V	Confused-inappropriate. Patient is able to respond to simple commands fairly consistently. However, with increased complexity of commands or lack of any external structure, responses are nonpurposeful, random, or fragmented. Demonstrates gross attention to the environment, but is highly distractible and lacks ability to focus attention to a specific task. With structure, may be able to converse on a social-automatic level for short periods of time. Verbalization is often inappropriate and confabulatory. Memory is severely impaired; often shows inappropriate use of objects; may perform previously learned tasks with structure but is unable to learn new information.
VI	Confused-appropriate. Patient shows goal-directed behavior, but is dependent on external input for direction. Follows simple directions consistently and shows carry-over for relearned tasks with little or no carry-over for new tasks. Responses may be incorrect due to memory problems but appropriate to the situation; past memories show more depth and detail than recent memory.
VII	Automatic-appropriate. Patient appears appropriate and oriented within hospital and home settings; goes through daily routine automatically, frequently robotlike with minimal-to absent confusion, but has shallow recall of activities. Shows carry-over for new learning, but at a decreased rate. With structure is able to initiate social or recreational activities; judgment remains impaired.
VIII	Purposeful and appropriate. Patient is able to recall and integrate past and recent events and is aware of and responsive to environment. Shows carry-over for new learning and needs no supervision once activities are learned. May continue to show a decreased ability relative to premorbid abilities, abstract reasoning, tolerance for stress, and judgment in emergencies or unusual

(a) Usually progress through levels in sequence and can plateau at any point.

(7) Amnesia.

    (a) Posttraumatic amnesia: inability to remember events occurring after the injury.

    (b) Retrograde amnesia: inability to remember events preceding the injury.

(8) Behavioral changes.

    (a) Inappropriate physical, verbal and sexual behaviors.

    (b) Irritable, easily frustrated.

    (c) Impulsivity with safety issues.

    (d) Depression.

b. Speech and communication impairments.

c. Sensory impairments and perceptual dysfunction.

d. Deconditioning from prolonged hospitalization.

e. Disuse atrophy, contractures and skin breakdown.

f. Motor impairments.

(1) Muscle tone.

    (a) Initial transient flaccidity with subsequent long-lasting spasticity.

    (b) Rigidity.

      • Decerebrate rigidity: UE and LE in extension; occurs with lesions of the brainstem.

      • Decorticate rigidity: UE in flexion and LE in extension; occurs with lesions above the brainstem.

⚐ Red Flag

  • The patient should always be placed out of obligatory synergy patterns in order to decrease the risk of contracture formation.

(2) Voluntary movement patterns.

    (a) Abnormal synergy patterns associated with cerebral lesion.

    (b) Ataxia and hypotonia associated with cerebellar lesion.

    (c) Extent of UE and LE involvement dependent upon extent of the infarct, etiology and vascular site.

g. Gait, locomotion and balance impairments will likely be bilateral.

3. Medical management.

a. Monitoring of intracerebral pressure.

b. Medication.

(1) Barbiturates to control cerebral edema and increased intracerebral pressure with severe injury.

(2) Botox or baclofen for spasticity.

(3) Various medications may be used for pain management.

c. Surgical intervention: hemorrhage or hematoma evacuation and decompression of skull.

4. Physical therapy management.

a. Issues to be addressed:

(1) Problems associated with acute rehabilitation:

    (a) Decreased arousal.

    (b) Development of secondary complications.

    (c) Poor understanding of injury and rehab by patient and family.

(2) Problems commonly associated with inpatient rehabilitation.

    (a) Decreased ROM and contracture development.

    (b) Posturing and increased tone.

    (c) Unresponsive or unaware of environment.

    (d) Primitive reflexes influence movement.

    (e) Decreased cardiovascular endurance.

    (f) Difficulty communicating.

b. Management with decreased response levels (LOCF I–III).

(1) Increase arousal and orientation.

    (a) Auditory, kinesthetic, visual and tactile stimulation.

    (b) Avoid overstimulation as patient may become agitated or shut down.

    (c) Avoid abstract concepts (humor, slang) that could be confusing to patient.

(2) Positioning.

    (a) PROM and proper positioning to decrease likelihood of contracture formation.

    (b) Static stretching or serial casting can be used to correct deformities.

    (c) Utilize positioning (side-lying and semi-prone) to inhibit the influence of primitive reflexes.

    (d) Prevent decubitus ulcer formation.

(3) Develop postural control.

    (a) Proximal stability (head and trunk control) before distal mobility.

    (b) Achieve a neutral pelvis, erect trunk and upright head.

    (c) Begin with manual contacts and maintained visual contact to assist with achievement of proper posturing.

    (d) Completing activities hand-over-hand provides both kinesthetic and proprioceptive feedback.

    (e) Utilize sitting activities to help orient patient to vertical and improve visual awareness of environment.

(4) Begin transfer training.

(5) Incorporate standing activities.

    (a) Lower extremity weight bearing helps slow development of osteoporosis.

    (b) Increases sensory input while completing ADL and functional tasks.

    (c) If necessary, begin with tilt table to slowly acclimate patient to upright standing.

(6) Patient and family education regarding PROM, sensory stimulation and positioning.

c. Management with mid-level recovery (LOCF IV–VI).

(1) Prevent overstimulation.

    (a) Maintain a calm and focused manner.

(b) Provide treatment in a closed environment: area with decreased distraction and minimal sensory stimuli (low lighting, quiet, etc.).

(c) Teach relaxation strategies.

(2) Provide consistency.

(a) Establish daily routine.

(b) Ensure all members of the team follow the behavior modification plan.

(c) Utilize clear feedback.

(d) Use daily journal or memory book to communicate with family.

(3) Utilize group treatment to facilitate peer modeling and reinforce appropriate behaviors.

(4) Plan multiple activities and allow patient some choice in selecting.

(5) Emphasize safety.

(6) Educate patient and family while preparing for discharge.

⮑ Red Flag

• Ensure safety of the patient and those around him/her if aggressive disinhibition (punching, biting, etc.) is present in patients at LOCF IV.

d. Management with high-level recovery (LOCF VII–VIII).

(1) Facilitate increasing independence.

(a) Begin working in open environments (community outings).

(b) Aid patient with reintegrating socially, cognitively and behaviorally.

(c) Patient and family education on socialization skills, behavioral control mechanisms and available support groups.

(2) Incorporate higher level balance activities, including protective and equilibrium reactions.

(3) Encourage cardiovascular conditioning and maintenance of an active lifestyle.

Spinal Cord Injury (SCI)

1. Basic information.

a. Partial or complete disruption of spinal cord resulting in paralysis, sensory loss, and altered autonomic function and altered reflex activity.

b. Spinal areas most frequently injured: C5, C7, T12 and Ll.

c. Traumatic causes: motor vehicle accident, falls, diving accidents, stab and gunshot wounds.

d. Nontraumatic causes: disc prolapsed, vascular insult, complications of osteoporosis or rheumatoid arthritis.

e. Mechanisms of injury.

(1) Flexion (most common lumbar injury).

(2) Flexion-rotation (most common cervical injury).

(3) Compression.

(4) Hyperextension.

f. Pathophysiology.

(1) Primary injury results in injury to the spinal cord and/or interruption of blood supply.

(2) Secondary sequelae: ischemia, edema, demyelination and/or necrosis of axons progressing to scar tissue formation.

2. Clinical picture.

a. Classification by level of injury: most distal uninvolved nerve root segment with normal function; muscles have a grade of at least 3+/5 or fair + function.

(1) Tetraplegia (quadriplegia).

(a) Injury occurs between C1 and C8 and involves all four extremities and trunk.

(b) Upper motor neuron injury.

(2) Paraplegia.

(a) Injury between TI and TI2-L1 involving both lower extremities and, to varying degrees, the trunk.

(b) Upper motor neuron injury.

(3) Cauda equina lesion.

(a) Lesion occurs below L1.

(b) Lower motor neuron injury.

b. Classification by degree of injury.

(1) Complete: no sensory or motor function below the level of lesion.

(2) Incomplete: preservation of some sensory or motor function below the level of injury (Table 3-26).

Table 3-26 ➤ TYPES OF INCOMPLETE SPINAL CORD INJURY

TYPE OF INCOMPLETE SPINAL CORD INJURY	DESCRIPTION OF KEY VARIABLES
Brown-Sequard Syndrome • Injury site: one half of spinal cord	• Loss of motor function, proprioception and vibration sense on side of injury. • Loss of pain and temperature on side opposite of injury.
Anterior cord syndrome • Injury site: anterior spinal cord or anterior spinal artery	• Loss of motor function, pain and temperature below the level of injury. • Retention of position sense and vibration below the level of injury.
Central cord syndrome • Injury site: center of the spinal cord	• More severe involvement of upper extremities than lower extremities. • Sensory deficits vary. • Bowel, bladder and sexual function may be spared. • Ambulation may be possible even with severely impaired upper extremity involvement.
Posterior cord syndrome • Rare • Injury site: posterior spinal cord or posterior spinal artery	• Loss of proprioception and vibration below the injury site. • Retention of motor function and pain perception below the injury site.

From O'Sullivan S, Schmidt T: Physical Rehabilitation: Assessment and Treatment, 4th ed, F.A. Davis, 2001, pg 893, with permission.

c. Spinal shock.
   (1) Transient period of reflex depression and flaccidity lasting several hours or up to 24 weeks.
   (2) Replaced by spasticity.
d. Spasticity.
   (1) More likely to develop with incomplete lesions.
   (2) Will not occur with cauda equina lesions (lower motor neuron lesions).
   (3) Irritating stimuli that may increase tone.
      (a) Blocked catheter.
      (b) Tight clothing or orthotic straps.
      (c) Environmental temperature.
      (d) Infection.
      (e) Decubitus ulcers.
e. Autonomic dysreflexia (hyperreflexia).
   (1) Occurs in patients with a spinal cord lesion above T6.
   (2) Emergency situation in which a noxious stimulus precipitates a pathologic autonomic reflex.
   (3) Symptoms.
      (a) Paroxysmal hypertension.
      (b) Bradycardia.
      (c) Headache.
      (d) Diaphoresis.
      (e) Flushing.
      (f) Diplopia.
      (g) Convulsions.
   (4) Management.
      (a) Elevate head.
      (b) Check for irritating stimuli (blocked catheter, tight ankle-foot orthosis [AFO]).
      (c) Treat as a medical emergency.

      ⚐ Red Flag
      • Failure to recognize the presence of autonomic dysreflexia can lead to drastic increases in blood pressure. If the patient's head is not elevated and the noxious stimuli removed, this places the patient at risk of CVA.

f. Heterotopic ossification.
   (1) Abnormal bone growth in the soft tissue.
   (2) Usually present in hips and knees.
   (3) Initial signs: swelling, pain, erythema and stiffness.
   (4) May lead to joint ankylosis if calcification occurs.

   ⚐ Red Flag
   • Care should be taken not to damage surrounding structures with PROM or stretching in the presence of heterotopic ossification.

g. Deep vein thrombosis (DVT).
   (1) Previously a test called the Homan's sign may have been used by the clinician to help determine the presence of a DVT. This test has since been shown to lack specificity and sensitivity and is likely not widely used.

   ⚐ Red Flag
   • The clinician must know the signs of DVT to decrease the risk of a pulmonary emboli occurring. These signs include dull ache, erythema and edema in the location of the DVT. If a DVT in the calf is suspected, the clinician should immediately notify the appropriate medical staff (inpatient—nurse; outpatient—physician, etc.).

h. Spinal cord dysesthesia.
   (1) Results from noxious stimuli (urinary tract infection [UTI], spasticity, bowel impaction, smoking).
   (2) TENS can be used to help decrease or resolve pain.
i. Bowel and bladder dysfunction.
   (1) UTIs are the most frequent complication of SCI.
   (2) Lesions above S2-4.
      (a) Result in a spastic or reflexive bladder.
      (b) Emptying is manually triggered by cutaneous stimuli (stroking the lower abdomen or pulling the pubic hairs).
   (3) Lesions of the cauda equina.
      (a) Result in a flaccid bladder.
      (b) Empty bladder by increasing intra-abdominal pressure (Valsalva's or Crede's maneuver).
   (4) Reflex bowel management programs involve high-fiber diet, suppositories and digital stimulation.
j. Sexual dysfunction.
   (1) Lesions above the cauda equina allow reflexive function that responds to physical stimulation.
   (2) Lesions of the cauda equina allow for psychogenic function that requires cognitive stimulation.
   (3) Both men and women retain the ability to reproduce.

3. **Medical management.**
a. Medication to limit posttraumatic ischemia and address secondary complications (spasticity, DVT, etc).
b. Fracture stabilization.
   (1) Surgical stabilization.
      (a) Restore alignment of the bony structures.
      (b) Decompress neural tissue.
      (c) Stabilize the spine to prevent further damage.
      (d) Improve potential for earlier mobilization.
   (2) Orthotic stabilization.
      (a) Cervical: halo is the most common but may see semirigid/rigid collars.
      (b) Thoracic/lumbar: thoracolumbosacral orthosis.
   (3) Combined surgical and orthotic stabilization.

4. **Physical therapy management.**
a. Reorient patient to vertical position using tilt table and wheelchair with use of an abdominal binder

and/or elastic lower extremity wraps to decrease venous pooling.

🏳 **Red Flag**
  • Check for signs and symptoms of orthostatic hypotension when beginning.

b. Improve cardiovascular endurance.
   (1) UE cycle ergometry.
   (2) Functional wheelchair activity training.
   (3) Functional electrical stimulation/LE ergometry.

   🏳 **Red Flag**
   Absolute contraindications to exercise (from the American College of Sports Medicine).
     • Autonomic dysreflexia.
     • Severe or infected skin on weight-bearing surfaces.
     • UTI.
     • Uncontrolled spasticity or pain.
     • Unstable fracture.
     • Insufficient ROM to perform exercises.
     • Uncontrolled hot or humid environment.

c. Improve respiratory capacity and functioning.
   (1) Respiratory function improves dramatically with full intercostal innervation.
   (2) Deep breathing exercises.
   (3) Respiratory muscle strengthening.
   (4) Proper respiratory hygiene: assisted cough, postural drainage, percussion, vibration and suctioning.

d. Integumentary integrity.
   (1) Maintain skin free of decubitus ulcers and other injury by maintaining proper schedule for positioning changes.
   (2) Pressure-relieving devices: wheelchair cushions and tilt-in-space wheelchair.
   (3) Patient education on pressure relief activities (push-ups, weight shifting) and proper skin inspection.

e. Maintain ROM and limit contracture formation via PROM and positioning.

🏳 **Red Flag**
  • Certain muscles may need strengthening, while others need to be allowed to shorten in order to preserve function via passive insufficiency (i.e., tenodesis grip).

f. Improve strength of all remaining innervated muscles.
   (1) Use selective strengthening during acute phase to reduce stress on spinal segments and increase function.
   (2) Resistive training to hypertrophy muscles in rehabilitation phase.

g. Promote maximum mobility in home and community environment.
   (1) Promote early return of functional mobility skills.
      (a) Emphasis on independent rolling and bed mobility.
      (b) Assumption of sitting.
      (c) Transfers.
      (d) Ambulation as indicated.
   (2) Improve sitting tolerance, postural control, symmetry and balance.
   (3) Promote wheelchair skills and independence in managing wheelchair parts.
   (4) Community reintegration outings.

h. Facilitate ambulation ability (Table 3-27).
   (1) Nonfunctional ambulators.
      (a) Stand to assist with transfers and bear weight on LE.
        • Relieve pressure on buttocks.
        • Allows weight bearing through LE bones.
        • Cardiopulmonary work.
      (b) Lesions of upper to mid-thoracic region.
   (2) Functional ambulators.
      (a) Ambulate independently in the home, with or without assistive device.
      (b) Lesions of low-thoracic region.
   (3) Community ambulators.
      (a) Ambulate throughout home and community, with or without device.
      (b) Must be able to do all components of community ambulation safely (cross street in appropriate time, ascend and descend stairs/curbs).
      (c) Lesions of lumbar region.

i. Provide psychological and emotional support.
   (1) Encourage socialization and motivation.
   (2) Promote independent problem solving, self-direction.

j. Provide patient and family education with focus on strategies to prevent skin breakdown, maintaining ROM, and strengthening to increase function.

Seizures

1. **Basic information: abnormal electrical event in the brain.**

2. **Clinical picture.**
   a. Partial seizures: focal lesions.
      (1) Simple partial seizures.
         (a) Consciousness is maintained.
         (b) Seizure is localized to one hemisphere.
      (2) Complex partial seizures.
         (a) Consciousness is altered or lost.
         (b) Both hemispheres involved.
         (c) Partial seizure secondarily generalized.
         (d) Partial or complex seizure transitions to tonic-clonic generalized seizure.
   b. Generalized seizures.
      (1) Diffuse EEG abnormalities with no evidence of localized onset.

Table 3-27 ➤ SCI FUNCTIONAL TABLE

NERVE ROOT LEVEL AND KEY MUSCLES INNERVATED	KEY MOVEMENTS AVAILABLE	ADL SUMMARY	W/C MOBILITY	TRANSFERS AND GAIT
C1–C3 • Face and neck	• Mouth and head	• Talking • Chewing • Sipping • Blowing	• Powered w/c with breath or chin control • Ventilator	• Total dependence • Respirator
C4 • Diaphragm • Trapezius	• Respiration • Scapular elevation	• Increased ability to use assistive devices that utilize scapular/head and mouth movement	• Power w/c with mouth or chin control	• Total dependence
C5 • Biceps • Deltoid	• Elbow flexion • Shoulder external rotation • Shoulder abduction to 90 degrees	• Self feeding • Some self care with UE assistive devices	• Powered w/c with hand controls • Limited manual w/c propulsion	• Can assist with transfers
C6 • Pectoralis major • Extensor carpi radialis • Teres major	• Shoulder flexion • Wrist extension	• Tenodesis grasp • Bed mobility with rails • Independent with pressure relief weight shifts	• Independent with manual w/c with projections • Will likely still use power w/c due to fatigue	• May be independent with sliding board transfers
C7 • Triceps • Latissimus dorsi • Extrinsic finger extensors • Flexor carpi radialis	• Elbow extension • Wrist flexion • Finger extension	• Independent living possible • Independent with: lateral push-up pressure relief • LE dressing • LE self-ROM	• Independent transfers	• Independent manual w/c propulsion
C8–T1 • Flexor carpi ulnaris • Extrinsic and intrinsic hand muscles	• Full innervation of upper extremities	• Full independence in activities requiring primarily UE use	• Negotiation of 2-4 inch curbs and wheelies in w/c	• Independent in w/c transfers
T1–T8 • Top half of intercostals	• Improved respiratory control	• Same as C8-T1 with improved respiratory and trunk control	• Negotiation of 6 inch curbs	• T6-T8 physiological standing with orthoses in parallel bars
T9–T12 • Abdominals	• Good trunk control	• Independence in all ADLs from a w/c level	• Independent	• Household ambulation with Bilateral KAFOs and assistive device
T12	• Same	• Same	• Will use w/c for primary means of mobility	• Community ambulation with Bilateral KAFOs and assistive device • No hip flexor function
L1, L2 • Quadratus lumborum • Iliopsoas and sartorius	• Hip hiking • Weak hip flexion	• Same	• Same	• Can be independent in community ambulation with Bilateral KAFOs and assistive devices
L3–L5 • L3-L4 iliopsoas strong • L4-L5 quadriceps, medial hamstrings strong	• Hip flexion • Knee extension	• Same	• Same • May continue to use w/c for efficient mobility	• Ambulation with bilateral AFOs and canes possible • No gluteus maximus function
S1–S2 • Plantar flexors • Gluteus maximus	• Plantar flexion • Hip extension	• Same	• Same	• May ambulate with articulated AFOs

(2) Absence seizure (old term: petit mal).
  (a) Conscious activity suddenly stops.
  (b) Mild motor manifestations may be present.
(3) Myoclonic seizure: repetitive muscle contractions in one part or the whole body.
(4) Atonic seizure: loss of consciousness without tonic muscular contractions.

(5) Tonic-clonic seizure (formerly called grand mal).
  (1) Loss of consciousness.
  (2) Cycling between rigidity (tonic) and rapid jerky movements (clonic).
c. Epilepsy.
  (1) Chronic disorder of recurrent seizures.

(2) Status epilepticus.
   (a) Continual, unprovoked recurrent seizures (>30 minutes).
   (b) Most common cause is sudden cessation of antiseizure medications.

☞ **Red Flag**
- Status epilepticus is a medical emergency and emergency procedures must be activated.
- Patients with seizures or epilepsy can have long-term neurological impairments from recurrent seizure activity.

3. **Medical management.**
  a. Medication: Dilantin, Tegretol, Valium, Klonopin.
  b. Surgical intervention: lobe resection or hemispherectomy.

4. **Physical therapy management.**
  a. Immediate management.
   (1) Protect from injury.
    (a) Stay with patient.
    (b) Assist to a surface that will prevent a fall.
    (c) Remove dangerous objects from the area.
    (d) Remove restrictive clothing but do not restrain limbs.
   (2) Roll onto side: may keep airway clear and prevent aspirating vomit.

☞ **Red Flag**
- It is important not to restrict the patient's movement or place anything in the patient's mouth.
  b. Monitoring.
   (1) Vital signs.
   (2) Note time and length of seizure and physical manifestations.
  c. Status epilepticus.
   (1) Medical emergency.
   (2) Prolonged seizing can lead to irreversible brain damage.
   (3) Patient/family education on proper medication usage.
  d. Promote routines for physical activity and emotional health.

Peripheral Nervous System (PNS) Disorders

1. **Basic information.**
  a. Pathology.
   (1) Wallerian degeneration: degeneration of the axon and myelin sheath distal to the site of axonal interruption.
   (2) Segmental demyelination: axons are preserved and remyelination restores function.
   (3) Axonal degeneration: degeneration of axon and myelin sheath.
  b. Neuropathies (peripheral neuropathy).
   (1) Overview.
    (a) Degenerative changes in peripheral nerves that produce sensory loss and motor weakness.
    (b) Caused by nutritional deficiencies, diabetes and alcohol abuse.
   (2) Mononeuropathy: involvement of a single nerve.
   (3) Polyneuropathy.
    (a) Bilateral symmetrical involvement of peripheral nerves, usually LEs more than UEs.
    (b) Stocking/glove distribution: distal segments earlier and more involved than proximal.
  c. Radiculopathy: involvement of nerve roots due to skeletal changes (soft tissue injuries).
  d. Traumatic nerve injury.
   (1) Neurapraxia (Class I).
    (a) Injury to nerve that causes a transient loss of function (e.g., compression).
    (b) Nerve dysfunction may be rapidly reversed or persist a few weeks.
   (2) Axonotmesis (Class 2).
    (a) Injury to nerve interrupting the axon and causing loss of function and degeneration distal to the lesion (e.g., crush injury).
    (b) Regeneration is possible.
   (3) Neurotmesis (Class 3).
    (a) Cutting of the nerve with severance of all structures and complete loss of function.
    (b) Reinnervation typically fails without surgical intervention.
  e. Entrapment syndrome.
   (1) Pressure on a nerve where it passes over a bony prominence or restricted opening.
   (2) Results in motor and sensory disturbances in the area distribution of the nerve.

2. **Clinical picture.**
  a. Symptoms.
   (1) Weakness/paresis of denervated muscle, hyporeflexia and hypotonia; rapid atrophy; fatigue.
   (2) Sensory loss corresponding to motor loss.
   (3) Autonomic dysfunction leading to vasodilation and loss of vasomotor tone (dryness, warm skin, edema).
   (4) Hyperexcitability of remaining fibers.
    (a) Sensory dysesthesias (hyperalgesia, paresthesias, burning).
    (b) Spasms and fasiculations.
   (5) Myalgia with inflammatory myopathies.
  b. Bell's palsy (facial paralysis).
   (1) Lower motor neuron (LMN) lesion involving the facial nerve (CNVII) resulting in unilateral facial paralysis.
   (2) Etiology: acute inflammatory process of unknown etiology resulting in compression of the nerve within the temporal bone.
   (3) Characteristics.

(a) Muscles of facial expression on one side are weakened or paralyzed.

(b) Loss of control of salivation or lacrimation.

(c) Sensation is normal.

(d) Onset is acute with maximum severity in few hours or days.

(e) Most recover fully in several weeks or months.

(4) Medical management: corticosteroids and analgesics.

(5) Physical therapy management.

(a) Electrical stimulation to maintain tone and support function of facial muscles.

(b) Provide active facial muscle exercises.

(c) Provide emotional support and reassurance.

↠ **Red Flag**

- Instruct patient not to "overdo it," as the nerve needs to rest.

c. Guillain-Barré syndrome (GBS).

(1) Polyneuritis with progressive muscular weakness that develops rapidly.

(2) Etiology.

(a) Unknown, but associated with an autoimmune attack.

(b) Usually occurs after recovery from an infectious illness.

(c) Evolves over a few days or weeks with slow recovery (months to a year) back to or near full functioning.

(3) Pathology: acute demyelination of both cranial and peripheral nerves.

(4) Clinical picture.

(a) Aerobic capacity and endurance may be severely limited, especially with pulmonary involvement.

(b) Integumentary integrity.

- Pain and paresthesias.
- Typically less sensory involvement than motor.

(c) Motor function.

- Motor paresis or paralysis: relative symmetrical distribution or weakness.
- Progresses from lower extremities to upper and from distal to proximal.
- May produce full tetraplegia with respiratory failure.
- Not uncommon to have residual bilateral foot-drop.

(d) Potential complications.

- Autonomic dysfunction.
- Respiratory failure and risk of pneumonia.
- Myalgia.
- Relapse.

(5) Physical therapy management.

(a) Ascending phase: patient is becoming weaker as the disease progresses.

- Monitor for signs of respiratory failure, increasing P_{CO_2}.
- Use pulse oximetry for O_2 saturation monitoring.
- Follow standard precautions to prevent infection.
- Facilitate coughing and airway clearance.
- Prevent indirect impairments associated with immobilization.
- Passive range of motion within pain tolerance.
- Positioning.
- Prevent injury to denervated muscles.

(b) Stabilization phase: early rehabilitation.

- Begins when patient is stable and no longer getting worse.
- Therapeutic pool or Hubbard's tank provides a medium to facilitate low-stress exercise.

↠ **Red Flag**

- Avoid overstretching and overuse of denervated muscles.

(c) Descending phase: beginning of extensive rehabilitation.

- Paralysis recedes and function returns.
- Provide muscle reeducation.
- PNF techniques: start with active and progress to resistive exercise.
- Functional training as recovery progresses.
- Teach energy conservation techniques and activity pacing.
- Improve cardiovascular fitness following prolonged bed rest and deconditioning.
- Provide emotional support and reassurance to patient and family.

↠ **Red Flag**

- Avoid overuse and fatigue, as this may prolong recovery.

d. Myasthenia gravis.

(1) Autoimmune neuromuscular disease.

(a) Decreased acetylcholine receptors.

(b) Ineffective postsynaptic membrane stimulation and poor transmission at the neuromuscular junction.

(2) Clinical picture.

(a) Fluctuating weakness.

- Increases with repeated muscle contractions.
- Usually affects eye movements or eyelids first.
- Progresses to oropharyngeal, facial, proximal and respiratory muscles.

(b) More noticeable in the proximal muscles.

- Muscles of trunk and extremities become involved in advanced cases.
- Ocular, facial and bulbar muscles commonly involved.

(c) Difficulty with swallowing.

(d) Usually improves with rest and anti-cholinesterase drugs.

(e) Variable course: some rapidly progressive with early death, and others with remissions and exacerbations.

⚑ Red Flag

• Myasthenic crisis is a life-threatening weakness of the respiratory muscles and requires immediate medical attention.

(f) Functional mobility skill difficulty: climbing stairs, rising from a chair, lifting.

(3) Physical therapy management.

(a) Monitor vital signs.

(b) Promote independence in functional mobility skills.

(c) Teach energy-conservation techniques.

(d) Promote optimal activity, with rest as indicated.

(e) Provide psychological and emotional support.

e. Postpolio syndrome.

(1) New onset of weakness and severe fatigue occurring an average of 25 years after recovery from acute poliomyelitis.

(2) Clinical picture.

(a) Severe long-lasting fatigue out of proportion with activity level and not relieved with rest.

(b) New onset of muscle weakness in muscles previously thought to be strong.

(c) New loss of functional abilities due to weakness.

(d) Slow, steady progression of dysfunction.

(e) Difficulty in concentration, memory and attention.

(f) Poor aerobic capacity.

(3) Physical therapy management.

(a) Aerobic capacity and endurance.

• Submaximal exercise can maintain and improve endurance.

• Maintain respiratory function via deep breathing exercises and postural drainage.

• Instruct in energy conservation techniques.

• Teach relaxation exercises to facilitate full relaxation periods.

(b) Strengthening exercises.

• Overuse will increase fatigue and joint pain.

• Partially denervated muscles will not respond to strengthening as innervated muscles would.

• Aquatic exercises programs can minimize fatigue with strengthening.

⚑ Red Flag

• Because of the concerns with overuse, the patient should stop exercising if pain, fatigue and/or weakness increase.

(c) Patient and family education regarding lifestyle modifications.

(d) Psychological support and reassurance.

f. Trigeminal neuralgia (tic douloureux).

(1) Neuralgia resulting from degeneration or compression of the trigeminal nerve (CNV).

(2) Clinical picture.

(a) Brief periods of stabbing and/or shooting pain along the nerve distribution.

(b) Autonomical dysfunction exacerbated by stress or cold and relieved by relaxation.

(c) May see increase in pain with chewing, talking, brushing teeth or movement of air across the face.

(3) Medical management: pain medication or surgery to section or permanently anesthetize nerve.

(4) Physical therapy management.

(a) TENS for pain relief.

(b) Symptomatic and supportive.

Application Concepts

• The PTA will likely be called upon to provide psychological support and reassurance with a variety of patients. It is important for the clinician to develop comfort in doing so.

• It is important for the PTA to know what type of medical management will be used with each diagnosis in order to determine the impact of such interventions on the rehabilitation of the patient.

• When possible, activities completed in rehabilitation should be active on the part of the patient to instill a sense of independence and success.

• The key to a successful rehabilitation program is patient education and developing functional activities based on the patient's goals.

Painful Neurological Conditions

Complex Regional Pain Syndrome (CRPS)

1. **An abnormal response of a peripheral nerve.**
   a. Previously known as reflex sympathetic dystrophy (RSD).
   b. Painful condition that can develop following trauma to a nerve.
   c. The process of the pathology is thought to facilitate or inhibit an overreaction of the sympathetic nervous system (SNS). Some studies show CNS dysfunction as well.
      (1) Injury at one somatic level initiates efferent activity of the sympathetic system affecting multiple levels.

2. **Variations.**
   a. CRPS I: painful syndrome developing following trauma to an area, no overt nerve injury.
      (1) Trauma may be planned (e.g., following shoulder surgery) or unplanned (e.g., following a fall on a knee).
   b. CRPS II: painful nerve syndrome developing following trauma to a peripheral nerve; also called *causalgia*.

3. **Etiology.**
   a. Origin may come from a variety of conditions.
      (1) Surgery.
      (2) Upper motor neuron (UMN) lesion secondary to a brain injury.

      (3) Cerebrovascular accident (CVA, the shoulder-hand syndrome occasionally seen following CVA).
      (4) Destructive lesion of CNS.
      (5) LMN disorder following peripheral nerve injury, neuropathies, entrapments.

4. **Clinical picture.**
   a. Begins with localized pain that is described as a burning sensation that occurs spontaneously; the level of pain is in excess of the stimulus.
   b. The syndrome progresses in three stages (Table 3-28).
   c. Manifestations of the stages.
      (1) Sensory impairments.
         (a) Pain that is out of proportion to the level of injury or insult.
            • Allodynia: touch that is typically non-painful (e.g., light touch, air movement, wearing a shirt) is interpreted as pain.
            • Hyperalgesia: increased level of sensitivity, lower pain threshold.
      (2) Vasomotor/thermal changes.
      (3) Tissue changes.
      (4) A progression of changes in the skin from dry and warm, to moist, to cool.
         (a) Trophic changes begin with increased hair and nail growth and progress to thin skin, loss of hair and thin, ridged nails.

Table 3-28 ➤ COMPLEX REGIONAL PAIN SYNDROME: CLINICAL STAGES

STAGE	TIME FRAME	TYPICAL SIGNS AND SYMPTOMS
Stage I	Begins up to 10-12 days following injury; lasts 1-6 months	Increasing pain that is characterized as burning or aching, is more severe than would be expected, pain response is generated by stimulus that is typically not painful. May present with edema. Affected limb is cooler or warmer. Skin: dry, increased hair growth, increased nail growth.
Stage II	Lasts approximately 3-6 months	Pain: worsens; is constant, burning, and aching. Abnormal painful sensations remain present; e.g. allodynia, hyperalgesia, hyperpathia. Edema spreads, causes joint stiffness. Skin: thin, glossy, cool, sweaty (hyperhydrosis); continued nail changes. Osteoporosis may be starting.
Stage III	Lasts up to 12 months and may continue after that.	Pain continues, may plateau. Edema hardens and continues to limit ROM. Muscles atrophy, contractures may be present. Skin: continued altered texture and temperature; fascia thickens potentially causing contractures. Osteoporosis and ankylosis progress. Depression may be a problem.

(5) Bone demineralization and ankylosis are major concerns.

(6) Edema.

5. Medical management.

a. Diagnosis is made by history and clinical examination; often delayed.

b. Diagnostic tests are aimed at determining secondary changes due to the CRPS.

(1) Radiography, thermography and Doppler flowmetry studies.

c. Limited or weak evidence for the effectiveness of:

(1) Stellate ganglion blocks or sympathectomy.

(2) Acupuncture.

(3) Corticosteroids and nonsteroidal anti-inflammatory drugs (NSAIDS).

(4) Amytriptyline to relieve depression and aid in sleep.

(5) Calcium channel blockers to help improve peripheral circulation.

d. Better evidence for the use of:

(1) Long-term intrathecal baclofen.

(2) Implanted dorsal column stimulation.

(a) Has been shown to help decrease pain perception and intensity.

6. Physical therapy management.

a. Education focusing on encouraging patient to use involved extremity or area as normally as possible.

b. Modalities for pain relief.

(1) Most effective when used in early stages.

(2) TENS is reported to be minimally effective.

(a) May be some evidence for high- and low-frequency stimulation application to the contralateral side.

c. Pool therapy may provide a medium to encourage movement, especially when the lower extremity is involved.

CHAPTER 3

chapter 4

Cardiac, Vascular and Lymphatic Physical Therapy

SUSAN B. O'SULLIVAN

Focus Areas for Content Review:

- Anatomy and physiology of the cardiac, vascular and lymphatic systems.
- Pathologies and conditions of the cardiac, vascular and lymphatic systems commonly seen in physical therapy.
- Physical therapy interventions; indications and contraindications, appropriate responses, PTA response to adverse reaction, effects of interventions on the cardiac, vascular and lymphatic systems.

- Cardiac, vascular and lymphatic systems tests and measures indicating patient ability to participate in and/or indication to discontinue intervention as well as to document the patient's progress toward the established goals.
- Principals of progression of intervention activities as related to cardiac, vascular and lymphatic systems conditions commonly encountered in physical therapy.

Anatomy and Physiology of the Cardiac, Vascular and Lymphatic Systems

The Heart and Circulation

1. Heart tissue.
   a. Pericardium: fibrous protective sac surrounding the heart.
   b. Epicardium: inner layer of the pericardium.
   c. Myocardium: heart muscle, major portion of the heart.
   d. Endocardium: smooth lining of the inner surface and cavities of the heart.

2. Heart chambers: four chambers arranged in pairs, functioning as pumps, working in sequence.
   a. Right atrium (RA): receives blood from systemic circulation, from the superior and inferior vena cavae.
   b. Right ventricle (RV): receives blood from the RA and pumps blood via the pulmonary artery to the lungs for oxygenation.
   c. Left atrium (LA): receives oxygenated blood from the lungs and the four pulmonary veins.
   d. Left ventricle (LV): receives blood from the LA and pumps blood via the aorta throughout the entire systemic circulation; walls of LV are thicker and stronger than the RV and form most of the left side and apex of the heart.

3. Heart valves.
   a. Atrioventricular valves: prevent backflow of blood into the atria during ventricular systole; valves close when ventricular walls contract.
      (1) Tricuspid valve (three cusps or leaflets): right heart valve.
      (2) Bicuspid valve or mitral valve (two cusps or leaflets): left heart valve.
   b. Semilunar valves: prevent backflow of blood from the aorta and pulmonary arteries into the ventricles during diastole.
      (1) Pulmonary valve: prevents right backflow.
      (2) Aortic valve: prevents left backflow.

4. Cardiac cycle: the rhythmic pumping action of the heart.
   a. Systole: the period of ventricular contraction. End-systole volume is the amount of blood in the ventricles after systole, about 50 mL.
   b. Diastole: the period of ventricular relaxation and filling of blood. End-diastole volume is the amount of blood in the ventricles after diastole, about 120 mL.
   c. Atrial contraction occurs during the last third of diastole and completes ventricular filling.

5. Coronary circulation.

a. Arteries: arise directly from aorta near aortic valve; blood circulates to myocardium during diastole.

(1) Right coronary artery (RCA): supplies right atrium, most of right ventricle and in most individuals the inferior wall of the left ventricle, atrioventricular node (AV) and bundle of His; 60% of the time supplies the sinoatrial (SA) node.

(2) Left coronary artery (LCA): supplies most of the left ventricle; has two main divisions:

(a) Left anterior descending artery (LAD): supplies the left ventricle and interventricular septum and in most individuals the inferior areas of the apex; it may also give off branches to the right ventricle.

(b) Circumflex artery (Circ): supplies blood to the lateral and inferior walls of the left ventricle and portions of the left atrium; 40% of the time supplies SA node.

b. Veins: parallel the arterial system; the coronary sinus receives venous blood from the heart and empties into the right atrium.

c. Distribution of blood supply varies from individual to individual.

6. Conduction.

a. Specialized conduction tissue: allows rapid transmission of electrical impulses in the myocardium (normal sinus rhythm, NSR).

(1) Nodal tissue.

(2) Purkinje fibers: specialized conducting tissue in both ventricles.

b. Sinoatrial (SA) node.

(1) Located in junction of superior vena cavae and right atrium.

(2) Main pacemaker of the heart, initiates the impulse.

(3) Has sympathetic and parasympathetic innervations affecting both the heart rate and strength of contraction.

c. Atrioventricular (AV) node.

(1) Located at the junction of the right atrium and right ventricle.

(2) Has sympathetic and parasympathetic innervations.

(3) Merges with bundle of His.

d. Purkinje tissue.

(1) Right and left bundle branches of the AV node are located on either side of intraventricular septum.

(2) Terminate in Purkinje fibers, specialized conducting tissue of the ventricles.

e. Conduction of heart beat.

(1) Origin is in the SA node; impulse spreads throughout both atria which contract together.

(2) Impulse stimulates AV node, is transmitted down the bundle of His to the Purkinje fibers; impulse spreads throughout the ventricles which contract together.

7. Myocardial fibers.

a. Muscle tissue: striated muscle fibers but with more numerous mitochondria; exhibits rhythmicity of contraction; fibers contract as a unit.

b. Myocardial metabolism is essentially aerobic; sustained by continuous oxygen delivery from the coronary arteries.

c. Smooth muscle tissue is found in the walls of the blood vessels.

8. Hemodynamics.

a. Stroke volume (SV): the amount of blood ejected with each myocardial contraction, about 70 mL.

b. Cardiac output (CO): the volume of blood discharged from the left or right ventricle per minute; approximately 4–6 L per minute in average adult.

c. Left ventricular end-diastolic pressure (LVEDP): pressure in the left ventricle during diastole.

d. Ejection fraction (EF): percentage of blood emptied from the ventricle during systole.

e. Atrial filling pressure: the difference between the venous and atrial pressures.

f. Diastolic filling time is decreased with increased heart rate with heart disease.

g. Myocardial oxygen demand (MVO_2) represents the energy cost to the myocardium.

(1) MVO_2 is increased with activity and increases with HR and/or BP.

Vascular System

1. Arteries: transport oxygenated blood from the heart. They decrease in size and become arterioles eventually ending as capillaries. Arteries have contractile abilities.

a. Arterial walls are thicker in order to tolerate strong blood flow pressures from the heart.

b. Influenced by elasticity and extensibility of vessel walls and by peripheral resistance, amount of blood in body.

c. Change in diameter when triggered by sympathetic activity of the autonomic nervous system (ANS), vasoconstriction or vasodilation.

2. Capillaries: minute blood vessels that connect the ends of arteries (arterioles) with the beginning of veins (venules).

a. Functions for exchange of nutrients and fluids between blood and tissues.

b. Capillary walls are thin, permeable.

3. Veins: transport dark, unoxygenated blood from peripheral tissues back to the heart.

a. Veins have larger capacity and thinner, weaker walls than arteries; greater number.

b. Veins have a one-way valve to prevent backflow of blood because they do not have contractile abilities.
  (1) Veins rely on movement of the surrounding muscles to squeeze blood back to the heart.
  (2) Venous reflux occurs when these valves do not function properly because of veins that are enlarged or weakened.
c. Venous system includes both superficial and deep veins (deep veins accompany arteries while superficial do not).
d. Venous circulation influenced by muscle contraction, gravity, respiration (increased return with inspiration), compliancy of right heart.

Lymphatic System

1. **The lymph system drains lymph from body tissues and returns it to the venous circulation.**
  a. Lymph travels from lymphatic capillaries and lymphatic vessels, through lymph nodes, to the right lymphatic and thoracic ducts before being returned to the bloodstream through the subclavian veins.
    (1) The lymph nodes contain macrophages to phagocytize (digest) bacteria and other pathogens.
    (2) Major lymph nodes are submaxillary, cervical, axillary, mesenteric, iliac, inguinal, popliteal and cubital.
  b. Lymph vessels rely on external forces, e.g., movement, muscle contraction, respiration, to pump fluid through the system. Lymph flow is also influenced by massage and gravity.
  c. Contributes to immune system response by digesting cellular debris and bacteria and producing antibodies.

Neurohumoral Influences

1. **Parasympathetic stimulation (cholinergic). This system aids in the body's recovery following sympathetic system activity.**
  a. Control located in medulla oblongata, cardio-inhibitory center.
  b. Via vagus nerve (CNX), cardiac plexus; innervates all myocardium; releases acetylcholine.
    (1) Slows rate and force of myocardial contraction; decreases myocardial metabolism.
    (2) Causes coronary artery vasoconstriction.

2. **Sympathetic stimulation (adrenergic). This system increases the body's cardiovascular, respiratory and neurologic system functions (fight-or-flight response).**
  a. Control located in medulla oblongata, cardio-acceleratory center.
  b. Via cord segments T1-4, upper thoracic to superior cervical chain ganglia; innervates all but ven-

tricular myocardium; releases epinephrine and norepinephrine.
  (1) Causes an increase in the rate and force of myocardial contraction and myocardial metabolism.
  (2) Causes coronary artery vasodilation.
c. The skin and peripheral vasculature receive only post ganglionic sympathetic innervations.
  (1) Causes vasoconstriction of cutaneous arteries; sympathetic inhibition must occur to obtain vasodilation.
d. Drugs that are used to stimulate sympathetic activity are called *beta-adrenergic agents;* drugs that are used to decrease sympathetic activity are called *beta-adrenergic blocking agents* (beta-blockers).

3. **Additional control mechanisms.**
  a. Baroreceptors (pressoreceptors): main mechanisms controlling heart rate.
    (1) Located in walls of aortic arch and carotid sinus, via vasomotor center.
    (2) Circulatory reflex: respond to changes in blood pressure.
      (a) Increased blood pressure (BP) results in parasympathetic stimulation, decreased rate and force of cardiac contraction; sympathetic inhibition, decreased peripheral resistance.
      (b) Decreased BP results in sympathetic stimulation, increased heart rate, blood pressure and vasoconstriction of peripheral blood vessels.
      (c) Increased right atrial pressure causes reflex acceleration of heart rate.
  b. Chemoreceptors.
    (1) Located in the carotid body.
    (2) Sensitive to changes in blood chemicals: O_2, CO_2, lactic acid.
      (a) Increased CO_2 or decreased O_2 or decreased pH (elevated lactic acid) results in an increase in heart rate.
      (b) Increased O_2 levels result in a decrease in heart rate.
  c. Body temperature.
    (1) Increased body temperature causes heart rate to increase.
    (2) Decreased body temperature causes heart rate to decrease.
  d. Ion concentrations changes' effect on the heart.
  Red Flag: These conditions pose a significant threat to the patient's response to and ability to participate in physical therapy interventions.
    (1) Hyperkalemia (increased potassium): ECG changes (widened PR interval and QRS, tall T waves), tachycardia (potentially leading to bradycardia), potential cardiac arrest.
    (2) Hypokalemia (decreased potassium): ECG changes (flattened T waves, prolonged PR and QT

intervals), hypotension, arrhythmias may progress to ventricular fibrillation.

(3) Hypercalcemia (increased calcium): hypertension, signs of heart block, cardiac arrest.

(4) Hypocalcemia (decreased calcium): arrhythmias, hypotension.

(5) Hypernatremia (increased sodium): hypertension, tachycardia, pitting edema, excessive weight gain.

(6) Hyponatremia (decreased sodium): hypotension, tachycardia.

4. Peripheral resistance.

a. Increased peripheral resistance increases arterial blood volume and pressure.

b. Decreased peripheral resistance decreases arterial blood volume and pressure.

c. Influenced by arterial blood volume: viscosity of blood and diameter of arterioles and capillaries.

Highlights—Cardiovascular System

- Four main arteries supply the different chambers of the heart. Interruption in any of the arteries can set off a cascade of cardiac events.
- Heart rhythm is controlled by specialized electrical conduction tissue within the myocardium, nodal tissue. Interruption in normal sinus rhythm can cause minor as well as significant cardiac events.
- The sympathetic and parasympathetic systems control vascular responses to activity, medications and changes in blood chemistry and volume.
- The vascular system is influenced by neurohumoral changes. Medications can be used to affect the vascular system thus, manage cardiovascular responses.
- Changes in ion (sodium, potassium, calcium, magnesium) concentration levels can significantly affect the cardiovascular system.

Cardiovascular System Assessment and Data Collection Techniques

The physical therapist assistant (PTA) must be aware of and be able to perform cardiac system data collection techniques to assess a patient's ability to participate in and respond to intervention. The PTA is also responsible to educate the patient throughout the rehabilitation process. The examination procedures and facts contained in this section fall within the scope of work for a physical therapist assistant and warrant review in preparation for the licensure examination and for practice.

Risk Factors

1. Positive risk factors (ACSM Risk Stratification in ACSM's Guidelines for Exercise Testing and Prescription, 7th ed, Philadelphia, Lippincott Williams & Wilkins, 2006).

a. Hypercholesterolemia.

b. Hypertension.

c. Cigarette smoking.

d. Impaired fasting glucose: fasting blood glucose of ≥110 mg/dL.

e. Obesity: persons with body mass index (BMI) of ≥30 kg/m^2 or waist girth of > 88–102 cm (35–40 inches).

(1) Persons with BMI of 25–29.9 kg/m^2 are considered overweight.

(2) BMI does vary depending on sex, race, age and athletic condition of the individual; comparisons across these spectrums can- not be made.

(3) Waist girth measurements male versus female with associated risk.

(a) Male waist girth measurements: >94 cm (37 inches) = increased risk and >102 cm (40 inches) = substantially greater risk for cardiac problems.

(b) Female waist girth measurements: >80 cm (31 inches) = increased risk and >88 cm (35 inches) = substantially greater risk for cardiac problems.

f. Sedentary life style.

g. Family history.

2. Negative risk factors.

a. High serum high-density lipoprotein (HDL) cholesterol: >60 mg/dL.

3. Other risk factors.

a. Past medical history: other diagnoses, surgeries, medications.

b. Social history: current living situation, family/social support, education level, employment, life style, risk factors.

c. Social habits: smoking, diet.

d. Past and present level of activity.

Pulse

1. Pulse: rhythmical throbbing of arterial wall as a result of each heartbeat; note rate and rhythm.

a. Influenced by force of contraction, volume and viscosity of blood, diameter and elasticity of vessels, emotions, exercise, blood temperature and hormones.

2. Palpate pulses; palpate for 30 seconds with regular rhythm, 1–2 minutes with irregular rhythm. **Red Flag: Use finger tips to palpate pulse; never use thumb.**
   a. Apical pulse or point of maximal impulse (PMI): patient is supine, palpate at fifth interspace, midclavicular vertical line (apex of the heart; may be displaced upward by pregnancy or high diaphragm; may be displaced laterally in congestive heart failure, cardiomyopathy, ischemic heart disease.
   b. Radial: palpate radial artery, radial wrist at base of thumb; most common monitoring site.
   c. Carotid: patient is lying down with head of bed elevated; palpate over carotid artery, on either side of anterior neck between sternocleidomastoid muscle and trachea.
      (1) Assess one side at a time to reduce the risk of bradycardia through stimulation of the carotid sinus baroreceptor which produces a reflex drop in pulse rate or blood pressure.
   d. Brachial: palpate over brachial artery, medial aspect of the antecubital fossa; used to monitor blood pressure. Best in infants.
   e. Femoral: palpate over femoral artery in inguinal region.
   f. Popliteal: palpate over popliteal artery, behind the knee with the knee slightly flexed.
   g. Pedal: palpate over dorsalis pedis artery, dorsal medial aspect of foot; used to monitor lower extremity circulation.

3. **Determine heart rate (HR).**
   a. Normal adult HR is 70 beats per minute (bpm); range 60–80 bpm.
   b. Pediatric: newborn average is 120 bpm; normal range 70–170 bpm.
   c. Tachycardia: >100 bpm. Exercise commonly results in tachycardia. Compensatory tachycardia can be seen with volume loss (surgery, dehydration).
   d. Bradycardia: <60 bpm.
   e. **Red Flag:** Rate of perceived exertion scale may be more appropriate than HR as measure of actual work (Box 4-1).

4. **Identify pulse abnormalities.**
   a. Irregular pulse: variations in force and frequency; may be due to arrhythmias, myocarditis.
   b. Weak, thready pulse: may be due to low stroke volume, cardiogenic shock.
   c. Bounding, full pulse: may be due to shortened ventricular systole and decreased peripheral pressure; aortic insufficiency.

Heart Sounds

1. **Auscultation: the process of listening for sounds within the body; stethoscope is placed directly on chest. Note intensity and quality of heart sounds.**

Box 4-1 ➤ BORG RATE OF PERCEIVED EXERTION SCALE

6 No exertion at all
7 Extremely light
8
9 Very light (easy walking slowly at a comfortable pace)
10
11 Light
12
13 Somewhat hard (quite an effort; patient feels tired but can continue)
14
15 Hard (heavy)
16
17 Very hard (very strenuous; patient is very fatigued)
18
19 Extremely hard (cannot continue for long at this pace)
20 Maximal exertion

2. **Auscultation landmarks:**
   a. Aortic valve: locate the 2nd right intercostal space at the sternal border.
   b. Pulmonic valve: locate the 2nd left intercostal space at the sternal border.
   c. Tricuspid valve: locate the 4th left intercostal space at the sternal border.
   d. Mitral valve: locate the 5th left intercostal space at the midclavicular area.

3. **S1 sound ("lub"): normal closure of mitral and tricuspid valves; marks beginning of systole. Decreased in first-degree heart block.**

4. **S2 sound ("dub"): normal closure of aortic and pulmonary valves; marks end of systole. Decreased in aortic stenosis.**

5. **Murmurs: extra sounds.**
   a. Systolic: falls between S1 and S2. May indicate valvular disease (e.g., mitral valve prolapse) or may be normal.
   b. Diastolic: falls between S2 and S1. Usually indicates valvular disease.
   c. Grades of heart murmurs: grade 1 (softest audible murmur) to grade 6 (audible with stethoscope off the chest).
   d. Thrill: an abnormal tremor accompanying a vascular or cardiac murmur; felt on palpation.

6. **Bruit: an adventitious sound or murmur (blowing sound) of arterial or venous origin; common in carotid or femoral arteries; indicative of atherosclerosis.**

7. **Gallop rhythm: an abnormal heart rhythm with three sounds in each cycle; resembles the gallop of a horse.**

Heart Rhythm

1. **Measured via electrocardiogram (ECG): 12-lead ECG provides information about rate, rhythm,**

conduction, areas of ischemia and infarct, hypertrophy, electrolyte imbalances.

2. **Normal cardiac cycle (normal sinus rhythm).**
   a. P wave: atrial depolarization.
   b. P-R interval: time required for impulse to travel from atria through conduction system to Purkinje fibers.
   c. QRS wave: ventricular depolarization.
   d. ST segment: beginning of ventricular repolarization.
   e. T wave: ventricular repolarization.
   f. QT interval: time for electrical systole.

3. **Calculate heart rate: count number of intervals between QRS complexes in a 6-second strip and multiply by 10.**

4. **Assess rhythm: regular or irregular.**

5. **Identify arrhythmias (dysrhythmias): abnormal, disordered rhythms.**
   a. Etiology: ischemic conditions of the myocardium, electrolyte imbalance, acidosis or alkalosis, hypoxemia, hypotension, emotional stress, drugs, alcohol, caffeine.
   b. Ventricular arrhythmias: originate from an ectopic focus in the ventricles (outside the normal conduction system).
      (1) Significant in adversely affecting cardiac output; ventricular fibrillation is a pulseless, emergency situation requiring emergency medical treatment: cardiopulmonary resuscitation (CPR), defibrillation, medications.
      (2) Premature ventricular contractions (PVCs): a premature beat arising from the ventricle; occurs occasionally in the majority of the normal population. On ECG: no P wave; a bizarre and wide QRS that is premature, followed by a long compensatory pause. Serious PVCs: >6 per minute, paired or in sequential runs, multifocal, very early PVC (R on T phenomena).
      (3) Ventricular tachycardia: a run of three or more PVCs occurring sequentially; very rapid rate (150–200 bpm); may occur paroxysmally (abrupt onset); usually the result of an ischemic ventricle. On ECG: wide, bizarre QRS waves, no P waves. Seriously compromised cardiac output.
      (4) Ventricular fibrillation: chaotic activity of ventricle originating from multiple foci; unable to determine rate. On ECG: bizarre, erratic activity without QRS complexes. No effective cardiac output; clinical death within 4–6 minutes.
   c. Atrial arrhythmias (supraventricular): rapid and repetitive firing of one or more ectopic foci in the atria (outside the sinus node).
      (1) On ECG, P waves are abnormal (variable in shape) or not identifiable (atrial fibrillation).
      (2) Rhythm may be irregular: chronic or occurring paroxysmally.

   (3) Rate: rapid with atrial tachycardia (140–250 bpm), atrial flutter (250–350 bpm); fibrillation (>300 bpm).
   (4) Cardiac output is usually maintained; may precipitate ventricular failure.
   d. Atrioventricular blocks: abnormal delays or failure to conduct through normal conducting system.
      (1) First-, second- or third- (complete) degree AV blocks; bundle branch blocks.
      (2) If ventricular rate is slowed, cardiac output decreased.
      (3) Third-degree, complete heart block is life threatening; requires medications (atropine), surgical implantation of pacemaker.
   e. **Red Flag:** careful consideration should be given to the specific arrhythmia prior to a patient's participation in physical therapy intervention.

6. **Holter monitoring: continuous ambulatory ECG monitoring via tape recording of cardiac rhythm for up to 24 hours.**
   a. Used to evaluate cardiac rhythm, transient symptoms, pacemaker function and effect of medications.
   b. Allows correlation of symptoms with activities (activity diary).

Blood Pressure (BP)

1. **Measure blood pressure (2003 Joint National Committee on Prevention, Detection, Evaluation and Treatment of High Blood Pressure Guidelines) (Table 4-1).**
   a. Normal adult BP: <120 mm Hg systolic; <80 mm Hg diastolic.
   b. Prehypertension: 120–139 mm Hg systolic; 80–89 mm Hg diastolic.
   c. Hypertension:
      (1) Stage 1: 140–159 mm Hg systolic; 90–99 mm Hg diastolic.
      (2) Stage 2: >160 mm Hg systolic; >100 mm Hg diastolic.
      (3) Majority of patients with hypertension are asymptomatic.
   d. Hypotension: a decrease in BP below normal; blood pressure is not adequate for normal perfusion/

Table 4-1 ➤ BLOOD PRESSURE CLASSIFICATION— ADULTS

CLASSIFICATION	SYSTOLIC BLOOD PRESSURE	DIASTOLIC BLOOD PRESSURE
Normal	<120 mm Hg	<80 mm Hg
Prehypertension	120–139	80–89
Stage 1 hypertension	140–159	90–99
Stage 2 hypertension	≥160	≥100

oxygenation of tissues. May be related to bed rest, drugs, arrhythmias, blood loss/shock or myocardial infarction (MI).

   e. Orthostatic hypotension: sudden drop in BP that accompanies change in position.
     (1) Take BP in lying (5 minutes). Repeat BP at 1 and 3 minutes after moving into standing or sitting position.
     (2) Common symptoms include light-headedness, dizziness and loss of balance.
     (3) Drop in systolic BP of >20 mm Hg or standing BP <100 mm Hg systolic BP is significant and should be reported.

   f. Pediatric BP.
     (1) Infants less than 2 years (95 percentile): 106–110 systolic; 59–63 diastolic.
     (2) Children 3–5 years: 113–116 systolic, 67–74 diastolic.

⮡ **2. Red Flag: Rate of Perceived Exertion scale may be more appropriate than BP as measure of actual work (see Box 4-1).**

Respiration

1. Determine rate, depth of breathing.
   a. Normal adult respiratory rate (RR) is 12–20 breaths per minute.
   b. Pediatric: newborn RR is between 30–60 breaths per minute.
   c. Tachypnea: an increase in rate of breathing, >20 breaths per minute.
   d. Hyperpnea: an increase in depth and rate of breathing.

2. Dyspnea: shortness of breath.
   a. Dyspnea on exertion (DOE): brought on by exercise or activity.
   b. Orthopnea: inability to breathe when in a reclining position.
   c. Paroxysmal nocturnal dyspnea (PND): sudden inability to breathe occurring during sleep.
   d. Dyspnea Scale:
     +1 mild, noticeable to patient but not observer.
     +2 mild, some difficulty, noticeable to observer.
     +3 moderate difficulty, but can continue.
     +4 severe difficulty, patient cannot continue.

3. Auscultation of the lungs: assess respiratory sounds:
   a. Normal breath sounds.
   b. Assess for adventitious sounds:
     (1) Crackles (rales): rattling, bubbling sounds; may be due to secretions in the lungs.
     (2) Wheezes: whistling sounds.

4. Assess cough: productive or nonproductive.

Measure Oxygen Saturation

1. Use pulse oximetry, an electronic device that measures the degree of saturation of hemoglobin with oxygen (SaO_2).

2. Provides an estimate of PaO_2 based on the oxyhemoglobin desaturation curve.

3. Hypoxemia: abnormally low amount of oxygen in the blood.

4. Hypoxia: low oxygen level in the tissues.
   a. Normal oxygen saturation is 98%, with no change during activity or exercise.
   b. Terminate activity if oxygen saturation drops below 90% for a healthy individual or below 86% for an individual with chronic lung disease.

Assess Pain

1. Chest pain may be cardiac or noncardiac in origin.

2. Ischemic cardiac pain (angina or myocardial infarction): diffuse, retrosternal pain; or a sensation of tightness, achiness, in the chest; associated with dyspnea, sweating, indigestion, dizziness, syncope, anxiety.
   a. Angina: sudden or gradual onset; occurs at rest or with activity; precipitated by physical or emotional factors, hot or cold temperatures; relieved by rest or nitroglycerin.
   b. Myocardial infarction pain: sudden onset; pain lasts for more than 30 minutes; may have no precipitating factors; not relieved by medications.
   c. Anginal Scale:
     1+ light, barely noticeable.
     2+ moderate, bothersome.
     3+ severe, very uncomfortable.
     4+ most severe pain ever experienced.
⮡ d. **Red Flag:** any complaints of pain resembling these symptoms should always be immediately regarded and reported to the appropriate individuals, e.g., physical therapist, nurse, physician.

3. Referred pain:
   a. Cardiac pain can refer to shoulders, arms, neck or jaw.
   b. Pain referred to the back can occur from dissecting aortic aneurysm.

Application Concept

Data Collection and the Patient with Cardiovascular System Conditions
- Perform tests to determine current cardiac conditions prior to, during and after physical therapy intervention.

- Determine patient heart rate via peripheral pulse, palpate with finger tips; may also be monitored through monitoring devices if the patient is in a cardiac unit or acute care environment.
- Note the quality of the pulse: weak, thready, bounding, regular or irregular, etc.
- Identify if pulse is within normal limits for this patient. Consider: age, medications. Also consider whether it is an appropriate reaction to intervention.
- Review the heart rhythm if patient is attached to ECG and recognize patterns that limit intervention.

- Take blood pressure; recognize norms, as well as appropriate and inappropriate changes based on intervention.
- Recognize signs and symptoms of intolerance to interventions.
- If a patient is taking certain cardiac medications they can artificially mask the patient's true HR and BP response during exercise. Use of the Borg RPE Scale may provide a more accurate representation of the patient's effort or work with activity.

Peripheral Vascular System Assessment and Data Collection Techniques

The physical therapist assistant must be aware of and be able to perform some vascular system data collection to assess a patient's ability to participate in and tolerance for physical therapy intervention. The examination procedures and facts contained in the section fall within the scope of knowledge for a physical therapist assistant and warrant review in preparation for the licensure examination and for practice. Though it is unlikely that the assistant will perform the tests listed in this section, it is important for patient care to know the implications of the results of these tests.

Observe and Assess Condition of Extremities

1. **Red Flag: Observe conditions listed below and recognize when changes of these conditions warrant modification or discontinuation of physical therapy intervention.**
   a. The PTA needs to know when immediate attention of the nurse or physician is required and when notification of the physical therapist is indicated.

2. **Observe for diaphoresis: excess sweating associated with decreased cardiac output.**

3. **Check arterial pulses: decreased or absent pulses associated with peripheral vascular disease (PVD); check bilaterally.**
   a. Lower extremity: position patient supine, check femoral, popliteal, dorsalis pedis, posterior tibial pulses. The PTA should be aware of these pulses, however may not routinely use these pulse points for monitoring patient response to intervention.
   b. Upper extremity: check radial, brachial and carotid pulses. The physical therapist assistant should be able to readily assess a patient using these pulse points.

c. Grading scale:
   4+ Bounding, very strong.
   3+ Normal, easy to palpate.
   2+ Diminished, palpable but not normal.
   1+ Weak pulse, difficult to palpate.
   0 Absent, unable to palpate.

4. **Observe skin color; use color changes to determine patient's response to intervention.**
   a. Cyanosis: bluish color related to decreased cardiac output or cold, especially lips, fingertips, nail beds.
   b. Pallor: absence of rosy color in light-skinned individuals, associated with decreased peripheral blood flow, PVD.
   c. Rubor: dependent redness with PVD.

5. **Palpate skin temperature.**

6. **Observe common skin changes that are associated with some cardiovascular conditions.**
   a. Clubbing: curvature of the fingernails with soft tissue enlargement at base of nail: associated with chronic oxygen deficiency, heart failure.
   b. Pale, shiny, dry skin, with loss of hair, associated with PVD.
   c. Abnormal pigmentation, ulceration, dermatitis, gangrene, associated with PVD.
   d. Temperature: decrease in superficial skin temperature is associated with poor arterial perfusion.

7. **Observe for and identify intermittent claudication: pain, cramping and fatigue occurring during exercise and relieved by rest, associated with PVD.**
   a. Related to arterial insufficiency: pain is typically in calf; may also be in thigh, hips or buttocks.
   b. Patient may experience pain at rest with severe decrease in arterial blood supply; typically in forefoot, worse at night.

8. Observe for and measure edema.
   a. Check girth measurements using a tape or volumetric measurements using a volumeter (useful with irregular body parts, such as hand or foot).
   b. Pitting edema (indentation): depression is maintained when finger is pressed firmly; grading scale:
   Mild   1+ <1/4" depth of depression.
   Moderate   2+ 1/4" to 1/2" depth of depression.
   Severe   3+ 1/2" to 1" depth of depression.
   c. Bilateral edema is associated with congestive heart failure.
   d. Unilateral edema is associated with local factors, thrombophlebitis, PVD.

Tests of Peripheral Venous Circulation

1. **Percussion test: determines competence of greater saphenous vein.**
   a. In standing, palpate one segment of vein while percussing vein approximately 20 cm higher.
   b. If pulse wave is felt by lower hand, the intervening valves are incompetent.

2. **Trendelenburg's test (retrograde filling test): determines competence of communicating veins and saphenous system.**
   a. Patient is positioned in supine with legs elevated to 60 degrees (empties venous blood).
   b. Tourniquet is then placed on proximal thigh (occludes venous flow in the superficial veins).
   c. Patient is then asked to stand.
   d. Examiner notes if veins fill in normal pattern; should take approximately 30 seconds.

3. **Doppler ultrasound: examination using an ultrasonic oscillator connected to earphones. The physical therapist assistant would not be responsible to perform this test, though should understand what it is.**
   a. Determines blood flow within a vessel; useful in both venous and arterial disease.
   b. Doppler probe placed over large vessel; ultrasound signal given transcutaneously; movement of blood causes an audible shift in signal frequency.
   c. Useful in locating nonpalpable pulses, measuring systolic BP in extremities.

4. **Air plethysmography (APG): pneumatic device calibrated to measure patency of venous system; volume.**

Tests of Peripheral Arterial Circulation

The physical therapist assistant may not be responsible to perform the tests in this section; however he or she should understand what they are and what the results indicate.

1. **Rubor of dependency. Check color changes in skin during elevation of foot followed by dependency (seated, hanging position).**
   a. With insufficiency, pallor develops in elevated position; reactive hyperemia (rubor of dependency) develops in dependent position.
   b. Changes that take longer than 30 seconds are also indicative of arterial insufficiency.

2. **Venous filling time. Check time necessary to refill veins after emptying.**
   a. With patient supine, leg elevated about 60° for 1 minute, then placed in dependent position. Note time for veins to refill.
   b. Greater than 10-15 seconds is indicative of arterial insufficiency.

3. **Examine for intermittent claudication: exercise-induced pain or cramping in the legs that is absent at rest. Usually calf pain, but may also occur in buttock, hip, thigh or foot.**
   a. Have the patient walk on level grade, 1 mile/hour, e.g., treadmill. Test is stopped with claudicatory pain.
   b. Note time of test. Use subjective ratings of pain to classify degree of claudication.
   Grade I: minimal discomfort or pain.
   Grade II: moderate discomfort or pain; patient's attention can be diverted.
   Grade III: intense pain; patient's attention cannot be diverted.
   Grade IV: excruciating and unbearable pain.
   c. Check for coldness, numbness or pallor in the legs or feet; loss of hair over anterior tibial area.
   d. Leg cramps may also result from diuretic use with hypokalemia.

Examine Lymphatic System

1. **Palpate superficial lymph nodes: cervical, axillary, epitrochlear, superficial inguinal.**

2. **Inspect for and measure edema. It is within the scope of the PTA to perform and record these data-collection procedures.**
   a. Visual inspection: note swelling, decreased range of motion, loss of functional mobility.
   b. Check girth measurements.

3. **Paresthesias may be present.**

4. **Lymphangiography (x-ray of lymph vessels) using radioactive agents.**
   a. Medical examination, not performed by physical therapy clinicians.
   b. Provides information about lymph flow, lymph node uptake and backflow.

Application Concepts

The PTA should recognize tests of peripheral venous circulation and tests of arterial circulation; however it generally falls outside the scope of a PTA to perform such tests. The PTA should, however:

- Recognize abnormal test results.
- Identify consequences of abnormal results and modify intervention as appropriate if necessary.

Diagnostic Tests

⚐ **Red Flag:** The physical therapist assistant should have an understanding of what these tests are; however he or she will not be required to perform them or interpret results.

Chest X-ray

1. Will reveal abnormalities of lung fields, overall cardiac shape and size (cardiomegaly), aneurysm.

Electrocardiogram (EKG, ECG)

1. Used to examine heart rhythm, heart rate, conduction delays and coronary perfusion.

2. Monitored in the room on a stationary monitor or via telemetry (radio transmission); telemetry allows continuous monitoring during physical activity.

3. ECG interpretation can be done by qualified clinicians. Changes in the ECG reading are indicative of the type of heart pathology the patient is experiencing.

Myocardial Perfusion Imaging

1. Used to diagnose and evaluate ischemic heart disease, myocardial infarction.

2. Can identify: areas or ischemia or infarct, myocardial blood flow, areas of stress-induced ischemia (exercise test), old infarcts.

Echocardiogram

1. Noninvasive test that uses ultrasound to visualize internal structures (size of chambers, movement of valves, septum, abnormal wall movement, left ventricular function).

2. Ejection fraction (EF, the amount of blood emptied from the ventricle during systole) can be measured; average 60-70%.

3. Stress echo an echocardiogram is performed during a stress test; provides information comparing left ventricular (LV) function and wall motion at rest and during exercise. The stress test is termed "positive" when it indicates worsening of LV function.

Cardiac Catheterization or Cath

1. Passage of a tiny tube, referred to as a central line, through heart into blood vessels with introduction of a contrast medium into coronary arteries and subsequent x-ray. A common type of central line is a Swan-Ganz catheter.
   a. Can be inserted through an artery in the patient's arm or leg.
   b. Provides information about anatomy of heart and great vessels, ventricular function, abnormal wall movements.
      (1) Measures central venous pressure (CVP), pulmonary artery pressure (PA), pulmonary capillary wedge pressures (PCWP).
   c. Allows determination of ejection fraction (EF).

Exercise Tolerance Test (ETT, exercise stress test, graded exercise test)

1. The patient is hooked up to an ECG machine and monitored as the individual is put through progressively increasing workloads.

2. The patient typically walks on a treadmill, pedals a stationary bike or an arm ergometer.

3. The work of the heart is measured in METS (metabolic equivalents). A MET represents the oxygen requirement of the body at rest.

Laboratory Tests and Values (Table 4-2)

Enzyme Changes Associated with Myocardial Infarction

1. Elevations in SGOT (serum glutamic-oxaloacetic transaminase) (peaks 24-48 hr).

2. Elevations CK or CPK (serum creatine phosphokinase) (peaks at 24 hr); CK-MB (serum creatine phosphokinase MB) is most sensitive when measured within 6-10 hours of onset of the MI.

3. Elevations in LDH (serum lactate dehydrogenase) (peaks 3-6 days).

Serum Lipids (Lipid Panel) (mg/dL)

1. Use to determine coronary risk

2. Cholesterol: desirable: <200, borderline: 200-230, high risk: >240.

3. High-density lipoprotein (HDL): low risk: >60, moderate risk: 35-60, high risk: <35.

4. Low density lipoprotein (LDL): >100 with multiple risk factors, >160 for low risk individuals.

5. Triglycerides: desirable: <165.

6. LDL/HDL ratio: low risk: 0.5-3.0, moderate risk: 3.0-6.0; high risk: >6.0.

CHAPTER 4

Table 4-2 ➤ LABORATORY TESTS & VALUES

NORMAL VALUES	CLINICAL SIGNIFICANCE	NORMAL VALUES	CLINICAL SIGNIFICANCE
Arterial Blood Gases (ABGs)		**Complete Blood Cell Count (CBC), adult values**	
$SaO_2 \geq 95\%$	SaO_2 below 88%–90% usually requires supplemental O_2	Leukocytes (WBCs) Male & Female: 5,000–10,000 cells/mm³	Indicative of status of immune system. ↑ in infection: bacterial, viral; inflammation, hematological malignancy, leukemia, lymphoma, drugs (corticosteroids) ↓ in aplastic anemia, B_{12} or folate deficiency With immunosuppression: ↑ risk of infection *Exercise considerations:* >5000 use light exercise only <5000 with fever exercise is contraindicated <1000 use mask, standard precautions
PaO_2 80–100 mm Hg	↑ in hyperventilation ↓ in cardiac decompensation, COPD and some neuromuscular disorders	Erythrocytes (RBCs) Male: 4.7–6.1 10⁶/mm³ Female: 4.2–5.4 10⁶/mm³	↑ in polycythemia ↓ in anemia
$PaCO_2$ 35–45 mm Hg	↑ in COPD ↓ in pregnancy, pulmonary embolism and anxiety	Erythrocyte Sedimentation Rate (ESR) Male up to 15 mm/hr Female up to 20 mm/hr	↑ in infection and inflammation: rheumatic or pelvic inflammatory disease, osteomyelitis Used to monitor effects of treatment (e.g., SLE, Hodgkin's disease)
pH, whole blood 7.35–7.45	below 7.35 is acidotic, above 7.45 is alkalotic ↑ in respiratory alkalosis: hyperventilation, sepsis, liver disease, fever ↑ in metabolic alkalosis: vomiting, potassium depletion, diuretics, volume depletion ↓ in respiratory acidosis: COPD, respiratory depressants, myasthenia ↓ in metabolic acidosis (bicarbonate deficit): increased acids (diabetes, alcohol, starvation); renal failure, increased acid intake and loss of alkaline body fluids	Hematocrit (Hct) % of RBC of the whole blood vol. Male 42%–52% Female 37%–47% (age-dependent)	↑ in erythrocytosis: dehydration and shock ↓ in severe anemias: cute hemorrhage *Exercise considerations:* >25% but less than normal: light exercise only <25% exercise is contraindicated

(Continued on following page)

Table 4-2 ➤ continued

NORMAL VALUES	CLINICAL SIGNIFICANCE	NORMAL VALUES	CLINICAL SIGNIFICANCE
Hemostasis (Clotting/Bleeding times)			
Prothrombin time (PT) 11–15 sec	Prolonged in factor X deficiency, hemorrhagic disease, cirrhosis, hepatitis drugs (warfarin) If clotting time is ↑ 2.5 times or more normal: physical therapy is contraindicated	Hemoglobin, total Male: 14–18 g/dL Female: 12–16 g/dL (age dependent)	↑ polycythemia, dehydration, shock ↓ in anemias, prolonged hemorrhage, RBC destruction (cancer, sickle cell disease) *Exercise considerations:* Low values (8–10 g/dL result in ↓ exercise tolerance, ↑ fatigue, and tachycardia: use light exercise only <8 g/dL exercise contraindicated
PTT 25–40 sec INR: Ratio of individual's PT to reference range 0.9–1.1 (ratio)	↑ in factor VIII, IX, and X deficiency INR <2 desirable INR >2: consult with MD for ↑ risk of bleeding INR >3 ↑ risk of hemarthrosis	Platelet count 150,000–450,000 cells/mm³	↑ chronic leukemia, hemoconcentration ↓ thrombocytopenia, acute leukemia, aplastic anemia, cancer chemotherapy *Exercise considerations:* <20,000: AROM, ADL only 20,000–30,000: use light exercise only 30,000–50,000: use moderate exercise
Bleeding time 2–10 min	↑ in platelet disorders: thrombocytopenia	Fibrinogen, plasma 175–433 mg/dL	↑ in inflammatory states, pregnancy, oral contraceptives ↓ in cirrhosis, hereditary diseases

Nicoll D, McPhee S, Chou T, Detmer W (eds) (1997). *Pocket Guide to Diagnostic Tests,* 2nd ed. Stamford CT, Appleton & Lange.
Goodman D, Boissonnault W (1998). *Pathology: Implications for the Physical Therapist,* Philadelphia, Saunders.
ADL, activities of daily living; AROM, active range of motion; COPD, chronic obstructive pulmonary disease; ESR, erythrocyte sedimentation rate; Hct, hematocrit; INR, international normalized ratio; PTT, partial thromboplastintin; RA, rheumatoid arthritis; SLE, systemic lupus erythematosus.

Signs and Symptoms of Cardiovascular Disease

➥ **Red Flag:** When treating patients the physical therapist assistant should be aware of these general signs and symptoms of cardiovascular compromise. The PTA is responsible to observe for these signs and symptoms, recognize them as potential adverse changes and to modify interventions and notify the physical therapist as appropriate. Table 4-3.

Chest Pain or Discomfort

1. Described as a tightness or pressure sensation in the chest.

Table 4-3 ➤ SIGNS AND SYMPTOMS OF CARDIOVASCULAR COMPROMISE

SIGNS AND SYMPTOMS	QUALITY
Chest pain	May be described as tightness or pressure. May radiate: neck, jaw, shoulder, upper trapezius area, upper back, arms.
Nausea	Vomiting may occur. Antacids may be taken to try and calm nausea.
Diaphoresis	Secondary to activation of the sympathetic nervous system.
Dyspnea	May occur at rest or with exertion; termed dyspnea on exertion (DOE).
Fatigue	Is out of proportion to amount of activity or work performed.
Pallor or Cyanosis	Due to decreased pumping ability of the heart.
Syncope	Transient loss of consciousness due to heart's impaired pumping ability.
Palpitations	May describe as a bumping, thud, flutter or a feeling of heart racing. Palpation will reveal a fast heart beat; it may be regular or irregular.
Peripheral edema	Typically seen bilaterally; secondary to failure of the right heart.
Claudication	May complain of pain or cramping in the lower extremities. Secondary to peripheral vascular disease.

2. Systemic complaints that may or may not be cardiac related can include chest pain that radiates to the neck jaw, shoulder or upper trap area, upper back or arms (most common left arm).

3. Symptoms may also include: nausea or vomiting, diaphoresis (sweating), dyspnea, fatigue, pallor. Some may mistake this as indigestion.
   a. May also be accompanied by weakness.

Palpitations

1. An irregular or very fast heart-beat.

2. Can indicate severe conditions such as coronary artery disease (CAD), cardiomyopathy, heart block, ventricular aneurysm, atrioventricular valve disease, mitral stenosis or aortic stenosis.
   a. It should also be noted that palpitations may be the result of conditions that are not cardiac related, e.g., anxiety, caffeine intake.

3. May be described as: a bump, thud, flutter, butterfly, a sensation of the heart racing.

4. The patient may complain of syncope or lightheadedness.

5. Palpation reveals: a skipped beat, rapid pulse, irregular pulse.

Dyspnea

1. Shortness of breath, breathlessness.

2. Can be the result of cardiac or pulmonary conditions. May also be the result of other, nonlife- threatening conditions as well.

3. Dyspnea on exertion (DOE) can be caused by left ventricular impairment, resulting in increased congestion of blood in the pulmonary system.

a. In the case of severe involvement, dyspnea may occur at rest as well.
b. Dyspnea increases as the severity of the pathology increases.

Cardiac Syncope

1. Lightheadedness or fainting.

2. Caused by a reduction in oxygen supply to brain secondary to impairment of the heart's pumping ability.

3. Conditions that may contribute to cardiac syncope include: arrhythmias, e.g. ventricular tachycardia or thostatic hypotension, CAD, vertebral artery insufficiency, hypoglycemia.

Fatigue

1. i.e., out of proportion to activity or the work performed.

Cyanosis

1. Often accompanied with cardiac involvement. Can also be associated with dysfunction of other systems.

Peripheral Edema

1. Commonly associated with right ventricular dysfunction or failure; typically occurs bilaterally.

Claudication

1. Cramping in the legs, leg pain.

2. Result of peripheral vascular disease (venous or arterial).

3. Can significantly limit ability to perform ADL by limiting tolerance to standing and walking.

Pathophysiology – Coronary Artery Disease (CAD)

Definition: A narrowing of the lumen of the coronary arteries from the atherosclerotic disease process. This results in ischemia to the myocardium which can progress to injury or death.

Atherosclerosis

1. Disease of moderate and large arteries; not limited to the coronary arteries, e.g., cerebrovascular disease – thickening of the arterial walls in the brain.

2. Characterized by thickening of the arterial wall from focal accumulation of lipids, platelets, monocytes, plaque and other debris.

3. Multiple risk factors are linked to atherosclerosis.
   a. Nonmodifiable risk factors: age, sex, race, family history of CAD.
   b. Modifiable risk factors: cigarette smoking, high blood pressure, elevated cholesterol levels and LDL levels, elevated blood homocystine, obesity, sedentary life style, obesity and stress.

c. Contributory diseases: diabetes.

d. Two or more risk factors multiply the risk of CAD.

Main Clinical Syndromes of CAD

1. **Ischemia leading to angina pectoris: substernal chest pain or pressure; may be accompanied by Levine sign (patient clenches fist over sternum; the Levine sign has a high diagnostic accuracy for ischemia).**

   a. Represents imbalance in myocardial oxygen supply and demand; brought on by:
      (1) Increased demands on heart: exertion, emotional stress, smoking, extremes of temperature especially cold, overeating, tachyarrhythmias.
      (2) Vasospasm: symptoms may be present at rest.

   b. Types of angina.
      (1) Stable angina: classic exertional angina; occurs at a predictable rate-pressure product, RPP (HR x BP), relieved with rest and/or nitroglycerin.
      (2) Unstable angina (preinfarction, crescendo angina): coronary insufficiency with risk for myocardial infarction or sudden death; pain is difficult to control; doesn't occur at predictable RPP.

2. **Myocardial infarction, MI: prolonged ischemia, injury and death of an area of the myocardium caused by occlusion of one or more of the coronary arteries.**

   a. Precipitating factors: atherosclerotic heart disease with thrombus formation, coronary vasospasm or embolism; cocaine toxicity.

3. **Heart failure, HF (cardiac failure): a condition in which the heart is unable to maintain adequate circulation of the blood to meet the metabolic needs of the body. Termed congestive heart failure (CHF) when edema is present. (Table 4-4).**

   a. Etiology: results from impairment of left ventricular functioning; from coronary artery disease, valvular disease, congenital heart disease, hypertension or infection.

   b. Physiological abnormalities: decreased cardiac output, elevated end diastolic pressures (preload); increased heart rate; impaired ventricular function which, over time, may progress to cardiomyopathy.

   c. Left heart failure (forward HF): blood is not adequately pumped into systemic circulation; due to an inability of left ventricle to pump, increases in ventricular end-diastolic pressure and left atrial pressures, with:
      (1) Increased pulmonary artery pressures and pulmonary edema.
      (2) Pulmonary signs and symptoms: cough, dyspnea or thopnea.
      (3) Weakness, fatigue.

Table 4-4 ➤ POSSIBLE CLINICAL MANIFESTATIONS OF CARDIAC FAILURE

Signs Associated With Right-Sided Heart Failure	
Nausea	Increase in RAP, CVP
Anorexia	Jugular venous distention
Weight gain	+ hepatojugular reflex
Ascites	Right ventricular heave
Right upper quadrant pain	Murmur of tricuspid insufficiency Hepatomegaly Peripheral edema

Signs Associated With Left-Sided Heart Failure	
Fatigue	Tachycardia
Cough	S_3 gallop
Shortness of breath	Crackles
DOE	Increased PAP, PAWP, SVR
Orthopnea	Laterally displaced PMI
PND	Left ventricular heave
Diaphoresis	Pulsus Alternans Confusion Decreased urine output Cheyne–Stokes respirations (advanced failure) Murmur of mitral insufficiency

RAP, right atrial pressure; CVP, central venous pressure; PAP, pulmonary artery pressure; PAWP, pulmonary artery wedge pressure; SVR, systemic vascular resistance; DOE, dyspnea on exertion; PND, paroxysmal nocturnal dyspnea; PMI, point of maximal impulse.

From Stillwell S, Randall E (1990). *Pocket Guide to Cardiovascular Care.* St. Louis, Mosby, p 19, with permission.

   d. Right heart failure (backward heart failure): blood is not adequately returned from the systemic circulation to the heart; due to failure of right ventricle, increased pulmonary artery pressures, with:
      (1) Peripheral edema: weight gain, venous stasis.
      (2) Nausea, anorexia.

   e. Compensated heart failure: symptoms are controlled by medical therapy.

   f. Sympathetic stimulation results in tachycardia.

   g. Decreased cardiac output results in prerenal failure.

4. **Sudden death.**

Medical and Surgical Management of Cardiovascular Disease

1. **Diet: low salt, low cholesterol, weight reduction.**

2. **Medical therapy: drugs aimed at reducing oxygen demand on the heart and increasing coronary blood flow.**

   a. Nitrates (nitroglycerin): decrease preload through peripheral vasodilation, reduce myocardial oxygen demand, reduce chest discomfort (angina); may also dilate coronary arteries, improve coronary blood flow.

b. Beta adrenergic blocking agents (e.g., propranolol/Inderal): reduce myocardial demand by reducing heart rate and contractility; control arrhythmias, chest pain; reduce blood pressure.

c. Calcium channel-blocking agents (e.g., diltiazem/Cardizem, Procardia): inhibit flow of calcium ions; decrease heart rate, decrease contractility, dilate coronary arteries, reduce BP, control arrhythmias, chest pain.

d. Antiarrhythmics (numerous drugs, 4 main classes): alter conductivity, restore normal heart rhythm, control arrhythmias and improve cardiac output, (e.g., Quinidine, Procainamide).

e. Antihypertensives (numerous drugs, 4 main types): control hypertension; goal is to maintain a diastolic pressure less than 90 mmHg; decrease afterload, reduce myocardial oxygen demand, (e.g., Propranolol, Reserpine).

f. Digitalis (cardiac glycosides): increases contractility and decreases heart rate; mainstay in the treatment of CHF, (e.g., Digoxin).

g. Diuretics: decrease myocardial work (reduce preload and afterload), control hypertension, (e.g., Lasix, Esidrix).

h. Aspirin: decreases platelet aggregation, may prevent myocardial infarction.

i. Tranquilizers: decrease anxiety, sympathetic effects.

j. Hypolipidemic agents (6 major cholesterol-lowering drugs): reduce serum lipid levels when diet and weight reduction are not effective, (e.g., Questran, Colestid, Zocor, Mevacor).

3. Activity restriction: acute MI, CHF: limited, generally to first 24 hours; or until patient is stable for 24 hours.

4. Surgical interventions.

a. Percutaneous transluminal coronary angioplasty (PTCA): under fluoroscopy, surgical dilation of a blood vessel using a small balloon-tipped catheter inflated inside the lumen; relieves obstructed blood flow in acute angina or acute MI; results in improved coronary blood flow, improved left ventricular function, anginal relief.

b. Intravascular stents: an endoprosthesis (pliable wire mesh) implanted post angioplasty to prevent restenosis and occlusion in coronary or peripheral arteries.

c. Coronary artery bypass graft (CABG): surgical circumvention of an obstruction in a coronary artery using an anastomosing graft (saphenous vein, internal mammary artery); multiple grafts may be necessary; results in improved coronary blood flow, improved left ventricular function, anginal relief.

d. Transplantation: used in end-stage myocardial disease, e.g., cardiomyopathy, ischemic heart disease, valvular heart disease.

(1) Heart and lung transplantation: involves removing both organs and replacing them with donor organs.

(2) Major problems post transplantation are: rejection, infection, complications of immunosuppressive therapy.

e. Ventricular assist device (VAD): an implanted device (accessory pump) that improves tissue perfusion and maintains cardiogenic circulation; used with severely involved patients, e.g., cardiogenic shock unresponsive to medications, severe ventricular dysfunction.

5. Thrombolytic therapy for acute myocardial infarction: medications administered to activate body's fibrinolytic system, dissolve clot and restore coronary blood flow, (e.g., Streptokinase, Tissue Plasminogen Activator [TPA], Urokinase).

Pathophysiology - Hypertension

Blood Pressure

1. Measure of tension exerted against arterial walls; regulated by blood flow and peripheral vascular resistance.

2. Blood flow is determined by cardiac output.

3. Blood pressure is determined by the resistance.

a. Resistance is primarily determined by the diameter of blood vessels; somewhat affected by viscosity of blood.

b. Increased peripheral resistance is the result of narrowing of arterioles.

↪ **Red Flag:** This is the most common characteristic of hypertension.

4. Prolonged hypertension leads to decreased elasticity of arterioles.

a. Elastic tissue is replaced with fibrous, collagen-based tissues that are not distensible.

b. This process increases resistance to blood flow through vessels.

c. This process also decreases blood flow to critical body tissues (kidney, heart, brain) and stimulates neurohumoral responses that increase blood pressure.

Clinical Manifestations

1. Hypertension is often asymptomatic, creating a significant health risk.

2. When symptoms are noticed they include:
   a. Headache.
   b. Vertigo.
   c. Flushed face.
   d. Blurred vision.
   e. Increased nocturnal urinary frequency.
   f. Increased blood pressure.

Medical Management

1. Prevention. (Box 4-2) Modifiable and Nonmodifiable Risk Factors for Hypertension.

2. Diet.
   a. Follow DASH diet (Dietary Approaches to Stop Hypertension) that includes:
      (1) High intake of fruits, vegetables and low-fat dairy products.
      (2) Avoidance of processed foods, e.g., sauces, gravies, prepackaged dinners, etc.
      (3) Decrease amount of sodium consumed.

3. Antihypertensive medications.
   a. These include: diuretics, adrenergic blockers, vasodilators, ACE inhibitors, calcium antagonists. (Appendix 4-I)

Data Collection

1. Ongoing blood pressure monitoring can help provide feedback regarding effectiveness of life style modifications and medical management.

Box 4-2 ➤ MODIFIABLE AND NONMODIFIABLE RISK FACTORS FOR HYPERTENSION

MODIFIABLE	NONMODIFIABLE
Sedentary life style	Family history of heart disease
Smoking	Age (>55 years)
Hypercholesterolemia, increased triglyceride levels	Gender
Long-term abuse of alcohol	Ethnicity
Obesity	
High sodium intake	
Diabetes mellitus	

2. Use of Borg RPE Scale (Box 4-1) may be necessary considering medications used that may potentially blunt HR and BP response to aerobic activity.

Physical Therapy Interventions

1. Patient education.
   a. Reinforce adherence to dietary and life style modifications.

2. Initiate aerobic conditioning program gradually.
   a. Aerobic program should include exercises that primarily use the lower extremities, e.g., walking, bicycling.
      (1) Monitor blood pressure before, during and after exercise.
   b. Intensity of programs can be beneficial when started at 65-70% of maximum heart rate and performed 3-4 times per week.
   c. Reinforce patient following medication regimen prescribed by physician.
   d. Identify possible side effects of specific medication with cardiac response.

Pathophysiology - Congestive Heart Failure

Definition

1. Inability of the heart to effectively pump enough blood to supply body needs. There are four main classifications. Congestive heart failure, left sided-heart failure, will be discussed here as it pertains to heart disease; other forms of heart failure are the result of pulmonary dysfunction. Refer to the chapter on Pulmonary Physical Therapy.

2. Systolic heart failure: heart fails to pump.

3. Diastolic failure: increased filling pressure required to maintain adequate cardiac output.

4. Left-sided heart failure: left ventricle cannot maintain cardiac output; true congestive heart failure.

5. Right-sided heart failure: right ventricular dysfunction due to left-sided failure or pulmonary disease; commonly associated with pulmonary embolism.

This table identifies common cardiac medications, their effects, and treatment considerations clinicians must keep in mind when working with patients who are taking these medications.

COMMON CARDIAC MEDICATIONS AND TREATMENT CONSIDERATIONS

DRUG CATEGORY (COMMON DRUG NAMES)	EFFECTS	TREATMENT CONSIDERATIONS
ACE inhibitors • enalapril (Vasotec) • ramipril (Altace) • catopril (Capoten) • lisinopril (Prinivil, Zertril)	Decrease blood pressure.	Watch for potential dizziness or orthostatic hypotension. NSAIDs can reduce or negate the effects of these medications; monitor patients closely for elevated blood pressure if taking.
Antiadrenergics • clonidine (Catapres) • guanadrel (Hylorel) • guanethidine (Ismelin) • methylodopa (Alodomet)	Decrease blood pressure without a selective receptor blockage.	
Calcium Channel Blockers • nifedipine (Procardia, Adalat) • verapamil (Calan, Isoptin) • amlodipine (Norvasc) • diltiazem (Cardizem) • Bepridil (Vascor)	Promote vasodilation. Decrease blood pressure and heart rate at rest and during exercise. They also help relieve anginal pain and coronary artery spasms.	Use perceived exertion scale (RPE) for monitoring physiological response to exercise. May reduce blood flow to heart muscle and create ischemic response. Monitor for orthostatic hypotension.
Alpha-Blockers • prazosin (Minipress) • doxazosin (Cardura) • labetalol (Trandate, Normodyne) • terazosin (Hytrin)	Decrease blood pressure	Monitor for signs of hypotension and reflex tachycardia; where heart rate increase to compensate for hypotension.
Beta-Blockers • acebutolol (Sectral, Tenormin) • metoprolol (Lopressor, Toprol) • propranolol (Inderal) • penbutolol (Levatol)	Decrease the force of the cardiac contraction, thereby decreasing the heart rate and create decreased demands on the heart and decrease blood pressure.	Use perceived exertion scale (RPE) for monitoring physiological response to exercise; monitoring heart rate is not useful. Watch for bradycardia and orthostatic hypotension. Can worsen asthma symptoms.
Diuretics • furosemide (Lasix) • digoxin (Lanoxin)	Increase blood pressure and heart rate at rest and during exercise to help increase cardiac contractility.	Can cause fluid and electrolyte imbalances; observe patients for muscle weakness or spasms, headache, and poor coordination. Monitor for bradycardia and orthostatic hypotension.
Nitrates • nitroglycerin (Nitrostat) • isosorbide dinitrate (Isordil, Diltrate)	Promote vasodilation. Increase heart rate and decrease blood pressure at reat.	Observe for dizziness, tachycardia, and orthostatic hypotension. Patients may complain of a headache.

ACE, angiotensin-converting enzyme; NSAIDs, nonsteroidal inti-inflammatory drugs; RPE, rate of perceived exertion.

Left Ventricular Failure

1. **Is a complication of hypertension and of ischemia.**
   a. Can develop as a result of the heart damage sustained from a heart attack or hypertension.

2. **It is the result of left ventricular inability to maintain enough blood supply for the body's needs. The process occurs in phases of compensatory techniques.**
   a. First phase: the left ventricle enlarges to hold more blood to pump. Eventually the ventricle enlarges to the point where the fibers are stretched so far they are no longer able to effectively pump.
      (1) Blood accumulates in the lungs (congestion); results in shortness of breath.
      (2) Eventually when totally saturated air spaces become flooded and blood seeps from the distended blood vessels; this is called *pulmonary edema* (or congestion).
   b. Second phase: the sympathetic system stimulates increased pumping action of the heart and an increased HR which ultimately results in hypertrophy of the heart.
      (1) This increased size of the heart demands more blood from the coronary arteries often resulting in ischemia and angina pectoris.
      (2) A cascade of sympathetic nervous system events begins.
   c. Third phase: further neurohumoral events take place to decreased blood to stimulate the kidneys to retain

water and increase sodium in an effort to increase blood volume.

   (1) This further increases edema and places increasing loads on the already compromised heart.

  d. Compensated CHF: the heart can manage these three phases to stabilize the system so effective cardiac output is maintained, termed *compensated CHF*.

  e. Fourth phase: decompensated CHF.

   (1) Mild to severe fluid overload leads to total heart failure.

   (2) Symptoms develop gradually; may not be apparent to the individual.

3. Signs and symptoms of left-sided heart failure.

  a. Dyspnea; extent to which it exists does not always correlate to extent of disease.

   (1) The time it takes to recover from periods of dyspnea can be used to measure progress or deterioration of patient's status.

  b. Fatigue and muscle weakness often develop.

   (1) Owing to weight gain, dyspnea and increased heart rate.

   (2) Inadequate cardiac output leads to decreased peripheral blood flow and tissue hypoxia.

  c. Increasing kidney dysfunction leads to decreased urine formation; this results in retained sodium and water in the system which further contributes to blood volume.

Right-sided Heart Failure

1. Right side of the heart fails to pump adequate blood supply to the lungs.

  a. Results in peripheral edema and venous congestion of the organs.

2. Signs and symptoms.

  a. Dependent edema: fluid retention as a result of body baroreceptors sensing decreased blood volume.

   (1) This stimulates the kidneys to retain fluid thus perpetuating the cycle.

  b. Jugular venous distension may develop.

  c. Cyanosis of the nail beds may be noted.

Medical Management of CHF

1. Echocardiogram used as diagnostic tool to determine left ventricle size and function. In addition to ECG, chest radiograph.

2. Arterial blood gases measured to determine oxygen saturation.

3. Diet modifications may include decreasing sodium and limited fluid intake.

4. Medications can be used to: decrease workload of the heart, increase muscle contraction, improve renal blood flow, ACE inhibitors and ACE inhibitors combined with vasodilators, diuretics, beta blockers.

5. Surgical management.

  a. CABG to correct underlying ischemia and infarct.

  b. Reconstruct dysfunctional heart valves.

  c. Cardiac transplant.

Prognosis

1. Prognosis is generally poor.

Physical Therapy Intervention

1. Goals of intervention are to improve physiological response to exercise as well as improve ability to perform physical activities.

  a. Monitor vital signs (O_2 saturation, RPE) prior to, during and following exercise bouts.

  b. Begin at mild to moderate intensity exercise, 40-60% VO_{2max} and gradually increase duration.

   (1) Maintain HR below 115 bpm.

  c. Include.

   (1) Extended warm up and cool down period.

   (2) Periods of rest and work as patient symptoms and vital signs. indicate. Interval training effective, especially for those with markedly limited exercise tolerance.

2. Activities should also include exercise to increase peripheral endurance and respiratory muscle training.

3. Avoid exercise immediately following a meal or administration of vasodilator medication.

Pathophysiology – Peripheral Vascular Disease (PVD) (Table 4-5)

Arterial Disease

1. **Arteriosclerosis obliterans (atherosclerosis): chronic, occlusive arterial disease of medium and large-sized vessels, the result of peripheral atherosclerosis.**
   a. Associated with hypertension and hyperlipidemia; patients may also exhibit CAD, cerebrovascular disease, diabetes.
   b. Pulses: decreased or absent.
   c. Color: pale on elevation, dusky red on dependency.
   d. Early stages, patients exhibit intermittent claudication. Pain is described as burning, searing, aching, tightness or cramping.
   e. Late stages, patients exhibit ischemia and rest pain; ulcerations and gangrene, trophic changes.
   f. Affects primarily the lower extremities.

2. **Thromboangiitis obliterans (Buerger's disease): chronic, inflammatory vascular occlusive disease of small arteries and also veins.**
   a. Occurs commonly in young adults, largely males, who smoke.
   b. Begins distally and progresses proximally in both upper and lower extremities.
   c. Patients exhibit paresthesias or pain, cyanotic cold extremities, diminished temperature sensation, fatigue, risk of ulceration and gangrene.

3. **Diabetic angiopathy: an inappropriate elevation of blood glucose levels and accelerated atherosclerosis.**
   a. Neuropathy a major problem.
   b. Neurotrophic ulcers, may lead to gangrene and amputation.

4. **Raynaud's disease or phenomenon: episodic spasm of small arteries and arterioles.**
   a. Abnormal vasoconstrictor reflex exacerbated by exposure to cold or emotional stress; tips of fingers develop pallor, cyanosis, numbness and tingling.
   b. Affects largely females.
   c. Occlusive disease is not usually a factor.

Table 4-5 ➤ CLINICAL MANIFESTATIONS OF PERIPHERAL VASCULAR DISEASES

	CHRONIC ARTERIAL INSUFFICIENCY	CHRONIC VENOUS INSUFFICIENCY
Etiology	Arteriosclerosis obliterans Atheroembolism	Thrombophlebitis trauma, vein obstruction
Risk factors	Smoking Diabetes mellitus Hyperlipoproteinemia Hypertension	Venous hypertension Varicose veins Inherited trait
Signs & Symptoms: determined by location and degree of vascular involvement		
Pain	Severe muscle Ischemia/intermittent claudication: worse with exercise, relieved by rest Rest pain indicates severe involvement Muscle fatigue, cramping, numbness paresthesias over time	Minimal to moderate steady pain aching pain in lower leg with prolonged standing or sitting (dependency) superficial pain along course of vein
Location of pain	Usually calf, lower leg or dorsum of foot may occur in thigh, hip or buttock	Muscle compartment tenderness
Vascular	Decreased or absent pulses pallor of forefoot on elevation, dependent rubor	Venous dilatation or varicosity edema: moderate to severe
Skin changes	Pale, shiny, dry Loss of hair Nail changes Coolness of extremity	Liposclerosis: dark, cyanotic thickened, brown may lead to stasis dermatitis, cellulites
Acute	Acute arterial obstruction: distal pain, paresthetic, pale, pulseless, sudden onset.	Acute thrombophlebitis (DVT): calf pain, aching, edema, muscle tenderness, 50% asymptomatic
Ulceration	May develop in toes or feet or areas of trauma; gangrene may develop	May develop at sides of ankles, especially medial malleolus; gangrene absent

DVT, deep vein thrombosis.
Adapted from: Bickley L, and Szilagyi P (2003). *Bates Guide to Physical Examination and History Taking,* 8th ed. Philadelphia, Lippincott Williams & Wilkins, pp 460–464.

Venous Disease

1. **Varicose veins: distended, swollen superficial veins; tortuous in appearance; may lead to varicose ulcers.**

2. **Superficial vein thrombophlebitis: clot formation and acute inflammation in a superficial vein. Localized pain; usually in saphenous vein.**

3. **Deep vein thrombophlebitis (DVT): clot formation and acute inflammation in a deep vein.**
   a. Usually occurs in lower extremity, associated with venous stasis (bed rest, lack of leg exercise), hyperactivity of blood coagulation and vascular trauma; early ambulation is prophylactic, helps eliminate venous stasis.
   b. Signs and symptoms: may be asymptomatic early; inflammation, tenderness, pain, swelling, warmth, skin discoloration.
   c. Homan's sign (test for DVT of calf veins): calf pain with dorsiflexion of ankle; limited diagnostic reliability.
   d. May precipitate pulmonary embolism: presents abruptly, with chest pain and dyspnea, also diaphoresis, cough, apprehension; requires emergency treatment, may be life threatening.
   e. Medical management: anticoagulation therapy, e.g., heparin; thrombolytic agents, (e.g., Streptokinase); bed rest.

4. **Chronic venous insufficiency (deep).**
   a. Pain: none to aching pain on dependency.
   b. Pulses: normal; difficult to take with edema.
   c. Color: normal or cyanotic on dependency.
   d. Venous valvular insufficiency: from fibroelastic degeneration of valve tissue, venous dilation.
   e. Muscle pump dysfunction.
   f. Edema, impairment of fibrinolysis; may lead to venous ulcer formation.
   g. Classification.
      Grade I: mild aching, minimal edema, dilated superficial veins.
      Grade II: increased edema, multiple dilated veins, changes in skin pigmentation.
      Grade III: venous claudication, severe edema, cutaneous ulceration.

Lymphatic Disease

1. **Lymphadenopathy: enlargement of nodes, with or without tenderness.**

2. **Lymphedema: excessive accumulation of fluid due to obstruction of lymphatics, causes swelling of the soft tissues in arms and legs.**

3. **Acute lymphangitis: acute bacterial infection spreading throughout lymph system; usually streptococcal.**

4. **Primary lymphatic disease: congenital.**

5. **Secondary lymphatic disease: acquired, due to trauma, surgery (radical mastectomy, femoral-popliteal by-pass), radiation or disease (malignancy, infection).**

Lymphedema Pathophysiology

Categories of Lymphedema

1. **Primary (idiopathic).**
   a. Thought to be the result of malformations of lymph nodes or lymph vessels at birth.
   b. Incidence unknown, less common than secondary, more common in females.

2. **Secondary (acquired).**
   a. Caused by some damage to one or more components of the lymph system.
   b. More prevalent than primary.
   c. Causes can include.
      (1) Surgery in area, e.g. abdominal, liposuction, hernia repair, total knee or total hip replacement.
      (2) Crush injuries or fractures.
      (3) Radiation treatment for cancer of the breast, prostate, bladder, uterus, etc.
      (4) Chronic venous insufficiency, due to long-standing fluid overload in area.
      (5) Complications of paralysis.
      (6) Disuse secondary to complex regional pain syndrome.
      (7) Filariasis (known as elephantiasis) caused by parasitic infection carried by a mosquito through a bite.

Stages

1. **There are three stages of lymphedema. Table 4-6.**
   a. One does not necessarily progress through all of the stages.

Table 4-6 ➤ STAGES OF LYMPHEDEMA

STAGE	CLINICAL PRESENTATION
Stage 1	Accumulation of protein-rich fluid in limb or area of trunk; pitting edema present. Edema will decrease with elevation of limb overnight. Edema increases with activity, heat or humidity.
Stage 2	Continued accumulation of protein-rich edema, nonpitting. Skin begins to toughen, connective scar tissue, fibrosis present. Edema is not reversible with elevation.
Stage 3	Continued accumulation of protein-rich edema, significant connective and scar tissue. Skin is resilient to touch, very tough, papillomas present, hyperkeratosis present. Edema is not reversible with elevation. Subject to infections due to build up of fluids.

Pathogenesis

1. Lymphedema is not a disease in itself, but a manifestation of a malfunctioning lymph system.

2. Inadequate transport of lymph volume through lymph system.

3. Valve safety system in lymph vessels become incompetent allowing accumulation of fluids in the system.
   a. May involve normal or abnormal amounts of fluid in system.
   b. Lymph system will attempt to create collateral vessels to repair itself; creates a constant state of inflammation.

4. Fibrotic state is created.
   a. Secondary to the constant inflammation.
   b. Delayed wound healing or infection.

5. Chronic lymphedema creates hypertrophied muscle wall in lymphatics, this decreases its effective pumping abilities.
   a. Macrophages become inactive and further contribute to waste and fluid accumulation.

Clinical Manifestations

1. Typically develop in the distal extremities.
   a. It can also manifest in the axilla, groin and trunk.

2. Signs and symptoms can include.
   a. Complaints of a heaviness or fullness, fatigue, stiffness and loss of ROM in affected region.
   b. Patient may complain of numbness or tingling.
   c. Patient may note that wrist watch or bracelet no longer fits, clothing becomes tight.
   d. Edema, typically pitting in the early stages.
   e. Edema that is not relieved by elevation.
   f. Delayed wound healing.

Tests and Measures

1. Patient history consistent with event potentially creating lymphedema.

2. Visual inspection of tissue integrity.
   a. Pitting or nonpittting, brawny or weeping edema.
   b. Fibrotic tissue changes.
   c. Girth and volumetric measurements.
   d. Range of available ROM.

Medical Management

1. No clear pharmaceutical management is available.
   a. There is some research in the area of medications and natural remedies that will lyse protein accumulation and stimulate macrophage activity.
   b. There is a concern regarding health risks to the liver.

2. Diuretics work if edema is secondary to sodium retention, however ineffective in lymphedema.
   a. Diuretics can add to further extracellular protein and increase fibrosis.

3. Surgical procedures are largely ineffective and typically only used treat severe involvement.

Physical Therapy Management and Intervention

1. See Section XIV.

Cardiac Rehabilitation

Exercise Tolerance Testing

1. **Exercise Tolerance Test (ETT), Graded Exercise Test.**
   a. Performed prior to exercise prescription to determine physiological responses during a measured exercise stress (increasing workloads); allows the determination of safe aerobic exercise levels without cardiac ischemia.
      (1) Serves as a basis for exercise prescription. Symptom-limited ETT is typically administered prior to start of Phase II outpatient cardiac rehabilitation program and following cardiac rehabilitation as an outcome measure.
         (a) Exercise level is set just below the level in which signs and symptoms of intolerance or ischemia begin.
   b. Testing modes.
      (1) Treadmill and cycle ergometry (leg or arm tests) allow for precise calibration of the exercise workload.
      (2) Step test (upright or sitting) can also be used for fitness screening, healthy population.
   c. ETT may be maximal or submaximal.
      (1) Maximal ETT: defined by target end-point heart rate.
         (a) Age-adjusted maximum heart rate (AAMHR): 220 minus age of individual.
         (b) Heart-rate range (Karvonen's formula): 60-80% (HR max - resting HR) + resting HR = target HR.
      (2) Submaximal ETT: symptom-limited, used to evaluate the early recovery of patients after MI, coronary bypass or coronary angioplasty.
   d. Continuous ETT: workload is steadily progressed usually in 2 or 3 minute stages.
   e. Discontinuous ETT: allows rest in between workloads/stages, used for patients with more pronounced CAD.

Exercise Prescription

1. **Indications and contraindications for entry into inpatient and outpatient exercise cardiac rehabilitation programs are identified in Box 4-3.**

2. **Expected responses during exercise and recovery.**
   a. HR: HR increases linearly as a function of increasing workload and oxygen uptake (VO_2), plateaus just before maximal oxygen uptake (VO_2 max).
   b. BP: systolic BP should rise with increasing workloads and VO_2; diastolic BP should remain about the same.

3. **Adverse responses to inpatient exercise. Exercises should be modified or stopped if any of the following are observed or noted:**
   a. Persistent dyspnea, sudden onset dyspnea.
   b. Dizziness or confusion.
   c. Onset of angina pain including discomfort in chest, arm or jaw and other signs and symptoms of cardiovascular insufficiency.
   d. Severe leg claudication.
   e. Excessive fatigue or muscle pain.
   f. Pallor, cold sweat.
   g. Ataxia, incoordination.
   h. Bone or joint pain/discomfort during or after exercise.
   i. Nausea or vomiting.
   j. Resting HR > 130 bpm or < 40 bpm.
   k. Increasing number of arrhythmias occurring.
   l. Increasing frequency of PVCs.
   m. Fall in systolic BP accompanied by other signs and symptoms of intolerance.
   n. Rise in systolic BP above 250 mm Hg, diastolic B/P > 115 mm Hg.
   o. Significant or dangerous changes in ECG.

4. **Monitoring during exercise participation.**
   a. Rating of perceived exertion (RPE).
      (1) Original Borg scale: rates exercise intensity using numbers from 6 to 20, with descriptors from very, very light to very, very hard.
      (2) RPE increases linearly with increasing exercise intensity and correlates closely to VO_2max and heart rate.
      (3) An important measure for individuals who do not exhibit the typical rise in HR with exercise (e.g., on medications that depress HR, beta blockers).
   b. Pulse oximetry: measure arterial oxygen saturation levels (SaO_2) before, during and after exercise.
      (1) Maintain levels at or above 86-90%.
   c. HR: use pulse points, a combination HR and SaO_2 monitor or telemetry.
   d. Monitor BP.

5. **Considerations following surgical procedures.**
   a. Restrictions following open chest procedures.
      (1) The patient is not allowed to pull themselves up in bed, roll to sidelying for bed transfers.
      (2) Use of hand hold assist versus assistive device may be necessary.

Box 4-3 ➤ CLINICAL INDICATIONS AND CONTRAINDICATIONS FOR INPATIENT AND OUTPATIENT CARDIAC REHABILITATION PROGRAMS

INDICATIONS

- Medically stable postmyocardial infarction.
- Stable angina.
- Coronary artery bypass graft surgery.
- Percutaneous transluminal coronary angioplasty (PTCA)
- Compensated congestive heart failure
- Cardiomyopathy
- Heart or other organ transplantation
- Other cardiac surgery including valvular and pacemaker insertion (including implantable cardioverter defibrillator)
- Peripheral arterial disease
- High-risk cardiovascular disease ineligible for surgical intervention sudden cardiac death syndrome
- End-stage renal disease
- At risk for coronary artery disease, with diagnoses of diabetes mellitus, dyslipidemia, hypertension, etc.
- Other patients who may benefit from structured exercise and/or patient education (based on physician referral and consensus of the rehabilitation team)

CONTRAINDICATIONS

- Unstable angina
- Resting systolic BP > 200 mm Hg or resting diastolic BP > 110 mm Hg evaluated on a case by case basis
- Orthostatic BP drop of > 20 mm Hg with symptoms
- Critical aortic stenosis (peak systolic pressure gradient of > 50 mm Hg with an aortic valve orifice area of < 0.75 cm^2 in an average size adult)
- Acute systemic illness or fever
- Uncontrolled atrial or ventricular dysrhythmias
- Uncontrolled sinus tachycardia (> 120 bpm)
- Uncompensated congestive heart failure
- Third degree A-V heart block (without pacemaker)
- Active pericarditis or myocarditis
- Recent embolism
- Thrombophlebitis
- Resting ST segment displacement (> 2 mm)
- Uncontrolled diabetes (resting glucose > 300 mg dL or > 250 mg dL with ketones present)
- Severe orthopedic problems that would prohibit exercise
- Other metabolic problems, such as acute thyroiditis, hyperkalemia, hypovolemia, etc.

From: American College of Sports Medicine, Guidelines for Exercise Testing and Prescription, 7th ed., Philadelphia, Lippincott Williams & Wilkins, 2006, p 176.

(3) No pushing, pulling or lifting anything > 5-10 pounds; for 6 weeks post-op.

(4) Limit shoulder (flexion, abduction) and trunk motions if sternum is unstable.

   (a) Chest is determined to be unstable if asynchronous chest movement occurs between the two sides. Therapist can evaluate this by placing their hands on the two chest sides and asking the patient to cough.

b. Instruct patient in splinting sternum by "hugging a pillow" during cough.

c. Scar mobilization can begin when scar(s) are fully healed; follow typical scar mobilization techniques.

d. Typical home discharge instructions.

   (1) No driving motorized vehicles e.g., golf cart, car; for 8 weeks post-op. Air bag precautions require sitting in rear seat.

   (2) Avoid soaking in the bath until incision is fully healed; avoid excessively hot water.

   (3) When bypass graft in leg is present avoid: crossing the legs, prolonged positions (sit, stand), elevate LE when possible.

   (4) Wear elastic stockings for 2 weeks following surgery when up.

   (5) Encourage walking; assists with managing edema in LE as well as helping increase development of collateral circulation.

   (6) Encourage balance between activity and rest.

   (7) Sexual relations can typically resume in 3-4 weeks following discharge when the patient feels comfortable.

6. Guidelines for exercise prescription.

a. Type (modality).

   (1) Cardiorespiratory endurance activities: walking, jogging or cycling recommended to improve exercise tolerance; can be maintained at a constant velocity; very low inter-individual variability.

(2) Dynamic arm exercise (arm ergometry): uses a smaller muscle mass, results in lower VO_2max (60-70% lower) than leg ergometry; at a given workload, HR will be higher, stroke volume lower; systolic and diastolic BPs will be higher.

(3) Other aerobic activities: swimming, cross-country skiing; less frequently used due to high inter-individual variability, energy expenditure related to skill level.

(4) Dancing, basketball, racquetball, competitive activities should not be used with high risk, symptomatic and low fit individuals.

(5) Early rehabilitation: activity is discontinuous (interval training), with frequent rest periods; continuous training can be used in later stages of rehabilitation.

(6) Warm-up and cool-down activities.
  (a) Gradually increase or decrease the intensity of exercise, promote circulatory and muscular adjustment to exercise.
  (b) Type: low intensity cardiorespiratory endurance activities, flexibility (ROM) exercises, functional mobility activities.
  (c) Duration: 5-10 minutes.
  (d) Abrupt beginning or cessation of exercise is not safe or recommended.

(7) Resistive exercises: to improve strength and endurance in clinically stable patients.
  (a) Usually prescribed in later rehabilitation, after a period of aerobic conditioning.
  (b) Moderate intensities are typically used (e.g., 40% of maximal voluntary contraction).
  (c) Monitor responses to resistive training using rate-pressure product (incorporates BP, a safer measure).
  (d) Precautions: carefully monitor BP, avoid breath-holding, Valsalva response (may dramatically increase BP and work of heart).
  (e) Contraindicated for patients with: poor left ventricular function, ischemic changes on EKG during ETT, functional capacity less than 6 METs, uncontrolled hypertension or arrhythmias. Table 4-7.

(8) Relaxation training: relieves generalized muscle tension and anxiety.
  (a) Usually incorporated following an aerobic training session and cool-down.
  (b) Assists in successful stress management and life-style modification.

b. Intensity: prescribed as percentage of functional capacity revealed on ETT, within a range of 40 to 85% depending upon initial level of fitness; typical training intensity is 60-70% of functional capacity; lower training intensities may necessitate an increase in training duration; most clinicians use a combination of HR, RPE and METs to prescribe exercise intensity

(eliminates problems that may be associated with individual measures).

(1) Heart rate.
  (a) Percentage of maximum heart rate achieved on ETT; without an ETT, 220 minus age is used (for upper extremity work, 220 minus age minus 11 is used). 70-85 % HR max closely corresponds to 60 to 80% of functional capacity or VO_2 max.
  (b) Estimated HR max is used in cases where submaximal ETT has been given.
  (c) Heart rate range or reserve (Karvonen's formula, see previous description). more closely approximates the relationship between HR and VO_2 max. Problems associated with use of HR alone to prescribe exercise intensity.
  (d) Beta blocking or calcium channel blocking medications: affects ability of HR to rise in response to an exercise stress.
  (e) Pacemaker: affects ability of HR to rise in response to an exercise stress.
  (f) Environmental extremes, heavy arm work, isometric exercise and Valsalva may affect HR and BP responses.

(2) Rating of Perceived Exertion, the original Borg RPE scale (6-20). Box 4-1.
  (a) RPE values of 12-13 (somewhat hard) correspond to 60% of HR range.
  (b) RPE of 16 (hard) corresponds to 85% of HR range.
  (c) Useful along with other measures of patient effort if beta-blockers or other HR suppressers are used.
  (d) Problems with use of RPE alone to prescribe exercise intensity.
    • Individuals with psychological problems (e.g., depression).
    • Unfamiliarity with RPE scale; may affect selection of ratings.

(3) METs or estimated energy expenditure (VO_2). Table 4-7.
  (a) 40-85% of functional capacity (maximal METs) achieved on ETT.
  (b) Problems associated with use of METs alone to prescribe exercise intensity.
    • With high intensity activities (e.g., jogging), need to adopt a discontinuous work pattern: walk 5 minutes; jog 3 minutes to achieve the desired intensity.
    • Varying skill level or stress of competition may affect the known metabolic cost of an activity.
    • Environmental stresses (heat, cold, high humidity, altitude, wind, changes in terrain such as hills) may affect the known metabolic cost of an activity.

Table 4-7 ➤ METABOLIC EQUIVALENT (MET) ACTIVITY CHART

INTENSITY (70-KG PERSON)	ENDURANCE PROMOTING	OCCUPATIONAL	RECREATIONAL
1.5–2 METS	Too low in energy level	Desk work, driving auto, calculating machine operation, light housework, polishing furniture, washing clothes	Standing, strolling (1 mph), flying, motorcycling, playing cards, sewing, knitting
2–3 METS	Too low in energy level unless capacity is very low	Auto repair, radio and television repair, janitorial work, bartending, riding lawn mower, light woodworking	Level walking (2 mph), level bicycling (5 mph), billiards, bowling, skeet shooting, shuffleboard, powerboat driving, golfing with power cart, canoeing, horseback riding at a walk
3–4 METS	Yes, if continuous and if target heart rate is reached	Brick laying, plastering, wheelbarrow (100 lb load), machine assembly, welding (moderate load), cleaning windows, mopping floors, vacuuming, pushing light power mower	Walking (3 mph), bicycling (6 mph), horseshoe pitching, volleyball (6–person, non–competitive), golfing (pulling bag cart), archery, sailing (handling small boat), fly fishing (standing in waders), horseback riding (trotting), badminton (social doubles)
4–5 METS	Recreational activities promote endurance; occupational activities must be continuous, lasting longer than 2 min	Painting, masonry, paperhanging, light carpentry, scrubbing floors, raking leaves, hoeing	Walking (3⅓ mph), bicycling (8 mph), table tennis, golfing (carrying clubs), dancing (foxtrot), badminton (singles), tennis (doubles), many calisthenics, ballet
5–6 METS	Yes	Digging garden shoveling light earth	Walking (4 mph), bicycling (10 mph), canoeing (4 mph), horseback riding (posting to trotting), stream fishing (walking in light current in waders), ice or roller skating (9 mph)
6–7 METS	Yes	Shoveling 10 times/min (4.5 kg or 10 lb), splitting wood, snow shoveling, hand lawn mowing	Walking (5 mph), bicycling (11 mph), competitive badminton, tennis (singles), folk and square dancing, light downhill skiing, ski touring (2.5 mph), water skiing, swimming (20 yd/min)
7–8 METS	Yes	Digging ditches, carrying 36 kg or 80 lb, sawing hardwood	Jogging (5 mph), bicycling (12 mph), horseback riding (gallop), vigorous downhill skiing, basketball, mountain climbing, ice hockey, canoeing (5 mph), touch football, paddleball
8–9 METS	Yes	Shoveling 10 time/min (5.5 kg or 14 lb)	Running (5.5 mph), bicycling (13 mph), ski touring (4 mph), squash (social), handball (social), fencing, basketball (vigorous), swimming (30 yd/min), rope skipping
10+ METS	Yes	Shoveling 10 times/min (7.5 kg or 16 lb)	Running (6 mph = 10 METS, 7 mph = 11.5 METS, 8 mph = 13.5 METS, 9 mph = 15 METS, 10 mph = 17 METS), ski touring (5+ mph), handball (competitive), squash (competitive), swimming (>40 yd/min)

METS, metabolic equivalents (of oxygen consumption).
From Fox, Naughton, Gorman. *Modern Concepts of Cardiovascular Disease* (1972). American Heart Association 4:25, with permission.

c. Duration.
 (1) Conditioning phase may vary from 15 to 60 minutes, depending upon intensity; the higher the intensity, the shorter the duration.
 (2) Average conditioning time is 20-30 minutes for moderate intensity exercise.
 (3) Severely compromised individuals may benefit from multiple, short exercise sessions spaced throughout the day (e.g., 3-10 minute sessions).
 (4) Warm-up and cool-down periods are kept constant, e.g., 5-10 minutes each.
d. Frequency.
 (1) Frequency of activity is dependent upon intensity and duration; the lower the intensity, the shorter the duration, the greater the frequency.
 (2) Average: 3-5 sessions/week for exercise at moderate intensities and duration, e.g., >5 METs.
 (3) Daily or multiple daily sessions for low intensity exercise, e.g., <5 METS.
e. Progression.
 (1) Modify exercise prescription if:
  (a) HR is lower than target HR for a given exercise intensity.
  (b) RPE is lower (exercise is perceived as easier) for a given exercise.
  (c) Symptoms of ischemia (e.g., angina) do not appear at a given exercise intensity.
 (2) Rate of progression depends on age, health status, functional capacity, personal goals and preferences.
 (3) As training progresses, duration is increased first, then intensity.
f. Consider reduction in exercise/activity with.
 (1) Acute illness: fever, flu.

(2) Acute injury or thopedic complications.

(3) Progression of cardiac disease: edema, weight gain, unstable angina.

(4) Overindulgence: e.g., food, caffeine, alcohol.

(5) Drugs: e.g., decongestants, bronchodilators, atropine, weight reducers.

(5) Environmental stressors: extremes of heat, cold, humidity; air pollution.

g. Exercise prescription for post-PTCA (percutaneous transluminal coronary angioplasty).

(1) Wait to exercise approximately 2 weeks post-PTCA to allow inflammatory process to subside.

(2) Use post-PTCA ETT to prescribe exercise.

h. Exercise prescription post-CABG (coronary artery bypass grafting).

(1) Limit upper extremity exercise while sternal incision is healing.

(2) Avoid lifting, pushing, pulling for 4 - 6 week post-surgery.

Phase 1: Inpatient Cardiac Rehabilitation (Acute)

Length of stay is commonly 3-5 days for uncomplicated MI (no post MI angina, malignant arrhythmias or heart failure).

1. **Exercise/activity goals and outcomes.**

a. Initiate early return to independence in activities of daily living, typically after 24 hours or until the patient is stable for 24 hours; monitor activity tolerance.

b. Counteract deleterious effects of bed rest: reduce risk of thrombi, maintain muscle tone, reduce orthostatic hypotension and maintain joint mobility.

c. Help allay anxiety and depression.

d. Provide medical surveillance.

e. Provide patient and family education.

f. Promote risk factor modification.

2. **Exercise/activity guidelines.**

a. Program components: ADLs, selected arm and leg exercises, early supervised ambulation.

b. Initial activities: are low intensity (2-3 METs) progressing to 3-5 METs by discharge; RPE in fairly light range; HR increase of 10-20 bmp above resting, depending on medications.

c. Short exercise sessions, 2-3 times a day; gradually duration is lengthened and frequency is decreased.

d. Post-surgical patients.

(1) Typically are progressed more rapidly than post-MI.

(2) Greater emphasis is placed on upper extremity ROM.

(3) Lifting activities are restricted, generally for 6 weeks.

e. ETT (thallium scan or symptom limited ETT): may be used to determine functional capacity prior to discharge, safely progress exercise intensity greater than 5 METs.

3. **Patient and family education goals.**

a. Improve understanding of cardiac disease, support risk factor modification.

b. Teach self-monitoring procedures, warning signs of exertional intolerance, e.g., persistent dyspnea, anginal pain, dizziness, etc.

c. Teach general activity guidelines, activity pacing, energy conservation techniques; home exercise program (HEP).

d. Teach cardiopulmonary resuscitation (CPR).

e. Provide emotional support.

4. **Home exercise program (HEP).**

a. Low-risk patients may be safe candidates for unsupervised exercise at home.

(1) Gradual increase in ambulation time: goal of 20–30 minutes, one to two times per day at 4–6 weeks post-MI.

(2) Upper and lower extremity mobility exercises.

b. Elderly, homebound patients with multiple medical problems may benefit from a home cardiac rehabilitation program.

c. Patients should be skilled in self-monitoring procedures.

d. Family training in CPR and AED (automated external defibrillator); emergency lifeline for some patients.

Phase 2: Outpatient Cardiac Rehabilitation (Subacute)

1. **Exercise/activity goals and outcomes.**

a. Improve functional capacity.

b. Progress toward full resumption of activities of daily living, habitual and occupational activities.

c. Promote risk-factor modification, counseling as to lifestyle changes.

d. Encourage activity pacing, energy conservation; stress importance of taking proper rest periods.

2. **Exercise/activity guidelines.**

a. Outpatient program: average of 36 visits allowed by most payers (three times a week for 12 weeks).

(1) Patients at risk for arrhythmias with exercise, angina and other medical problems benefit from outpatient programs with availability of ECG monitoring, trained personnel and emergency support.

(2) Group camaraderie and support of program participants may assist in risk-factor modification and lifestyle changes.

(3) Frequency: three to four sessions/week.

(4) Duration: 30–60 minutes with 5–10 minutes of warm-up and cool down.

(5) Programs may offer a single mode of training (e.g., walking) or multiple modes using a circuit training approach (e.g., treadmill, cycle ergometer, arm ergometer); strength training.

(6) Patients are gradually weaned from continuous monitoring to spot checks and self-monitoring.

(7) Suggested exit point: 9 METS functional capacity (5 METS capacity is needed for safe resumption of most daily activities).

b. Strength training is a recent addition to phase 2 programs.

(1) Guidelines: after 3 weeks' cardiac rehab, 5 weeks' post-MI or 8 weeks' post-CABG.

(2) Begin with use of elastic bands and light weights (1–3 lb).

(3) Progress to moderate loads, 12–15 comfortable repetitions.

3. **Patient and family education goals: progression of phase 1 goals.**

Phase 3: Community Exercise Programs (Postacute, Postdischarge from Phase 2 Program)

1. **Exercise/activity goals and outcomes.**
   a. Improve and/or maintain functional capacity.
   b. Promote self-regulation of exercise programs.
   c. Promote life-long commitment to risk-factor modification.

2. **Exercise/activity guidelines.**
   a. Location: community centers, YMCA or clinical facilities.
   b. Entry level criteria: functional capacity of 5 METS, clinically stable angina, medically controlled arrhythmias during exercise.
   c. Progression is from supervised to self-regulation of exercise.
   d. Progression to 50%–85% of functional capacity, three to four times/week, 45 minutes or more/session.
   f. Regular medical check-ups and periodic ETT generally required.
   g. Utilize motivational techniques to maintain compliance with exercise programs, life-style modification.
   h. Discharge typically in 6–12 months.

3. **Patient and family education goals: progression from phase 1 goals.**

Exercise Prescription for Patients Requiring Special Considerations

1. **Congestive heart failure (CHF).**
   a. Patients demonstrate significant ventricular dysfunction, decreased cardiac output, low functional capacities. Functional classification of the stages of heart failure (New York Heart Association).
      (1) Class I: mild; no limitation in physical activity (up to 6.5 METS); comfortable at rest or dinary activity does not cause undue fatigue, palpitation, dyspnea or anginal pain.
      (2) Class II: mild; slight limitation in physical activity (up to 4.5 METS); comfortable at rest or dinary physical activity results in fatigue, palpitation, dyspnea or anginal pain.
      (3) Class III: moderate; marked limitation of physical activity (up to 3 METS); comfortable at rest, less than ordinary activity causes fatigue, palpitation, dyspnea or anginal pain.
      (4) Class IV: severe; unable to carry out any physical activity (1.5 METS) without discomfort; symptoms of ischemia, dyspnea, anginal pain present even at rest; increasing with exercise.
   b. Criteria for exercise training.
      (1) Medically stable.
      (2) Exercise capacity >3 METS.
      (3) Exercise-induced ischemia and arrhythmias poor prognostic indicators.
   c. Exercise training.
      (1) Use low intensities: (40%–60% functional capacity); gradually increasing durations, with frequent rest periods (interval training).
      (2) Monitor with RPE (ratings of 12–14), ECG, BP, signs of exertional intolerance (dyspnea, fatigue); HR response may be impaired (most patients on digoxin); HR limited to resting HR + 10–20 bpm; exercise HR >115 bpm generally contraindicated.
      (3) Exercise may exacerbate CHF: check for delayed responses of weight gain, edema lower extremities.
      (4) Patients with CHF (capacities <6 METS) are not candidates for resistance training.
      (5) Respiratory muscle training. Monitoring SaO_2 via pulse oximetry is advisable in some cases.
   d. Emphasis on training in energy conservation, self-monitoring techniques.

2. **Cardiac Transplant.**
   a. Patients may present with:
      (1) Exercise intolerance due to extended inactivity and convalescence.
      (2) Side effects from immunosuppressive drug therapy: hyperlipidemia, hypertension, obesity, diabetes, leg cramps.

CHAPTER 6

(3) Decreased lower extremity strength.

(4) Increased fracture risk owing to long-term corticosteroid use.

b. HR alone is not an appropriate measure of exercise intensity (heart is denervated). Use RPE, METS, dyspnea scale.

c. Use longer periods of warm-up and cool-down because the physiological responses to exercise and recovery take longer.

3. Pacemakers and automatic implantable cardioverter defibrillators (AICDs): devices programmed to pace heart rate (pacemaker) and/or deliver an electric shock if HR exceeds set limit (defibrillator).

a. Should know setting for HR limit.

b. ST segment changes may be common.

c. Avoid UE aerobic or strengthening exercises initially after implant.

d. Electromagnetic signals (antitheft devices) may cause devices to fire (defibrillator) or slow down or speed up (pacemaker).

4. Diabetes.

a. Patients demonstrate problems controlling blood glucose, with associated cardiovascular disease, renal disease, neuropathy, peripheral vascular disease and ulceration and/or autonomic dysfunction.

b. Exercise testing.

(1) May need to use submaximal ETT tests; maximal tests precluded with autonomic neuropathy.

(2) With PVD/peripheral neuropathy, may need to shift to arm ergometry.

c. Exercise training.

(1) Use principles of exercise prescription: intensities of 40%–85% functional capacity.

(a) Insulin-dependent diabetes: daily exercise recommended, with shorter durations (20–30 minutes).

(b) Non–insulin-dependent diabetes: five times/week recommended, with longer durations (40–60 minutes).

(2) Exercise effects: lowers blood glucose levels; overall less insulin required.

(3) Hypoglycemia may result with too much insulin (most common response to exercise).

(a) Carefully monitor for signs of hypoglycemia: acute fatigue, restlessness, marked irritability and weakness; in severe cases, mental disturbances, delirium, coma (a life-threatening situation).

(b) Control by eating carbohydrate snacks prior to or during prolonged exercise or by self-blood glucose monitoring and placing insulin in a nonexercising body part (e.g., abdominal wall).

(4) Poorly controlled diabetes: lack adequate insulin, may lead to impaired glucose transport, ketosis, hyperglycemia (too much blood sugar).

(5) Proper footwear is important, especially with changes associated with diabetic feet.

(6) Jogging, jarring activities are contraindicated in cases of advanced diabetic retinopathy.

Possible Effects of Physical Training/ Cardiac Rehabilitation

1. Decreased HR at rest and during exercise; improved HR recovery after exercise.

2. Increased stroke volume.

3. Increased myocardial oxygen supply and myocardial contractility; myocardial hypertrophy.

4. Improved respiratory capacity during exercise.

5. Improved functional capacity of exercising muscles.

6. Reduced body fat, increased lean body mass; successful weight reduction requires multifactorial interventions.

7. Decreased serum lipoproteins (cholesterol, triglycerides).

8. Improved glucose tolerance.

9. Improved blood fibrinolytic activity and coagulability.

10. Improvement in measures of psychological status and functioning: self-confidence and sense of well-being.

11. Increased participation in exercise; improved outcomes with adherence to rehabilitation programming.

a. Decreased angina in patients with CAD: anginal threshold is raised secondary to decreased myocardial oxygen consumption.

b. Reduced total and cardiovascular mortality in patients following myocardial infarction.

c. Decreased symptoms of heart failure, improved functional capacity in patients with left ventricular systolic dysfunction.

d. Improved exercise tolerance and function in patients with cardiac transplantation.

Peripheral Vascular Disease Management

Rehabilitation Guidelines for Arterial Disease

1. Encourage risk factor modification: cessation of smoking, weight control, glucose and lipid control.

2. Avoid excessive strain, protection of extremities from injury and extremes of temperature.

3. Bed rest may be required if gangrene, ulceration, acute arterial disease are present.

4. Exercise training for patients with PVD: may result in improved functional capacity, improved peripheral blood flow and muscle oxidative capacity.
   a. Consider interval training (multistage discontinuous protocol) with frequent rests.
   b. Walking program, moderate intensity (40%–70% VO_2max) and duration, two to three times/day, 3–7 days/week.
   c. Exercise to the point of pain, not beyond. Use scale for subjective ratings for pain. Record time of pain onset.
   d. Non–weight-bearing exercise (cycle ergometry, arm ergometry) may be necessary in some patients; less effective in producing a peripheral conditioning effect.
   e. Well fitting shoes essential; with insensitive feet, teach techniques of proper foot inspection and care.
   f. Beta-blockers for treatment of hypertension or cardiac disorders may decrease time to claudication or worsen symptoms
   g. Pentoxifylline, dipyridamole, aspirin and warfarin may improve time to claudication.
   h. High risk for CAD.

5. Lower extremity exercise.
   a. Modified Buerger-Allen exercises: postural exercises plus active plantar and dorsiflexion of the ankle; active exercises improve blood flow during and after exercise; effects less pronounced in patients with PVD.
   b. Resistive calf exercises: most effective method of increasing blood flow.

6. Medical treatment.
   a. Medications to decrease blood viscosity, prevent thrombus formation (e.g., heparin).
   b. Vasodilators: controversial.
   c. Calcium channel blockers in vasospastic disease.

7. Surgical management.
   a. Atherectomy, thromboembolectomy, laser therapy.
   b. Revascularization: angioplasty or bypass grafting.
   c. Sympathectomy: results in permanent vasodilation, improvement of blood flow to skin.
   d. Amputation when gangrene is present.

Rehabilitation Guidelines for Venous Disease

1. Deep vein thrombophlebitis (DVT). Early stages may be asymptomatic; symptomatic patients demonstrate dull ache, pain, tenderness in calf; may also see slight edema or fever.
   a. Acute: patients on bed rest until signs of inflammation have subsided; elevation of involved leg.
   b. Anticoagulation medications.
   c. Exercise therapy contraindicated during acute phase; increases pain, potential to dislodge clot, progress to pulmonary embolism, potentially fatal.
   d. Ambulation permitted (with elastic stockings) after local tenderness and swelling resolve.

2. Chronic venous insufficiency (CVI).
   a. Varies by severity.
   b. Focus on activation of "muscle pump"; venous stasis associated with prolonged bed rest or sitting with legs in dependent position contributory to development of DVT.
      (1) Active and active-resistive lower extremity exercises: emphasis on muscle pump exercises (dorsiflexion/plantarflexion, foot circles.
      (2) Periodic elevation of extremities, massage to improve flow.
      (3) Consider cycle ergometry in sitting or attached to foot of bed.
      (4) Early ambulation as soon as patient is able to get out of bed, three to four times/day.
   c. Pressure wrapping: compression stockings.
   d. Manual lymphatic drainage (MLD).
   e. Exercise including ROM.
   f. Intermittent pneumatic compression: contraindicated in acute thrombophlebitis.
   g. Patient education: meticulous skin care.
   h. Severe conditions with dermal ulceration: may require surgery (ligation and vein stripping, vein grafts, valvuloplasty).

CHAPTER 2

Rehabilitation Guidelines for Lymphatic Disease

Patient Education

1. Advise individuals at risk of signs and symptoms.

2. Early intervention increases favorable results.

3. Educate individuals in mechanisms to reduce edema (Box 4-4).

Complete Decongestive Therapy (CDT)

1. Phase I.
   a. Skin care.
   b. Manual lymphatic drainage (MLD) by skilled practitioner; e.g. Vodder techniques, modifications by Asdonk, Leduc, Fodi.
      (1) Performed on a daily basis.

Box 4-4 ➤ PATIENT EDUCATION FOR LYMPHEDEMA MANAGEMENT

Prevention and Maintenance Techniques
- Avoid dependent positions for extended periods of time.
- Avoid sitting cross-legged.
- When traveling, break long distances up by getting up and walking (car, plane, train). Elevate affected extremity on window ledge, dashboard, another seat when able.
- Maintain water intake.
- Maintain ideal body weight.
- Perform muscle-pumping exercises routinely.
- Avoid lifting and carrying heavy loads; e.g., carrying large brief case or suitcase, shoulder bag or backpack.
- Avoid vigorous, repetitive tasks; e.g., lifting weights.
- Avoid wearing restrictive clothing; e.g., elastic bands on socks and sleeves. Be careful of tight jewelry; e.g., rings, wrist watch, bracelet.
- Wear compressive garments, especially when traveling.
- Monitor sodium intake in diet.

Skin Care
- Keep skin clean and moisturize. Use caution as some moisturizers have a high petroleum content and can damage or breakdown the latex fibers in compression garments.
- Pat skin dry versus rubbing dry.
- Pay careful attention to avoid infections any time integrity of skin is compromised; e.g., scrape, insect bite, blister.
- Avoid exposure to harsh chemicals (e.g., cleaning agents) by wearing gloves.
- Protect feet; wear properly fitting shoes and socks.
- Use caution with shaving; an electric razor is a good choice.
- Use caution when trimming nails.
- Avoid hot baths, whirlpools and saunas secondary to the increase in core temperature and related superficial vasodilation.

   (2) Drainage is performed by clearing trunk quadrants first, followed by limb drainage starting at the proximal segments first and continuing to more distal segments in a successive manner. Direction of strokes is in direction of flow—toward the trunk.
      (a) **Red Flag:** Lymphatic system is very superficial; excess pressure can occlude superficial capillaries and prevent lymphatic resorption of excess fluids.
      (b) Specialized strokes are used for fibrous areas.
   c. Short-stretch compression bandages are used during treatment phase.
   d. Compression garments are fitted at end of phase I.
   e. Patient education for self-massage and self-care techniques.

2. Phase II—self-management.
   a. Skin care.
   b. Compression garment use during day.
   c. Exercise.
   d. Lymphedema bandaging at night.
   e. MLD as needed.
   f. Compression pumps.
      (1) **Red Flag:** Pressures higher than 45 mm Hg are contraindicated as they can cause lymphatic collapse.

General Exercise Program Guidelines

1. Begin exercise with trunk musculature first, then incorporate extremity exercise.

2. Perform exercise with compression bandages or garment in place.

3. Include aerobic conditioning.
   a. At lower intensity when lymphedema is present, 40%–50% max target HR.
   b. At higher intensity when lymphedema reduced, up to 80% max target HR.
   c. **Red Flag:** Avoid strenuous activities.
      (1) Running, jogging, stair climbing.
      (2) Sports requiring ballistic movements (e.g. tennis, racquetball).
   d. Activities with lower risk.
      (1) Brisk walking, tai chi, cross country skiing, snowshoeing, swimming.

4. Include active ROM and gentle stretching.

5. Include low-intensity resistance exercise. Wear compression garment.

6. Include deep breathing and diaphragmatic breathing activities.

Lymphatic Drainage Exercise Guidelines

1. Pumping exercises designed to follow a sequence to move lymph away from congested areas.
   a. Exercise focuses first on proximal body areas and progress to more distal areas; effectively following the premise of decongesting proximally prior to moving distally.
   b. The exercises are performed with the body parts in an elevated position.
   c. Compressive dressings or garments are worn.
   d. Diaphragmatic breathing is combined with exercise.

2. Schedule.
   a. Perform exercise twice daily.
   b. Allow 20–30 minutes to complete.
   c. Follow lymph drainage exercises with elevation for 30 minutes.
   d. Include low-intensity cardiovascular activity two to three times per week.

3. Exercise routines.
   a. Upper extremity, perform with affected extremity elevated, supine position.
      (1) Initiate several deep breaths using diaphragmatic breathing.
      (2) Begin with active ROM activities of the shoulder; e.g., circumduction, horizontal abduction/adduction, shoulder press.
      (3) Include isometric activities of shoulder musculature; e.g. hand press.
      (4) Progress to distal musculature: active elbow, forearm, wrist, finger exercises.
      (5) Include light isometric elbow, wrist, hand activities; e.g., flexion, extension, fist clenching.
      (6) Rest with extremity elevated for 20–30 minutes.
   b. Lower extremity, performed with extremity elevated, supine position with wall at feet for support if needed.
      (1) Initiate several deep breaths using diaphragmatic breathing.
      (2) Begin with active hip flexion, extension and rotation sliding feet along wall, include hip rotations.
      (3) Single and bilateral knee-to-chest activities.
      (4) Include isometrics: gluteal sets, extension press against wall, adductor press.
      (5) Reciprocal hip flexion and extension away from wall, hip and knee flexion and extension.
      (8) Active ankle plantarflexion, dorsiflexion and circumduction.
      (9) Rest with LEs elevated for 20–30 minutes.

4. Signs and symptoms of over-doing it.
   a. Aching or throbbing feeling of the limb.
   b. Congested, full feeling in limb.
   c. Discomfort in the lymph nodal area.
   d. Pain.
   e. Change in skin color.

APPENDIX A

Sample Exercise Programs per MET Level

Level I: 1.0–1.5 METS

1. Exercises.
   a. Passive/active assistive ROM (AAROM) to larger joints, active ROM (AROM) smaller joints (ankles, knees, hands, wrists).
   b. Diaphragmatic breathing.
   c. Use of incentive spirometer every hour for surgical patients.

2. Activities: feed self, turn self, wash hands and face, use commode, sit on edge of bed with feet supported (10–15 minutes, one to times times/day as tolerated; ensure 1-hour rest between activities.

Level II: 1.5–2.5 METS

1. Exercises (may add in prone activities).
   a. Continue diaphragmatic breathing.
   b. Incorporate active exercises or larger joints (may need to limit shoulder elevation to 90 degrees).
   c. Use of incentive spirometer every hour for surgical patients.

2. Activities.
   a. Sit in chair, for meals, as tolerated.
   b. May bathe entire body, with assistance for legs and back.
   c. Ensure rest between activities.
   d. Use commode.
   e. Sit on edge of bed with feet supported 10–15 minutes, one to two times/day.
   f. Ensure 1 hour of rest between activities.

Level III: 2.5–3.5 METS

1. Exercises.
   a. Continue diaphragmatic breathing with surgical patients.
   b. Warm up exercises: active knee, ankle and shoulder movements.
   c. Cervical AROM.
   d. Walk 100–150 feet each walk, gradually increase the distance. A minimum of three walks/day is desired.

2. Activities.
   a. Use bathroom.
   b. Shave or apply makeup.
   c. May wash at sink.
   d. Up in room, as tolerated.
   e. Ensure rest between activities.

Level IV: 3.5–4.5 METS

1. Warm-Up Exercises:
   a. Continue diaphragmatic breathing exercises with surgical patients.
   b. Marching in place.
   c. Trunk rotation and side bending.
   d. Shoulder elevation to 90 degrees.

2. Exercise.
   a. Walk 150–250 feet, three times a day.

3. Activities.
   a. May shower if permitted (surgical heart patients shower seventh day if incision is intact and dry and there are no stitches or staples).
   b. Continue previous activities.
   c. Ensure rest periods between activities.

Level V: 4.5–5.5 METS

1. Exercises (in standing).
   a. Continue level IV warm-up.
   b. Walk 250–350 feet, three times/day.
   c. Walk up and down 10 steps slowly with a pause every fifth step. Walk should be timed and time and distance slowly increased.

2. Activities.
   a. Continue previous activities, increase as tolerated within heart rate and activity guidelines.

Pulmonary Physical Therapy

JULIE ANN STARR, PT, MS, CCS

Focus Areas for Content Review:
- Anatomy and physiology of the pulmonary system.
- Most common pathologies and diseases of the pulmonary system.
- Physical therapy interventions: indications and contraindications, appropriate physiological response, PTA response to adverse

reaction, effects of interventions on pulmonary and other systems.
- Pulmonary system tests and measures indicating patient ability to participate in and/or indication to discontinue intervention.

Pulmonary Anatomy and Physiology

Bony Thorax

1. Anterior border is the sternum: manubrium, body, xiphoid process. The lateral borders of the trachea run perpendicularly into the suprasternal notch. The angle of Louis (sternal angle), the bony ridge between the manubrium and body, is the point of anterior attachment of the second rib and tracheal bifurcation.

2. Lateral border is the ribcage. Ribs 1–6, termed true or costosternal ribs, have a single anterior costochondral attachment to the sternum. Ribs 7–10, termed false or costochondral ribs, share costochondral attachments before attaching anteriorly to the sternum. Ribs 11 and 12 are termed floating or costovertebral ribs, as they have no anterior attachment.

3. Posterior border is the vertebral column, T1 through T12.

4. Shoulder girdle can affect the motion of the thorax. Provides attachments for accessory muscles of ventilation.

Internal Structures

1. Upper airways.
   a. Nose or mouth: entry point into the respiratory system. The nose filters, humidifies and warms air.

   b. Pharynx: common area used for both respiratory and digestive systems.
   c. Larynx: connects the pharynx to trachea, including the epiglottis and vocal cords.

2. Lower airways.
   a. The conducting airways, trachea to terminal bronchioles, transport air only. No gas exchange occurs.
   b. The respiratory unit: respiratory bronchioles, alveolar ducts, alveolar sacs and alveoli. Diffusion of gas occurs through all of these structures.

3. Lung structures.
   a. Right lung divides into three lobes by the oblique and horizontal fissure lines. Each lobe divides into segments, totaling 10 segments.
   b. Left lung divides into two lobes by a single oblique fissure line. Each lobe divides into segments, totaling 8 segments.

4. Pleura.
   a. Parietal pleura covers the inner surface of the thoracic cage, diaphragm and mediastinal border of the lung.
   b. Visceral pleura wraps the outer surface of the lung, including the fissure lines.
   c. Intrapleural space is the potential space between the two pleura that maintains the approximation of the

ribcage and lungs, allowing forces to be transmitted from one structure to another.

Muscles of Ventilation

1. **Primary muscles of inspiration produce a normal resting tidal volume.**
   a. Primary muscle of inspiration is the diaphragm. The diaphragm is made of two hemidiaphragms, each with a central tendon. When the diaphragm is at rest, the hemidiaphragms are arched high into the thorax. When the muscle contracts, the central tendon is pulled downward, flattening the dome. The result is a protrusion of the abdominal wall during inhalation.
   b. Additional primary muscles of inspiration are portions of the intercostals.

2. **Accessory muscles of inspiration are used when a more rapid or deeper inhalation is required or in disease states. The upper 2 ribs are raised by the scalenes and sternocleidomastoid. The rest of the ribs are raised by levator costarum and serratus. By fixing the shoulder girdle, the trapezius, pectorals and serratus can become muscles of inspiration.**

3. **Expiratory muscles of ventilation.**
   a. Resting exhalation results from a passive relaxation of the inspiratory muscles and the elastic recoil tendency of the lung. Normal abdominal tone holds the abdominal contents directly under the diaphragm, assisting the return of the diaphragm to the normal high-domed position.
   b. Expiratory muscles, used when a quicker and/or fuller expiration is desired, as in exercise or in disease states. These are quadratus lumborum, portions of the intercostals, abdominal muscles, lower iliocostalis and serratus posterior inferior.

4. **Special populations: patients who lack functional abdominal musculature: e.g. patients with spinal cord injury. Due to the lack of abdominal musculature, the resting position of the diaphragm is lower in the thorax, decreasing inspiratory reserve. The more upright the body position, the lower the diaphragm and the lower the inspiratory capacity. The more supine, the more advantageous the position of the diaphragm. An abdominal binder may be helpful in providing support to the abdominal viscera, thereby assisting ventilation. Care must be taken not to constrict the thorax with the abdominal binder.**

Ventilation

1. **Refers to the movement of gas in and out of the pulmonary system**

2. **Volumes (Figure 5-1).**
   a. Tidal volume (TV): volume of gas inhaled (exhaled) during a normal resting breath.

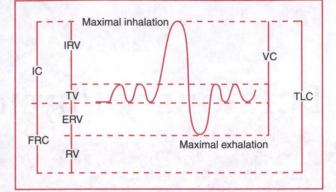

Figure 5-1 • Lung volumes and capacities. IRV = inspiratory reserve volume; TV = tidal volume; ERV = expiratory reserve volume; RV = residual volume; IC = inspiratory capacity; FRC = functional residual capacity, VC = vital capacity; TLC = total lung capacity.
(From O'Sullivan S, Schmidt T: Physical Rehabilitation: Assessment and Treatment. 5th ed, FA Davis, 2001:447, with permission.)

   b. Inspiratory reserve volume (IRV): volume of gas that can be inhaled beyond a normal resting tidal inhalation.
   c. Expiratory reserve volume (ERV): volume of gas that can be exhaled beyond a normal resting tidal exhalation.
   d. Residual volume (RV): volume of gas that remains in the lungs after ERV has been exhaled.

3. **Capacities: two or more lung volumes added together.**
   a. Inspiratory capacity (IRV + TV): the amount of air that can be inhaled from right endexpiratory pressure (REEP).
   b. Vital Capacity (IRV + TV + ERV): the amount of air that is under volitional control, conventionally measured as a forced expiratory vital capacity (FVC).
   c. Functional Residual Capacity (ERV + RV): the amount of air that resides in the lungs after a normal resting tidal exhalation.
   d. Total lung capacity (IRV + TV + ERV + RV): the total amount of air that is housed within the thorax during a maximum inspiratory effort.

4. **Flow rates.**
   a. Forced expiratory volume in 1 second (FEV1): the amount of air exhaled during the first second of FVC. In the healthy, at least 75% of the FVC is exhaled within the first second (FEV1/FVC $\times$ 100 >75%).
   b. Forced expiratory flow rate (FEF 25%–75%) is the slope of a line drawn between the points 25% and 75% of exhaled volume on a forced vital capacity exhalation curve. This flow rate is more specific to the smaller airways and shows a more dramatic change with disease than FEV1.

Respiration

1. The diffusion of gas across the alveolar-capillary membrane

2. Arterial oxygenation: the ability of arterial blood to carry oxygen.
   a. Partial pressure of oxygen in the atmosphere (Pao_2) at sea level is 760 mm Hg (barometric pressure) $\times$ 21% = 159.6 mm Hg.
   b. The partial pressure of oxygen in the arterial blood, Pao_2, depends on the integrity of the pulmonary system, the circulatory system and the Pao_2. In health, Pao_2 at room air is 95–100 mm Hg. Hypoxemia: Pao_2 less than 90. Hyperoxemia: Pao_2 >100.
   c. Fraction of oxygen in the inspired air (Fio_2) is the percentage of oxygen in air based on a total of 1.00. The Fio_2 of room air, approximately 21% oxygen, is written as 0.21. Supplemental oxygen increases the percentage (>21%) of oxygen in the patient's atmosphere. Supplemental oxygen is usually prescribed when the Pao_2 falls below 55–60 mm Hg.

3. Alveolar ventilation: ability to remove carbon dioxide from the pulmonary circulation and maintain pH.
   a. pH indicates the concentration of free-floating hydrogen ions within the body. Normal range for pH is 7.36–7.44.
      (1) A pH <7.36 is considered acidic (respiratory acidosis).
      (2) A pH >7.44 is considered alkaline (respiratory alkalosis).
   b. Removal, or retention, of CO_2 by the respiratory system alters the pH of the body.
      (1) An increase in the $Paco_2$ decreases the body's pH.
      (2) A decrease in the $Paco_2$ raises the body's pH.
   c. $PaCO_2$: the partial pressure of carbon dioxide within the arterial blood, in health, 36–44 mm Hg. Hypercapnea is a $Paco_2$ greater than 44 mm Hg. Hypocapnea is a $Paco_2$ <36 mmHg. Removal or retention of CO_2 by the respiratory system alters the pH of the body with an inverse relationship. An increase in the $Paco_2$ decreases the body's pH. A decrease in the $Paco_2$ raises the body's pH.
   d. HCO_3^-: amount of bicarbonate ions within the arterial blood, normally 23–30 mEq/mL. Removal or retention of HCO_3^- alters the pH of the body with a direct relationship. An increase in bicarbonate ions increases the body's pH. A decrease in bicarbonate ions decreases the body's pH.

Ventilation (VE) and Perfusion (blood flow or Q). Optimal respiration occurs when ventilation and perfusion (blood flow to the lungs) are matched. Different ventilation and perfusion relationships exist.

1. Effects of body position on ventilation perfusion relationship. Gravity affects the distribution of ventilation and perfusion.
   a. Upright position.
      (1) Perfusion is gravity dependent; i.e., more pulmonary blood is found at the base of the lung.
      (2) Ventilation. At the static point of REEP, the apical alveoli are fuller than those at the base. During the dynamic phase of inspiration, more air will be delivered to the less filled alveoli at the bases, making the greater change in VE at the bases.
   b. Other body positions. Every body position creates these zones: gravity independent, middle and gravity dependent. The gravity independent area of the lung, despite the position of the body, will act as dead space. The gravity dependent area of the lung will act as a shunt. Body positions can be used for a variety of treatment goals: draining secretions, increasing ventilation, or to optimize ventilation perfusion relationships.

Control of Ventilation

1. A complex system controls the cycle of ventilation

2. Receptors (baroreceptors, chemoreceptors, irritant receptors, stretch receptors) within the body assist in adjusting the ventilatory cycle by sending information to the controller.

3. Central control centers (cortex, pons, medulla and autonomic nervous system) evaluate the receptors' information and send a message out to the ventilatory muscles to alter the respiratory cycle in order to maintain adequate alveolar ventilation and arterial oxygenation.

4. Ventilatory muscles institute the changes deemed necessary by the central controllers.

Physical Therapy Examination

Pertinent Information from Pulmonary Assessment (performed by the PT)

1. **Patient interview.**
   a. Information is gathered by the physical therapist available to the PTA for intervention purposes.
      (1) The information is gathered from the medical records, patient's family and patient history.

2. **Present illness.**
   a. Initial onset and progression of primary problem.
   b. Factors which exacerbate or improve the condition: positions, rest, medications, activities.

3. **Findings from patient history.**
   a. The PTA should review the patient's history before the initial treatment; discuss any questions with the PT as necessary.
   b. Occupational history.
      (1) Be aware of past and present exposures to environmental toxins and specific diseases such as asbestosis, silicosis, pneumoconiosis.
   c. Past medical history that would alter treatment plans.
      (1) Heart disease.
      (2) Long-term steroid use.
   d. Current medications that could alter vital sign responses.
      (1) Beta blockers.
      (2) Bronchodilators.
      (3) Steroids.
   e. Social habits.
      (1) Issues that may need to be addressed while the PTA provides treatment to the patient.
         (a) Smoking history.
         (b) Alcohol consumption.
         (c) Recreational drug use.
         (d) Functional activities during periods of wellness, as well as with present illness.
   f. Cough and sputum production.
      (1) Note any changes in production while providing treatment to the patient.
         (a) Notify the PT if there is a change in the patient's baseline status.
            • Color of the sputum (white to yellow to green to red).
            • Viscosity of the sputum (from thin to thick).
            • Production/amount of sputum (minimal to greater amounts).
   g. Family history of pulmonary disease, such as cystic fibrosis.

Tests and Measures

1. **Vital signs.** See Table 5-1 for normal values.
   a. Temperature: normal (afebrile) 98.6°F, (37°C). Core temperature increase indicates infection.
   b. Heart rate (HR): normal 60–100 bpm; tachycardia: HR >100 bpm; bradycardia: HR <60 bpm.
   c. Respirations.
      (1) Rate: in health is 12–20 breaths per minute. Tachypnea is a rate greater than 20 breaths per minute. Apnea means no respirations.
      (2) Rhythm: regular or irregular.
      (3) Amplitude: shallow, deep.
   d. Blood pressure.

2. **Observation.**
   a. Peripheral edema seen in gravity dependent areas and jugular venous distension indicates possible heart failure. Right ventricular hypertrophy and dilation (cor pulmonale) are common sequelae to chronic lung disease.
   b. Body positions. Stabilizing the shoulder girdle places the thorax in the inspiratory position and allows the additional recruitment of muscles for inspiration (pectorals).
   c. Color: cyanosis, an acute sign of hypoxemia, is a bluish tinge to nail beds and the areas around eyes and mouth.
   d. Digital clubbing: a sign of chronic hypoxemia. The configuration of the distal phalanx of fingers or toes becomes bulbous.

3. **Auscultation.**
   a. Intensity of inspiration and expiration will be quieter at the bases than the apex.
      (1) Vesicular (normal breath sound): a soft rustling sound heard throughout all of inspiration and the beginning of expiration.

Table 5-1 ➤ NORMAL VALUES FOR INFANTS AND ADULTS

PARAMETER	INFANT	ADULT
Heart Rate	120 bpm	60–100 bpm
Blood Pressure	75/50 mm Hg	<120/80 mm Hg
Respiratory Rate	40 br/min	12–20 br/min
Pao_2	75–80 mm Hg	80–100 mm Hg
$Paco_2$	34–54 mm Hg	35–45 mm Hg
pH	7.26–7.41	7.35–7.45
Tidal Volume	20 mL	500 mL

Table 5-2 ➤ INTERPRETATION OF ABNORMAL ACID-BASE BALANCE

TYPE	pH	PaCO$_2$	HCO$_3$	CAUSES	SIGNS AND SYMPTOMS
Respiratory alkalosis	↑	↓	WNL	Alveolar hyperventilation	Dizziness, syncope, tingling, numbness, early tetany
Respiratory acidosis	↓	↑	WNL	Alveolar hypoventilation	Early: anxiety, restlessness, dyspnea, headache. Late: confusion, somnolence, coma
Metabolic alkalosis	↑	WNL	↑	Bicarbonate ingestion, vomiting, diuretics, steroids, adrenal disease	Vague symptoms: weakness, mental dullness, possibly early tetany
Metabolic acidosis	↓	WNL	↓	Diabetic, lactic, or uremic acidosis, prolonged diarrhea	Secondary hyperventilation (Kussmaul's breathing), nausea, lethargy, and coma

From Rothstein J, Roy S, Wolf S. The four basic conditions of acid-base balance. In: The Rehabilitation Specialist's Handbook, 2nd ed, FA Davis, Philadelphia, 1998:529, with permission.

(2) Bronchial: a more hollow, echoing sound normally found only over the right superior anterior thorax. This corresponds to an area over the right main stem bronchus. All of inspiration and most of expiration are heard with bronchial breath sounds.

(3) Decreased: a very distant sound not normally heard over a healthy thorax; allows only some inspiration to be heard. Often associated with obstructive lung diseases.

b. Adventitious (extra) sounds. According to the American Thoracic Society, there are only two adventitious breath sounds:

(1) Crackles (also termed *rales, crepitations*): a crackling sound heard usually during inspiration that indicates pathology (atelectasis, fibrosis, pulmonary edema).

(2) Wheezes: a musical pitched sound, usually heard during expiration caused by airway obstruction (asthma, chronic obstructive pulmonary disease [COPD], foreign body aspiration). With severe airway constriction, as with croup, wheezes may be heard on inspiration as well.

4. Radiographic examination.

a. Chest x-rays (CXRs): a two-dimensional radiographic film to detect the presence of abnormal material (exudates, blood) or a change in pulmonary parenchyma (fibrosis, collapse).

b. Computerized axial tomography (CT or CAT scan): a computer-generated picture of a cross-sectional plane of the body.

c. Ventilation perfusion (V/Q) scan: matches the ventilation pattern of the lung to the perfusion pattern to identify the presence of pulmonary emboli.

d. Fluoroscopy: continuous x-ray beam allows observation of diaphragmatic excursion.

5. Laboratory tests: See Table 5-1 for normal values.

a. Arterial blood gas (ABG) analysis indicates the adequacy of:

(1) Alveolar ventilation by determining pH, bicarbonate ion and partial pressure of carbon dioxide.

Table 5-2 presents the four basic conditions of acid-base balance and the PaCO$_2$, pH and HCO$_3^-$ values that accompany each condition.

(2) Arterial oxygenation by determining the partial pressure of oxygen in relation to the fraction of inspired oxygen.

b. Electrocardiogram: see chapter 4 on Cardiovascular Physical Therapy for discussion.

c. Sputum studies:

(1) Gram's stain: immediate identification of the category of bacteria (gram negative or gram positive) and its appearance (pairs, chains, etc.).

(2) Culture and sensitivity: identifies the specific bacteria as well as the organism's susceptibility to various antibiotics. Results available within a few days.

(3) Cytology: reports the presence of cancer cells in sputum.

d. Pulmonary function tests (PFTs): evaluate lung volumes, capacities and flow rates. Used to diagnose disease, monitor progression and determine the benefits of medical management. Refer to Figure 5-2 for changes with disease states. Refer to Table 5-3 for classification of respiratory impairments including PFT predicted values.

e. Blood values

(1) White blood cell count (WBC) normal values: 4,000–11,000.

(2) Hematocrit (Hct) normal values: 35–48.

(3) Hemoglobin (Hgb) normal values: 12–16.

6. Bronchoscopy: endoscope used to view, biopsy, wash, suction and/or brush the interior aspects of the tracheobronchial tree.

7. Exercise tolerance tests (ETT) (Graded Exercise Test). See also chapter 4 on Cardiovascular Physical Therapy.

a. Evaluates an individual's cardiopulmonary response to gradually increasing exercise.

b. Determines the presence of exercise-induced bronchospasm by testing pulmonary function, particularly FEV1 before and after ETT.

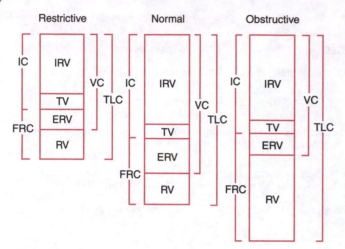

ERV = Expiratory reserve volume
FRC = Functional residual capacity
IC = Inspiratory capacity
IRV = Inspiratory reserve volume

RV = Residual volume
TLC = Total lung capacity
TV = Tidal volume

Figure 5-2 • Lung volumes of a healthy pulmonary system compared with the lung volumes and capacities found in restrictive and obstructive pulmonary disease.
(From Rothstein J, Roy S, Wolf S. The four basic conditions of acid-base balance. In: The Rehabilitation Specialist's Handbook, 2nd ed, FA Davis, Philadelphia, 1998:529, with permission.)

Table 5-4 ➤ GRADED EXERCISE TEST TERMINATION CRITERIA

1. Maximal shortness of breath.
2. A fall in Pao_2 of >20 mm Hg or a Pao_2 <55 mm Hg.
3. A rise in $Paco_2$ of >10 mm Hg or >65 mm Hg.
4. Cardiac ischemia or arrhythmias.
5. Symptoms of fatigue.
6. Increase in diastolic blood pressure readings of 20 mm Hg, systolic hypertension >250 mm Hg, decrease in blood pressure with increasing workloads.
7. Leg pain.
8. Total fatigue.
9. Signs of insufficient cardiac output.
10. Reaching a ventilatory maximum.

From Brannon, F, et al: Cardiopulmonary Rehabilitation: Basic Theory and Application. 3rd ed, FA Davis, 1998: 300, with permission.

c. Documents the need for supplemental oxygen during an exercise program by analyzing arterial blood gas values throughout the ETT. ABGs also provide a criterion for test termination. If arterial blood sampling is unavailable, pulse oximetry can be used to monitor the percent saturation of oxygen within the arterial blood. Table 5-4 presents criteria for test termination for patients with pulmonary disease.

Table-3 ➤ CLASSES OF RESPIRATORY IMPAIRMENT

	CLASS 1 0% IMPAIRMENT	CLASS 2 20–30% IMPAIRMENT	CLASS 3 40–50% IMPAIRMENT	CLASS 4 60–90% IMPAIRMENT
Roentgenographic appearance	Usually normal but there may be evidence of healed or inactive chest disease including, e.g., minimal nodular silicosis or pleura scars	May be normal or abnormal	May be normal but usually is not	Usually is abnormal
Dyspnea	When it occurs, it is consistent with the circumstances or activity	Does not occur at rest and seldom occurs during the performance of the usual activities of daily living. The patient can keep pace with persons of same age and body build on level ground without breathlessness but not on hills or stairs	Does not occur at rest but does occur during the usual activities of daily living. However, the patient can walk a mile at his own pace without dyspnea although he cannot keep pace on level ground with others of the same age and body build	Occurs during such activities as climbing one flight of stairs or walking 100 yards on level ground, on less exertion, or even at rest
Tests of ventilatory function FEV1, FCV, MMV	Not <85% of predicted	70–85% of predicted	55–70% of predicted	<55% of predicted
Arterial oxygen saturation	Not applicable	Not applicable	Usually 88%* or greater at rest and after exercise	Usually less than 88% at rest and after exercise

*88% saturation corresponds to an arterial PO_2 of 58 mm Hg, assuming the arterial pH is in the normal range.
From Guides to the evaluator of permanent impairment; the respiratory system. JAMA, 1965;194: 919, with permission.

Physical Dysfunction/Impairments

Acute Diseases

1. **Bacterial pneumonia.**
   a. Description: An intra-alveolar bacterial infection. Gram-positive bacteria are usually acquired in the community. Pneumococcal pneumonia (streptococcal) is the most common type of gram-positive pneumonia. Gramnegative bacteria usually develop in a host who has underlying chronic debilitating conditions, severe acute illness and recent antibiotic therapy. Gram-negative infections result in early tissue necrosis and abscess formation. Common infecting organisms: *Klebsiella, Haemophilus Influenza, Pseudomonas Aeruginosa, Proteus, Serratia.*
   b. Pertinent physical findings.
      (1) Shaking chills.
      (2) Fever.
      (3) Chest pain if pleuritic involvement.
      (4) Cough becoming productive of purulent, blood-streaked or rusty sputum.
      (5) Decreased or bronchial breath sounds and/or crackles.
      (6) Tachypnea.
      (7) Increased white blood cell count.
      (8) Hypoxemia, hypocapnea initially, hypercapnea with increasing severity.
      (9) CXR confirmation of infiltrate.

2. **Viral pneumonia.**
   a. Description: An interstitial or intra-alveolar inflammatory process caused by viral agents (influenza, adenovirus, cytomegalovirus, herpes, parainfluenza, respiratory syncytial virus, measles).
   b. Pertinent physical findings.
      (1) Recent history of upper respiratory infection.
      (2) Fever.
      (3) Chills.
      (4) Dry cough.
      (5) Headaches.
      (6) Decreased breath sounds and/or crackles.
      (7) Hypoxemia and hypercapnea.
      (8) Normal white blood cell count.
      (9) CXR confirmation of interstitial infiltrate.

3. **Aspiration pneumonia.**
   a. Description: aspirated material causes an acute inflammatory reaction within the lungs. Usually found in patients with impaired swallowing (dysphagia), fixed neck extension, intoxication, impaired consciousness, neuromuscular disease and recent anesthesia.
   b. Pertinent physical findings.
      (1) Symptoms begin shortly after aspiration event (hours).
      (2) Cough may be dry at the onset, progress to producing putrid secretions.
      (3) Dyspnea.
      (4) Tachypnea.
      (5) Cyanosis.
      (6) Tachycardia.
      (7) Wheezes and crackles with decreased breath sounds.
      (8) Hypoxemia, hypercapnea in severe cases.
      (9) Chest pain over the involved area.
      (10) Fever.
      (11) WBC count shows varying degrees of leukocytosis.
      (12) CXR initially shows pneumonitis. Chronic aspiration shows necrotizing pneumonia with cavitation.

4. **Tuberculosis (TB).**
   a. Description: *Mycobacterium tuberculosis* infection spread by aerosolized droplets from an untreated infected host. Incubation period: 2–10 weeks. Primary disease lasts approximately 10 days to 2 weeks. Postprimary infection is reactivation of dormant tuberculous bacillus which can occur years after the primary infection. Two weeks on appropriate antituberculin drugs renders the host noninfectious. During the infectious stage, the patient must be isolated from others in a negative pressure room. Anyone entering the room must wear a protective TB mask and follow universal precautions. If the patient leaves the negative pressure room, then the patient must wear the specialized mask to keep from infecting others. Medication is taken for prolonged periods: 3–12 months. There is an increased incidence of TB in the patient population infected by HIV.
   b. Pertinent physical findings of primary disease can be unnoticed as it causes only mild symptoms: slight nonproductive cough, low-grade fever and possible CXR changes consistent with primary disease.
   c. Pertinent physical findings of post primary infection are characterized by:
      (1) Fever.
      (2) Weight loss.
      (3) Cough.
      (4) Hilar adenopathy: enlargement of the lymph nodes surrounding the hilum.
      (5) Night sweat.
      (6) Crackles.

(7) Hemoptysis: blood-streaked sputum.

(8) WBC shows increased lymphocytes.

(9) CXR shows upper lobe involvement with air-space densities, cavitation, pleural involvement and parenchymal fibrosis.

5. **Pneumocystis carinii pneumonia.**

   a. Description: pulmonary infection caused by a protozoan in immunocompromised hosts. Most often found in patients following transplantation, neonates or patients infected with HIV.

   b. Pertinent physical findings.

      (1) Insidious progressive shortness of breath.

      (2) Nonproductive cough.

      (3) Crackles.

      (4) Weakness.

      (5) Fever.

      (6) CRX shows interstitial infiltrates.

      (7) Complete blood count (CBC) shows no evidence of infection.

6. **SARS (severe acute respiratory syndrome).**

   a. Definition: An atypical respiratory illness caused by a coronovirus. Initial outbreak in southern mainland China with worldwide spread to other areas such as Singapore, Toronto, Vietnam and Hong Kong.

   b. Pertinent physical findings:

      (1) High temperature.

      (2) Dry cough.

      (3) Decreased white blood cells, decreased platelets and decreased lymphocytes.

      (4) Increased liver function tests.

      (5) Abnormal CXR with borderline breath sounds changes.

7. **Refer to Table 5-2, Transmission-Based Precautions.**

Chronic Obstructive Diseases

1. **Chronic obstructive pulmonary disease (COPD).**

   a. Description: according to the Global Initiative for Obstructive Lung Disease (GOLD): COPD is a disease state characterized by airflow limitation that is not fully reversible. The airflow limitation is usually both progressive and associated with an abnormal inflammatory response of the lungs to noxious particles or gases.

   b. Stages.

      (1) Stage 0 (at risk).

         (a) Normal spirometry.

         (b) Chronic symptoms (cough, sputum production).

      (2) Stage 1 (mild).

         (a) FEV1/FVC <70%.

         (b) FEV1 > = 80% predicted.

         (c) With or without chronic symptoms.

   (3) Stage 2 (moderate).

      (a) FEV1/FVC <70%.

      (b) 50% <FEV1<80% predicted.

      (c) With or without chronic symptoms.

   (4) Stage 3 (severe).

      (a) FEV1/FVC <70%.

      (b) 30% <FEV1 <50%.

      (c) With or without chronic symptoms.

   (5) Stage 4 (very severe).

      (a) FEV1/FVC <70%.

      (b) FEV1 <30% predicted.

      (c) FEV1 <50% with chronic respiratory failure symptoms.

      (d) PaO_2 <60.

      (e) $PaCO_2$ > 50.

      (f) Cor pulmonale.

      (g) Increased jugular venous distention.

   c. Physical findings: findings increase in severity as the stage of disease advances.

      (1) Cough/sputum production/hemoptysis.

      (2) Dyspnea on exertion.

      (3) Breath sounds decreased with adventitious sounds.

      (4) Increased respiratory rate (RR).

      (5) Weight loss/anorexia.

      (6) Increased A-P diameter of chest wall.

      (7) Cyanosis.

      (8) Clubbing.

      (9) Postures to structurally elevate shoulder girdle.

      (10) CXR showing hyperinflation, flattened diaphragms, hyperlucency.

      (11) ABG changes of hypoxemia, hypercapnea.

      (12) PFTs showing obstructive disease, such as decreased FEV1, decreased FVC, increased FRC and RV and decreased FEV1/FVC ratio.

2. **Asthma.**

   a. Description: increased reactivity of the trachea and bronchi to various stimuli (allergens, exercise and cold); manifests by widespread narrowing of the airways due to inflammation, smooth muscle constriction and increased secretions that are reversible in nature. Even during remission, some degree of airway inflammation is present.

   b. Pertinent physical findings during exacerbation:

      (1) Wheezing, possible crackles and decreased breath sounds.

      (2) Increased secretions of variable amounts.

      (3) Dyspnea.

      (4) Increased accessory muscle use.

      (5) Anxiety.

      (6) Tachycardia.

      (7) Tachypnea.

      (8) Hypoxemia.

      (9) Hypocapnea. Responding to hypoxemia, there is an increased respiratory rate and minute ventilation. This will decrease $PaCO_2$. With severe

airway constriction, an increase in minute ventilation cannot occur and hypercapnea can be found.

 (10) Cyanosis.

 (11) PFTs show impaired flow rates.

 (12) CXR shows hyperlucency and flattened diaphragms during exacerbation.

3. Cystic fibrosis (CF).

a. Description: a genetically inherited disease characterized by thickening of secretions of all exocrine glands, leading to obstruction (pancreatic, pulmonic, gastrointestinal, etc.). CF may present as an obstructive, restrictive or mixed disease. Clinical signs of CF include: meconium ileus, frequent respiratory infections, especially Staph Aureus and Pseudomonas Aeruginosa, inability to gain weight despite adequate caloric intake. Diagnosis is made by a positive sweat electrolyte test.

b. Pertinent physical findings with exacerbation of disease:

 (1) Onset of symptoms usually in early childhood.

 (2) Dyspnea, especially on exertion.

 (3) Productive cough.

 (4) Hypoxemia, hypercapnea.

 (5) Cyanosis.

 (6) Clubbing.

 (7) Use of accessory muscles of ventilation.

 (8) Tachypnea.

 (9) Crackles, wheezes and/or decreased breath sounds.

 (10) Abnormal PFTs showing an obstructive pattern, restrictive pattern or both.

 (11) CXR shows increased markings, findings of bronchiectasis and/or pneumonitis.

4. Bronchiectasis.

a. Description: a chronic congenital or acquired disease characterized by dilatation of the bronchi and excessive sputum production.

b. Pertinent physical findings.

 (1) Cough and expectoration of large amounts of mucopurulent secretions.

 (2) Frequent secondary infections.

 (3) Hemoptysis.

 (4) Crackles, decreased breath sounds.

 (5) Cyanosis.

 (6) Clubbing.

 (7) Hypoxemia.

 (8) Dyspnea.

 (9) CXR which shows increased bronchial markings with interstitial changes. Bronchograms can outline bronchial dilatation but are rarely needed.

5. Hyaline membrane disease (also called respiratory distress syndrome [RDS]).

a. Description: alveolar collapse in a premature infant resulting from lung immaturity, inadequate level of pulmonary surfactant.

b. Pertinent physical findings within a few hours of birth:

 (1) Respiratory distress.

 (2) Crackles.

 (3) Tachypnea.

 (4) Hypoxemia.

 (5) Cyanosis.

 (6) Accessory muscle use.

 (7) Expiratory grunting, flaring nares.

 (8) CXR shows a classic granular pattern ("ground glass") caused by distended terminal airways and alveolar collapse.

c. Physical therapy considerations: The increased work of breathing that handling a premature infant might cause must be carefully weighed against any possible benefit that physical therapy might have.

6. Bronchopulmonary dysplasia.

a. Description: an obstructive pulmonary disease, often a sequela of premature infants with respiratory distress syndrome; results from high pressures of mechanical ventilation, high fractions of inspired oxygen (FiO_2) and/or infection. The lungs show areas of pulmonary immaturity and dysfunction due to hyperinflation.

b. Pertinent physical findings.

 (1) Hypoxemia, hypercapnea.

 (2) Crackles, wheezing and/or decreased breath sounds.

 (3) Increased bronchial secretions.

 (4) Hyperinflation.

 (5) Frequent lower respiratory infections.

 (6) Delayed growth and development.

 (7) Cor pulmonale.

 (8) CXR shows hyperinflation, low diaphragms, atelectasis and/or cystic changes.

Chronic Restrictive Diseases

1. Different etiologies typified by difficulty expanding the lungs causing a reduction in lung volumes

2. Restrictive disease due to alterations in lung parenchyma and pleura.

a. Description: fibrotic changes within the pulmonary parenchyma or pleura, as a result of idiopathic pulmonary fibrosis, asbestosis, radiation pneumonitis, oxygen toxicity.

b. Pertinent physical findings:

 (1) Dyspnea.

 (2) Hypoxemia, hypocapnea (hypercapnea appears with severity).

 (3) Crackles.

 (4) Clubbing.

 (5) Cyanosis.

 (6) PFTs reveal a reduction in vital capacity, functional residual capacity and total lung capacity.

(7) CXR show reduced lung volumes, diffuse interstitial infiltrates and/or pleural thickening.

3. Restrictive disease due to alterations in the chest wall.
a. Description: restricted motion of bony thorax, with diseases such as ankylosing spondylitis, arthritis, scoliosis, pectus excavatum, arthrogryposis or the integumentary changes of the chest wall such as thoracic burns or scleroderma.
b. Pertinent physical findings:
(1) Shallow, rapid breathing.
(2) Dyspnea.
(3) Hypoxemia, hypocapnea (hypercapnea with increasing severity).
(4) Cyanosis.
(5) Clubbing.
(6) Crackles.
(7) Reduced cough effectiveness.
(8) PFTs show reduced vital capacity, functional residual capacity and total lung capacity.
(9) CXR show reduced lung volumes, atelectasis.

4. Restrictive disease due to alterations in the neuromuscular apparatus.
a. Description: decreased muscular strength results in an inability to expand the ribcage, with multiple sclerosis, muscular dystrophy, Parkinson's disease, spinal cord injury or cardiovascular accident (CVA).
b. Pertinent physical findings:
(1) Dyspnea.
(2) Hypoxemia, hypocapnea (hypercapnea with increasing severity).
(3) Decreased breath sounds, crackles.
(4) Clubbing.
(5) Cyanosis.
(6) Reduced cough effectiveness.
(7) PFTs show reduced vital capacity and total lung capacity.
(8) CXR show reduced lung volumes, atelectasis.

Bronchogenic Carcinoma

1. Refers to a tumor which arises from the bronchial mucosa.

2. Characteristics: smoking and occupational exposures are the most frequent causal agents.
a. Cell types are: Small cell carcinoma (oat cell) and non small cell carcinoma (squamous cell, adenocarcinoma and large cell undifferentiated).
b. Secondary changes due to the tumor include obstruction or compression of an airway, blood vessel or nerve.
c. Local metastases are found in the pleura, chest wall and mediastinal structures. Common distant metastases are found in lymph nodes, liver, bone, brain and adrenals.

3. Pertinent physical findings with pulmonary involvement.
a. Unexplained weight loss.
b. Hemoptysis.
c. Dyspnea.
d. Weakness.
e. Fatigue.
f. Wheezing.
g. Pneumonia with productive cough due to airway compression.
h. Hoarseness with compression of the laryngeal nerve.
i. Atelectasis or bacterial pneumonia with nonproductive cough due to airway obstruction.

4. Management of bronchogenic cancer.
a. Chemotherapy.
b. Radiation therapy.
c. Surgical resection if possible.

5. Physical therapy considerations.
a. Pneumonias that develop behind a completely obstructed bronchus cannot be cleared with physical therapy techniques. Hold treatment and inform the supervising physical therapist until palliative therapy reduces the tumor size and relieves the bronchial obstruction.
b. Possible fractures from thoracic bone metastasis with chest compressive maneuvers and coughing.
c. Ecchymosis (bruising) in patients with low platelet count.
d. Fatigue which restricts other necessary activities.

Trauma

1. Rib fracture, flail chest.
a. Description: fracture of the ribs usually due to blunt trauma. Flail chest is two or more fractures in two or more adjacent ribs.
b. Pertinent physical findings:
(1) Shallow breathing.
(2) Splinting due to pain (especially with deep inspiration or cough).
(3) Crepitation may be felt during the ventilatory cycle over fracture site.
(4) Paradoxical movement of the flail section during the ventilatory cycle (inspiration, the flail section is pulled inward; exhalation, the flail moves outward).
(5) Confirmation by chest x-ray.

2. Pleural injury.
a. Pneumothorax.
(1) Description: air in the pleural space, usually through lacerated visceral pleura from a rib fracture or ruptured bullae.
(2) Pertinent physical findings all increase with the severity of injury.

(a) Chest pain.

(b) Dyspnea.

(c) Tracheal and mediastinal shift away from injured side.

(d) Absent or decreased breath sounds.

(e) Increased tympany with mediate percussion.

(f) Cyanosis.

(g) Respiratory distress.

(h) Confirmation by CXR.

b. Hemothorax.

(1) Description: blood in the pleural space usually from a laceration of the parietal pleura.

(2) Pertinent physical findings: all increase with the severity of injury.

(a) Chest pain.

(b) Dyspnea.

(c) Tracheal and mediastinal shift away from side of injury.

(d) Absent or decreased breath sounds.

(e) Cyanosis.

(f) Respiratory distress.

(g) Confirmation by CXR.

(h) May have signs of blood loss.

3. Lung contusion.

a. Description: Blood and edema within the alveoli and interstitial space due to blunt chest trauma with or without rib fractures.

b. Pertinent physical findings: all increase with the severity of injury.

(1) Cough with hemoptysis.

(2) Dyspnea.

(3) Decreased breath sounds and/or crackles.

(4) Cyanosis.

(5) Confirmation by CXR of ill-defined patchy densities.

Miscellaneous

1. Pulmonary edema.

a. Description: excessive seepage of fluid from the pulmonary vascular system into the interstitial space; may eventually cause alveolar edema.

(1) Cardiogenic: results from increased pressure in the pulmonary capillaries associated with left ventricular failure, aortic valvular disease, or mitral valvular disease.

(2) Non cardiogenic: results from an increased permeability of the alveolar capillary membranes due to inhalation of toxic fumes, hypervolemia, narcotic overdose or adult respiratory distress syndrome (ARDS).

b. Pertinent physical findings:

(1) Crackles.

(2) Tachypnea.

(3) Dyspnea.

(4) Hypoxemia.

(5) Peripheral edema if cardiogenic.

(6) Cough with pink, frothy secretions.

(7) CXR shows increased vascular markings, hazy opacities in gravity dependent areas of the lung showing a typical butterfly pattern. Atelectasis is possible if the surfactant lining is removed by alveolar edema.

2. Pulmonary emboli.

a. Description: a thrombus from the peripheral venous circulation becomes embolic and lodges in the pulmonary circulation. Small emboli do not necessarily cause infarction.

b. Pertinent physical findings without infarction.

(1) History consistent with pulmonary emboli: deep vein thrombosis, oral contraceptives, recent abdominal or hip surgery, polycythemia, prolonged bed rest.

(2) Sudden onset of dyspnea.

(3) Tachycardia.

(4) Hypoxemia.

(5) Cyanosis.

(6) Auscultatory findings may be normal or show crackles and decreased breath sounds.

(7) Ventilation-perfusion scan showing perfusion defects with concomitant normal ventilation.

c. Added pertinent physical findings consistent with pulmonary infarction.

(1) Chest pain.

(2) Hemoptysis.

(3) CXR shows decreased vascular markings, high diaphragm, pulmonary infiltrate and/or pleural effusion.

3. Pleural effusion.

a. Description: excessive fluid between the visceral and parietal pleura. The main causes of pleural effusion are increased pleural permeability to proteins from inflammatory diseases (pneumonia, rheumatoid arthritis, systemic lupus), neoplastic disease, increased hydrostatic pressure within pleural space (CHF), decrease in osmotic pressure (hypoproteinemia), peritoneal fluid within the pleural space (ascites, cirrhosis) or interference of pleural reabsorption from tumor invading pleural lymphatics.

b. Pertinent physical findings:

(1) Decreased breath sounds over effusion; bronchial breath sounds may be present around the perimeter of the effusion. Pleural friction rub may be possible with inflammatory process.

(2) Mediastinal shift away from large effusion.

(3) Breathlessness with large effusions.

(4) CXR shows fluid in the pleural space in gravity dependent areas of the thorax if greater than 300 mL.

(5) Pain and fever only if the pleural fluid is infected (empyema).

4. Atelectasis.

a. Description: collapsed or airless alveolar unit, caused by hypoventilation secondary to pain during the ventilatory cycle (pleuritis, postoperative pain or rib fracture), internal bronchial obstruction (aspiration, mucus plugging), external bronchial compression (tumor or enlarged lymph nodes), low tidal volumes (narcotic overdose, inappropriately low ventilator settings) or neurological insult.

b. Pertinent physical findings.
   (1) Decreased breath sounds.
   (2) Dyspnea.
   (3) Tachycardia.
   (4) Increased temperature.
   (5) CXR with plate-like streaks.

Physical Therapy Intervention

Physical Therapist Assistant's Role

1. Follow the plan of care established by the supervising physical therapist and make appropriate decisions regarding the continuation or discontinuation of each treatment session based on:

   a. Chart review prior to initiating treatment. Assess pertinent changes in any lab values or patient condition, withhold care and report to physical therapist as indicated.

   b. Collect tests and measures to determine appropriateness of initiating the plan interventions.

   c. Patient response to intervention. Notify supervising physical therapist if altered response than would be expected.

2. Monitor appropriate vital signs and oxygen saturation.

3. Respond appropriately to emergency situations per facility protocol.

Manual Secretion Removal Techniques

1. Postural drainage: placing the patient in varying positions for optimal gravity drainage of secretions and increased expansion of the involved segment (Figure 5-3).

   a. Indications for the use of postural drainage.
      (1) Increased pulmonary secretions.
      (2) Aspiration.
      (3) Atelectasis or collapse.

   b. Considerations prior to the use of the postural drainage positions (Table 5-5). These considerations are not intended to imply absolute danger with their use, but rather a possible need for position modification.

   c. Procedure.
      (1) Explain procedure to the patient.
      (2) Place patient in the appropriate postural drainage position.
      (3) Observe for signs of intolerance.
      (4) Duration of procedure can be up to 20 minutes per postural drainage position. Typically, the duration equals the duration of the other manual techniques which are being used in conjunction with postural drainage.

2. Percussion: a force rhythmically applied with the assistant's cupped hands to the specific area of the chest wall that corresponds to the involved lung segment. Percussion is used to increase the amount of secretions cleared from the tracheobronchial tree. It is usually used in conjunction with postural drainage.

   a. Indications for the use of percussion.
      (1) Excessive pulmonary secretions.
      (2) Aspiration.
      (3) Atelectasis or collapse due to mucus plugging obstructing the airways.

   b. Considerations to weigh the possible benefits of percussion against possible detriments prior to the application of this technique are listed in Table 5-6. Modification of the technique may be necessary for patient tolerance.

Table 5-5 ➤ CONSIDERATIONS PRIOR TO THE USE OF POSTURAL DRAINAGE

Precautions to the use of Trendelenburg's position (head of bed tipped down 15–18 degrees)	
Circulatory system	Pulmonary edema, congestive heart failure, hypertension.
Abdominal problems	Obesity, ascites, pregnancy, hiatal hernia, nausea and vomiting, recent food consumption.
Neurological system	Recent neurosurgery, increased intracranial pressure, aneurysm precautions.
Pulmonary system	Shortness of breath.
Precautions to the use of sidelying position	
Circulatory system	Axillofemoral bypass graft
Musculoskeletal system	Humeral fractures, need for hip abduction brace, other situations that make sidelying uncomfortable e.g., arthritis, shoulder bursitis.

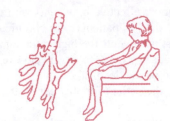

UPPER LOBES Apical Segments

Bed or drainage table flat.

Patient leans back on pillow at 30° angle against therapist.

Therapist claps with markedly cupped hand over area between clavicle and top of scapula on each side.

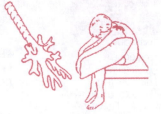

UPPER LOBES Posterior Segments

Bed or drainage table flat.

Patient leans over folded pillow at 30° angle.

Therapist stands behind and claps over upper back on both sides.

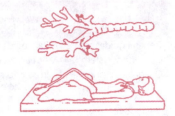

UPPER LOBES Anterior Segments

Bed or drainage table flat.

Patient lies on back with pillow under knees.

Therapist claps between clavicle and nipple on each side.

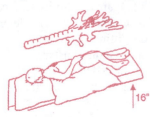

RIGHT MIDDLE LOBE

Foot of table or bed elevated 16 inches.

Patient lies head down on left side and rotates ¼ turn backward. Pillow may be placed behind from shoulder to hip. Knees should be flexed.

Therapist claps over right nipple area. In females with breast development or tenderness, use cupped hand with heel of hand under armpit and fingers extending forward beneath the breast.

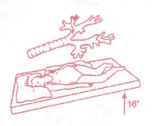

LEFT UPPER LOBE Lingular Segments

Foot of table or bed elevated 16 inches.

Patient lies head down on right side and rotates 1/4 turn backward. Pillow may be placed behind from shoulder to hip. Knees should be flexed.

Therapist claps with moderately cupped hand over left nipple area. In females with breast development or tenderness, use cupped hand with heel of hand under armpit and fingers extending forward beneath the breast.

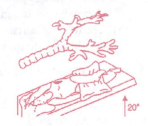

LOWER LOBE Anterior Basal Segments

Foot of table or bed elevated 20 inches.

Patient lies on side, head down, pillow under knees.

Therapist claps with slightly cupped hand over lower ribs. (Position shown is for drainage of left **ant**erior basal segment. To drain the right anterior basal segment, patient should lie on his left side in same posture.)

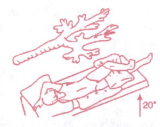

LOWER LOBES Lateral Basal Segments

Foot of table or bed elevated 20 inches.

Patient lies on abdomen, head down, then rotates ¼ turn upward. Upper leg is flexed over a pillow for support.

Therapist claps over uppermost portion of lower ribs. (Position shown is for drainage of right lateral basal segment. To drain the left lateral basal segment, patient should lie on his right side in the same posture.)

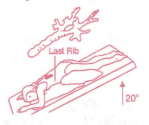

LOWER LOBES Posterior Basal Segements

Foot of table or bed elevated 20 inches.

Patient lies on abdomen, head down, with pillow under hips. Therapist claps over lower ribs close to spine on each side.

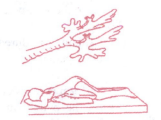

LOWER LOBES Superior Segments

Bed or table flat.

Patient lies on abdomen with two pillows under hips.

Therapist claps over middle of back at tip of scapula on either side of spine.

Figure 5-3 • Positions used for postural drainage.
(From Rothstein J, Roy S, Wolf S. The four basic conditions of acid-base balance. In: The Rehabilitation Specialist's Handbook, 2nd ed, FA Davis, Philadelphia, 1998:534–535, with permission.)

c. Procedure:
(1) Explain procedure to the patient.
(2) Place patient in the appropriate postural drainage position.
(3) Cover the area to be percussed with a light-weight cloth to avoid erythema.
(4) Percuss over area of thorax which corresponds to the involved lung segment. The duration of per-

Table 5-6 ➤ CONSIDERATIONS PRIOR TO THE USE OF PERCUSSION AND SHAKING

General guidelines	Pain made worse by the technique.
Circulatory system	Aneurysm precautions, hemoptysis.
Coagulation disorders	Increased partial thromboplastin time (PTT), increased prothrombin time (PT), decreased platelet count (<50,000), or medications that interfere with coagulation.
Musculoskeletal system	Fractured rib, flail chest, degenerative bone disease, bone metastases.

cussion depends on the patient's needs and tolerance. Three to five minutes of percussion per postural drainage position with clinically assessed improvement is a guideline.

(5) The force of percussion is one that causes the patient's voice to quiver.

3. **Shaking (Vibration): following a deep inhalation, shaking is a bouncing maneuver applied to the rib cage throughout exhalation. Shaking hastens the removal of secretions from the tracheobronchial tree. Commonly used following percussion in the appropriate postural drainage position. Modification of this technique may be necessary for patient tolerance.**

   a. Indications for the use of shaking.
      (1) Excessive pulmonary secretions.
      (2) Aspiration.
      (3) Atelectasis or collapse of an airway from mucus plugging.

   b. Considerations prior to the application of shaking are similar to those of percussion (Table 5-6).

   c. Procedure:
      (1) Explain procedure to the patient.
      (2) Place patient in the appropriate postural drainage position.
      (3) Perform percussion, if appropriate.
      (4) As the patient inhales deeply, the assistant's hands are placed so that fingers are parallel to the ribs.
      (5) As the patient exhales, the assistant's hands provide a jarring, bouncing motion to the ribcage below.
      (6) The duration of shaking depends on the patient's needs, tolerance and clinical improvement. Five to ten deep inhalations with the shaking technique are generally acceptable practice. Any more than 10 would risk hyperventilation (increased VE resulting in decreased Pa_{CO_2}) and less than 5 might be ineffective.

4. **Airway clearance techniques.**

   a. Cough: the patient should be asked to cough in the upright sitting position, if possible, after each area of lung has been treated. Coughing is effective in clearing secretions from the major central airways.

   b. Huff: huffing is more effective in patients with collapsible airways, such as patients with chronic obstructive diseases; it prevents the high intrathoracic pressure which causes premature airway closure.
      (1) Ask patient to inhale deeply.
      (2) Immediately, the patient forcibly expels the air saying "ha, ha."

   c. Assisted cough: the assistant's hand(s) (or fist) becomes the force behind the patient's exhaled air. Assisted cough is used when the patient's abdominal muscles cannot generate effective cough (e.g., spinal cord injury). The amount of force by the assistant is dependent upon patient tolerance and abdominal sensation.
      (1) Position the patient against a solid surface; supine with head of bed flat or in Trendelenburg's position, or sitting with wheelchair against the wall or against the assistant.
      (2) The assistant's hand is placed below the patient's subcostal angle (similar to hand placement for the Heimlich maneuver).
      (3) The patient inhales deeply.
      (4) As the patient attempts to cough, the assistant's hand pushes inward and upward, assisting the rapid exhalation of air.
      (5) Any secretions raised should be removed by a suction catheter if expectoration is problematic.

Independent Secretion Removal Techniques

1. **Active cycle of breathing: an independent program used to assist in the removal of the more peripheral secretions that coughing alone may not clear.**

   a. Breathe in a controlled diaphragmatic fashion.

   b. Perform thoracic expansion exercises (with or without percussion and shaking). These are deep inhalations with a hold at the top if possible.

   c. Controlled diaphragmatic breathing. The patient is now to decide what is needed next. If there are no secretions felt to be mobilized at this time, then the patient returns to step b, then c and reassesses the situation. If the patient believes there to be secretions that can be cleared, the patient moves on to step d, e and f.

   d. Inhale a resting tidal volume. Contract the abdominal muscles to produce one or two forced expiratory huffs from mid to low lung volume to raise secretions.

   e. Huff from high lung volume or cough to clear.

   f. Controlled diaphragmatic breathing.

   g. Repetition of these cycles is continued until secretions are in large airways.

2. **Autogenic drainage: an independent program used to sense peripheral secretions and clear them without the tracheobronchial irritation from coughing. The amount of time spent in each of the following**

phases is determined by where the patient feels the secretions.

   a. The unstick phase: quiet breathing at low lung volumes to affect peripheral secretions.

   b. The collect phase: breathing at mid lung volumes to affect secretions in the middle airways.

   c. The evacuation phase: breathing from mid to high lung volumes to clear secretions from central airways. This phase replaces coughing as the means to clear secretions.

   d. Repeat the steps which correspond to the area of retained secretions until all secretions are removed from the airways.

3. The FLUTTER device: an independent program using an external device that vibrates the airways on exhalation to improve airway clearance.

   a. The patient breathes in through the nose or around the mouthpiece of the flutter device.

   b. A 3-second hold at the top of inhalation.

   c. Rapid forced exhalations through the FLUTTER device.

   d. Repeat between 4 and 10 times.

   e. Huff or cough to clear secretions.

   f. Repeat until all secretions are removed from the airways.

4. Low-pressure positive expiratory pressure (PEP) mask: an independent exercise program that uses positive expiratory resistance via face mask to assist in the removal of airway secretions. Low-pressure PEP measures 10–20 cm H_2O.

   a. Seated, the patient breathes at tidal volumes with mask in place.

   b. After approximately 10 breaths, the mask is removed for coughing and clearing of secretions.

   c. The sequence is repeated until all secretions are removed from the airways.

5. High-pressure positive expiratory pressure (PEP) mask: an independent exercise program for patients with unstable airways that uses the high expiratory pressures via face mask to assist in the removal of airway secretions. High-pressure PEP uses the point of PEP between 50 and 120 cm H_2O where the patient is able to exhale a larger FVC with the mask than without.

   a. Seated, the patient breathes at tidal volumes with mask in place.

   b. After approximately 10 breaths, huffing from high to low lung volumes is performed with the mask in place.

   c. The sequence is repeated until all secretions are removed from the airways.

Breathing Exercises

1. Diaphragmatic breathing is used to increase ventilation, improve gas exchange, decrease work of
breathing, facilitate relaxation, maintain or improve mobility of chest wall, prevent pulmonary compromise.

   a. Used with postoperative patients, post trauma patients and patients with obstructive or restrictive pulmonary lung diseases.

   b. Procedure:

     (1) Explain procedure to patient.

     (2) Position the patient semireclined (e.g., semi-Fowler's position).

     (3) Place the assistant's hand gently over the subcostal angle of the patient's thorax.

     (4) Apply gentle pressure throughout the exhalation phase of breathing.

     (5) Increase to firm pressure at the end of exhalation.

     (6) Ask the patient to inhale against the resistance of the assistant's hand.

     (7) Release pressure allowing a full inhalation.

     (8) Progress to independence of assistant's hand, in upright sitting, standing, walking and stair climbing.

2. Segmental breathing is used to improve ventilation to hypoventilated lung segments, alter regional distribution of gas, maintain or restore functional residual capacity, maintain or improve mobility of chest wall and prevent pulmonary compromise.

   a. Used with patients who have pleuritic, incisional or posttrauma pain that is causing a decreased movement in a portion of the thorax (splinting) and are at risk for developing atelectasis.

   b. Segmental breathing is inappropriate in cases of intractable hypoventilation until the medical situation is resolved (palliative therapy to reduce bronchogenic tumor size or a chest tube to reduce a pneumothorax).

   c. Procedure:

     (1) Explain procedure to the patient.

     (2) Position the patient to facilitate inhalation to a certain segment, such as postural drainage positions, upright sitting.

     (3) Apply gentle pressure to the thorax over the area of hypoventilation during exhalation.

     (4) Increase to firm pressure just prior to inspiration.

     (5) Ask the patient to breathe in against the resistance of the assistant's hands.

     (6) Release resistance allowing a full inhalation.

3. Sustained maximal inspiration (SMI) is used to increase inhaled volume, sustain or improve alveolar inflation, maintain or restore functional residual capacity.

   a. Used in acute situations for patients with posttrauma pain, postoperative pain, acute lobar collapse.

   b. Procedure:

     (1) Inspire slowly through nose or pursed lips to maximal inspiration.

(2) Hold maximal inspiration for 3 seconds.

(3) Passively exhale the volume.

(4) Incentive spirometers (devices used to measure and encourage deep inspiration) can assist the patient in achieving maximal inspiration during SMI.

4. **Pursed lip breathing is used to reduce the respiratory rate, increase tidal volume, reduce dyspnea, decrease mechanical disadvantage of an impaired ventilatory pump, improve gas mixing at rest for patients with COPD and facilitate relaxation.**

a. Primarily used for patients with obstructive disease who experience dyspnea at rest or with minimal activity/exercise, or who use an ineffective breathing pattern during activity/exercise.

b. Procedure:

(1) Slowly inhale through nose or mouth.

(2) Passively exhale through pursed lips (position the mouth as if blowing out candles). Increases intrabronchial pressure.

(3) Additional hand pressure from the assistant applied to abdomen can be used to gently prolong expiration.

(4) Abdominal muscle contraction can be used judiciously to increase exhaled volume. Care must be taken not to increase intrathoracic pressure which might produce airway collapse.

5. **Abdominal strengthening can be used when abdominal muscles are too weak to provide an effective cough. Abdominal splinting can be used when the abdominal muscles cannot provide the necessary support for the abdominal contents needed for passive exhalation, with high thoracic and cervical spinal cord injuries. It is important to ensure that the binder does not restrict inspiration.**

a. Glossopharyngeal breathing (air gulping) can also be taught to assist coughing.

Pre- and Postsurgical Care

1. **Preoperative teaching and treatment decrease the number and severity of postoperative pulmonary complications.**

a. Goals and outcomes:

(1) Determine baseline cardiopulmonary function.

(2) Treat any existing condition which may alter postoperative course.

(3) Educate patient and family regarding postoperative course and physical therapy treatment.

(4) Enhance compliance postoperatively.

b. Physical therapy considerations:

(1) Familiarize the patient with the therapist and department.

(2) Extract pertinent patient information from medical record and physical examination.

(3) Demonstrate secretion removal techniques used postoperatively.

(4) Teach breathing exercises, splinting, incentive spirometry.

(5) Describe postoperative course, e.g., site of incision, monitoring and therapeutic devices, levels of discomfort, treatment times and hospital guidelines for visitors. Information is tailored to the patient's inquiries and level of understanding.

(6) Perform secretion removal techniques as required.

2. **Postoperative physical therapy sessions decrease the number and severity of pulmonary complications.**

a. Description: prevent postoperative pulmonary complications.

(1) Remove any residual secretions.

(2) Improve aeration.

(3) Gradually increase activity.

(4) Return to baseline pulmonary functioning.

b. Pertinent physical findings of postoperative pulmonary complications:

(1) Increased temperature.

(2) Increase in white blood cell count.

(3) Change in breath sounds from the preoperative evaluation.

(4) Abnormal chest x-ray.

(5) Decreased expansion of the thorax.

(6) Shortness of breath.

(7) Change in cough and sputum production.

c. Physical therapy considerations:

(1) Determine need for pain management.

(2) Choose appropriate intervention based on the individual patient's needs.

(a) Secretion removal techniques.

(b) Breathing exercises to improve aeration, incentive spirometry.

(c) Early mobilization.

Activities for Increasing Functional Abilities

1. **General conditioning. A prescription for exercise can be written to improve cardiopulmonary fitness based on the results of an exercise tolerance test. Refer to Chapters 4 and 10 for more in-depth discussion.**

a. Mode. Any type of aerobic activity which allows a graded workload can be used. Usually, a circuit program of multiple activities (bike, walking, arm ergometry, etc.) is used because patients with pulmonary disease may be quite deconditioned. Patient preference should enter into the decision-making process for mode of exercise.

b. Intensity. Using the test data in Karvonen's formula ([maximum heart rate – resting heart rate] [40%–85%] + resting heart rate) results in safe range for exercise intensity. Most patients with pulmonary disorders will work in the upper end of the target heart rate range. Ratings of perceived exertion scale are also used to monitor exercise intensity.

c. Duration. Using a high intensity for exercise, the patient may need an intermittent exercise program with rest periods for tolerance. Progression is directed first towards a duration of 20–30 minutes of continuous exercise before an increase in intensity is considered.

d. Frequency. The goal is 20–30 minutes of exercise three to five times per week. If the duration is less than 20–30 minutes, exercise must be performed more frequently (five to seven times per week).

2. Inspiratory muscle trainers (IMTs) load the muscles of inspiration by breathing through a series of graded aperture openings. By increasing strength and endurance of muscles of ventilation, the patient will have increased efficiency of ventilatory muscles, decreased work of breathing and decreased possibility of respiratory muscle fatigue,.Whether or not this has translated into improved functional abilities has been cause for debate and has yet to be conclusively proven.

a. IMT is appropriate for patients with decreased compliance, decreased intrathoracic volume, resistance to airflow, alteration in length tension relationship of ventilatory muscles, decreased strength of the respiratory muscles.

b. Procedure:
(1) Explain procedure to patient with emphasis on maintenance of respiratory rate and tidal volume during training sessions.
(2) Determine maximum inspiratory pressure (MIP).
(3) Choose an aperture opening which requires 30%–40% of MIP (intensity) and allows 15–30 minutes' training per session.
(4) Ask patient to breathe through device while maintaining respiratory rate and tidal volume for at least 15 minutes.
(5) Progression initially focused on increasing du-

ration to 30 minutes, then increasing intensity by using smaller apertures.

3. Paced breathing (activity pacing) is used to spread out the metabolic demands of an activity over time by slowing its performance.

a. Used with patients who becomes dyspneic during the performance of an activity or exercise.

b. Procedure:
(1) Break down any activity into manageable components that can be performed within the patient's pulmonary system's abilities.
(2) Inhale at rest.
(3) Upon exhalation with pursed lips, complete the first component of the desired activity.
(4) Stop the activity and inhale at rest.
(5) Upon exhalation with pursed lips, complete next component of activity.
(6) Repeat steps (4) and (5) until activity is accomplished in full without shortness of breath. For example, stair climbing can be done ascending one or more stairs on the exhalation phase of breathing; cease activity and breathe in at rest, then more stairs on exhalation, followed by another inhalation at rest and so on.

4. Energy conservation. The energy consumption of many activities of daily living can be decreased with some careful thought and planning, making seemingly impossible tasks possible. For example, showering is difficult for the patient with pulmonary disease given the activity and the hot humid environment that accompanies the task. With a shower seat, hand-held shower and use of a terrycloth robe after showering, the patient does not have to stand, hold the breath as often, nor dry off in the humid environment, thus reducing the energy cost of the activity.

Medical and Surgical Management of Pulmonary Disease

Surgical Management

1. Types of surgeries to remove diseased lung portions.
a. Pneumonectomy: removal of a lung.
b. Lobectomy: removal of a lobe of a lung.
c. Segmental resection: removal of a segment of a lobe.
d. Wedge resection: removal of a portion of a segment of a lobe.
e. Lung volume reduction surgery (LVRS), or pneumectomy, removes large emphysematous, nonfunc-

tioning areas of the lung in order to restore more normal thoracic mobility and improve gas exchange of the healthier remaining lung.

2. Types of incisions.
a. Midsternotomy. The sternum is cut in half lengthwise and the rib cage retracted. Used in most heart surgeries. The sternum is wired together at the close of surgery; therefore, physical therapy should encourage full upper extremity range of motion postoperatively.

CHAPTER 5

b. Thoracotomy. Used for most lung resections. The incision follows the path of the fourth intercostal space. Full range of motion should be encouraged postoperatively.

Medical Management

1. **Bronchodilator agents:**
   a. Beta-2 agonists (sympathomimetics): mimics the activity of the sympathetic nervous system which will produce bronchodilation. Also can cause increase in heart rate and blood pressure. Giving these topically through a metered-dose inhaler (MDI), reduces unwanted systemic effects. Most of the drugs in this category are termed *rescue drugs* as they are to be used primarily for immediate relief of breakthrough symptoms of chest tightness, wheezing and shortness of breath. Examples of rescue beta-2 agonists are Ventolin, Alupent, Maxair and Albuterol. Newer treatment options include a beta-2 agonist for maintenance. They are long-acting inhaled bronchodilators that may decrease the need for rescue drugs and decrease the need for inhaled anti-inflammatories. An example of this type of beta-2 maintenance drug is Serevent.
   b. Anticholinergics: inhibit the parasympathetic nervous system. Inhibiting the parasympathetic system can also cause an increase in heart rate and blood pressure along with bronchodilation. Side effects can include lack of sweating, dry mouth and delusions. These drugs are administered by MDI with minimal side effects. They should be used on a regular schedule to maintain bronchodilation. An example of this category of drug is Atrovent.
   c. Methylxanthines: produce smooth muscle relaxation, but their use is limited due to the serious toxicity of increased blood pressure, increased heart rate, arrhythmias, gastrointestinal distress, nervousness, headache and seizures. Blood levels need to be drawn to ensure medication effect without causing toxicity. Examples are aminophylline and theophylline.

2. **Anti-inflammatory agents: used to decrease mucosal edema, decrease inflammation and reduce airway reactivity.**
   a. Steroids: These drugs are used for maintenance of airway and should be taken on a regularly scheduled basis. They are not to be used for the acute onset with breakthrough symptoms. These drugs can be administered systemically or topically (MDI). Side effects of systemic administration are increased blood pressure, sodium retention, muscle wasting, osteoporosis, GI irritation and hypercholesteremia. The main side effect of inhaled steroids is thrush, a fungal infection of the mouth and throat. Examples are Vanceril (MDI), Azmacort (MDI), prednisone (po—by mouth) and Solumedral (IV).
   b. Leukotriene receptor antagonist: blocks leukotrienes that are released in an allergic reaction. Inhibits airway edema and smooth muscle contraction without being a steroid. It has additive benefits when used in conjunction with other anti-inflammatories. An example of this drug is montelukast (Singulair).
   c. Cromolyn sodium: an antiallergic drug. Prevents release of mast cells (i.e., histamine) after contact with allergens. Used prophylactically to prevent exercise-induced bronchospasm and severe bronchial asthma via oral inhalation. It is not to be used as a rescue drug during acute situations. Frequent inhalation can result in hoarseness, cough, dry mouth and bronchial irritation. Symptoms of overdosage include paradoxical bronchospasm. Brand names include Intal.

3. **Antibiotics: to control infection.**
   a. Categories: culture and sensitivity results are used to prescribe the most effective antibiotic.
      (1) Penicillins.
      (2) Erythromycins.
      (3) Tetracyclines.
      (4) Cephalosporins.
      (5) Aminoglycosides.
   b. Side effects:
      (1) Allergic reactions, stomach cramps, nausea, vomiting and diarrhea.

Intensive Care Unit Management

Definition

1. Physical therapy is employed in the ICU for pulmonary care (secretion removal or improved aeration) and early mobility (range of motion, positioning, therapeutic exercise, transfers and ambulation). The following provides a brief description of some equipment frequently encountered when treating a patient in the ICU.

Mechanical Ventilation

1. Maintain an adequate VE for patients who cannot do so independently. Requires intubation with an endotracheal (oral), nasotracheal (nasal) or tracheal (through a tracheostomy directly into the trachea) tube. Endotracheal and nasotracheal tubes are only taped into place. Tracheal tube may be sutured in

place. Tubes or mechanical ventilation pose no contraindications to physical therapy treatment. A patient who is intubated can ambulate using a mechanical resuscitator bag to maintain ventilation. It is sometimes easier to use a stationary device, e.g., peddler, to exercise a patient who needs a ventilator. When moving a patient who is intubated, care should be taken that excessive tension is not placed on the tube. Alteration in the placement of the tube (either a drop inward or a pull outward) could be detrimental to optimal ventilation. If tube movement is suspected, a nurse or respiratory therapist should check the placement of tube. If the tube is dislodged, a physician, often an anesthesiologist, needs to replace the tube.

Chest Tubes

1. Used to evacuate air or fluid trapped in the intrapleural space. The chest tubes are sutured in place, making them secure. There are no contraindications to physical therapy treatment with a chest tube. If the chest tube is connected to a suction device, mobility is limited only by the length of the tubing. Portable suction machines can be used to allow increased mobility. If the tube is dislodged during treatment, cover the defect and seek assistance.

IVs: Intravenous catheters used to deliver medications

1. There are no contraindications to physical therapy treatment with IV lines; however, the upper extremity should not be raised above the level of the IV medication for any length of time or backflow of blood may occur. Rolling IV poles allow for mobility. Most IV pumps have a battery back-up system to allow the patient to be mobile.

Arterial Lines

1. Catheters that are placed within the arterial system, usually the radial artery. The tubing is connected to a pressure pack that exceeds arterial pressure so the line does not back up with blood. Caution to maintain patency during moving is warranted. These lines limit mobility only by the length of the tubing. If this line becomes dislodged, immediate firm pressure needs to be applied to or above the arterial insertion site to stop bleeding.

Monitors/Oscilloscopes

1. Continuous ECG with a reported heart rate.

2. Blood pressure reading: either periodic, using noninvasive cuff (NIBP) or continuous, using a transducer attached to the arterial line (ABP).

3. Continuous oxygen saturation (Sao_2) with pulse wave. Sao_2 is the percent saturation of oxygen in the arterial blood. It is a noninvasive measurement that relates to the Pao_2 on the S-shaped curve called the oxyhemoglobin desaturation curve. Normal levels are 98%–100% saturated. The pulse oximeter utilizes a finger sensor (or an ear sensor) to obtain a consistent reading.

Supplemental Oxygen

1. Increases the Fio_2 (up to 1.0) of the patient's environment. A portable oxygen cylinder attached to the oxygen delivery device (cannula, mask or even a manual resuscitator bag attached to the endotracheal tube) can be used during mobility training to provide supplemental oxygen for the patient. Supplemental oxygen is indicated if Sao_2 is less than 88% or Pao_2 is less than 55 mm Hg regardless of activity level. Monitor the patient's Sao_2 to assure adequate oxygenation with increased activity. Oxygen must be prescribed by a physician. It is considered a form of medication.

chapter 6

Integumentary Physical Therapy

SUSAN B. O'SULLIVAN and
BRIDGET BRAUNS

Focus Areas for Content Review:

- Anatomy and physiology of the integumentary system.
- Pathologies and injuries of the integumentary system commonly seen in physical therapy.
- Physical therapy interventions; indications and contraindications, appropriate responses, PTA response to adverse reaction, effects of interventions on the integumentary system.
- Integumentary tests and measures indicating patient ability to participate in and/or indication to discontinue intervention as well as to document the patient's progress toward the established goals.
- Principals of progression of intervention activities as related to conditions of the integumentary system commonly encountered in physical therapy.

Integumentary System

Skin or Integument

1. **External covering of the body, the largest organ system of the body (15%–20% of body weight).**

2. **Functions of skin.**
   a. Protection of underlying body structures against injury or invasion.
   b. Insulation of body.
   c. Maintenance of homeostasis: fluid balance, regulation of body temperature.
   d. Aids in elimination: small amounts of urea and salt are excreted in sweat.
   e. Synthesizes vitamin D.
   f. Receptors in dermis give rise to cutaneous sensations.

3. **Consists of three layers.**
   a. Epidermis: outer, most superficial layer; contains no blood vessels. Comprised of five layers of stratified epithelium.
      (1) Stratum corneum is outermost, horny layer, comprised of nonliving cells.
      (2) Stratum lucidum is composed of three to five layers of dead flattened keratinocytes. This layer is found where epidermis is thicker: the palms of the hands and soles of feet. It is not found in thinner skin, such as eyelids.
      (3) Stratum granulosum is the granular layer. It is one to five cells thick and lies beneath the stratum lucidum if present; otherwise, it lies beneath the stratum corneum.
      (4) Stratum spinosum is found below the stratum granulosum; often called the prickly layer.
      (5) Stratum basale, or stratum germinativum, is the innermost layer. These active cells respond to extracellular matrix, growth factors, hormones and vitamins. Melanocytes are found in this layer responsible for skin pigmentation.
   b. Dermis (corium): inner layer comprised primarily of collagen and elastin fibrous connective tissues. Mucopolysaccharide matrix and elastin fibers provide elasticity and strength to skin. Contains lymphatics, blood vessels, nerves and nerve endings, sebaceous and sweat glands.
   c. Subcutaneous tissues: underneath dermis; consists of loose connective and fat tissues; provides insulation, support and cushion for skin; stores energy for skin.
   d. Underneath subcutaneous layer: muscles and fascia.

4. **Appendages of the skin.**
   a. Hair.
      (1) Terminal hair: coarse, thick, pigmented; e.g., scalp, eyebrows.

(2) Vellus hair: short, fine; e.g., arms, chest.
b. Nails: nail plate, lunula (whitish moon), proximal nail fold/cuticle, lateral nail folds.
c. Sebaceous glands: secrete fatty substance through hair follicles; on all skin surfaces except palms and soles.
d. Sweat glands.
   (1) Eccrine glands: widely distributed, open on skin, help control body temperature.
   (2) Apocrine glands: found in axillary and genital areas, open into hair follicles; stimulated by emotional stress.

Circulation

1. **Blood flows through arteries to capillaries of the skin.**
   a. Increased blood flow with an increase in oxyhemoglobin to skin capillaries causes reddening of the skin.
   b. Peripheral cyanosis is due to reduced blood flow to skin and loss of oxygen to tissues (changes to deoxyhemoglobin) and results in a darker and bluish color.
   c. Central cyanosis is due to reduced oxygen level in the blood; causes include advanced lung disease, congenital heart disease and abnormal hemoglobins.

Common Skin Disorders

Dermatitis (eczema)

1. **Inflammation of the skin with itching, redness, skin lesions.**

2. **Causes.**
   a. Allergic or contact dermatitis: e.g., poison ivy, harsh soaps, chemicals, adhesive tape.
   b. Actinic: photosensitivity, reaction to sunlight, ultraviolet.
   c. Atopic: etiology unknown, associated with allergic, hereditary or psychological disorders.

3. **Stages.**
   a. Acute: red, oozing, crusting rash; extensive erosions, exudate, pruritic vesicles.
   b. Subacute: erythematous skin, scaling, scattered plaques.
   c. Chronic: thickened skin, increased skin marking secondary to scratching; fibrotic papules and nodules; postinflammatory pigmentation changes. Course can be relapsing.

4. **Precaution or contraindication to some physical therapy modalities (e.g., paraffin, electrical stimulation); avoid use of alcohol.**

5. **Medical management aimed at inflammation: topical or systemic therapy.**

6. **Daily care includes hydration and lubrication of skin.**

Bacterial Infections

1. **Bacteria typically enter through portals in the skin; e.g., abrasions or puncture wounds.**

2. **Impetigo: superficial skin infection caused by staphylococci or streptococci; associated with inflammation, small pus-filled vesicles, itching; contagious; common in children and the elderly.**

3. **Cellulitis: suppurative inflammation of cellular or connective tissue in or close to the skin.**
   a. Tends to be poorly defined and widespread.
   b. Streptococcal or staphylococcal infection common; can be contagious.
   c. Skin is hot, red and edematous.
   d. Management: antibiotics; elevation of the part; cool, wet dressings.
   e. If untreated, lymphangitis, gangrene, abscess and sepsis can occur.
   f. The elderly and individuals with diabetes, wounds, malnutrition or on steroid therapy are at increased risk.

4. **Abscess: a cavity containing pus and surrounded by inflamed tissue.**
   a. The result of a localized infection.
   b. Commonly a staphylococcal infection.
   c. Healing typically facilitated by draining or incising the abscess.

5. **Methicillin-resistant *Staphylococcus aureus* (MRSA) can be prevalent in hospitals and chronic care facilities. Community-acquired MRSA can attack athletic teams, school or prison populations.**
   a. Infection by MRSA can result in infections not responsive to usual antibiotic therapy.
   b. Can be life threatening if infection becomes systemic.
   c. PTA should ensure that standard precautions are in place: all wounds are covered and any wound that does not seem to be responding to usual treatments should be reported.

Viral Infections

1. Herpes 1 (herpes simplex): itching and soreness followed by vesicular eruption of the skin on the face or mouth; a cold sore or fever blister.

2. Herpes 2: common cause of vesicular genital eruption.
   a. Spread by sexual contact.
   b. In newborns, may cause meningoencephalitis and may be fatal.

3. Herpes zoster (shingles): caused by varicella-zoster virus (chicken pox); reactivation of virus lying dormant in cerebral ganglia or ganglia of posterior nerve roots.
   a. Pain and tingling affecting spinal or cranial nerve dermatome; progresses to red papules along distribution of infected nerve; red papules progressing to vesicles develop along a dermatome.
   b. Usually accompanied by fever, chills, malaise, GI disturbances.
   c. Ocular complications with CNIII involvement: eye pain, corneal damage, loss of vision with CNV involvement.
   d. Postherpetic neuralgic pain: may be intermittent or constant, lasts weeks, occasionally intractable pain lasting for months or years.
   e. Management: no curative agent, antiviral drugs slow progression, symptomatic treatment for itching and pain; e.g., systemic corticosteroids.
   f. Contagious to individuals who have not had chicken pox.
   g. Heat or ultrasound contraindicated: can increase severity of symptoms.

4. Warts: common, benign infection by human papillomaviruses (HPVs).
   a. Transmission is through direct contact; autoinoculation is possible.
   b. Common warts: on skin, especially hands and fingers.
   c. Plantar wart: on pressure points of feet.
   d. Management: cryotherapy, acids, electrodesiccation and curettage, over-the-counter medications.

5. Contagious, observe standard precautions.

Fungal Infections

1. Ringworm (tinea corporis): fungal infection involves the hair, skin or nails; forms ring-shaped patches with vesicles or scales; itchy; transmission is through direct contact. Treated with topical or oral antifungal drugs (e.g., griseofulvin).

2. Athlete's foot (tinea pedis): fungal infection of foot, typically between the toes; causes erythema, inflammation, pruritus, itching and pain. Treated with antifungal creams. Can progress to bacterial infections, cellulitis if untreated.

3. Transmission is person-to-person or animal-to-person; observe standard precautions.

Parasitic Infections

1. Caused by insect and animal contacts.

2. Scabies (mites) burrow into skin causing inflammation, itching and possibly pruritus. Treated with scabicide.

3. Lice (pediculosis): a parasite that can affect head, body, genital area; bite marks, redness and nits. Treatment with special soap or shampoo.

4. Transmission is person-to-person or can be sexually transmitted. Avoid direct contact; observe standard precautions.

Immune Disorders of the Skin

1. Psoriasis: chronic disease of skin with erythematous plaques covered with a silvery scale; common on ears, scalp, knees, elbows and genitalia.
   a. Common complaints: itching and pain from dry cracked lesions.
   b. Variable course: exacerbations and remissions are common.
   c. May be associated with psoriatic arthritis, joint pain, particularly of small distal joints.
   d. Etiological factors: hereditary, associated immune disorders, certain drugs.
   e. Precipitating factors: trauma, infection, pregnancy and endocrine changes; cold weather, smoking, anxiety and stress.
   f. Management: no cure; topical preparations (corticosteroids, occlusive ointments, coal tar); systemic drugs (methotrexate).
   g. Physical therapy intervention: long-wave ultraviolet light; combination UV light with oral photosensitizing drugs (psoralen).

2. Lupus erythematosus: chronic, progressive inflammatory disorder of connective tissues; characteristic red rash with raised, red, scaly plaques. Forms include:
   a. Discoid lupus erythematosus (DLE): affects only skin; flare-ups with sun exposure; lesions can resolve or cause atrophy, permanent scarring, hypopigmentation or hyperpigmentation.
   b. Systemic lupus erythematosus (SLE): chronic, systemic inflammatory disorder affecting multiple organ systems including skin, joints, kidneys, heart,

nervous system, mucous membranes; can be fatal; commonly affects young women. Symptoms can include fever, malaise and characteristic butterfly rash across bridge of nose, skin lesions, chronic fatigue, arthralgia, arthritis, skin rashes, photosensitivity, anemia, hair loss, Raynaud's phenomenon.

  c. Management: no cure; topical treatment of skin lesions (corticosteroid creams); salicylates or indomethacin with fever and joint pain; immunosuppressive agents (cytotoxic agents) with life-threatening disease.

  d. Observe for side effects of corticosteroids: edema, weight gain, acne, hypertension, bruising, purplish stretch marks; long-term use of corticosteroids is associated with increased susceptibility to infection (immunosuppressed patient), osteoporosis, myopathy, tendon rupture, diabetes, gastric irritation, low potassium.

3. **Scleroderma: a chronic, diffuse disease of connective tissues causing fibrosis of skin, joints, blood vessels and internal organs (GI tract, lungs, heart, kidneys). Usually accompanied by Raynaud's phenomenon. Progressive systemic sclerosis (PSS) is a relatively rare autoimmune form.**

  a. Skin is taut, firm, edematous, firmly bound to subcutaneous tissues.

  b. Limited disease/skin thickening: symmetrical skin involvement of distal extremities and face, slow progression of skin changes, late visceral involvement.

  c. Diffuse disease/skin thickening: symmetrical, widespread skin involvement of distal and proximal extremities, face, trunk; rapid progression of skin changes with early appearance of visceral involvement.

  d. Management: no specific therapy; supportive therapy can include corticosteroids, vasodilators, analgesics immunosuppressive agents.

  e. Physical therapy slows development of contracture and deformity.

  f. Precautions with sclerosed skin, sensitive to pressure; acute hypertension may occur, stress regular BP checks.

4. **Polymyositis (PM): a disease of connective tissue characterized by edema, inflammation and degeneration of the muscles; dermatitis is associated with some forms.**

  a. Affects primarily proximal muscles: shoulder and pelvic girdles, neck, pharynx; symmetrical distribution.

  b. Etiology unknown; autoimmune reaction affecting muscle tissue with degeneration and regeneration, fiber atrophy; inflammatory infiltrates.

  c. Rapid, severe onset: may require ventilatory assistance, tube feeding.

  d. Cardiac involvement: may be fatal.

  e. Managemnt: medication (corticosteroids and immunosuppressants).

  f. Precautions: additional muscle fiber damage with too much exercise; contractures and pressure ulcers from inactivity, prolonged bed rest.

Skin Cancer

1. **Benign tumors.**

  a. Seborrheic keratosis: proliferation of basal cells leading to raised lesions, typically multiple lesions on trunk of older individuals; untreated unless causing irritation, pain; can be removed with cryotherapy.

  b. Actinic keratosis: flat, round or irregular lesions, covered by dry scale on sun-exposed skin. Precancerous: can lead to squamous cell carcinoma.

  c. Common mole (benign nevus): proliferation of melanocytes, round or oval shape, sharply defined borders, uniform color, <6 mm, flat or raised. Can change into melanoma: signs include new swelling, redness, scaling, oozing or bleeding.

2. **Malignant tumors.**

  a. Basal cell carcinoma: slow growing epithelial basal cell tumor, characterized by raised patch with ivory appearance; has rolled border with indented center. Rarely metastasizes, common on face, in fair-skinned individuals. Associated with prolonged sun exposure.

  b. Squamous cell carcinoma: has poorly defined margins; presents as a flat red area, ulcer or nodule. Grows more quickly, common on sun-exposed areas, face and neck, back of hand. Can be confined (in situ) or invasive to surrounding tissues; can metastasize.

  c. Malignant melanoma: tumor arising from melanocytes (cells that produce melanin); superficial spreading melanoma (SSM) most common type.

    (1) Clinical manifestations: "ABCDs," asymmetry (uneven edges, lopsided), borders (irregular, poorly defined edges), color (variations or changes in color, black brown, red or white), diameter (larger than 6 mm). Irritation, itching or tenderness can be seen.

    (2) Risk factors: family history, intense sun exposure, individuals with fair skin and freckles.

    (3) Treatment is surgical resection. Prognosis depends on extent of invasion.

  d. Kaposi's sarcoma (KS): lesions of endothelial cell origin with red or dark purple/blue macules that progress to nodules or ulcers; associated with itching and pain.

    (1) Common on lower extremities; may involve internal structures producing lymphatic obstruction.

    (2) Increased incidence in individuals of central European descent and with AIDS-associated immunodeficiency.

Skin Trauma

1. Contusion: injury in which skin is not broken (a bruise). Characterized by pain, swelling and discoloration. Immediate application of cold may limit effects.

2. Ecchymosis: bluish discoloration of skin caused by extravasations of blood into the subcutaneous tissues; the result of trauma to underlying blood vessels or fragile vessel walls.

3. Petechiae: tiny red or purple spots on the skin that result from tiny hemorrhages within the dermal or submucosal layers; pinpoint.

4. Abrasion: scraping away of skin as a result of injury or mechanical abrasion (e.g., dermabrasion).

5. Laceration: an irregular tear of the skin producing a torn, jagged wound.

Assessment of Integumentary Integrity

Tissue Assessment

1. Techniques include observation, palpation, photographic assessment and thermography.

2. Pruritus: itching, common in diabetes, drug hypersensitivity, hyperthyroidism.

3. Urticaria: smooth, red, elevated patches of skin (hives); indicative of an allergic response to drugs or infection.

4. Rash: local redness and eruption on the skin, typically accompanied by itching; seen in inflammation, skin diseases, chronic alcoholism, vasomotor disturbances, pyrexia, medications; e.g., diaper rash, heat rash, drug rash.

5. Xeroderma: excessive dryness of skin with shedding of epithelium; can indicate deficiency of thyroid function, diabetes.

6. Edema: can indicate anemia, venous or lymphatic obstruction, inflammation; cardiac, circulatory or renal decompensation.
   a. Determine activities and postures that aggravate or relieve edema.
   b. Palpation, volume and girth measurements.

7. Changes in nails.
   a. Clubbing: thickened and rounded nail end with spongy proximal fold; indicative of chronic hypoxia secondary to heart disease, lung cancer, cirrhosis.
   b. White spots seen with trauma to nails.

8. Changes in skin pigmentation, tissue mobility, skin turgor and texture.
   a. Wrinkling may be due to aging or prolonged immersion in water, dehydration.
   b. Blistering.

9. Changes in skin color.
   a. Cherry red: indicative of carbon monoxide poisoning.
   b. Cyanosis: slightly bluish, grayish, slate-like discoloration.
      (1) Indicative of lack of oxygen (hemoglobin); can indicate congestive heart failure, advanced lung disease, congenital heart disease, venous obstruction.
      (2) Observe lips, oral mucosa, tongue for blue color (central causes) or nails, hands, feet (peripheral causes).
   c. Pallor (lack of color, paleness).
      (1) Can indicate anemia, internal hemorrhage, lack of exposure to sunlight.
      (2) Temporary pallor seen with arterial insufficiency and syncope, chills, shock, vasomotor instability or nervousness.
   d. Yellow: indicates jaundice, liver disease: look for yellow color in sclerae of eyes, lips, skin. With increased carotene intake (carotenemia), look for yellow color of palms, soles and face.
   e. Liver spots: brownish yellow spots may be due to aging, uterine and liver malignancies, pregnancy.
   f. Brown: increased pigmentation, sometimes associated with venous insufficiency.

10. Changes in skin temperature: correlates with internal temperature unless skin is exposed to local heat or cold.
   a. Assess with backs of fingers for generalized warmth or coolness.
      (1) Abnormal heat can indicate febrile condition, hyperthyroidism, mental excitement, excessive salt intake.
      (2) Abnormal cold can indicate poor circulation or obstruction; e.g., vasomotor spasm, venous or arterial thrombosis, hypothyroidism.
   b. Assess temperature of reddened areas: local warmth may indicate inflammation or cellulitis.

11. Hidrosis.

    a. Moist skin (hyperhidrosis), increased perspiration, can indicate fevers, pneumonic crisis, drugs, hot drinks, exercise.

    b. Dry skin (hypohidrosis) can indicate dehydration, ichthyosis or hypothyroidism.

    c. Cold sweats: can indicate great fear, anxiety, depression or disease (AIDS).

12. Changes in hair: note quality, texture, distribution.

    a. Alopecia: hair loss.

    b. Hypothyroidism sees thinning hair; hyperthyroidism sees silky hair.

Application Concept

The PTA should continuously be aware of changes in the appearance of tissues while working with patients/clients and report any changes noted to the patient (as appropriate) and physical therapist.

Physical Therapy Intervention for Impaired Integumentary Integrity

Patient/Client-Related Instruction

1. Enhance disease awareness, healthy behaviors.

2. Assist patient to avoid harsh soaps, known irritants, temperature extremes, exacerbating factors or triggers.

3. Enhance ADLs, functional mobility and safety.

4. Enhance self-management of symptoms.

Infection Control Practices

1. See Box 7-1.

Therapeutic Exercise

1. Strengthening and ROM exercises.

2. Aerobic conditioning.

3. Body mechanics, postural awareness training.

4. Gait, locomotion and balance training.

5. Aquatic therapy.

Functional Training

1. ADL training (basic and instrumental).

2. Activity pacing and energy conservation; stress management.

3. Skin and joint protection techniques.

4. Instruct in safe use of assistive and adaptive devices.

5. Prescription, application and training in use of orthotic, protective or supportive devices.

Dressings and Topical Agents (see section on wound care)

Electrotherapeutic Modalities

1. Refer to Chapter 11 Therapeutic Modalities for details.

2. Electrical muscle stimulation (EMS).

3. High-voltage pulsed current (HVPC).

4. Transcutaneous electrical nerve stimulation (TENS): relief of pain.

Physical Agents and Therapeutic Modalities

1. Refer to Chapter 11 Therapeutic Modalities for details

2. Sound agents: ultrasound, phonophoresis.

3. Hydrotherapy: aquatic therapy, whirlpool tanks.

4. Light agents: ultraviolet.

5. Mechanical modalities: compression therapies.

Burns

Tissue Injury or Destruction

1. Results from thermal, chemical, electrical or radioactive agents.

Pathophysiology

1. Burn wound consists of three zones.

2. Zone of coagulation: area of greatest damage is closest to the heat source, cells are irreversibly injured, cell death occurs, full-thickness damage has occurred.

3. Zone of stasis: involves the vascular system in the area, cells are injured; may die without specialized treatment, usually within 24–48 hours.

4. Zone of hyperemia: minimal cell injury; cells should recover, superficial partial thickness burn.

Degree of Burn

1. Burns are classified by severity, layers of skin damaged.

2. Superficial burn (first-degree burn): damage is to epidermis only.
   a. Characterized by erythema, slight edema, tenderness; no blistering.
   b. Full healing in 3–7 days.

3. Superficial partial thickness burn (second-degree burn): epidermis and upper layers of dermis are damaged.
   a. Characterized by blisters, inflammation, severe pain.
   b. Healing in 7–21 days.

4. Deep partial-thickness burn (second-degree burn): severe damage to epidermis and dermis with injury to nerve endings, hair follicles and sweat glands.
   a. Characterized by red or white appearance, edema, blistering, severe pain.
   b. Healing occurs through scar formation and reepithelialization, in 21–28 days.

5. Full-thickness burn (third-degree burn): complete destruction of epidermis, dermis and subcutaneous tissues, may extend into muscle.
   a. Characterized by white, gray or black (charred) appearance; dry surface, edema, eschar (scab or dry crust); little pain (nerve endings are destroyed).
   b. Removal of eschar; grafting is necessary due to destruction of dermal and epidermal tissue.
   c. Risk of infection is increased.
   d. Hypertrophic scarring and wound contracture are likely to develop without preventive measures.
      (1) Hypertrophic scar: a raised scar that stays within the boundaries of the burn wound; characteristically red, raised, firm.
      (2) Keloid scar: a raised scar that extends beyond the boundaries of the original burn wound; red, raised, firm.

5. Subdermal burn (fourth-degree burn): complete destruction of epidermis, dermis, subcutaneous tissues; also involves muscle and bone; e.g., electrical burn, prolonged contact with flame.
   a. Extensive tissue damage; destruction of vascular system, may lead to additional necrosis.
   b. Course unpredictable.
   c. Requires extensive surgery; amputation may be necessary.
   d. Additional complications likely with electrical burns; e.g., ventricular fibrillation, acute kidney damage, spinal cord damage.

Extent of Burned Area

1. Rule of Nines for estimating burn area (estimates are for adult patients).
   a. Head and neck: 9%.
   b. Anterior trunk: 18%.
   c. Posterior trunk: 18%.
   d. Arms: each 9%.
   e. Legs: each 18%.
   f. Perineum: 1%.

2. Percentages vary by age (growth) for children: use Lund-Browder charts for estimating body areas.

3. Classification by percentage of body area burned.
   a. Critical: 10% of body with third-degree burns and 30% or more with second-degree burns; complications common: e.g., respiratory involvement, smoke inhalation.
   b. Moderate: less than 10% with third-degree burns and 19%–30% with second-degree burns.
   c. Minor: less than 2% with third-degree burns and 15% with second-degree burns.

Complications of Burn Injury

1. Infection: leading cause of death; gangrene may develop.

2. Shock.

3. Pulmonary complications.
   a. Smoke inhalation injury from inhalation of hot gases, smoke poisoning; results in pulmonary edema and airway obstruction; suspect with burns of the face, singed nose hairs.
   b. Restrictive lung disease from burns of the trunk.
   c. Pneumonia.

4. Metabolic complications: increased metabolic and catabolic activity results in weight loss, negative nitrogen balance and decreased energy.

5. Cardiac and circulatory complications: fluid and plasma loss results in decreased cardiac output.

Burn Healing

1. Epidermal healing: retention of viable cells allows for epithelialization to occur (epithelial cells grow and proliferate, migrate to cover the wound).
   a. Protection of epithelial cells is critical.
   b. Loss of sebaceous glands can result in drying and cracking of wound; protection with moisturizing creams important.

2. Dermal healing: results in scar formation (injured tissue is replaced by connective tissue); scars are initially red or purple, later become white.
   a. Inflammatory phase: characterized by redness, edema, warmth, pain, decreased ROM motion; lasts 3–5 days.
   b. Proliferative phase: fibroblasts form scar tissue (deeper tissues); characterized by wound contraction; reepithelialization may occur at wound surface if viable cells remain.
   c. Maturation phase: scar tissue remodeling lasts up to 2 years.
      (1) Hypertrophic scar may result.
      (2) Keloid scar may result; more common in young women and those with dark skin.

Emergency Burn Management

1. Immersion of burned part in cold water (if less than half the body burned and injury is immediate); cold compresses may also be used.

2. Cover burn with sterile bandage or clean cloth; no ointments or creams.

Medical Management

1. Asepsis and wound care.
   a. Removal of charred clothing.
   b. Wound cleansing.

   c. Topical medications (antibacterial agents): can be applied without dressings (open technique); reapplied daily.
      (1) Silver nitrate: acts only on surface organisms; applied with wet dressings; requires frequent dressing changes.
      (2) Silver sulfadiazine: common topical agent.
      (3) Sulfamylon (mafenide acetate): penetrates through eschar.
   d. Occlusive dressings (closed technique): dressings are applied on top of a topical agent.
      (1) Prevents bacterial contamination, prevents fluid loss and protects the wound.
      (2) May additionally limit ROM.

2. Establish and maintain airway, adequate oxygenation and respiratory function.

3. Monitor.
   a. Arterial blood gases, serum electrolyte levels, urinary output, vital signs.
   b. Gastrointestinal function: provide nutritional support.

4. Pain relief; e.g., morphine sulfate.

5. Prevention and control of infection.
   a. Tetanus prophylaxis.
   b. Antibiotics.
   c. Isolation, sterile techniques.

6. Fluid replacement therapy.
   a. Prevention and control of shock.
   b. Postshock fluid and blood replacement.

7. Surgery.
   a. Primary excision: surgical removal of the eschar.
   b. Grafts: closure of the wound.
      (1) Allograft (homograft): use of other human skin; e.g., cadaver skin; temporary grafts for large burns, used until autograft is available.
      (2) Xenograft (heterograft): use of skin from other species; e.g., pigskin; a temporary graft.
      (3) Biosynthetic grafts: combination of collagen and synthetics.
      (4) Cultured skin: laboratory grown from patient's own skin.
      (5) Autograft: use of the patient's own skin.
      (6) Split-thickness graft: contains epidermis and upper layers of dermis from donor site.
      (7) Full-thickness graft: contains epidermis and dermis from donor site.
   c. Surgical resection of scar contracture; e.g., Z-plasty (a surgical incision in the form of the letter Z used to lengthen a burn scar).

Physical Therapy Interventions, Goals and Outcomes

1. Burn wound care. Infection control techniques at all times.

a. Immersion in hydrotherapy tank.
(1) Debridement: the excision of loose, charred, dead skin.
(2) Wet removal of dressings.
(3) ROM exercises, early mobilization.
(4) Anti-infection agents are added to assist in infection control.
b. Sharp debridement: excision of eschar using sterilized surgical instruments (forceps, scalpel, scissors).
c. Autolytic dressings or enzyme use are other selective means to help remove eschar.

2. Rehabilitation: prevent or reduce the complications of immobilization.
a. Exercises to promote deep breathing and chest expansion; ambulation to prevent pneumonia.
b. Positioning and splinting to prevent or correct deformities.
(1) Anterior neck: common deformity is flexion; stress hyperextension; position with firm (plastic) cervical orthosis.
(2) Shoulder: common deformity is adduction and internal rotation; stress abduction, flexion and external rotation; position with an axillary splint (airplane splint).
(3) Elbow: common deformity is flexion and pronation; stress extension and supination; position in extension with posterior arm splint.
(4) Hand: common deformity is a claw hand (intrinsic minus position); stress wrist extension (15 degrees), MP flexion (70 degrees), PIP and DIP extension, thumb abduction (intrinsic plus posi-

tion); position in intrinsic plus position with resting hand splint.
(5) Hip: common deformity is flexion and adduction; stress hip extension and abduction; position in extension, abduction, neutral rotation.
(6) Knee: common deformity is flexion; stress extension; position in extension with posterior knee splint.
(7) Ankle: common deformity is plantar flexion; stress dorsiflexion; position with foot-ankle in neutral with splint or plastic ankle-foot orthosis.
c. Edema control: elevation of extremities, active ROM.
d. Active and passive exercise to promote full ROM.
(1) Combine with dressing changes, hydrotherapy; medication doses.
(2) Postgrafting: discontinue exercise for 3–5 days to allow grafts to heal.
e. Massage to help reduce scar formation; e.g., deep friction massage.
f. Resistive and strengthening exercises to correct loss of muscle mass and strength.
g. Increase activity tolerance and cardiovascular endurance; e.g., ambulation.
h. Promote independence in activities of daily living, all functional mobility skills.
i. Elastic supports to help control edema; pressure garments to help prevent hypertrophic scarring or keloid formation.
j. Management of chronic pain.

3. Provide emotional support.

Wounds

Venous Ulcer (Table 6-1)

1. Etiology: associated with chronic venous insufficiency; valvular incompetence history of DVT, venous hypertension.

Table 6-1 ➤ DIFFERENTIATION AMONG WOUND TYPES

ULCERS	ARTERIAL	VENOUS	NEUROPATHIC
Etiology	Atherosclerosis Thromboangiitis obliterans	Venous hypertension, Valvular incompetence	Peripheral vascular disease
Location	Tips of toes; pressure points; areas of trauma	Medial malleolus; between ankles and knees	Plantar surface over metatarsal head Repetitive to toes and sides of the feet
Wound Base	Pale or necrosis	Dark red; may be covered with fibrin slough	Red
Drainage	Minimal	Moderate to large amounts	Moderate to large amounts
Wound Edges	Well defined	Poorly defined, irregular	Well defined, sometimes associated with callus formation
Other	Infection common, painful, pulses diminished/absent, pallor on elevation, ruddy in a dependent position	Edema, hyperpigmentation, stasis dermatitis, good pulses	Infection common

CHAPTER 6

2. Location: can occur anywhere in lower leg; common over area of medial malleolus, sometimes lateral.

3. Clinical features.
   a. Pulses: normal.
   b. Pain: none to dull, aching pain in dependent position.
   c. Color: normal or cyanotic in dependent position. Dark pigmentation may appear, liposclerosis (thick, tender, indurated, fibrosed tissue).
   d. Temperature: normal.
   e. Edema: present, often marked.
   f. Skin changes: pigmentation, stasis dermatitis may be present; thickening of skin as scarring develops.
   g. Ulceration: may develop, especially medial ankle; wet, with large amount of drainage. Gangrene absent.

4. Staging for venous, arterial and diabetic ulcers uses partial- and full-thickness classifications.

Arterial Ulcer (see Table 6-1)

1. Etiology: associated with chronic arterial insufficiency, arteriosclerosis obliterans, atheroembolism, history of minor nonhealing trauma.

2. Location: can occur anywhere in lower leg; common in small toes, feet, on bony areas of trauma (shin).

3. Clinical features.
   a. Preceded by signs of arterial insufficiency; pulses poor or absent.
   b. Pain: often severe, intermittent claudication, nocturnal pain, progressing to pain at rest.
   c. Color: pale on elevation; dusky rubor on dependency.
   d. Temperature: cool.
   e. Skin changes: trophic changes (thin, shiny, atrophic skin); loss of hair on foot and toes; nails thickened.
   f. Ulceration: of toes or feet; can be deep.
   g. Gangrene: black gangrenous skin adjacent to ulcer can develop.

4. Staging for venous, arterial and diabetic ulcers uses partial- and full-thickness classifications.

Diabetic Ulcer

1. Etiology: diabetes associated with arterial disease and peripheral neuropathy; caused by repetitive trauma on insensitive skin.

2. Location: occurs where arterial ulcers usually appear or where peripheral neuropathy appears (plantar aspect of foot).

3. Clinical features.
   a. Pain: typically not painful; burning/tingling, pins and needles or shooting; sensory loss usually present.
   b. Pulses: may be present or diminished.
   c. Absent ankle jerks with neuropathy.
   d. Sepsis common; gangrene may develop.

4. Staging for venous, arterial and diabetic ulcers uses partial- and full-thickness classifications.

Pressure Ulcer

1. Etiology: lesions caused by unrelieved pressure resulting in ischemic hypoxia and damage to underlying tissue.

2. Contributory factors: prolonged pressure, shear forces, friction, repetitive stress, nutritional deficiency and maceration (softening associated with excessive moisture).

3. Risk factors.
   a. Elderly, debilitated or immobilized individuals.
   b. Decrease blood flow from hypotension or microvascular disease: diabetes, atherosclerosis.
   c. Neurologically impaired skin: decreased sensation.
   d. Cognitive impairment.

4. Clinical features.
   a. Location: occurs over bony prominences; i.e., sacrum, heels, trochanter, lateral malleoli, ischial areas, elbows.
   b. Color: red, brown/black or yellow.
   c. Localized infection.
   d. Pain: can be painful if sensation intact.
   e. Inflammatory response with necrotic tissue: hyperemia, fever, increased WBC.
   f. If left untreated, will progress from superficial simple erosion to involvement of deep layers of skin and underlying muscle and bone.

5. Graded by stages of severity (tissue damage) (Table 6-2).

Assessment of Wounds

1. Observation and documentation.
   a. Identify location of wound: use specific anatomical landmarks.
   b. Assess and document size: (length, width, depth, wound area).
      (1) Use clear film grid superimposed on wound for size.
      (2) Insert sterile cotton tip applicator into deepest part of wound for depth; indicate gradations of depth from shallow to deep.

Table 6-2 ➤ STAGING OF PRESSURE ULCERS

STAGE	CHARACTERISTICS
Stage I	Intact skin with nonblanchable redness of a localized area usually over a bony prominence. This area may be painful, firm, soft, warmer or cooler compared to adjacent tissue.
Stage II	Partial-thickness loss of dermis presenting as a shallow open ulcer with a red wound base, without slough. May also present as an intact or open/ruptured serum-filled blister. Do not use this stage to describe skin tears, tape burns, perineal dermatitis, maceration or excoriation.
Stage III	Full-thickness tissue loss. Subcutaneous fat may be visible but bone, tendon or muscle is not exposed. Slough may be present but does not obscure the depth of tissue loss. May include tunneling and undermining.
Stage IV	Full-thickness tissue loss with exposed tendon, muscle or bone. Slough and eschar may be present on parts of the base. Tunneling and undermining are often present.
Deep Tissue Injury	Purple or maroon localized area of discolored intact skin or blood-filled blister due to damage of underlying tissue due to pressure and or shear. The tissue may be painful, firm, mushy, boggy, warmer or cooler to adjacent tissue.
Unstageable	Full-thickness tissue loss in which the base of the ulcer is covered by slough and/or eschar. Until enough slough and/or eschar can be removed to expose the base of the wound, the true depth and, therefore, the stage of the wound cannot be determined.

c. Identify presence, size and location of any tunneling (rimming or undermining): underlying tissue destruction beneath intact skin.
  (1) Sinus tracts (communication with deeper structures); associated with unusual or irregular borders.
  (2) Sinogram (radiographic imaging studies) may be ordered.
d. Describe wound exudate (drainage).
  (1) Type: serous (watery serum), purulent (containing pus), sanguineous (containing blood).
  (2) Amount: dry, moderate or high exudate.
  (3) Odor.
  (4) Consistency: e.g., macerated ulcer (softened tissues due to high fluid environment).
e. Identify color and tissues involved.
  (1) Clean red wounds: healthy granulating wounds (in need of protection); absence of necrotic tissue.
  (2) Yellow wounds: include slough (necrotic or dead tissue), fibrous tissue.
  (3) Black wounds: covered with eschar (dried necrotic tissue).
  (4) Indolent ulcer: ulcer that is slow to heal; not painful.
f. Determine girth.
  (1) Use circumferential measurements of both involved and noninvolved limbs; referenced to bony landmarks.

(2) Use volumetric measurements: measure water displacement from filled volumeter.
g. Observe periwound tissue.
  (1) Halo of erythema, warmth and swelling may indicate infection (cellulitis).
  (2) Maceration of surrounding tissues due to moisture (urine, feces) or wound drainage increases risk for wound deterioration and enlargement.
  (3) Trophic changes may indicate poor arterial nutrition.
  (4) Cyanosis may indicate arterial insufficiency.
h. Examine for signs of infection.
  (1) Bacterial culture: is to identify colonization and infection; culture wound site only.
  (2) Observations, palpation.
i. Photographic records of wound appearance aid narrative descriptions. Use marker pen to outline wound edges on transparent dressing with a calibrated grid to provide a measuring scale.

Wound Care

1. **Infection control.**
  a. Wounds are cultured; antibiotic treatment regimen prescribed.
    (1) Topical antimicrobial agents: e.g., silver nitrate, silver sulfadiazine, erythromycin, gentamicin, neomycin, triple antibiotic, Silvasorb gel.
    (2) Anti-inflammatory agents: e.g., corticosteroids, hydrocortisone, ibuprofen, indomethacin.
    (3) Topical anesthetics and analgesics: e.g., lidocaine, lignocaine.
  b. Hand washing of health care practitioners.
  c. Sterile technique.
  d. Vacuum-assisted closure (VAC).
    (1) An open-cell foam dressing placed into the wound.
    (2) Controlled subatmospheric pressure (typically 125 mm Hg below ambient pressure) is applied via specialized device.
    (3) Helps to control chronic edema, increases localized blood flow and removes infectious material.

2. **Surgical intervention.**
  a. Indicated for excising of ulcer, enhancing vascularity and resurfacing wound (grafts) and preventing sepsis and osteomyelitis.
  b. May be indicated for stages III and IV ulcers.

3. **Hyperbaric oxygen therapy (HBO).**
  a. Patient breathes 100% oxygen in a sealed, full-body chamber with elevated atmospheric pressure (between 2.0 and 2.5 atmospheres absolute, ATA).
  b. Hyperoxygenation reverses tissue hypoxia and facilitates wound healing owing to enhanced solubility of oxygen in the blood.

c. Contraindicated in untreated pneumothorax and some antineoplastic medications (e.g., doxorubicin, disulfiram, cisplatin, mafenide acetate).

4. Wound cleansing: removal of loose cellular debris, metabolic wastes, bacteria and topical agents that retard wound healing.

a. Cleanse wounds initially and at each dressing change.

b. Normal saline (0.9% NaCl) recommended for most ulcers; nontoxic effects in wound.

c. Cleansing topical agents: contain surfactants that lower surface tension. Limited use, may be toxic to healing tissues; e.g., povidone-iodine solution, sodium hypochlorite solution, Dakin's solution, acetic acid solution, hydrogen peroxide.

d. Delivery systems.

(1) Minimal mechanical force: cleansing with gauze, cloth or sponge.

(2) Irrigation.

(a) Using syringe, squeezable bottle with tip or battery-powered irrigation device (pulsatile lavage); loosens wound debris and removes it by suction.

(b) Safe and effective irrigation pressures range from 4 to 15 psi.

(3) Hydrotherapy (i.e., whirlpool).

(a) Indicated for ulcers with large amounts of exudate, slough and necrotic tissue.

(b) Increases circulation; assists in debridement of wounds or removal of dressings.

(c) Discontinue whirlpool when ulcer is clean.

e. Do not use harsh soaps, alcohol-based products or harsh antiseptic agents; may erode skin.

5. Wound debridement: removal of necrotic or infected tissue that interferes with wound healing (Table 6-3).

a. Allows examination of ulcer, determination of extent of wound.

b. Decreases bacterial concentration in wound; improves wound healing.

c. Decreases spread of infection; i.e., cellulitis or sepsis.

6. Wound dressings: topical products that protect the wound from contamination and trauma, permit application of medications, absorb drainage, debride necrotic tissue and enhance healing (Table 6-4).

Table 6-3 ➤ METHODS OF DEBRIDEMENT

Debridement classifications: physiology or methodologic approaches used.

Physiological methods (classified as selective or nonselective):

Selective debridement removes only nonviable tissue from the wound.

Nonselective debridement removes both viable and nonviable tissue.

Methodologic method:

Methodologic debridement is based on the actual mechanism of action, autolysis, chemical, mechanical or sharp.

Debridement is indicated for any chronic or acute wound when necrotic tissue, foreign bodies or infection is present and the goal for treatment is to heal the wound and /or control infection.

DEBRIDEMENT	DEFINITION	INDICATION	CONTRAINDICATIONS	DRESSING EXAMPLES
Autolytic	Selective, natural physiological process, body uses own white blood cells and enzymes to soften and break down necrotic tissue.	Noninfected wound with minimal to moderate amount of necrotic tissue	Infected wounds, Immuno-compromised patients	Hydrogels, hydrocol-loids, hydrofibers, hy-dropolymers, alginates and foams
Mechanical	Nonselective, an external force that is great enough to separate or break up the adhesive forces between the necrotic tissue and the wound base.	Moderate to large amounts of necrotic tissue.	Clean and granulating wounds	Scrubbing, wet to dry and irrigation
Chemical	Nonselective and selective, removing necrotic tissue from the wound base through a chemical process	Small to moderate amounts of necrotic tissue.	Clean and granulating wounds.	Mesalt, santyl, Dakin's solution and maggot
Sharp	Selective, removing necrotic tissue from a wound using sterile instruments such as forceps, scalpel, scissor or laser.	Large amounts of necrotic tissue.	Patients who are not candidates for surgical debridement because of comorbidities, associated risk factors and complications of anesthesia.	N/A
Surgical	The most efficient method of debridement. Is nonselective and performed by the physician or surgeon using sterile instruments (scalpel, scissors, forceps, hemostat, silver nitrate sticks) in a one-time operative procedure performed in an operating room. Patient may be anesthetized.	Advancing cellulitis with sepsis. Immunocompromised individuals. Surgical wound closure.	Individuals who are not appropriate candidates for a surgical procedure.	N/A

Table 6-4 ➤ CHARACTERISTICS OF COMMON WOUND DRESSINGS

CATEGORY	FUNCTION	DESCRIPTION	EXAMPLES	INDICATIONS	PRECAUTIONS	USAGE
Gauze	Absorption minimal-heavy; packing material	Woven or nonwoven. Comes in variety of sizes (2 x 2, 4 x 4), also in strips for use in tunneling or undermining	Curity, Kerlix, Nu-gauze	Partial- and full-thickness wounds, infected wounds, cavities or tracts	Adheres to tissue, may lint or shred if cut	Dressing change is dependent on saturation. Fluff the gauze to avoid tight packing.
Impregnated gauze	Provides wound with moisture, antimicrobial medications, nutrients, packing material	Woven sponges impregnated with agents	Mesalt, Xeroform, Hydrogel sponges, Curasalt, Vaseline gauze	Partial to full thickness wounds	Can provide too much moisture	Monitor to avoid maceration.
Alginates	Heavy to moderate absorption, packing	Natural fiber, derived from algae. Available in rope and sheets	Aquacel, Restore, Sorbsan, Calci-Care, Hydrofiber, AlgiSite M	Full thickness wounds, cavities, tunnels and undermined areas. Infected wounds, with or without slough	Not for nondraining wounds	Loosely pack into a wound, a secondary dressing is required.
Nonadherent; composites	Minimal absorption	Impermeable barrier	Telfa island dressing, Alldress, Medipore pad, soft cloth adhesive	Partial- and shallow full-thickness wounds	Not suitable if causes bleeding or needs soaking to remove	Must remove a paper backing.
Foam	Minimal to heavy absorption	Nonadherent, semipermeable foam that maintains a moist environment	Allevyn, Lyofoam, Flexzan, PolyMem	Partial-to full-thickness wounds, Infected wounds	Not suitable for dry or wounds covered with eschar	Dressing should be 2-3 cm larger than the wound.
Hydrocolloid	Minimal to moderate absorption	Impermeable barrier, adhesive, comes in a variety of shapes and sizes	Duoderm, Replicare, Tegasorb	Partial- to full-thickness wounds	Not recommended for immunosuppressed patients, anaerobic infected wounds, or sites subjected to incontinence	Dressing must have a 2- to 3-cm overlap from the margin of the wound.
Hydrogel	Hydrates the wound	Water- or glycerin-based amorphous gel or sheet	Hypergel sheet, Curasol, Intrusive gel	Partial- to full-thickness wounds, wounds that are dry to minimal drainage	Not suitable for draining wounds; monitor periwound tissue for maceration	Sheets are available with or without adhesive covers
Film/transparent	Protect the wound, minimal drainage	Thin and transparent, occlusive, adhesive dressing	Op-Site, CarraFilm, Polyskin II, Tegaderm film	Partial-thickness wounds	Not suitable for infected, heavy draining wounds	Must allow 4- to 5-cm overlap from wound margin to the surrounding tissue
Antimicrobial	Control or disease bioburden	Comes available in powder, ointments, gels and sheets	Acticoat, Iodosorb gel, Silvasorb gel, Arglaes powder	Partial- to full-thickness wounds, odorous and infected wounds	Not a substitute for systemic antibiotics	Read package insert for specific usage instructions
Negative pressure therapy (NPWT)	Reduces interstitial edema, controls drainage, for both acute and chronic wounds, promotes wound healing	Comes available in black or white sponge, which is placed inside the wound sealed with drape and attached to subatmospheric pressure by way of an evacuation tube connected to a computerized pump	KCI-VAC, vacuum-assisted closure	Full-thickness wounds, partial-thickness burns	Not suitable for cancer in the wound margins, or untreated osteomyelitis. Patients with active bleeding, clotting disorders	Dressings changes done two to three times per week

a. Moisture-retentive (occlusive) wound dressings: maintain a moist environment; wound tissue fluid is maintained in contact with tissues and cells; facilitates autolytic debridement, wound healing (reepithelialization) with less pain.
   (1) Alginate dressings: e.g., Sorbsan, Algisite, Restore, Aquacel, Hydrofiber.
   (2) Transparent film dressings: e.g., Tegaderm, OpSite.
   (3) Foam dressings: e.g., LYOfoam, PolyMen, Allevyn.
   (4) Hydrogel dressings: e.g., Curasol, Hypergel, Elastogel.
   (5) Hydrocolloid dressings: e.g., DuoDerm, Restore, Tegasorb.
b. Gauze dressings.
   (1) Standard gauze (not impregnated).
   (2) Impregnated gauze: e.g., Vaseline Petroleum Gauze, Curasalt, Mesalt, Xeroform.
c. Semirigid dressings: Unna boot is a pliable, non-stretchable dressing impregnated with ointments; e.g., zinc oxide, calamine and gelatin.

7. **Edema management.**
   a. Leg elevation and exercise (ankle pumps).
   b. Compression therapy: to facilitate movement of excess fluid from lower extremity.
      (1) Compression wraps: elastic or tubular bandages.
      (2) Paste bandages; e.g., Unna boot.
      (3) Compression stockings; e.g., Jobst.
      (4) Compression pump therapy.
      (5) Manual lymphatic drainage techniques.

8. **Electrical stimulation for wound healing.**
   a. Uses capacitive coupled electrical current to transfer energy to a wound, improve circulation, facilitate debridement, enhance tissue repair.
   b. Continuous waveform application with direct current.
   c. High-voltage pulsed current (HVPC).
   d. Microcurrent electrical stimulation (MENS).
   e. Alternating/biphasic current.

9. **Nutritional considerations.**
   a. Delayed wound healing associated with malnutrition and poor hydration.
   b. Provide adequate hydration: eight 8-oz glasses of non-caffeine fluids per day unless contraindicated.
   c. Provide adequate nutrition: frequent high-calorie/high-protein meals; energy intake (25–35 kcal/kg/body weight) and protein (1.5–2.5 gm/kg body weight).
   d. Patients with trauma stress and burns require higher intakes.

10. **Injury prevention or reduction.**
    a. Daily, comprehensive skin inspection, paying particular attention to bony prominences (e.g., sacrum, coccyx, trochanter, ischial tuberosities, medial or lateral malleolus).
    b. Therapeutic positioning to relieve pressure and allow tissue reperfusion.
       (1) In bed: turning or repositioning schedule every 2 hours during acute and rehabilitation phases.
       (2) In wheelchair: wheelchair push-ups every 15 minutes.
    c. Use techniques to ensure skin protection, avoid friction, shear or abrasion injury.
       (1) Lifting, not dragging.
       (2) Use of turning and draw sheets; trapeze, manual or electric lifts.
       (3) Use of cornstarch, lubricants, pad protectors, thin film dressings or hydrocolloid dressings over friction risk sites.
       (4) Use of transfer boards for sliding wheelchair transfers.
    d. Pressure-relieving devices (PRDs).
       (1) Reduce tissue interface pressures.
       (2) Static devices: use if patient can assume a variety of positions; examples include foam, air or gel mattress overlays, water-filled mattresses, pillows or foam wedges, protective padding (heel-relief boots).
       (3) Dynamic devices: use if patient cannot assume a variety of positions; examples include alternating pressure air mattresses, fluidized air or high-air-loss bed.
       (4) Seating supports: use for chair-bound or wheelchair-bound patients; examples include cushions made out of foam, gel, air or some combination.
    e. Avoid restrictive clothing, clothing with rough textures, hard fasteners, studs, etc. Avoid tight-fitting shoes, socks, splints and orthoses.
    f. Avoid maceration injury.
       (1) Prevent moisture accumulation and temperature elevation where skin contacts support surface.
       (2) Incontinence management strategies: use of absorbent pads, brief or panty pad; scheduled toileting and prompted voiding; ointments, creams and skin barriers prophylactically in perineal and perianal areas.
    g. Patient and caregiver education.
       (1) Mechanisms of pressure ulcer development.
       (2) Daily skin inspection.
       (3) Avoidance of prolonged positions.
       (4) Repositioning, weight shifts, lifts.
       (5) Safety awareness during self-care.
       (6) Safety awareness with use of devices and equipment.
       (7) Importance of ongoing activity/exercise program.

chapter *7*

Other Systems and Conditions: Immune, Hematological, Gastrointestinal, Endocrine, Metabolic and Bariatrics

SUSAN B. O'SULLIVAN

Focus Areas for Content Review:

- General anatomy and physiology of the immune, hematological, gastrointestinal, endocrine and metabolic systems.
- Pathologies and injuries of these systems commonly encountered in physical therapy. How these conditions impact the patient's ability to participate in physical therapy.
- Physical therapy interventions; indications and contraindications, appropriate responses, PTA response to adverse reaction, effects of interventions on the these systems.

- Problems associated with obesity.
- Physical therapy interventions to address problems associated with obesity and implication of obesity on the provision of physical therapy interventions.
- Psychological issues and disorders and their impact on the provision of physical therapy interventions.

The Immune System

Overview

1. **Anatomy and physiology of the immune system.**
   a. The immune system consists of immune cells, central immune structures where immune cells are produced (the bone marrow and thymus) and the peripheral immune structures (lymph nodes, spleen and other accessory structures).
   b. There are several different types of immune cells:
      (1) An antigen (immunogen) is a foreign molecule that elicits the immune response. Antibodies or immunoglobulins are the proteins that are engaged to tag antigens.
      (2) Lymphocytes (T and B lymphocytes) are the primary cells of the immune system.
      (3) Macrophages are the accessory cells that process and present antigens to the lymphocytes.
      (4) Cytokines are molecules that link immune cells with other tissues and organs.
      (5) CD molecules (e.g., CD4 helper cells) serve as master regulators of the immune response by

influencing the function of all other immune cells.
      (6) Recognition of foreign threat from self (autoimmune responses) is mediated by major histocompatibility complex (MHC) membrane molecules.
   c. The thymus is the primary central gland of the immune system. It is located behind the sternum above the heart and extends into the neck region to the lower edge of the thyroid gland.
      (1) It is fully developed at birth and reaches maximum size at puberty. It then decreases in size and is slowly replaced by adipose tissue.
      (2) It produces mature T lymphocytes.
   d. The lymph system is a vast network of capillaries, vessels, valves, ducts, nodes and organs that functions to produce, filter and convey various lymph and blood cells.
      (1) Lymph nodes are small areas of lymphoid tissue connected by lymphatic vessels throughout the body. High concentrations are found in the axilla, groin and along the great vessels of the neck, thorax and abdomen.

(2) Lymph nodes function to filter the lymph and trap antigens. Lymphocytes, monocytes and plasma cells are formed in lymph nodes.

e. The spleen is a large lymphoid organ located in the upper left abdominal cavity between the stomach and the diaphragm.

   (1) It functions to filter antigens from the blood and produce leukocytes, monocytes, lymphocytes and plasma cells in response to infection.

   (2) In the embryo the spleen produces red and white blood cells; after birth, only lymphocytes are produced unless severe anemia exists.

2. The immune response is the coordinated response of the body's cells and molecules that provide protection from infectious disease (bacteria, viruses, fungi, parasites) and foreign substances (plant pollens, poison ivy resin, insect venom, transplanted organs). It also defends against abnormal cells produced by the body (cancer cells).

a. The innate immune response is the natural resistance to disease and consists of rapidly activated phagocytes (macrophages, neutrophils, natural killer cells, dendritic cells). Barriers also provide a natural defense (skin, mucous membranes) as do inflammation and fever (antimicrobial molecules).

b. The adaptive immune response includes the slower-acting defenses mediated by the lymphocytes.

c. Repeat exposure activates immunological memory producing more rapid and efficient responses.

d. When the immune response is excessive, the result causes allergies or autoimmune responses.

3. Immunodeficiency diseases.

a. Characterized by depressed or absent immune responses.

b. Primary immunodeficient disorders result from a defect in T cells, B cells or lymphoid tissues.

   (1) Congenital disorders are a failure of organs to develop and produce mature lymphocytes.

   (2) Severe combined immunodeficiency disease (SCID).

c. Secondary immunodeficiency disorders result from underlying pathology or treatment that depresses the immune system, resulting in failure of the immune response.

   (1) Diseases include leukemia, bone marrow tumor, chronic diabetes, renal failure, cirrhosis, cancer treatment (chemotherapy, radiation therapy).

   (2) Organ transplant, graft versus host disease.

4. Autoimmune diseases.

a. Characterized by immune system responses directed against the body's normal tissues; self-destructive processes impair body function.

b. Can be organ specific: Hashimoto's thyroiditis.

c. Can be systemic (nonorgan-specific): systemic lupus erythematosus (SLE), fibromyalgia.

d. Etiology is unknown; possible factors include genetic predisposition, hormonal changes, environment, viral infection and stress.

Acquired Immunodeficiency Syndrome (AIDS)

1. Caused by the human immunodeficiency virus (HIV-1 or HIV-2).

2. Loss of immune system function.

a. Opportunistic infections: most common is *Pneumocystis carinii* pneumonia; also oral and esophageal candidiasis, cytomegalovirus infection, cryptococcus, atypical mycobacteriosis, chronic herpes simplex, toxoplasmosis, *Mycobacterium tuberculosis*.

b. Malignancies: most common is Kaposi's sarcoma; also non-Hodgkin's lymphoma; primary brain lymphoma.

c. Neurological disease: focal encephalitis (central nervous system [CNS] toxoplasmosis); cryptococcal meningitis; AIDS dementia complex; herpes zoster.

3. Pathophysiology.

a. Reduction of CD4+ helper T cells, resulting in CD4+ T lymphocytopenia; a major defect in the immune system.

b. A retrovirus: replicates in reverse fashion, i.e., the RNA code is transcribed into DNA.

4. Transmission is through contact with infected body fluids (blood, saliva, semen, cerebrospinal fluid, breast milk, vaginal/cervical secretions).

a. High-risk behaviors for HIV transmission.

   (1) Unprotected sexual contact.

   (2) Contaminated needles: sharing, frequent injection of IV drugs; transfusions (exposure to contaminated blood is no longer a major risk).

   (3) Maternal-fetal transmission in utero or at delivery; contaminated breast milk.

b. Low-risk behaviors for HIV transmission.

   (1) Occupational transmission: needle sticks.

   (2) Casual contact: kissing.

c. AIDS cannot be contacted through respiratory inhalation, skin contact or human waste (urine, feces, sweat or vomit).

5. Diagnosis: based on clinical findings and systemic evidence of HIV infection and absence of other known causes of immunodeficiency.

a. AIDS-related complex (ARC): presence of acute symptoms secondary to immune system deficiency; early/middle AIDS.

   (1) May include recurrent fever and chills, night sweats, swollen lymph glands, loss of appetite, weight loss, diarrhea, persistent fatigue, infections, apathy and depression.

   (2) May last weeks or months; a precursor to full-blown AIDS.

b. AIDS: exhibits some or all of the symptoms of ARC, general failure to thrive and also:

(1) Opportunistic infections.

(2) Headaches, blurred vision, dyspnea, dry cough, oral or skin lesions, dysphagia, dementia, seizures and focal neurological signs.

c. Deconditioning, anxiety and depression are common.

d. Laboratory evidence.

(1) HIV-1 antibody test (enzyme-linked immunosorbent assay [ELISA]): 30,000–50,000 copies of HIV per milliliter.

(2) Absolute T4 (CD4) cell counts per deciliter of blood: normal CD4 counts: 800–1200/mL; symptomatic AIDS CD4 counts: 200–500/mL.

6. Clinical course.

a. May exhibit brief early nonspecific viral infection and then remain asymptomatic for many years.

b. There is no cure. Combination therapies may extend life. Prognosis is poor without treatment, or with long-standing disease with secondary infections.

7. Medical interventions.

a. Multidrug (antiviral) therapy; three main groups of anti-AIDS drugs:

(1) Nucleoside reverse transcriptase inhibitors (NRTIs); e.g., AZT (azidothymidine).

(2) Protease inhibitors.

(3) Nonnucleoside reverse transcriptase inhibitors (NNRTIs).

(4) Initiated for symptomatic patients with AIDS, patients with CD4 counts fewer than 500, newly infected individuals.

(5) Common adverse effects of antiviral therapy include rash, nausea, headaches, dizziness, muscle pain, weakness, fatigue and difficulty sleeping. With hepatotoxicity, signs of carpal tunnel syndrome may be seen.

b. Symptomatic treatment.

(1) Education to prevent the spread of infection and disease.

(2) Treat opportunistic infections; prophylactic vaccinations.

(3) Maintain nutritional status.

(4) Provide supportive care for management of fatigue, e.g., energy conservation techniques, self-care.

(5) Respiratory management as needed.

(6) Provide skin care.

(7) Maintain functional mobility and safety; prevent disability.

(8) Provide supportive care, e.g., emotional support for patients and families.

8. Physical therapy goals, outcomes and interventions.

a. Observe universal AIDS/HIV precautions for healthcare workers.

b. Exercise has a positive effect on the immune system, reduces stress level and pain, improves cardiovascular endurance and strength (disuse effects common).

c. Exercise recommendations.

(1) Moderate aerobic exercise training.

(2) Strength training.

(3) Avoid exhaustive exercise with symptomatic individuals.

(4) During acute stages of opportunistic infections, reduce exercise to mild levels.

d. Teach activity pacing: balancing rest with activity, scheduling strenuous activities during periods of high energy.

e. Teach energy conservation: analysis and modification of daily activities to reduce energy expenditure.

f. Teach stress management, relaxation training (e.g., meditation and mindfulness, tai chi chuan, yoga).

g. Neurological rehabilitation for patients with involvement of the CNS: refer to chapter 3 on Neuromuscular Physical Therapy.

Chronic Fatigue Syndrome (CFS)

1. A complex syndrome characterized by disabling fatigue accompanied by various other complaints. Also called chronic fatigue and immune dysfunction syndrome (CFIDS)

2. Pathophysiology and clinical characteristics.

a. Etiology: unknown, viral cause suspected; often preceded by flu-like symptoms.

b. Immunological abnormalities present.

c. Neuroendocrine changes.

3. Diagnosis by exclusion: must have the two major criteria and either eight symptom criteria or six symptom criteria with at least two physical criteria (Centers for Disease Control and Prevention [CDC] case definition).

a. Major criteria:

(1) New onset of persistent or relapsing fatigue; must be present for at least 6 months; does not resolve with bed rest and reduces daily activity by at least 50%.

(2) Exclusion of other chronic conditions.

b. Symptom criteria:

(1) Profound or prolonged fatigue; inability to recover from normal exercise.

(2) Low-grade fever or chills.

(3) Sore throat: nonexudative pharyngitis.

(4) Lymph node pain and tenderness.

(5) Muscle weakness.

(6) Muscle discomfort or myalgia.

(7) Sleep disturbances (insomnia or hypersomnia).

(8) Headaches.

(9) Migratory arthralgias without joint swelling or redness.

(10) Cognitive impairments: photophobia, impaired memory, difficulty thinking, inability to concentrate, irritability, confusion.

(11) Main symptom complex develops over a few hours or days.

c. Deconditioning, anxiety and depression are common.

d. More common in women than men; younger ages (20s and 30s).

e. Limited recovery: only 5%–10% recover completely.

4. Medical interventions:

a. Antiviral agents in clinical trials.

b. Supportive and symptomatic treatment; symptoms may persist for months or years.

   (1) Analgesics and anti-inflammatory nonsteroidal medications for myalgia and arthralgia.

   (2) Nutritional support.

   (3) Psychological support and counseling; antidepressants.

5. Physical therapist assistant assessment.

a. Assess exercise tolerance levels. Vital signs may reveal fluctuations in HR and BP; orthostatic hypotension is common. If deconditioned, dyspnea with exercise.

b. Assess posture. Postural stress syndrome (poor posture) and movement adaptation syndrome (inefficient movement patterns) may be present and can contribute to chronic pain.

c. Assess activity levels and degree of fatigue. Objective measure: Modified Fatigue Impact Scale.

d. Monitor for depression and degree of emotional support present.

6. Physical therapy goals, outcomes and interventions.

a. Activities are reduced when fatigue is maximal; bed rest contraindicated other than for sleep.

b. Graded exercise program: short duration, gradually increasing intensity; components include stretching, strengthening, aerobic training (e.g., walking).

c. Avoid overexertion.

d. Teach activity pacing: balancing rest with activity; scheduling strenuous activities during periods of high energy.

e. Teach energy conservation: analysis and modification of daily activities to reduce energy expenditure.

f. Teach stress management, relaxation training (e.g., meditation and mindfulness, tai chi chuan, yoga).

g. Refer to support group.

Fibromyalgia Syndrome (FMS)

1. A chronic pain syndrome affecting muscles and soft tissues (nonarticular rheumatism).

2. Pathophysiology/clinical characteristics.

a. Etiology unknown; viral cause suspected, multifactorial.

b. Immunological and neurohormonal abnormalities are present; genetic factor (autosomal dominant).

3. Characterized by myalgia (muscle pain), generalized aching, persistent fatigue (mental and physical), sleep disturbances with generalized morning stiffness and multiple tender points (trigger points).

a. Additional signs and symptoms: visual problems, mental and physical fatigue, spasm, cold intolerance, headaches, irritable bladder or bowel, cognitive problems (impaired memory, decreased attention and concentration), restless legs, atypical patterns of numbness and tingling (sensitivity amplification).

b. Anxiety and depression are common.

c. Triggering events: emotional stress/anxiety trauma, hyperthyroidism, infection.

d. More common in women (75%–80% of cases) than men.

4. Medical management.

a. Diagnosis by exclusion. Presence of 11 of 18 specified tender points (Copenhagen Fibromyalgia Syndrome definition).

b. Anti-inflammatory agents, muscle relaxants, pain medications.

c. Nutritional support.

d. Psychological support and counseling; antidepressants.

5. Physical therapy goals, outcomes and interventions.

a. See recommendations for chronic fatigue syndrome.

b. Patient typically demonstrates exercise intolerance. Daily exercise is important. Focus is on aerobic training, mild to moderate intensities.

c. Teach protection strategies to avoid overuse syndromes.

d. Aquatic therapy is ideal to decrease pain and increase cardiovascular conditioning and strength.

e. Teach techniques for taking control: self-responsibility for health, education, coping strategies, keeping a journal.

f. Work and work environment adjustments.

g. Refer to support group.

Infectious Diseases

Staphylococcal Infections

1. *Staphylococcus aureus* (SA) is a common bacterial pathogen.

2. Typically begins as localized infection; entry is through skin portal, e.g., wounds, ulcers, burns.

3. Bacterial invasion and spread is through bloodstream or lymphatic system to almost any body location: e.g., heart valves, bones (acute staphylococcus osteomyelitis), joints (bacterial arthritis), skin (cellulitis, furuncles and carbuncles, ulcers), respiratory tract (pneumonia), bowel (enterocolitis).

4. Infection produces suppuration (pus formation) and abscess.

5. Medical interventions.
   a. Laboratory diagnosis to confirm pathogen.
   b. Antibiotic therapy; determine antibiotic sensitivity. Antibiotic resistance is common.
   c. Drainage of abscesses.
   d. Skin infections that are untreated can become systemic; sepsis can be lethal.

6. Infection control procedures: refer to section III.

7. Methicillin-resistant Staphylococcus aureus (MRSA) is an antibiotic-resistant strain.
   a. MRSA is resistant to all penicillins (especially methicillin) and cephalosporins.
   b. It is found in about 1% of the population.
   c. Hospitalized patients with MRSA infections are isolated and standard mask-gown-gloves precautions required.
   d. Community acquired MRSA [CA-MRSA] can impact athletic teams, school populations, prison populations and those engaging in male on male sex.

8. Vancomycin-resistant Staphylococcus aureus (VRSA) is resistant to vancomycin and can be a life-threatening infection.

Streptococcal Infections

1. a common bacterial pathogen.

2. Types:
   a. Group A streptococcus (*Streptococcus pyogenes*): pharyngitis, rheumatic fever, scarlet fever, impetigo, necrotizing fasciitis (gangrene), cellulitis and myositis.
   b. Group B streptococcus (*Streptococcus agalactiae*): neonatal and adult streptococcal B infections.
   c. Group C streptococcus (*Streptococcus pneumoniae*): pneumonia, otitis media, meningitis, endocarditis.

3. Medical interventions:
   a. Laboratory diagnosis to confirm pathogen.
   b. Antibiotic therapy; antibiotic resistance common.
   c. Skin infections that are untreated can become systemic.

Hepatitis

1. Inflammation of the liver; may be caused by viral or bacterial infections; chemical agents (alcohol, drugs, toxins).

2. Types:
   a. Hepatitis A virus (HAV, acute infectious hepatitis).
      (1) Transmission is primarily through fecal-oral route; contracted through contaminated food or water, infected food handlers.
      (2) Prevention: good personal hygiene, hand washing, sanitation, immunization (vaccine).
   b. Hepatitis B virus (HBV, serum hepatitis).
      (1) Transmission from blood, body fluids or body tissues, through blood transfusion, oral or sexual contact or contaminated needles.
      (2) Prevention: education, use of disposable needles, screening of blood donors, precautions for health care workers, immunization (vaccine).
   c. Hepatitis C virus (HCV, non-A, non-B).
      (1) Transmission is same as for HBV (posttransfusion is most common route).

3. Clinical manifestations: may be mild or severe (life threatening).
   a. Clinical signs and symptoms:
      (1) Initial (preicteric phase): low-grade fever, anorexia, nausea, vomiting, fatigue, malaise, headache, abdominal tenderness and pain.
      (2) Jaundice (icteric) phase: fever, jaundice, enlarged liver with tenderness, abatement of earlier symptoms.
      (3) Elevated lab values: hepatic transaminases and bilirubin.
   b. Course: variable.
      (1) Acute: may last from several weeks to months.
      (2) Chronic: HBV and HCV may lead to chronic liver infection, including necrosis, cirrhosis and liver failure.

4. Medical interventions:
   a. No specific treatment for acute viral hepatitis; treatment is symptomatic: e.g., IV fluids, analgesics.
   b. Chronic hepatitis: interferon is the main therapy.

Tuberculosis (TB)

1. An airborne infectious disease caused by the bacillus *Mycobacterium tuberculosis.*

2. Most commonly affects the respiratory system; may also affect the gastrointestinal and genitourinary systems, bones, joints, the nervous system and skin.

3. Course: may be acute, generalized or chronic, localized.

4. Signs and symptoms:
   a. Pulmonary: productive cough, rales, dyspnea, pleuritic pain and hemoptysis.
   b. Systemic: fatigue, low-grade fever, night sweats, anorexia and weight loss.

5. Medical interventions:
   a. Chemotherapy: a combination of daily drugs; incidence of drug-resistant strains is increasing.
   b. Isolation and bed rest (limited with advent of chemotherapy).
   c. Adequate diet.

6. Pulmonary precautions: instruct patient in infection control measures. Transmission is through:
   a. Respiratory droplets or sputum: use tissues to cover nose and mouth when coughing or sneezing; disposable containers for sputum, tissues.
   b. Soiled dressings.

Center for Disease Control and Prevention (CDC) Guidelines for Isolation Precautions

Standard Precautions

1. Include a group of infection prevention practices that apply to all patients regardless of suspected or confirmed infection status (Box 7-1).

2. Standard Precautions combine major features of:
   a. Universal Precautions.
   b. Body Substance Isolation.

3. Based on the principle that all blood, body fluids, secretions, excretions except sweat, nonintact skin and mucous membranes may contain transmissible infections agents.

Physical Therapy-Related Infection Control

1. Purpose: to destroy bacteria, infectious organisms.

2. Sterilization: the total destruction of all microorganisms by exposure to chemical or physical agents; required for all objects introduced into the body: scalpels, catheters, etc.
   a. Autoclaving: sterilization of instruments by heat (250–270°F) and water pressure; contraindicated with heat-sensitive articles.
   b. Boiling water (212°F): kills nonspore-forming organisms.
   c. Ionizing radiation: used to sterilize some medications, plastics or sutures.
   d. Dry heat: prolonged exposure to high heat in ovens.
   e. Gaseous: ethylene oxide, formaldehyde gas.

3. Disinfection: the reduction of the number of microorganisms; typically used on surfaces or equipment, e.g., respiratory and hydrotherapy equipment.
   a. Ultraviolet light: used for air and surface disinfection; harmful to unprotected skin and eyes.
   b. Filtration: used for water or air purification.
   c. Physical cleaning.
      (1) Ultrasonic: disinfects instruments.
      (2) Washing with an antimicrobial product: used to disinfect hands and surfaces.
   d. Chemicals:
      (1) Chlorination: used for water disinfection, filtration systems; also used for food surface sanitizing.
      (2) Iodines: used in hydrotherapy when filtering system not possible; provides full bactericidal activity when organic matter (skin, feces, urine) is present.
      (3) Phenols: general disinfectants.
      (4) Quaternary ammonia compounds, e.g., Zephiran.
      (5) Formaldehyde (5%).
   e. Hydrotherapy disinfection.
      (1) Drain and clean tanks after every patient.
      (2) Scrub pumps and equipment (e.g., drains, agitator unit) with a germicidal detergent; e.g., sodium hypochlorite (bleach), povidone-iodine, chlorazene (Chloramine-T).
      (3) Rinse before refilling.

Box 7-1 ➤ STANDARD PRECAUTIONS*

Standard Precautions include a group of infection prevention practices that apply to all patients, regardless of suspected or confirmed infection status, in any setting in which healthcare is delivered. These include hand hygiene; use of gloves, gown, mask, eye protection or face shield, depending on the anticipated exposure; and safe injection practices. Also, equipment or items in the patient environment likely to have been contaminated with infectious body fluids must be handled in a manner to prevent transmission of infectious agents (e.g., wear gloves for direct contact, contain heavily soiled equipment, properly clean and disinfect or sterilize reusable equipment before use on another patient). The application of Standard Precautions during patient care is determined by the nature of the health care worker (HCW)–patient interaction and the extent of anticipated blood, body fluid or pathogen exposure. For some interactions (e.g., performing venipuncture), only gloves may be needed; during other interactions (e.g., intubation), use of gloves, gown and face shield or mask and goggles is necessary. Education and training on the principles and rationale for recommended practices are critical elements of Standard Precautions because they facilitate appropriate decision-making and promote adherence when HCWs are faced with new circumstances. An example of the importance of the use of Standard Precautions is intubation, especially under emergency circumstances when infectious agents may not be suspected, but later are identified (e.g., severe acute respiratory syndrome [SARS]–coronavirus [CoV], *Neisseria meningitides*). Standard Precautions are also intended to protect patients by ensuring that healthcare personnel do not carry infectious agents to patients on their hands or via equipment used during patient care.

A.1. New Elements of Standard Precautions Infection control problems that are identified in the course of outbreak investigations often indicate the need for new recommendations or reinforcement of existing infection control recommendations to protect patients. Because such recommendations are considered a standard of care and may not be included in other guidelines, they are added here to Standard Precautions. Three such areas of practice that have been added are Respiratory Hygiene/Cough Etiquette, safe injection practices and use of masks for insertion of catheters or injection of material into spinal or epidural spaces via lumbar puncture procedures (e.g., myelogram, spinal or epidural anesthesia). While most elements of Standard Precautions evolved from Universal Precautions that were developed for protection of healthcare personnel, these new elements of Standard Precautions focus on protection of patients.

A.1.a. Respiratory Hygiene/Cough Etiquette The transmission of SARS-CoV in emergency departments by patients and their family members during the widespread SARS outbreaks in 2003 highlighted the need for vigilance and prompt implementation of infection control measures at the first point of encounter within a healthcare setting (e.g., reception and triage areas in emergency departments, outpatient clinics and physician offices). The strategy proposed has been termed Respiratory Hygiene/Cough Etiquette and is intended to be incorporated into infection control practices as a new component of Standard Precautions. The strategy is targeted at patients and accompanying family members and friends with undiagnosed transmissible respiratory infections, and applies to any person with signs of illness including cough, congestion, rhinorrhea or increased production of respiratory secretions when entering a healthcare facility. The term *cough etiquette* is derived from recommended source control measures for *Mycobacteria tuberculosis*. The elements of Respiratory Hygiene/Cough Etiquette include (1) education of healthcare facility staff, patients and visitors; (2) posted signs, in language(s) appropriate to the population served, with instructions to patients and accompanying family members or friends, (3) source control measures (e.g., covering the mouth/nose with a tissue when coughing and prompt disposal of used tissues, using surgical masks on the coughing person when tolerated and appropriate); (4) hand hygiene after contact with respiratory secretions; and (5) spatial separation, ideally > 3 feet, of persons with respiratory infections in common waiting areas when possible. Covering sneezes and coughs and placing masks on coughing patients are proven means of source containment that prevent infected persons from dispersing respiratory secretions into the air. Masking may be difficult in some settings (e.g., pediatrics, in which case, the emphasis by necessity may be on cough etiquette. Physical proximity of < 3 feet has been associated with an increased risk for transmission of infections via the droplet route (e.g., *N. meningitidis* and group A streptococcus and therefore supports the practice of distancing infected persons from others who are not infected. The effectiveness of good hygiene practices, especially hand hygiene, in preventing transmission of viruses and reducing the incidence of respiratory infections both within and outside healthcare settings is summarized in several reviews.

These measures should be effective in decreasing the risk of transmission of pathogens contained in large respiratory droplets (e.g., influenza virus, adenovirus, *Bordetella Pertussis,* and *Mycoplasma pneumoniae*. Although fever will be present in many respiratory infections, patients with pertussis and mild upper respiratory tract infections are often afebrile. Therefore, the absence of fever does not always exclude a respiratory infection. Patients who have asthma, allergic rhinitis or chronic obstructive lung disease also may be coughing and sneezing. While these patients often are not infectious, cough etiquette measures are prudent.

Healthcare personnel are advised to observe Droplet Precautions (i.e., wear a mask) and hand hygiene when examining and caring for patients with signs and symptoms of a respiratory infection. Healthcare personnel who have a respiratory infection are advised to avoid direct patient contact, especially with high-risk patients. If this is not possible, then a mask should be worn while providing patient care.

Recommendations
IV. Standard Precautions

Assume that every person is potentially infected or colonized with an organism that could be transmitted in the healthcare setting and apply the following infection control practices during the delivery of healthcare.

IV.A. Hand Hygiene

IV.A.1. During the delivery of healthcare, avoid unnecessary touching of surfaces in close proximity to the patient to prevent both contamination of clean hands from environmental surfaces and transmission of pathogens from contaminated hands to surfaces.

IV.A.2. When hands are visibly dirty, contaminated with proteinaceous material or visibly soiled with blood or body fluids, wash hands with either a nonantimicrobial soap and water or an antimicrobial soap and water.

IV.A.3. If hands are not visibly soiled, or after removing visible material with nonantimicrobial soap and water, decontaminate hands in the clinical situations described in IV.A.2.a–f. The preferred method of hand decontamination is with an alcohol-based hand rub. Alternatively, hands may be washed with an antimicrobial soap and water. Frequent use of an alcohol-based hand rub immediately following hand washing with nonantimicrobial soap may increase the frequency of dermatitis. Perform hand hygiene:

   IV.A.3.a. Before having direct contact with patients.

   IV.A.3.b. After contact with blood, body fluids or excretions, mucous membranes, nonintact skin or wound dressings.

   IV.A.3.c. After contact with a patient's intact skin (e.g., when taking a pulse or blood pressure or lifting a patient).

   IV.A.3.d. If hands will be moving from a contaminated body site to a clean body site during patient care.

   IV.A.3.e. After contact with inanimate objects (including medical equipment) in the immediate vicinity of the patient.

   IV.A.3.f. After removing gloves.

(Continued on following page)

Box 7-1 ➤ continued

IV.A.4. Wash hands with nonantimicrobial soap and water or with antimicrobial soap and water if in contact with spores (e.g., *Clostridium difficile* or *Bacillus anthracis*) is likely to have occurred. The physical action of washing and rinsing hands under such circumstances is recommended because alcohols, chlorhexidine, iodophors, and other antiseptic agents have poor activity against spores.

IV.A.5. Do not wear artificial fingernails or extenders if duties include direct contact with patients at high risk for infection and associated adverse outcomes (e.g., those in intensive care units [ICUs] or operating rooms).

   IV.A.5.a. Develop an organizational policy on the wearing of nonnatural nails by healthcare personnel who have direct contact with patients outside of the groups specified above.

IV.B. Personal protective equipment (PPE)

IV.B.1. Observe the following principles of use:

   IV.B.1.a. Wear PPE, as described in IV.B.2–4, when the nature of the anticipated patient interaction indicates that contact with blood or body fluids may occur.

   IV.B.1.b. Prevent contamination of clothing and skin during the process of removing PPE.

   IV.B.1.c. Before leaving the patient's room or cubicle, remove and discard PPE.

IV.B.2. Gloves

   IV.B.2.a. Wear gloves when it can be reasonably anticipated that contact with blood or other potentially infectious materials, mucous membranes, nonintact skin, or potentially contaminated intact skin (e.g., of a patient incontinent of stool or urine) could occur.

   IV.B.2.b. Wear gloves with fit and durability appropriate to the task.

      IV.B.2.b.i. Wear disposable medical examination gloves for providing direct patient care.

      IV.B.2.b.ii. Wear disposable medical examination gloves or reusable utility gloves for cleaning the environment or medical equipment.

   IV.B.2.c. Remove gloves after contact with a patient and/or the surrounding environment (including medical equipment) using proper technique to prevent hand contamination. Do not wear the same pair of gloves for the care of more than one patient. Do not wash gloves for the purpose of reuse since this practice has been associated with transmission of pathogens.

   IV.B.2.d. Change gloves during patient care if the hands will move from a contaminated body site (e.g., perineal area) to a clean body site (e.g., face).

IV.B.3. Gowns

   IV.B.3.a. Wear a gown that is appropriate to the task to protect skin and prevent soiling or contamination of clothing during procedures and patient-care activities when contact with blood, body fluids, secretions or excretions is anticipated.

      IV.B.3.a.i. Wear a gown for direct patient contact if the patient has uncontained secretions or excretions.

      IV.B.3.a.ii. Remove gown and perform hand hygiene before leaving the patient's environment.

   IV.B.3.b. Do not reuse gowns, even for repeated contacts with the same patient.

   IV.B.3.c. Routine donning of gowns upon entrance into a high-risk unit (e.g., ICU, neonatal intensive care unit [NICU], hematopoietic stem cell transplantation [HSCT] unit) is not indicated.

IV.B.4. Mouth, nose, eye protection.

   IV.B.4.a. Use PPE to protect the mucous membranes of the eyes, nose and mouth during procedures and patient-care activities that are likely to generate splashes or sprays of blood, body fluids, secretions and excretions. Select masks, goggles, face shields and combinations of each according to the need anticipated by the task performed.

IV.B.5. During aerosol-generating procedures (e.g., bronchoscopy, suctioning of the respiratory tract [if not using in-line suction catheters], endotracheal intubation) in patients who are not suspected of being infected with an agent for which respiratory protection is otherwise recommended (e.g., *M. tuberculosis*, SARS or hemorrhagic fever viruses), wear one of the following: a face shield that fully covers the front and sides of the face, a mask with attached shield or a mask and goggles (in addition to gloves and gown).

IV.C. Respiratory Hygiene/Cough Etiquette

IV.C.1. Educate healthcare personnel on the importance of source control measures to contain respiratory secretions to prevent droplet and fomite transmission of respiratory pathogens, especially during seasonal outbreaks of viral respiratory tract infections (e.g., influenza, respiratory syncytial virus [RSV], adenovirus, parainfluenza virus) in communities.

IV.C.2. Implement the following measures to contain respiratory secretions in patients and accompanying individuals who have signs and symptoms of a respiratory infection, beginning at the point of initial encounter in a healthcare setting (e.g., triage, reception and waiting areas in emergency departments, outpatient clinics and physician offices).

   IV.C.2.a. Post signs at entrances and in strategic places (e.g., elevators, cafeterias) within ambulatory and inpatient settings with instructions to patients and other persons with symptoms of a respiratory infection to cover their mouths/noses when coughing or sneezing, use and dispose of tissues and perform hand hygiene after hands have been in contact with respiratory secretions.

   IV.C.2.b. Provide tissues and no-touch receptacles (e.g., foot pedal–operated lid or open, plastic-lined waste basket) for disposal of tissues.

   IV.C.2.c. Provide resources and instructions for performing hand hygiene in or near waiting areas in ambulatory and inpatient settings; provide conveniently located dispensers of alcohol-based hand rubs and, where sinks are available, supplies for hand washing.

   IV.C.2.d. During periods of increased prevalence of respiratory infections in the community (e.g., as indicated by increased school absenteeism, increased number of patients seeking care for a respiratory infection), offer masks to coughing patients and other symptomatic persons (e.g., persons who accompany ill patients) upon entry into the facility or medical office and encourage them to maintain special separation, ideally a distance of at least 3 feet, from others in common waiting areas.

      IV.C.2.d.i. Some facilities may find it logistically easier to institute this recommendation year-round as a standard of practice.

IV.D. Patient placement

(Continued on following page)

IV.D.1. Include the potential for transmission of infectious agents in patient placement decisions. Place patients who pose a risk for transmission to others (e.g., uncontained secretions, excretions or wound drainage, infants with suspected viral respiratory or gastrointestinal infections) in a single-patient room when available.

IV.D.2. Determine patient placement based on the following principles:

- Route(s) of transmission of the known or suspected infectious agent
- Risk factors for transmission in the infected patient
- Risk factors for adverse outcomes resulting from a hospital-acquired infection (HAI) in other patients in the area or room being considered for patient placement
- Availability of single-patient rooms
- Patient options for room sharing (e.g., cohorting patients with the same infection)

IV.E. Patient-care equipment and instruments/devices

IV.E.1. Establish policies and procedures for containing, transporting and handling patient-care equipment and instruments/devices that may be contaminated with blood or body fluids.

IV.E.2. Remove organic material from critical and semicritical instrument/devices, using recommended cleaning agents before high-level disinfection and sterilization to enable effective disinfection and sterilization processes.

IV.E.3. Wear PPE (e.g., gloves, gown), according to the level of anticipated contamination, when handling patient-care equipment and instruments/devices that are visibly soiled or may have been in contact with blood or body fluids.

IV.F. Care of the environment

IV.F.1. Establish policies and procedures for routine and targeted cleaning of environmental surfaces as indicated by the level of patient contact and degree of soiling.

IV.F.2. Clean and disinfect surfaces that are likely to be contaminated with pathogens, including those that are in close proximity to the patient (e.g., bed rails, over bed tables) and frequently touched surfaces in the patient-care environment (e.g., door knobs, surfaces in and surrounding toilets in patients' rooms) on a more frequent schedule compared to that for other surfaces (e.g., horizontal surfaces in waiting rooms).

IV.F.3. Use Environmental Protection Agency (EPA)–registered disinfectants that have microbiocidal (i.e., killing) activity against the pathogens most likely to contaminate the patient-care environment. Use in accordance with manufacturer's instructions.

> **IV.F.3.a.** Review the efficacy of in-use disinfectants when evidence of continuing transmission of an infectious agent (e.g., rotavirus, *C. difficile*, norovirus) may indicate resistance to the in-use product and change to a more effective disinfectant as indicated.

IV.F.4. In facilities that provide healthcare to pediatric patients or have waiting areas with child play toys (e.g., obstetric/gynecology offices and clinics), establish policies and procedures for cleaning and disinfecting toys at regular intervals. *Category IA*

Use the following principles in developing this policy and procedures:

- Select play toys that can be easily cleaned and disinfected.
- Do not permit use of stuffed furry toys if they will be shared.
- Clean and disinfect large stationary toys (e.g., climbing equipment) at least weekly and whenever visibly soiled.
- If toys are likely to be mouthed, rinse with water after disinfection; alternatively wash in a dishwasher.
- When a toy requires cleaning and disinfection, do so immediately or store in a designated labeled container separate from toys that are clean and ready for use.

IV.F.5. Include multiuse electronic equipment in policies and procedures for preventing contamination and for cleaning and disinfection, especially those items that are used by patients, those used during delivery of patient care and mobile devices that are moved in and out of patient rooms frequently (e.g., daily).

> **IV.F.5.a.** No recommendation for use of removable protective covers or washable keyboards. *Unresolved issue*

IV.G. Textiles and laundry

IV.G.1. Handle used textiles and fabrics with minimum agitation to avoid contamination of air, surfaces and persons.

IV.G.2. If laundry chutes are used, ensure that they are properly designed, maintained and used in a manner to minimize dispersion of aerosols from contaminated laundry.

IV.H. Safe injection practices: see CDC website

IV.I. Infection control practices for special lumbar puncture procedures: see CDC website

IV.J. Worker safety. Adhere to federal and state requirements for protection of healthcare personnel from exposure to bloodborne pathogens.

*Date last modified: October 12, 2007.

*Excerpt with modifications from Centers for Disease Control and Prevention, the *Guideline for Isolation Precautions: Preventing Transmission of Infectious Agents in Healthcare Settings 2007*. PDF (1.33MB / 219 pages), downloaded 9.15.08. http://www.cdc.gov/ncidod/dhqp/gl_isolation_standard.html

4. **Antisepsis: procedures that inhibit or destroy microorganisms on skin or living tissue.**
   a. Antiseptic solutions: alcohol, iodines; e.g., povidone-iodine (Betadine).
   b. Quaternary ammonia compounds (0.1%); e.g., Zephiran.
   c. Mercurials (0.1%).
   d. Germicidal soaps: used for bacteriostatic action (e.g., pHisoHex).
   e. Antibacterial additives to whirlpools, tubs, tanks or pools.

Hematological System

Overview

1. **Composition of blood.**
   a. Plasma comprises about 55% of total blood volume and is the liquid part of blood and lymph; it carries the cellular elements of blood through the circulation.
      (1) Plasma is composed of about 91% water, 7% proteins and 2%–3% other small molecules.
      (2) Electrolytes in plasma determine osmotic pressure and pH balance and are important in the exchange of fluids between capillaries and tissues.
      (3) Carries nutrients and waste products and hormones.
      (4) Plasma proteins include albumin, globulins and fibrinogen.
      (5) Serum is plasma without the clotting factors.
   b. Erythocytes or red blood cells (RBCs) comprise about 45% of the total blood volume and contain the oxygen-carrying protein hemoglobin responsible for transporting oxygen.
      (1) RBCs are produced in the marrow of the long bones and controlled by hormones (erythropoietin). RBCs are time-limited, surviving for approximately 120 days.
      (2) Normal RBC count is 4.2–5.4×10^6 for men and 3.6–5.0×10^6 for women. RBC count varies with age, activity and environmental conditions.
   c. Leukocytes or white blood cells (WBCs) comprise about 1% of the total blood volume and circulate through the lymphoid tissues.
      (1) Leukocytes function in immune processes as phagocytes of bacteria, fungi and viruses. They also aid in capturing toxic proteins resulting from allergic reactions and cellular injury.
      (2) Leukocytes are produced in the bone marrow.
      (3) There are five types of leukocytes: lymphocytes and monocytes (agranulocytes) and neutrophils, basophils and eosinophils (granulocytes).
      (4) Normal WBC count is 4.4–11.3×10^3.

2. **Hematopoiesis: the normal function and generation of blood cells in the bone marrow.**
   a. Production, differentiation and function of blood cells is regulated by cytokines and growth factors (chemical messengers) acting on blood-forming cells (pluripotent stem cells).
   b. Disorders of hematopoiesis include aplastic anemia and leukemias.

3. **Blood screening tests.**
   a. Complete blood count (CBC) determines the number of red blood cells, white blood cells and platelets per unit of blood.
   b. White cell differential count determines the relative percentages of individual white cell types.
   c. Erythrocyte sedimentation rate (ESR) is the rate of red blood cells that settle out in a tube of unclotted blood, expressed in millimeters per hour.
      (1) Elevated ESR indicates the presence of inflammation.
      (2) Normal values are 1–13 mm/hour for men and 1–20 mm/hour for women.

4. **Hemostasis is the termination or arrest of blood flow by mechanical or chemical processes. Mechanisms include vasospasm, platelet aggregation and thrombin and fibrin synthesis.**
   a. Blood clotting requires platelets produced in bone marrow, von Willebrand factor produced by the endothelium of blood vessels and clotting factors produced by the liver using vitamin K.
   b. Fibrinolysis is clot dissolution that prevents excess clot formation.

5. **Hypercoaguability disorders are caused by:**
   a. Increased platelet functions as seen in atherosclerosis, diabetes mellitus, elevated blood lipids and cholesterol.
   b. Accelerated activity of the clotting system as seen in congestive heart failure, malignant diseases, pregnancy and use of oral contraceptives, immobility.

6. **Hypocoagulopathy (bleeding) disorders are caused by:**
   a. Platelet defects as seen in bone marrow dysfunction, thrombocytopenia, thrombocytopathia.
   b. Coagulation defects as seen in hemophilia and von Willebrand disease.
   c. Vascular disorders as seen in hemorrhagic telangiectasia, vitamin C deficiency, Cushing's disease, senile purpura.

7. **Shock is an abnormal condition of inadequate blood flow to the body tissues. It is associated with hypotension, inadequate cardiac output and changes in peripheral blood flow resistance.**
   a. Hypovolemic shock is caused by hemorrhage, vomiting or diarrhea. Loss of body fluids also occurs with dehydration, Addison's disease, burns and pancreatitis or peritonitis.
   b. Orthostatic changes may develop characterized by a drop of systolic blood pressure of 10–20 mm Hg or more. Pulse and respirations are increased.

c. Progressive shock is associated with restlessness and anxiety, weakness, lethargy, pallor with cool, moist skin and fall in body temperature.

d. Vital functions must be carefully monitored and restored as quickly as possible. The patient should be placed supine or in a modified Trendelenburg's position to aid venous return.

8. **Physical examination of patients with hematological disorders reveals typical signs and symptoms.**
   a. Easy bruising with spontaneous petechiae and purpura of the skin.
   b. External hematomas may also be present (e.g., thrombocytopenia).

9. **Long-term use of certain drugs (steroids, non-steroidal anti-inflammatory drugs [NSAIDs]) can lead to bleeding and anemia.**

10. **Red Flags: Physical therapy interventions.**
   a. Use extreme caution with manual therapy and use of some modalities (e.g., mechanical compression).
   b. Strenuous exercise is contraindicated due to the risk of increased hemorrhage.

Anemia

1. **Decrease in hemoglobin levels in the blood: normal range is 12–16 g/dL for woman and 13.5–18 g/dL for men.**

2. **Causes:**
   a. Decrease in RBC production: nutritional deficiency (iron, vitamin B, folic acid); cellular maturation defects, decreased bone marrow stimulation (hypothyroidism), bone marrow failure (leukemia, aplasia and neoplasm) and genetic defect.
   b. Destruction of RBCs: autoimmune hemolysis, sickle cell disease, enzyme defects, parasites (malaria), hypersplenism, chronic diseases (rheumatoid arthritis, tuberculosis, cancer).
   c. Loss of blood (hemorrhage): trauma, wound, bleeding, peptic ulcer, excessive menstruation.

3. **Clinical symptoms:**
   a. Fatigue and weakness with minimal exertion.
   b. Dyspnea on exertion.
   c. Pallor or yellow skin of the face, hands, nail beds and lips.
   d. Tachycardia.
   e. Bleeding of gums, mucous membranes or skin in the absence of trauma.
   f. Severe anemia can produce hypoxic damage to liver and kidney, heart failure.

4. **Medical intervention.**
   a. Variable, depends on causative factors.
   b. Transfusion.
   c. Nutritional supplements.

5. **Physical therapy intervention.**
   a. **Red Flag:** Patients with anemia exhibit decreased exercise tolerance.
      (1) Exercise should be instituted gradually with physician approval.
      (2) Perceived exertion levels should be used (RPE ratings).

Sickle Cell Disease

1. **Group of inherited, autosomal recessive disorders; erythrocytes, specifically hemoglobin S (Hb S) are abnormal. RBCs are crescent or sickle-shaped instead of biconcave.**

2. **Sickle cell trait: heterozygous form of sickle cell anemia characterized by abnormal red blood cells. Individual are carriers and do not develop the disease. Counseling is important, especially if both parents have the trait.**

3. **Characteristics.**
   a. Chronic hemolytic anemia (sickle cell anemia): hemoglobin is released into plasma with resultant reduced oxygen delivery to tissues, results from bone marrow aplasia, hemolysis, folate deficiency or splenic involvement.
   b. Vaso-occlusion from misshapen erythrocytes: results in ischemia, occlusion and infarction of adjacent tissue.
   c. Chronic illness that can be fatal.

4. **Sickle cell crisis: acute episodic condition occurring in children with sickle cell anemia.**
   a. Pain: acute and severe from sickle cell clots formed in any organ, bone or joint.
      (1) Acute abdominal pain from visceral hypoxia.
      (2) Painful swelling of soft tissue of the hands and feet (hand-foot syndrome).
      (3) Persistent headache.
   b. Bone and joint crises: migratory, recurrent joint pain; extremity and back pain.
   c. Neurological manifestations: dizziness, convulsions, coma, paresthesias, cranial nerve palsies, blindness, nystagmus.
   d. Coughing, dyspnea, tachypnea may occur.
   e. Vascular complications: stroke, chronic leg ulcers, bone infarcts, avascular necrosis of femoral head.
   f. Renal complications: enuresis, nocturia, hematuria, renal failure.
   g. Anemic crisis: characterized by rapid drop in hemoglobin levels.
   h. Aplastic crisis: characterized by severe anemia; associated with acute viral, bacterial or fungal infection. Increased susceptibility to infection.
   i. Splenic sequestration crisis: liver and spleen enlargement, spleen atrophy.

CHAPTER 7

5. **Medical interventions.**
   a. Immediate transfusion of packed red cells in acute anemic crisis.
   b. Analgesics or narcotics as needed for pain.
   c. Short-term oxygen therapy in severe anoxia.
   d. Hydration, electrolyte replacement.
   e. Antibiotics for infection control.
   f. Oral anticoagulants to relieve pain of vaso-occlusion; associated with increased risk of bleeding.
   g. Splenectomy may be considered.
   h. Bone marrow transplant in severe cases.
   i. Uremia may require renal transplantation or hemodialysis.

6. **Physical therapy goals, outcomes and interventions.**
   a. Pain control: application of warmth is soothing (e.g., hydrotherapy).
   ☞b. **Red Flag:** Cold is contraindicated as it increases vasoconstriction and sickling.
   c. Relaxation techniques.
   d. Emotional support and counseling of family.
   e. Patient and family education: avoidance of stressors that can precipitate a crisis.

Hemophilia

1. **Pathophysiology: a group of hereditary bleeding disorders.**
   a. Inherited as a sex-linked recessive disorder of blood coagulation; affects males, females are carriers.
   b. Clotting factor VIII deficiency (hemophilia A) is most common; classic hemophilia.
   c. Clotting factor IX deficiency (hemophilia B or Christmas disease).
   d. Level of severity and rate of spontaneous bleeds varies by percentage of clotting factor in blood: mild, moderate, severe.
   e. Bleeding is spontaneous or a result of trauma; may result in internal hemorrhage and hematuria.
   f. Hemarthrosis (bleeding into joint spaces) most common in synovial joints: knees, ankles, elbows, hips.
      (1) Joint becomes swollen, warm and painful with decreased range of motion (ROM).
      (2) Long-term results can include chronic synovitis and arthropathy leading to bone and cartilage destruction.
   g. Hemorrhage into muscles often affects forearm flexors, gastrocnemius/soleus and iliopsoas.
      (1) Produces pain.
      (2) Decreases movement.

2. **Medical interventions.**
   a. Blood infusion, factor replacement therapy.
   b. Use of acetaminophen (Tylenol), not aspirin, for pain management.
   c. Rest, ice, elevation, functional splinting and no weight-bearing during an acute bleed.

   d. HIV or hepatitis transmission a possible transfusion result (before current purification techniques).

3. **Complications:**
   a. Joint contractures.
      (1) Hip, knee, elbow flexion; ankle plantar flexion.
   b. Muscle weakness around affected joints.
   c. Leg-length discrepancies.
   d. Postural scoliosis.
   e. Decreased aerobic fitness.
   f. Gait deviations:
      (1) Equinus gait.
      (2) Lack of knee extensor torque.
   g. Activities of daily living (ADL) deficiencies; e.g., elbow contractures could affect dressing ability.

4. **Physical therapy examination.**
   a. Clinical signs and symptoms of acute bleeding episodes: decreased ROM, stiffening, pain, swelling, tenderness, heat, prickling or tingling sensations.
   b. Goniometry.
   c. Joint deformities; e.g., genu valgum, rearfoot/forefoot.
   d. Muscle strength; girth.
   e. Functional mobility skills, gait.
   f. Pain.
   g. Activities of daily living.

5. **Physical therapy interventions: acute stage.**
   a. RICE: rest, ice, compression, elevation.
   b. Maintain position, prevent deformity.

6. **Physical therapy interventions: subacute stage after hemostasis.**
   a. Factor replacement best done just before treatment.
   b. Isometric exercise and aquatic therapy early.
   c. Pain management: transcutaneous electrical nerve stimulation (TENS), massage, relaxation techniques, ice, biofeedback.
   d. Active assistive exercise progressing to active, isokinetic and open chain resistive exercises.
      (1) Passive ROM rarely, if ever, used.
      (2) Closed chain exercise may put too much compressive force through joint.
      (3) Important to strengthen hip, knee, elbow extensors and ankle dorsiflexors.
   e. Contracture management.
      (1) Manual traction, mobilization techniques, serial casting, dynamic splinting during the day, resting splints at night.
   ☞(2) **Red Flag:** Passive stretching rarely used due to risk of myositis ossificans.
   f. Functional and gait training as needed.
      (1) Protective use of helmets or pads for very young boys during ambulation and play.
      (2) Temporary use of ambulatory aids as needed.
      (3) Foot orthoses, shoe inserts and adhesive taping for ankle or foot problems.

7. Physical therapy interventions: chronic stage.
   a. Daily home exercise program to maintain or increase joint function, aerobic fitness and strength.
   b. Outpatient physical therapy as necessary.

c. Appropriate recreational activities or adaptive physical education if at school.

8. Emotional support for patients and families.

Cancer

Overview

1. Characteristics: involves all body organs; invasive.
   a. Etiology: unknown; multiple factors are implicated:
      (1) Carcinogens: chemical (e.g., asbestos, smoking or oral tobacco), radiation (e.g., x-rays, sun exposure), or viral (e.g., herpes simplex; AIDS/immune system depression).
      (2) Genetic factors: hereditary.
      (3) Dietary factors: obesity, high-fat diet, diet low in vitamins A, C, E.
      (4) Psychological factors: chronic stress.
   b. Early warning signs.
      (1) Unusual bleeding or discharge.
      (2) A lump or thickening of any area; e.g., breast.
      (3) A sore that does not heal.
      (4) A change in bladder or bowel habits.
      (5) Hoarseness or persistent cough.
      (6) Indigestion or difficulty swallowing.
      (7) Change in size or appearance of a wart or mole.
      (8) Unexplained weight loss.
   c. Classification (staging): delineates extent and prognosis of disease.
   d. Incidence: second leading cause of death in United States.
   e. Prognosis: aggressive treatments have resulted in higher cure rates, increased survival times.
   f. Quality of life (maintaining normal function and life styles) is an important issue.

2. Terminology/pathologies.
   a. Tumor or neoplasm: an abnormal growth of new tissue that is nonfunctional and competes for vital blood supply and nutrients.
   b. Benign tumor (neoplasm): localized, slow growing, usually encapsulated; not invasive.
   c. Malignant tumors (neoplasms): invasive, rapid growth giving rise to metastases; can be life threatening.
      (1) Carcinoma: a malignant tumor originating in epithelial tissues; e.g., skin, stomach, colon, breast, rectum. Carcinoma in situ is a premalignant neoplasm that has not invaded the basement membrane.
      (2) Sarcoma: a malignant tumor originating in connective and mesodermal tissues; e.g., muscle, bone, fat.
      (3) Lymphoma: affecting the lymphatic system; e.g., Hodgkin's disease, lymphatic leukemia.
      (4) Leukemias and myelomas: affecting the blood (unrestrained growth of leukocytes) and blood-forming organs (bone marrow).
   d. Metastasis: movement of cancer cells from one body part to another; spread is via lymphatic system or bloodstream.

3. Staging: describes extent of disease.
   a. Primary tumor (T).
   b. Regional lymph node involvement (N).
   c. Metastasis (M).
   d. Numbers used to denote extent of involvement, from 1–4 (least involvement to most involvement; e.g., T2, N1, M1).

4. Medical interventions: curative versus palliative (relief of symptoms, e.g., pain); can be used alone or in combination.
   a. Surgery:
      (1) Can be curative (tumor removal following biopsy) or palliative (to relieve pain, correct obstruction).
      (2) Often used in combination with chemotherapy or radiation therapy.
      (3) Can result in significant functional deficits and weakness, edema.
   b. Radiation therapy:
      (1) Destroys cancer cells, inhibits cell growth and division.
      (2) Can be used preoperatively to shrink tumors, prevent spread.
      (3) Can be used postoperatively to kill/prevent residual cancer cells from metastasizing.
   c. Chemotherapy:
      (1) Drugs can be given orally, subcutaneously, intramuscularly, intravenously, intrathecally (within the spinal canal).
      (2) Usually intermittent doses to allow for bone marrow recovery.

d. Biotherapy (immunotherapy):
  (1) Strengthens host's ability to fight cancer cells.
  (2) Agents can include interferons, interleukin-2, cytokine.
  (3) Bone marrow (stem cell) transplant; follows high doses of chemotherapy or radiation that destroys both cancer cells and bone marrow cells.
  (4) Monoclonal antibodies.
  (5) Hormonal therapy.

e. **Red Flags:** Local and systemic effects of cancer therapy.
  (1) With radiation therapy, can see radiation sickness, immunosuppression, fibrosis, burns, delayed wound healing, edema, hair loss, central nervous system (CNS) effects.
  (2) With chemotherapy, can see gastrointestinal symptoms (anorexia, nausea, vomiting, diarrhea, ulcers and hemorrhage), bone marrow suppression, skin rashes, neuropathies, phlebitis and hair loss.
  (3) With biotherapy (immunotherapy), can see fever, chills, nausea, vomiting, anorexia, fatigue, fluid retention.
  (4) With hormonal therapy, can see gastrointestinal symptoms, hypertension, steroid-induced diabetes and myopathy, weight gain, hot flashes and sweating, altered mental status, impotence.

5. **Hospice care: care for the terminally ill patient and family.**
  a. Multidisciplinary focus.
  b. Palliative care provided at home or in a hospice center.
  c. Provision for supportive services: emotional, physical, social, spiritual, financial.

Physical Therapy Considerations for Intervention

1. **The physical therapist will be responsible for systems review and patient evaluation.**

2. **The physical therapist assistant should be aware for signs and symptoms identified in this section and immediately report suspicious findings or new complaints to the physical therapist.**

3. **Pain: monitor typical pain pattern and any changes.**
  a. Cancer pain syndrome: cancer-related pain is a common experience; e.g., nerve or nerve root compression, ischemic response to blockage of blood supply, bone pain. Sympathetic signs and symptoms may accompany moderate to severe pain; e.g., tachycardia, hypertension, tachypnea, nausea, vomiting.
  b. Pain at site distal to initial tumor site may suggest metastasis.

c. Iatrogenic pain may result from surgery, radiation or chemotherapy.

4. **Lung, breast, prostate, thyroid and lymphatic cancers commonly metastasize to bone. Pathological fractures, pain and muscle spasms may result.**

5. **Red Flags: Paraneoplastic syndrome. Signs and symptoms are produced at a site distant from the tumor or its metastasized sites, from ectopic hormone production by tumor cells or metabolic abnormalities from secretion of tumor vasoactive products.**
  a. Cushing's syndrome can result from small cell cancer of the lung.
  b. Symptoms can result from cancer stimulation of antibody production; e.g., anorexia, malaise, diarrhea, weight loss, fever, progressive muscle weakness (type II atrophy), diminished deep tendon reflexes (DTRs), myositis, joint pain.
  c. Neurological syndromes can include cerebellar degeneration, peripheral neuropathy, myasthenia gravis, etc.

6. **Red Flags: Adverse side effects of cancer treatment:**
  a. With immunosuppressed patient monitor vital signs, physiological responses to exercise carefully; may see elevated HR and BP, dyspnea, pallor, sweating, fatigue. Patient is easily fatigued with minimal exertion.
  b. Muscle atrophy and weakness: secondary to high doses of steroids in many chemotherapy protocols; weakness may also result from disuse, or tumor compression/invasion.
  c. ROM deficits: particularly with high dose radiation around joints.
  d. Hematological disruptions:
    (1) White blood cell suppression (leukopenia); increased susceptibility to infection.
    (2) Platelet suppression (thrombocytopenia): increased bleeding.
    (3) Red blood cell suppression (anemia): diminished aerobic capacity.

Physical Therapy Goals, Outcomes and Interventions

1. **Educate patient and family about disease process, rehabilitation goals, process and expected outcomes.**

2. **Identify and support patient and family.**
  a. Assist in coping mechanisms.
  b. Assist through the grieving process.

3. **Provide for proper positioning to prevent or correct deformities, maintain skin integrity; provide for overall patient comfort.**

4. **Edema control: elevation of extremities, active ROM, massage; postoperative compression (elastic bandages, pressure garments).**

5. **Pain control.**
   a. TENS stimulation: may not control deep cancer pain; effective for postoperative pain.
   b. Massage.

6. **Maintain or correct loss of range of motion: active-assisted/stretching, active ROM exercises.**

7. **Maintain or correct loss of muscle mass and strength.**
   a. Isometric and light weight isotonic strengthening exercises safe for most patients with cancer.
   b. **Red Flags:** Patients with significant bony metastases, osteoporosis, or low platelet counts (<20,000).
      (1) Active ROM (AROM), ADL exercise only.
      (2) Weight-bearing may be restricted; provide appropriate ambulatory aids, orthoses.
      (3) High risk of vertebral compression and other fractures with metastatic disease. Use light exercise only.

8. **Maintain or increase activity tolerance and cardiovascular endurance; e.g., cycle ergometry, ambulation, energy conservation techniques.**
   a. Following prolonged bed rest or inactivity: careful examination, gradual exercise and activity progression; submaximal aerobic exercise is indicated.
   b. Monitor fatigue levels. Use activity pacing, carefully balance activity and rest periods; use short sessions throughout the day. Teach energy conservation techniques.
   c. Precaution with patients who are anemic: may experience decreased aerobic capacity.
   d. Precaution with certain types of chemotherapy (e.g., Adriamycin): may experience cardiac side effects.
   e. Precaution with severe bony metastases, weakness: light aerobic exercise (cycling, swimming) may be indicated.

9. **Maintain or increase independence.**
   a. Activities of daily living, e.g., self-care.
   b. Functional mobility skills; e.g., bed mobility, transfers and ambulation.
   c. Coordination, balance and safety.

10. **Specific considerations for exercise programs:**
    a. Postmastectomy:
       (1) Focus is on restoration of pain-free full ROM of the shoulder, prevention/reduction of edema, restoration of function.
       (2) Early postoperative exercise is stressed: some protocols as early as day one.
    b. Postbone marrow transplant.
       (1) Experience prolonged hospitalization and inactivity: average is 30 days; prolonged chemotherapy and radiotherapy, strict isolation.
       (2) Focus is on restoration of function, overcoming the effects of deconditioning.
       (3) **Red Flag:** Exercise is contraindicated in patients with platelet counts 20,000 or less; use caution with counts 20–50,000.

11. **Therapeutic Modalities. Refer to chapter 11 on Therapeutic Modalities.**
    a. Thermal agents (hot packs, paraffin baths, fluidotherapy, infrared lamps) and deep heating agents (ultrasound, diathermy).
       Red Flags:
       (1) Do not use directly over tumor.
       (2) Do not use over dysvascular tissue, i.e., tissue exposed to radiation therapy.
       (3) Do not use with individuals with decreased sensitivity to temperature or pain in affected area.
       (4) Do not use in areas of increased bleeding or hemorrhage, typically the result of corticosteroid therapy.
       (5) Do not use with acute injury, inflammation, open wounds.
    b. Cryotherapy:
       Red Flags:
       (1) Do not use with patients with insensitivity to cold, or delayed wound healing.
       (2) Do not use over dysvascular tissue, i.e., tissue exposed to radiation therapy.
    c. Hydrotherapy with agitation:
       Red Flags:
       (1) Do not use over dysvascular tissue, i.e., tissue exposed to radiation therapy.
       (2) Do not use with individuals with decreased sensitivity to temperature or pain in affected area.
       (3) Do not use in areas of increased bleeding or hemorrhage or open wounds.
       (4) Risk of cross infection is high with immunosuppressed patients.

Gastrointestinal System

Overview

1. **The gastrointestinal (GI) tract is a long hollow tube extending from the mouth to the anus. Ingested foods and fluids are broken down into molecules that are absorbed and used by the body, while waste products are eliminated.**
   a. The upper GI tract consists of the mouth, esophagus, stomach and functions for ingestion and initial digestion of food.
   b. The middle GI tract is the small intestine (duodenum, jejunum and ileum). The major digestive and absorption processes occur here.
   c. The lower GI tract consists of the large intestine (cecum, colon and rectum) with primary functions that include absorption of water and electrolytes, storage and elimination of waste products.
   d. Accessory organs aid in digestion by producing digestive secretions and include the salivary glands, liver and pancreas.

2. **GI motility propels food and fluids through the GI system and is provided by rhythmic, intermittent contractions (peristaltic movements) of smooth muscle (except for pharynx and upper one-third of the esophagus).**

3. **Neural control is achieved by the autonomic nervous system (ANS). Both sympathetic and parasympathetic plexuses extend along the length of the GI wall. Vagovagal (mediated by the vagus nerve) reflexes control the secretions and mobility of the GI tract.**

4. **Major GI hormones include cholecystokinin, gastrin and secretin.**

5. **Signs and symptoms common to many types of GI disorders.**
   a. Nausea and vomiting. Nausea is an unpleasant sensation that signals stimulation of medullary vomiting center and often precedes vomiting. Vomiting is the forceful oral expulsion of abdominal contents.
      (1) Nausea and vomiting can be triggered by many different causes including food, drugs, hypoxia, shock, inflammation of abdominal organs, distention, irritation of the GI tract and motion sickness.
      (2) Prolonged vomiting can produce fluid and electrolyte imbalance and can result in pulmonary aspiration and mucosal or GI damage.
   b. Diarrhea is the passage of frequent watery unformed stools. The amount of fluid loss determines the severity of the illness.
      (1) Dehydration, electrolyte imbalance, dizziness, thirst and weight loss are common complications of prolonged diarrhea.
      (2) Numerous conditions can trigger diarrhea including infectious organisms (*Escherichia coli*, rotavirus, *Salmonella*), dysentery, diabetic enteropathy, irritable bowel syndrome, hyperthyroidism, neoplasm and diverticulitis. Diet, medications and strenuous exercise can also cause diarrhea.
   c. Constipation is a decrease in normal elimination with excessively hard, dry stools and difficult elimination.
      (1) Constipation causes increased bowel pressure and lower abdominal discomfort.
      (2) Many different factors can trigger constipation including a diet lacking in bulk and fiber, inadequate consumption of fluids, sedentary life style, increasing age and drugs (opiates, antidepressants, calcium channel blockers, anticholinergics).
      (3) Numerous conditions can cause constipation including hypothyroidism, diverticular disease, irritable bowel syndrome, Parkinson's disease, spinal cord injury, tumors, bowel obstruction and rectal lesions.
      (4) Obstipation is intractable constipation with resulting fecal impaction, the retention of hard, dry stools in the rectum and colon. Impaction can cause partial or complete bowel obstruction. The patient may exhibit a history of watery diarrhea, fecal soiling and fecal incontinence. Removal of the fecal mass is indicated.
      (5) **Red Flag:** Constipation can cause abdominal pain and tenderness in the anterior hip, groin or thigh regions.
      (6) Constipation may develop as a result of muscle guarding and splinting, for example, the patient with low back pain.
   d. Anorexia is the loss of appetite with an inability to eat. It is associated with anxiety, fear and depression along with a number of different disease states and drugs.
      (1) Anorexia nervosa is a disorder characterized by prolonged loss of appetite and inability to eat. Individuals exhibit emaciation, emotional disturbance concerning body image and fear of gaining weight. It is common in adolescent girls who may also exhibit amenorrhea.

e. Dysphagia refers to difficulty in swallowing.
   (1) Patients experience choking, coughing or abnormal sensations of food sticking in the back of the throat or esophagus.
   (2) Numerous conditions can cause dysphagia including lesions of the CNS (stroke, Alzheimer's disease, Parkinson's disease), strictures and esophageal scarring, swelling, cancer and scleroderma.
   (3) Achalasia is a condition in which the lower esophageal sphincter fails to relax and food is trapped in the esophagus.
f. Heartburn is a painful burning sensation felt in the esophagus in the mid-epigastric area behind the sternum or in the throat.
   (1) It is typically caused by reflux of gastric contents into the esophagus.
   (2) Certain foods (fatty foods, citrus foods, chocolate, peppermint, alcohol, coffee, caffeine), increased abdominal pressure (food, tight clothing, back supports, pregnancy) and certain positions/movements (bending over or lying down after a large meal) can aggravate heartburn.
g. Abdominal pain is common in GI conditions. It is the result of inflammation, ischemia and mechanical stretching. Visceral pain can occur in the epigastric region (T3-5 sympathetic nerve distribution; the periumbilical region (T10 sympathetic nerve distribution); and the lower abdominal region (T10-L2 sympathetic nerve distribution).
h. **Red Flags:** Referred GI pain patterns:
   (1) Visceral pain from the esophagus can refer to the mid-back.
   (2) Mid-thoracic spine pain (nerve-root pain) can appear as esophageal pain.
   (3) Visceral pain from the liver, diaphragm, or pericardium can refer to the shoulder.
   (4) Visceral pain from the gallbladder, stomach, pancreas or small intestine can refer to the mid-back and scapular regions.
   (5) Visceral pain from the colon, appendix or pelvic viscera can refer to the pelvis, low back or sacrum.
i. GI bleeding is evidenced by blood appearing in vomitus or feces.
   (1) It can result from erosive gastritis, peptic ulcers, prolonged use of NSAIDs and chronic alcohol use.
   (2) Occult or hidden blood can only be revealed by stool testing.
j. Abdominal pain is generally aggravated by coughing, sneezing or straining.

Esophagus

1. **Gastroesophageal reflux disease (GERD) is caused by reflux or backward movement of gastric contents of the stomach into the esophagus, producing heartburn.**
   a. Results from failure of the lower esophageal sphincter to regulate flow of food from the esophagus into the stomach and increased gastric pressure.
   b. The diaphragm that surrounds the esophagus and oblique muscles also contribute to anti-reflux function.
   c. Over time, acidic gastric fluids (pH <4) damage the esophagus producing reflux esophagitis.
   d. Heartburn commonly occurs 30-60 minutes after eating and at night when lying down (nocturnal reflux).
   e. **Red Flags:**
      (1) Atypical pain may present as head and neck pain.
      (2) Chest pain is sometimes mistaken for heart attack; it is unrelated to activity.
      (3) Respiratory symptoms can occur including wheezing and chronic cough due to microaspiration, laryngeal injury and vagus-mediated bronchospasm. Hoarseness can also result from chronic inflammation of the vocal cords.
   f. Complications include strictures and Barrett's esophagus (a precancerous state).
   g. Physical therapy interventions:
      (1) Positional changes from full supine to modified, more upright position are indicated.
      (2) Valsalva's is contraindicated.
   h. Lifestyle modifications include avoiding large meals and certain foods; sleeping with head elevated; medications include acid-suppressing proton pump inhibitors, PPIs (e.g., Prilosec); H-2 blockers (e.g. Zantac, Tagamet) and antacids (e.g., Tums). In severe cases, surgery is an option.

2. **Hiatal hernia is the protrusion of the stomach upward through the diaphragm (rolling hiatal hernia) or displacement of both the stomach and gastroesophageal junction upward into the thorax (sliding hiatal hernia).**
   a. May be congenital or acquired.
   b. Symptoms include heartburn from GERD.
   c. Conservative or symptomatic treatment is the same as for GERD. Surgery may be indicated.

Stomach

1. **Gastritis is inflammation of the stomach mucosa. Gastritis can be acute or chronic.**
   a. Acute gastritis is caused by severe burns, aspirin or other NSAIDs, corticosteroids, food allergies or viral or bacterial infections. Hemorrhagic bleeding can occur.
   b. Symptoms include anorexia, nausea, vomiting and pain.

c. Chronic gastritis occurs with certain diseases such as peptic ulcer (*Helicobacter pylori* bacterial infection), stomach cancer and pernicious anemia or with autoimmune disorders (thyroid disease, Addison's disease).

d. **Red Flag:** Patients taking NSAIDs long term should be monitored carefully for stomach pain, bleeding, nausea or vomiting.

e. Management is symptomatic and includes avoiding irritating substances (caffeine, nicotine, alcohol), dietary modification and medications include acid-suppressing PPIs, H-2 blockers and antacids.

2. **Peptic ulcer disease refers to ulcerative lesions that occur in the upper GI tract in areas exposed to acid-pepsin secretions. It can affect one or all layers of the stomach or duodenum.**

a. It is caused by a number of factors including bacterial infection (*H. pylori*), acetylsalicylic acid (aspirin) and NSAIDs, excessive secretion of gastric acids, stress and heredity.

b. Symptoms include epigastric pain which is described as gnawing, burning or cramp-like. Pain is aggravated by change in position and absence of food in the stomach and relieved by food or antacids.

c. Complications include hemorrhage. Bleeding may be sudden and severe or insidious, with blood in vomitus or stools. Symptoms can include weakness, dizziness or other signs of circulatory shock.

d. Management includes use of antibiotics for treatment of *H. pylori* along with acid-suppressing drugs (PPIs, H-2 blockers and antacids). Dietary modification including avoidance of stomach irritants is indicated. Surgical intervention is indicated for perforation and uncontrolled bleeding.

e. **Red Flags:**
   (1) Pain from peptic ulcers located on the posterior wall of the stomach can present as radiating back pain. Pain can also radiate to the right shoulder.
   (2) Stress and anxiety can increase gastric secretions and pain.

Intestines

1. **Malabsorption syndrome is a complex of disorders characterized by problems in intestinal absorption of nutrients (fat, carbohydrates, proteins, vitamins, calcium and iron).**

a. Can be caused by gastric or small bowel resection (short-gut syndrome) or a number of different diseases including cystic fibrosis, celiac disease, Crohn's disease, chronic pancreatitis and pernicious anemia. Malabsorption can also be drug induced (NSAID gastroenteritis).

b. Deficiencies of enzymes (pancreatic lipase) and bile salts are contributing factors.

c. Symptoms can include anorexia, weight loss, abdominal bloating, pain and cramps, indigestion and steatorrhea (abnormal amounts of fat in feces). Diarrhea can be chronic and explosive.

d. **Red Flags:**
   (1) Iron-deficiency anemia.
   (2) Easy bruising and bleeding due to lack of vitamin K.
   (3) Muscle weakness and fatigue due to lack of protein, iron, folic acid and vitamin B.
   (4) Bone loss, pain and predisposition to develop fractures from lack of calcium, phosphate and vitamin D.
   (5) Neuropathy including tetany, paresthesias, numbness and tingling from lack of calcium, vitamins B and D, magnesium, potassium.
   (6) Muscle spasms from electrolyte imbalance and lack of calcium.
   (7) Peripheral edema.

2. **Inflammatory bowel disease (IBD) refers to two related chronic inflammatory intestinal disorders, Crohn's disease (CD) and ulcerative colitis (UC). Both diseases result in inflammation of the bowel and are characterized by remissions and exacerbations.**

a. Symptoms include abdominal pain, frequent attacks of diarrhea, fecal urgency and weight loss.
   Red Flags:
   (1) Joint pain (reactive arthritis) and skin rashes can occur. Pain can be referred to the low back.
   (2) Complications can include intestinal obstruction and corticosteroid toxicity (low bone density, increased fracture risk).
   (3) Intestinal absorption is disrupted and nutritional deficiencies are common.
   (4) Chronic IBD can lead to anxiety and depression.

b. Crohn's disease involves a granulomatous type of inflammation that can occur anywhere in the GI tract. Areas of adjacent normal tissue called *skip lesions* are present.

c. Ulcerative colitis involves an ulcerative and exudative inflammation of the large intestine and rectum. It is characterized by varying amounts of bloody diarrhea, mucus and pus. Skip lesions are absent.

3. **Irritable bowel syndrome (IBS) is characterized by abnormally increased motility of the small and large intestines. IBS is also known as spastic colon, nervous or irritable colon.**

a. IBS is associated with emotional stress and certain foods (high fat content or roughage, lactose intolerance). No structural or biochemical abnormalities have been identified.

b. Symptoms include persistent or recurrent abdominal pain that is relieved by defecation. Patients may experience constipation or diarrhea, bloating, abdominal cramps, flatulence, nausea and anorexia.

c. Stress reduction and medications to reduce anxiety or depression are important components of treatment.

d. Regular physical activity is effective in reducing stress and improving bowel function.

4. **Diverticular disease is characterized by pouch-like herniations (diverticula) of the mucosal layer of the colon through the muscularis layer.**
   a. Diverticulosis refers to pouchlike herniations of the colon, especially the sigmoid colon.
      (1) Symptoms are minimal but can include rectal bleeding.
      (2) Dietary factors (lack of dietary fiber), lack of physical activity and poor bowel habits contribute to its development.
      (3) Diverticulosis can lead to diverticulitis.
   b. Diverticulitis refers to inflammation of one or more diverticula. Fecal matter penetrates diverticula and causes inflammation and abscess.
      (1) Symptoms include pain and cramping in the lower left quadrant, nausea and vomiting, slight fever and an elevated WBC.
      (2) Complications include bowel obstruction, perforation with peritonitis and hemorrhage.
   c. **Red Flag:** Patients may complain of back pain.
   d. Regular exercise is an important component of treatment.

5. **Appendicitis is an inflammation of the vermiform appendix. As the condition progresses, the appendix becomes swollen and gangrenous and perforates. Perforation can be life-threatening and lead to the development of peritonitis.**
   a. Pain is abrupt in onset, localized to the epigastric or periumbilical area and increases in intensity over time.
   b. Rebound tenderness (Blumberg's sign) is present in response to depression of the abdominal wall at a site distant from the painful area.
   c. Point tenderness is located at McBurney's point, the site of the appendix located 1.5–2.0 inches above the anterior superior iliac spine in the right lower quadrant.
   d. **Red Flag:** Immediate medical attention is required.
   e. Elevations in WBC count ($>20,000/mm^3$) are indicative of perforation. Surgery is indicated.

6. **Peritonitis is inflammation of the peritoneum, the serous membrane lining the walls of the abdominal cavity.**
   a. Peritonitis results from bacterial invasion and infection of the peritoneum. Common agents include *E. coli, Bacteroides, Fusobacterium* and streptococci.
   b. A number of different factors can introduce infecting agents including penetrating wounds, surgery, perforated peptic ulcer, ruptured appendix, perforated diverticulum, gangrenous bowel, pelvic inflammatory disease and gangrenous gallbladder.
   c. Symptoms include abdominal distension, severe abdominal pain, rigidity from reflex guarding, rebound tenderness, decreased or absent bowel sounds, nausea and vomiting and tachycardia.
   d. Elevated WBC count, fever, electrolyte imbalance and hypotension are common.
   e. Peritonitis can lead to toxemia and shock, circulatory failure and respiratory distress.
   f. Treatment is aimed at controlling inflammation and infection and restoring fluid and electrolyte imbalances. Surgical intervention may be necessary to remove an inflamed appendix or close a perforation.

Rectum

1. **Rectal fissure is a tear or ulceration of the lining of the anal canal. Constipation and large, hard stools are factors.**

2. **Hemorrhoids (piles) are varicosities in the lower rectum or anus caused by congestion of the veins in the hemorrhoidal plexus.**
   a. Hemorrhoids can be internal or external (protruding from the anus).
   b. Symptoms include local irritation, pain, rectal itching.
   c. Prolonged bleeding can result in anemia.
   d. Straining with defecation, constipation and prolonged sitting contribute to discomfort.
   e. Pregnancy increases the risk of hemorrhoids.
   f. Treatment includes topical medications to shrink the hemorrhoid, dietary changes, sitz baths and local hot or cold compresses and ligation or surgical excision.

Genital/Reproductive System

Overview

1. Female Reproductive System

2. External genitalia, located at the base of the pelvis, consist of the mons pubis, labia majora, labia minora, clitoris and perineal body.

3. The urethra and anus are in close proximity to the external genital structures and cross-contamination is possible.

4. The internal genitalia consist of the vagina, the uterus and cervix, the fallopian tubes and paired ovaries.

5. Sexual and reproductive functions.
   a. The ovaries store female germ cells (ova) and produce female sex hormones (the estrogens and progesterone) under control of the hypothalamus (gonadotropin-releasing hormone) and the anterior pituitary gland (gonadotropic follicle-stimulating and luteinizing hormones).
   b. Sex hormones influence the development of secondary sex characteristics, regulate the menstrual cycle (ovulation), maintain pregnancy (fertilization and implantation, gestation) and influence menopause (cessation of the menstrual cycle).
      (1) Estrogens decrease the rate of bone resorption.
      ▷ **Red Flag:** Osteoporosis and risk of bone fracture increase dramatically after menopause.
      (2) Estrogens increase production of the thyroid and increase high-density lipoproteins (a protective effect against heart disease).
      ▷ **Red Flag:** Heart disease and stroke risk increases after menopause.

6. The breasts are mammary tissues located on the anterior chest wall between the 3rd and 7th ribs.
   a. Breast function is related to production of sex hormones and pregnancy, producing milk for infant nourishment.

Pregnancy: Normal

1. Pregnancy weight gain: average 20–30 lb.

2. Physical therapists teach childbirth education classes.
   a. Relaxation training: e.g., Jacobsen's progressive relaxation, relaxation response, mental imagery, yoga.
   b. Breathing management: slow, deep, diaphragmatic breathing; Lamaze techniques; avoidance of Valsalva's maneuver.
   c. Provide information about pregnancy and childbirth.

3. Common changes with pregnancy and physical therapy interventions:
   a. Postural changes: kyphosis with scapular protraction, cervical lordosis and forward head; lumbar lordosis; postural stress may continue into postpartum phase with lifting and carrying the infant.
      (1) Postural evaluation.
      (2) Teach postural exercises to stretch, strengthen and train postural muscles.
      (3) Teach pelvic stabilization exercises, e.g., posterior pelvic tilt.
      (4) Teach correct body mechanics, e.g., sitting, standing, lifting, ADLs.
      (5) Limit certain activities in the third trimester, e.g., supine position to avoid inferior vena cava compression, bridging.
   b. Balance changes: center of gravity shifts forward and upward as the fetus develops; with advanced pregnancy, there will be a wider base of support, increased difficulty with walking and stair climbing, rapid challenges to balance.
      (1) Teach safety strategies.
   c. Ligamentous laxity secondary to hormonal influences (relaxin).
      (1) Joint hypermobility (e.g., sacroiliac joint), pain.
      (2) Predisposition to injury, especially in weight-bearing joints of lower extremities and pelvis.
      (3) May persist for some time after delivery; teach joint protection strategies.
   d. Muscle weakness: abdominal muscles are stretched and weakened as pregnancy develops; pelvic floor weakness with advanced pregnancy and childbirth. Stress incontinence secondary to pelvic floor dysfunction (experienced by 80% of women).
      (1) Teach exercises to improve control of pelvic floor, maintain abdominal function.
      (2) Stretching exercises to reduce muscle cramping.
      (3) Avoid Valsalva's maneuver: may exacerbate condition.
   e. Urinary changes: pressure on bladder causes frequent urination; increased incidence of reflux, urinary tract infections.
   f. Respiratory changes: elevation of the diaphragm with widening of thoracic cage; hyperventilation, dyspnea may be experienced with mild exercise during late pregnancy.
   g. Cardiovascular changes: increased blood volume; increased venous pressure in the lower extremities; increased heart rate and cardiac output, decreased blood pressure due to venous distensibility.

(1) Teach safe progression of aerobic exercises.
  (a) Exercise in moderation, with frequent rests.
  (b) Stress use of familiar activities, avoidance of unfamiliar.
  (c) Postpartum: emphasize gradual return to previous level of activity.
(2) Stress gentle stretching, adequate warm-ups and cool-downs.
(3) Teach ankle pumps for lower extremity edema (late stage pregnancy); elevate legs to assist in venous return.
(4) Wear loose, comfortable clothing.

h. Altered thermoregulation: increased basal metabolic rate; increased heat production.

Pregnancy-Related Pathologies

1. **Diastasis recti abdominis.**
   a. Lateral separation or split of the rectus abdominis; separation from mid-line (linea alba) >2 cm is significant; associated with loss of abdominal wall support, increased back pain.
   b. Physical therapy interventions
     (1) Teach protection of abdominal musculature: avoid abdominal exercises; e.g., full sit-ups or bilateral straight-leg raising.
     (2) Resume abdominal exercises when separation is <2 cm: teach safe abdominal strengthening exercises; e.g., partial sit-ups (knees bent), pelvic tilts; utilize hands to support abdominal wall.

2. **Pelvic floor disorders: the result of weakening of pelvic floor muscles (pubococcygeal [PCP] muscles).**
   a. PC muscles normally function to support the vagina, urinary bladder and rectum and help maintain continence of the urethra and rectum.
   b. Weakness or laxity of PC muscles typically results from overstretching during pregnancy and childbirth. Further loss of elasticity and muscle tone during later life can result in partial or total organ prolapse.
     (1) Cystocele: the herniation of the bladder into the vagina.
     (2) Rectocele: the herniation of the rectum into the vagina.
     (3) Uterine prolapse: the bulging of the uterus into the vagina.
   c. PC muscles can also go into spasm.
   d. Symptoms include pelvic pain (perivaginal, perirectal and lower abdominal quadrant), urinary incontinence and pain with sexual intercourse.
     Red Flag: Pain can radiate down the posterior thigh.
   e. Surgical correction is often required, depending on degree of prolapse.
   f. Physical therapy intervention (pelvic floor rehabilitation).

   (1) Observe for urinary frequency and urgency, painful urination, painful defecation, low back and perineal pain with prolapse.
   (2) Teaching pelvic floor exercises (Kegel's exercises) to strengthen the PC muscles is indicated.
   (3) Postural education and muscle reeducation, pelvic mobilization and stretching of tight LE muscles are also important components.

3. **Low back and pelvic pain.**
   a. Physical therapy interventions.
     (1) Teach proper body mechanics.
     (2) Balance rest with activity.
     (3) Emphasize use of a firm mattress.
     (4) Massage, modalities for pain (no deep heat).

4. **Sacroiliac dysfunction secondary to postural changes; ligamentous laxity.**
   a. Symptoms include posterior pelvic pain, pain in buttocks; may radiate into posterior thigh or knee.
   b. Associated with prolonged sitting, standing or walking.
   c. Physical therapy interventions.
     (1) External stabilization, e.g., sacroiliac support belt may help reduce pain.
     (2) Avoid single-limb weight-bearing: may aggravate sacroiliac dysfunction.

5. **Varicose veins: may produce discomfort or pain.**
   a. Physical therapy interventions.
     (1) Elevate extremities; avoid crossing legs which may press on veins.
     (2) Use of elastic support stockings may help.

6. **Preeclampsia: pregnancy-induced acute hypertension after the 24th week of gestation.**
   a. May be mild or severe.
   b. Evaluate for symptoms of hypertension, edema, sudden excessive weight gain, headache, visual disturbances or hyperreflexia.
   c. Initiate prompt physician referral.

7. **Cesarean childbirth.**
   a. Surgical delivery of the fetus by an incision through the abdominal and uterine wall; indicated in pelvic disproportion, failure of the birth process to progress, fetal or mother distress, or other complications.
   b. Physical therapy interventions.
     (1) Postoperative TENS can be used for incisional pain; electrodes are placed parallel to the incision.
     (2) Prevent postsurgical pulmonary complications: assist patient in breathing, coughing.
     (3) Postcesarean exercises.
       (a) Gentle abdominal exercises; provide incisional support with pillow.
       (b) Pelvic floor exercises: labor and pushing is typically present before surgery.
       (c) Postural exercises; precautions about heavy lifting for 4–6 weeks.
     (4) Ambulation.
     (5) Prevent incisional adhesions: friction massage.

Renal and Urological Systems

Overview

1. **Anatomy.**
   a. Kidneys are paired, bean-shaped organs located outside of the peritoneal cavity (retroperitoneal) in the posterior upper abdomen on each side of the vertebral column at the level of T12–L2.
   b. Each kidney is multilobular; each lobule is composed of more than a million nephrons (the functional units of the kidney).
   c. Each nephron consists of a glomerulus that filters the blood and nephron tubules. Water, electrolytes and other substances vital for function are reabsorbed into the bloodstream, while other waste products are secreted into the tubules for elimination.
   d. The renal pelvis is a wide, funnel-shaped structure at the upper end of the urethra that drains the kidney into the lower urinary tract (bladder and urethra).
   e. The bladder is a membranous sac that collects urine and is located behind the symphysis pubis.
   f. The ureter extends from the renal pelvis to the bladder and moves urine via peristaltic action.
   g. The urethra extends from the bladder to an external orifice for elimination of urine from the body.
   h. In females, proximity of the urethra to vaginal and rectal openings increases the likelihood of urinary tract infection (UTI).

2. **Functions of the kidney.**
   a. Regulates the composition and pH of body fluids through reabsorption and elimination; controls mineral (sodium, potassium, hydrogen, chloride and bicarbonate ions) and water balance.
   b. Eliminates metabolic wastes (urea, uric acid and creatinine) and drugs/drug metabolites.
   c. Assists in blood pressure regulation through rennin-angiotensin-aldosterone mechanisms and salt and water elimination.
   d. Contributes to bone metabolic function by activating vitamin D and regulating calcium and phosphate conservation and elimination.
   e. Controls the production of red blood cells in the bone marrow through the production of erythropoietin.
   f. The glomerular filtration rate (GFR) is the amount of filtrate that is formed each minute as blood moves through the glomeruli and serves as an important gauge of renal function.
      (1) Regulated by arterial blood pressure and renal blood flow.
      (2) Measured clinically by obtaining creatinine levels in blood and urine samples.
      (3) Normal creatinine clearance is 115–125 mL/min.
   g. Blood urea nitrogen (BUN) is urea produced in the liver as a by-product of protein metabolism that is eliminated by the kidneys.
      (1) BUN levels are elevated with increased protein intake, gastrointestinal bleeding and dehydration.
      (2) BUN-creatinine ratio is abnormal in liver disease.

3. **Normal values of urine (urinalysis findings):**
   a. Color: yellow-amber.
   b. Clarity: clear.
   c. Specific gravity: 1.010–1.025 with normal fluid intake.
   d. pH: 4.6–8.0; average is 6 (acid).
   e. Protein: 0–8 mg/dL.
   f. Sugar: 0.

Urinary Regulation of Fluids and Electrolytes

1. **Homeostasis regulated through thirst mechanisms and renal function via circulating antidiuretic hormone (ADH)**

2. **Fluid imbalances: daily fluid requirements vary based on presence or absence of sweating, air temperature, fever, etc.**
   a. Dehydration: excessive loss of body fluids; fluid output exceeds fluid intake.
      (1) Causes: poor intake; excess output: profuse sweating, vomiting and diarrhea, diuretics; closely linked to sodium deficiency.
      (2) Observe for: poor skin turgor, dry mucous membranes, headache, irritability, postural hypotension, incoordination, lethargy, disorientation.
      (3) May lead to uremia and hypovolemic shock (stupor and coma).
      (4) Decreased exercise capacity, especially in hot environments.
   b. Edema: an excess of body fluids with expansion of interstitial fluid volume.
      (1) Causes.
         (a) Increased capillary pressure: heart failure, kidney disease, premenstrual retention, pregnancy, environmental heat stress; venous obstruction (liver disease, acute pulmonary edema, venous thrombosis).

(b) Decreased colloidal osmotic pressure: decreased production or loss of plasma proteins (protein-losing kidney disease, liver disease, starvation, malnutrition).

(c) Increased capillary permeability: inflammation, allergic reactions, malignancy, tissue injury, burns.

(d) Obstruction of lymphatic flow.

(2) Observe for swelling of the ankles and feet, weight gain; headache, blurred vision; muscle cramps and twitches.

(a) Edema can be restrictive, producing a tourniquet effect.

(b) Tissues are susceptible to injury and delayed healing.

(c) Pitting edema occurs when the amount of interstitial fluid exceeds the absorptive capacity of tissues.

2. **Potassium imbalance: normal serum level is 3.5–5.5 mEq/L.**
   a. Hypokalemia: decreased potassium in the blood.
      (1) Muscle weakness and fatigue, leg cramps; hyporeflexia.
      (2) Postural hypotension, dizziness, arrhythmias, ECG abnormalities: flat T wave, prolonged Q-T interval; depressed S-T segment, U wave appears; arrhythmias.
      (3) Respiratory distress.
      (4) Irritability, confusion, depression.
      (5) Gastrointestinal: nausea and vomiting, anorexia, diarrhea.
   b. Hyperkalemia: excess of potassium in the blood; common in acute renal failure.
      (1) Muscle weakness, flaccid paralysis.
      (2) Tachycardia and later bradycardia; arrhythmias; ECG changes: tall, peaked T wave, prolonged P-R interval and QRS duration.
      (3) Gastrointestinal: nausea, diarrhea, abdominal cramps.

3. **Sodium imbalance: normal serum level is 134–145 mEq/L.**
   a. Hyponatremia: decreased sodium in the blood.
      (1) Muscle weakness and twitching.
      (2) Hypotension, tachycardia; progressive circulatory collapse and shock.
      (3) Anxiety, headaches, restlessness, convulsions.
      (4) Respiratory: cyanosis with severe sodium deficiency.
      (5) Skin: cold, clammy, decreased turgor.
   b. Hypernatremia: excess of sodium in the blood.
      (1) Circulatory congestion: pitting edema, excessive weight gain, ultimately pulmonary edema with dyspnea, respiratory arrest.
      (2) Hypertension, tachycardia.
      (3) Agitation, restlessness, convulsions.
      (4) Flushed skin, sticky mucous membranes.

4. **Calcium imbalance.**
   a. Hypocalcemia: decreased calcium in the blood.
      (1) Muscle cramps, tetany, spasms.
      (2) Paresthesias (tingling and numbness).
      (3) Anxiety, irritability, twitching, convulsions.
      (4) Arrhythmias, hypotension.
   b. Hypercalcemia: excess of calcium in the blood.
      (1) Decreased muscle tone, weakness, bone pain, pathological fractures.
      (2) Drowsiness, lethargy, headaches, irritability, confusion.
      (3) Heart block, cardiac arrest, hypertension.
      (4) Anorexia, nausea, weight loss, lethargy.

5. **Magnesium imbalance.**
   a. Hypomagnesemia: decreased magnesium.
      (1) Hyperirritability, confusion, delusions, hallucinations, convulsions.
      (2) Tetany, leg and foot cramps.
      (3) Arrhythmias, vasomotor changes (vasodilation and hypotension), occasionally hypertension.
   b. Hypermagnesemia: increased magnesium.
      (1) Hyporeflexia, muscle weakness, flaccid paralysis.
      (2) Respiratory muscle paralysis.
      (3) Drowsiness, flushing, lethargy, confusion, diminished sensorium.
      (4) Bradycardia, weak pulse, hypotension, heart block and cardiac arrest.

6. **Acid-base balance: balance of acids and bases in the body (normally a ratio of 20 base to 1 acid; normal serum pH is 7.35–7.45 [slightly alkaline]); regulated by blood buffer systems (the lungs and the kidneys).**
   a. Metabolic acidosis: a depletion of bases or an accumulation of acids; blood pH falls below 7.35.
      (1) Causes: diabetes, renal insufficiency or failure, diarrhea.
      (2) Observe for: hyperventilation (compensatory), deep respirations, weakness, muscular twitching, malaise, nausea, vomiting and diarrhea, headache, dry skin and mucous membranes, poor skin turgor.
      (3) May lead to stupor and coma (death).
   b. Metabolic alkalosis: an increase in bases or a reduction of acids; blood pH rises above 7.45.
      (1) Causes: excess vomiting, excess diuretics, hypokalemia; peptic ulcer and excessive intake of antacids.
      (2) Observe for: hypoventilation (compensatory), depressed respirations; dysrhythmias; prolonged vomiting, diarrhea, weakness, muscle twitching, irritability, agitation, convulsions and coma (death).
   c. Respiratory acidosis: CO_2 retention, impaired alveolar ventilation.
      (1) Causes: hypoventilation, drugs/oversedation, chronic pulmonary disease (e.g., emphysema,

asthma, bronchitis, pneumonia) or hypermetabolism (sepsis, burns).

(2) Observe for: dyspnea, hyperventilation cyanosis, restlessness, headache.

(3) May lead to disorientation, stupor and coma, death.

d. Respiratory alkalosis: diminished CO_2, alveolar hyperventilation.

(1) Causes: anxiety attack with hyperventilation; hypoxia (emphysema, pneumonia); impaired lung expansion; congestive heart failure (CHF); pulmonary embolism; diffuse liver or CNS disease; salicylate poisoning; extreme stress (stimulation of respiratory center).

(2) Observe for: tachypnea, dizziness, anxiety, difficulty concentrating, numbness and tingling, blurred vision, diaphoresis, muscle cramps, twitching or tetany, weakness- arrhythmias, convulsions.

Renal and Urological Disorders

1. **Urinary tract infections (UTIs): infection of the urinary tract with microorganisms.**
    a. Lower UTI: cystitis (inflammation and infection of the bladder) or urethritis (inflammation and infection of the urethra).
        (1) Usually secondary to ascending urinary tract infections; may also involve kidneys and ureters.
        (2) Associated with symptoms of urinary frequency, urgency, burning sensation during urination. Urine may be cloudy and foul smelling. Pain is noted in suprapubic, lower abdominal or groin areas, depending on site of infection.
    b. Upper UTI: pyelonephritis (inflammation and infection of one or both kidneys).
        (1) Associated with symptoms of systemic involvement: fever, chills, malaise, headache, tenderness and pain over kidneys (back pain), tenderness over the costovertebral angle (Murphy's sign). Symptoms also include frequent and burning urination; nausea and vomiting may occur.
        (2) Palpitation or percussion over the kidney typically causes pain.
        (3) Can be acute or chronic; generally more serious than lower UTI.
    c. Increased risk of UTI in persons with autoimmunity, urinary obstruction and reflux, neurogenic bladder and catheterization, diabetes and kidney transplantation. Older adults and women are also at increased risk for UTI.

2. **Renal cystic disease: renal cysts are fluid-filled cavities that form along the nephron and can lead to renal degeneration or obstruction.**
    a. Types include polycystic, medullary sponge, acquired and simple renal cysts.

b. Symptoms can include pain, hematuria and hypertension. Fever can occur with associated infection. Cysts can rupture, producing hematuria. Simple cysts are generally asymptomatic.

3. **Obstructive disorders: developmental defects, renal calculi, prostatic hyperplasia or cancer, scar tissue from inflammation, tumors and infection, tumors.**
    a. Pressure build-up backwards from site of obstruction; can result in kidney damage. Dilation of ureters and renal pelves may be used to reduce obstruction. Observe for pain, signs and symptoms of UTI and hypertension.
    b. Renal calculi (kidney stones): crystalline structures formed from normal components of urine (calcium, magnesium, ammonium phosphate, uric acid and cystine).
        (1) Etiological influences include concentration of stone components in urine and a urinary environment conducive to stone formation.
        (2) Symptoms include renal colic pain (pain from a stone lodged in the ureter made worse by stretching the collecting system). Pain may radiate to the lower abdominal quadrant, bladder and perineal areas (scrotum in the male and labia in the female). Nausea and vomiting are common and the skin may be cool and clammy.
        (3) Extracorporeal shock wave lithotripsy (ESWL) is used to break up stones into fragments to allow for easy passage.
        (4) Treatment/prevention can also include increased fluid intake, thiazide diuretics, dietary restriction of foods high in oxalate, acidification or alkalinization of urine depending on type of stone.

4. **Renal failure:**
    a. Acute renal failure: sudden loss of kidney function with resulting elevation in serum urea and creatinine.
        (1) Etiology: may be due to circulatory disruption to kidneys, toxic substances, bacterial toxins, acute obstruction or trauma.
    b. Chronic renal failure: progressive loss of kidney function leading to end-stage failure.
        (1) Etiology: may result from prolonged acute urinary tract obstruction and infection, diabetes, systemic lupus erythematosus, uncontrolled hypertension.
        (2) Uremia: an end-stage toxic condition resulting from renal insufficiency and retention of nitrogenous wastes in blood; symptoms can include anorexia, nausea and mental confusion.
        (3) **Red Flags:** May lead to multisystem abnormalities and failure.
            (a) Dizziness, headaches, anxiety, memory loss, inability to concentrate, convulsions and coma.
            (b) Hypertension, dyspnea on exertion, heart failure.

    (c) Chronic pain: ischemic leg pain, painful cramps.

    (d) Edema: peripheral edema, pulmonary edema.

    (e) Muscle weakness: peripheral neuropathy, cramping, restless legs.

    (f) Skeletal: osteomalacia, osteoporosis, bone pain, fracture.

    (g) Skin: pallor, ecchymosis, pruritus, dry skin.

    (h) Anemia, tendency to bleed easily.

    (i) Decreased endurance; functional losses.

    (j) Autonomic nervous system dysfunction: decreased heart rate, blood pressure; orthostatic hypotension.

c. Dialysis: process of diffusing blood across a semipermeable membrane for the purposes of removal of toxic substances; maintains fluid, electrolyte and acid-base balance in presence of renal failure; peritoneal or renal (hemodialysis).

   (1) Dialysis disequilibrium: symptoms of nausea, vomiting, drowsiness, headache and seizures; the result of rapid changes after beginning dialysis.

   (2) Dialysis dementia: signs of cerebral dysfunction (e.g., speech difficulties, mental confusion, myoclonus, seizures, eventually death); the result of long-standing years of dialysis treatment.

   (3) Locate dialysis shunts: taking BP at the shunt site is contraindicated.

   (4) Locate peritoneal catheters (if used): avoid trauma to area.

   (5) Examine for multisystem dysfunction: vital signs, strength, sensation, ROM, function and endurance.

d. Transplantation is a major treatment choice (renal allograft).

5. Urinary incontinence: inability to retain urine; the result of loss of sphincter control; may be acute (due to transient causes, e.g., cystitis) or persistent (e.g., stroke, dementia).

a. Types:

   (1) Stress incontinence: sudden release of urine due to.

    (a) Increases in intra-abdominal pressure; e.g., cough, laugh, exercise, straining, obesity.

    (b) Weakness and laxity of pelvic floor musculature, sphincter weakness, e.g., postpartum incontinence, menopause, damage to pudendal nerve.

   (2) Urge incontinence: bladder begins contracting and urine is leaked after sensation of bladder fullness is perceived; an inability to delay voiding to reach toilet due to.

    (a) Detrusor muscle instability or hyperreflexia, e.g., stroke.

    (b) Sensory instability: hypersensitive bladder.

   (3) Overflow incontinence: bladder continuously leaks secondary to urinary retention (an overdistended bladder or incomplete emptying of bladder) due to:

    (a) Anatomical obstruction, e.g., prostate enlargement.

    (b) Acontractile bladder, e.g., spinal cord injury, diabetes.

    (c) Neurogenic bladder, e.g., multiple sclerosis, suprasacral spinal lesions.

   (4) Functional incontinence: leakage associated with inability or unwillingness to toilet due to.

    (a) Impaired cognition (dementia); depression (e.g., Alzheimer's disease).

    (b) Impaired physical functioning, e.g., stroke.

    (c) Environmental barriers.

b. Management.

   (1) Dietary management: control of food and beverages that aggravate the bladder or incontinence, e.g., limit citrus fruit or juices, caffeine, chocolate; control fluid intake.

   (2) Medical management.

    (a) Identify and treat acute, reversible problems, e.g., cystometry.

    (b) Drug therapy for urge, stress and overflow incontinence, e.g., estrogen with phenylpropanolamine.

    (c) Control of medications that may aggravate incontinence, e.g., diuretics for CHF, anticholinergic or psychotropic drugs.

    (d) Catheterization: used for overflow incontinence and other types if unresponsive to other treatments and skin integrity is threatened; associated with high rates of urinary tract infection.

    (e) Surgery: bladder neck suspension, removal of prostate obstructions; suprapubic cystostomy.

   (3) Bladder training: prompted voiding to restore a pattern of voiding.

    (a) Involves toileting schedule: taking patient to bathroom at regular intervals.

    (b) May also include intermittent catheterization, e.g., for patients with over-distention, persistent retention (e.g., multiple sclerosis).

c. Examination.

   (1) Symptoms of incontinence: onset and duration, urgency, frequency, timing of episodes/causative factors.

   (2) Strength of pelvic floor muscles using a perineometer.

   (3) Functional mobility, environmental factors.

d. Physical therapy goals, outcomes and interventions for stress and urge incontinence.

   (1) Teach pelvic floor muscle exercises (pubococcygeus muscle): used to treat stress incontinence.

(a) Kegel's exercises: active, strengthening exercises; type 1 works on holding contractions, progressing to 10-second holds, rest 10 seconds between contractions; type 2 works on quick contractions to shut off flow of urine, 10–80 repetitions a day. Avoid squeezing buttocks or contracting abdominals (bearing down).

(b) Functional electrical stimulation: for muscle reeducation if patient is unable to initiate active contractions.

(c) Biofeedback: uses pressure recordings to reinforce active contractions, relax bladder.

(d) Progressive strengthening: use of weighted vaginal cones for home exercises or pelvic floor exerciser.

(e) Incorporating Kegel's exercises into everyday life: with lifting, coughing, changing positions, etc.

(2) Provide behavioral training.

(a) Record keeping: patients are asked to keep a history of their voiding (voiding diary).

(b) Education: regarding anatomy, physiology, reasons for muscle weakness, incontinence; avoidance of Valsalva's maneuver, heavy resistance exercises.

(3) Functional mobility training as needed. Ensure independence in sit-to-stand transitions, ambulation and safe toilet transfers.

(4) Environmental modifications as needed: toilet rails, raised toilet seat, or commode, etc.

(5) Maintain adequate skin condition.

(a) Teach appropriate skin care, maintain toileting schedule.

(b) Adequate protection: adult diapers, underpads.

(6) Provide psychological support: emotional and social consequences of incontinence are significant.

Endocrine and Metabolic Systems

Overview of the Endocrine System

1. **The endocrine system uses hormones (chemical messengers) to relay information to cells and organs and regulate many of the body functions (digestion, use of nutrients, growth and development, electrolyte and water balance and reproductive functions). The hypothalamus and pituitary gland along with the nervous system comprise the central network that exerts control over many other glands in the body with wide-ranging functions. Endocrine functions are also closely linked with the immune system.**

a. Hormones bind to specific receptor sites which are linked to specific systems and functions.

b. The hypothalamus controls release of pituitary hormones (corticotropin-releasing hormone [CRH], thyrotropin-releasing hormone [TRH], growth hormone–releasing hormone [GHRH], somatostatin).

c. The anterior pituitary gland controls the release of growth hormone (GH), adrenocorticotropic hormone (ACTH), follicle-stimulating hormone (FSH), luteinizing hormone (LH) and prolactin.

d. The posterior pituitary gland controls the release of antidiuretic hormone (ADH) and oxytocin.

e. The adrenal cortex controls the release of mineral corticosteroids (aldosterone), glucocorticoids (cortisol), adrenal androgens (dehydroepiandrosterone (DHEA) and androstenedione.

f. The adrenal medulla controls the release of epinephrine and norepinephrine.

g. The thyroid controls the release of triiodothyronine and thyroxine. Thyroid C cells control the release of calcitonin.

h. The parathyroid glands control the release of parathyroid hormone (PTH).

i. The pancreatic islet cells control the release of insulin, glucagons and somatostatin.

j. The kidney controls the release of 1,25-dihydroxyvitamin D.

k. The ovaries control the release of estrogen and progesterone.

l. The testes control the release of androgens (testosterone).

Diabetes Mellitus (DM)

1. **Definitions: a complex disorder of carbohydrate, fat and protein metabolism caused by deficiency or absence of insulin secretion by the beta cells of the pancreas or by defects of the insulin receptors. May be nephrogenic. Possible viral/autoimmune and genetic etiology. (Represents 5%–10% of DM.)**

a. Signs and symptoms of uncontrolled DM:

(1) Elevated blood sugar (hyperglycemia).

(2) Elevated sugar in urine (glycosuria).

(3) Presence of ketone bodies in the urine, the byproducts of fat metabolism (ketonuria).

(4) Excessive excretion of urine (polyuria).

(5) Excessive thirst (polydipsia).

(6) Excessive hunger (polyphagia) and weight loss (usually type 1).

(7) Fatigue and weakness.

(8) Blurred vision.

(9) Irritability.

(10) Numbness and tingling in the hands and feet.

(11) Prolonged healing times (cuts, bruises, infections).

b. Type 1 diabetes mellitus (T1DM). Also known as juvenile-onset diabetes. Characteristics include:

(1) Decrease in size and number of islet cells resulting in inadequate insulin production.

(2) Long preclinical period, often with abrupt onset of symptoms around the age of puberty.

(3) Etiology: caused by autoimmune abnormalities, genetic causes or environmental causes.

(4) Insulin dependent: requires insulin delivery by injection, insulin pump or inhalation.

(5) Prone to ketoacidosis. Presence of ketone bodies in the urine, the by-products of fat metabolism (ketonuria).

c. Type 2 diabetes mellitus (T2DM) results from inadequate utilization of insulin (insulin resistance) and progressive beta cell dysfunction; also known as adult-onset or maturity-onset diabetes. (Represents 90%–95% of DM cases.) Characteristics include:

(1) Gradual onset; may have familial pattern.

(2) Usually not insulin dependent.

(3) Individual is not prone to ketoacidosis (may form ketones with stress).

(4) Etiology: a progressive disease caused by a combination of factors, including:

(a) Insulin resistance in muscle and adipose tissue.

(b) Progressive decline in pancreatic insulin production.

(c) Excessive hepatic glucose production.

(d) Inappropriate glucagon secretion.

(5) Linked to obesity in older adults (typically over the age of 40). Can occur in nonobese individuals with increased percentage of body fat in the abdominal area.

d. Metabolic syndrome (insulin resistance syndrome, syndrome X).

(1) Leads to type 2 diabetes.

(2) Characterized by three or more of the following:

(a) Abdominal obesity: waist circumference >35 inches in women or >40 inches in men.

(b) Elevated triglycerides 150 mg/dL or higher.

(c) Low high-density lipoproteins (HDLs) or being on medicine to treat low HDLs: HDL level <40 mg/dL in men or 50 mg/dL in women.

(d) Elevated blood pressure: systolic BP 130 mm Hg or higher and/or diastolic pressure 85 mm Hg or higher.

(e) Fasting plasma glucose level >110 mg/dL. A level between 100 and 125 mg/dL is considered prediabetes.

e Secondary diabetes: associated with other conditions (pancreatic disease, hormonal disease, drugs and chemical agents).

f. Impaired glucose tolerance (IGT): asymptomatic or borderline diabetes with abnormal response to oral glucose test. Ten to 15% of individuals will convert to type 2 diabetes within 10 years.

g. Gestational diabetes mellitus (GDM): glucose intolerance associated with pregnancy; most likely in third trimester.

2. Red Flags: Signs and symptoms of hypoglycemia (low blood sugar):

a. Rapid onset (minutes).

b. Glucose is low: <60 mg/dL. Results from failure to eat after taking insulin, excessive insulin; can be precipitated by exercise.

c. CNS changes: labile, irritable, headache, blurred vision, slurred speech, difficulty concentrating, confusion, incoordination.

d. Sympathetic changes: diaphoresis, pallor, piloerection, tachycardia, heart palpitations, nervousness and irritability, weakness, shakiness/trembling, hunger.

e. Hypoglycemic coma: a loss of consciousness that results from an abnormally low blood sugar level.

f. First aid: If patient is awake, give sugar (juice, candy bar). If unresponsive, call for help; intravenous glucose is required.

3. Red Flags: Signs and symptoms of hyperglycemia (abnormally high blood sugar).

a. Gradual onset (days).

b. Glucose is high: >250 mg/dL. Results from untreated diabetes.

c. CNS changes: dulled senses, confused, diminished reflexes, paresthesias.

d. Thirst.

e. Flushed, signs of dehydration.

f. Nausea/vomiting, abdominal pain.

g. Deep, rapid respirations.

h. Pulse: rapid, weak.

i. Fruity odor to the breath.

j. Weakness.

k. Hyperglycemic coma: a diabetic coma caused by hyperosmolarity of extracellular fluid and dehydration; can lead to death.

4. Complications associated with long-term diabetes and poor glucose control.

a. Microvascular disease.

(1) Retinopathy.

(2) Renal disease.

(3) Polyneuropathy.

b. Macrovascular disease: dyslipidemia (accelerated atherosclerosis).

(1) Stroke (CVA).

(2) Myocardial infarcion (MI).

(3) Peripheral arterial disease (PAD).

c. Integumentary impairments: including degenerative connective tissue changes; anhidrosis; increased risk of ulcers and infections.

d. Musculoskeletal impairments:

(1) Joint stiffness and increased risk of contractures.

(2) Increased risk of adhesive capsulitis of shoulder, tenosynovitis, plantar fasciitis.

(3) Increased risk of osteoporosis.

e. Neuromuscular impairments:

(1) Diabetic polyneuropathy.

(a) Symmetrical; stocking and glove distribution.

(b) Distal (long nerves first) progressing to proximal.

(c) Altered sensations; paresthesias, shooting pain; loss of protective sensations.

(d) Motor weakness: foot/ankle weakness initially with balance and gait impairments.

(2) Diabetic autonomic neuropathy (DAN).

(a) Cardiovascular autonomic neuropathy (CAN): resting tachycardia; exercise intolerance with abnormal HR, BP and cardiac output responses; exercise-induced hypoglycemia; postural hypotension.

(b) Integumentary: anhidrosis, abnormal sweating, dry skin, heat intolerance.

(c) Gastrointestinal: gastroparesis, GERD, diarrhea, constipation.

(d) Metabolic: abnormal or delayed responses to hypoglycemia; lack of awareness of hypoglycemia.

f. Kidney impairments including kidney failure.

g. Vision impairments including diabetic retinopathy (associated with chronic hyperglycemia) and diabetic macular edema.

h. Liver impairments including fatty liver disease (steatosis).

5. Diagnosis.

a. Symptoms of diabetes plus casual plasma glucose concentration >200 mg/dL (11.2 mmol/L). "Causal" is defined as any time of day, without regard to time since last meal.

b. Fasting plasma glucose test (FPG) ≥126 mg/dL (7 mmol/L). Fasting is defined as no caloric intake for at least 8 hours.

6. Medical goals and interventions.

a. Maintain insulin glucose homeostasis.

(1) Frequent monitoring of blood glucose levels.

(2) Dietary control: weight reduction, control of carbohydrate, protein, fat and calorie intake.

(3) Oral hypoglycemic agents to lower blood glucose; indicated for type 2 diabetes.

(4) Insulin to lower blood glucose via injections, infusion pump, or intraperitoneal dialysis for patients with renal failure. Indicated for type 1 diabetes or for more severe type 2 diabetes.

(5) Maintenance of normal lipid levels.

(6) Control of hypertension, exercise, physical fitness.

b. Health promotion.

7. Physical therapy goals, outcomes and interventions.

a. Exercise.

(1) Outcomes of exercise include improved glucose tolerance, increased insulin sensitivity, decreased glycosylated hemoglobin and decreased insulin requirements. Additional outcomes include improved lipid profiles, BP reduction, weight management, increased physical work capacity and improved well-being.

(2) Response to exercise is dependent upon adequacy of disease control.

b. Exercise testing is recommended prior to exercise due to increased cardiovascular risk.

c. Exercise prescription—cardiovascular training (ACSM Guidelines, 2006).

(1) Intensity: 50%–80% of Vo_2max or heart rate reserve (HRR).

(2) Frequency: 3–4 days/week.

(3) Duration: 20–60 minutes.

d. Exercise prescription — resistance training (ACSM Guidelines, 2006).

(1) Lower resistance, 40%–60% of 1 repetition max.

(2) One set of exercises for major muscle groups with 10–15 repetitions (progress to 15–20 repetitions).

(3) Minimum frequency 2 days/week; at least 4 hours between sessions.

(4) Proper technique: minimize sustained gripping, static work and Valsalva's maneuver (essential to decrease risk of hypertensive response).

e. Flexibility exercises.

f. Balance exercises.

g. **Red Flags:** Exercise precautions:

(1) Monitor glucose levels prior to and following exercise. Have carbohydrate snack readily available during exercise.

(2) Observe for signs and symptoms of hypoglycemia (Box 7-2). Do not exercise if blood glucose is <70 mg/dL.

(3) Do not exercise when blood glucose level is >300 mg/dL or poorly controlled (Box 7-3).

(4) Do not exercise without eating at least 2 hours before exercise.

Box 7-2 ➤ SIGNS AND SYMPTOMS OF HYPOGLYCEMIA (LOW BLOOD SUGAR)

Glucose is low: < 70 mg/dL or a rapid drop in glucose. Onset is rapid (minutes)

Early signs and symptoms:

Pallor

Shakiness/trembling

Sweating

Excessive hunger

Tachycardia and palpitations

Fainting or feeling faint

Dizziness

Fatigue and weakness

Poor coordination and unsteady gait

Late signs and symptoms:

Nervousness and irritability

Headache

Blurred or double vision

Slurred speech

Drowsiness

Inability to concentrate, confusion, delusions

Loss of consciousness and coma

Response: If patient is awake, provide sugar (juice, candy bar, glucose tablets and gel).

If patient unresponsive, seek immediate medical treatment; glucagon injection or intravenous glucose is required

(5) Do not exercise without adequate hydration. Maintain hydration during exercise session.

(6) Do not exercise alone. Some patients may require close supervision.

(7) Do not exercise if urine test is positive for ketones.

(8) Do not inject short-acting insulin in exercising muscles or sites close to exercising muscles, as insulin is absorbed more quickly.

(9) Do not exercise patients with poorly controlled complications, e.g., cardiovascular disease, hypertension, retinopathy, neuropathy, nephropathy.

Box 7-3 ➤ SIGNS AND SYMPTOMS OF HYPERGLYCEMIA (ABNORMALLY HIGH BLOOD SUGAR)

Glucose is high: > 300 mg/dL. Gradual onset (days).

Weakness

Increased thirst

Dry mouth

Frequent, scant urination

Decreased appetite, nausea/vomiting, abdominal tenderness

Dulled senses, confusion, diminished reflexes, paresthesias

Flushed, signs of dehydration

Deep, rapid respirations

Pulse: rapid, weak

Fruity odor to the breath (acetone breath)

Hyperglycemic coma

Response: seek immediate medical treatment

Table 7-1 ➤ OBESITY AND ASSOCIATED COMPLICATIONS

Cardiovascular diseases; atherosclerosis, hypertension	Type 2 Diabetes Mellitus
Osteoarthritis	Metabolic syndrome
Sleep apnea	Stroke
Liver disease	Cancer

(10) Do not exercise in extreme environmental temperatures (very hot or cold).

h. Emphasize proper diabetic foot care: good footwear, hygiene.

i. Patient and family education.

   (1) Control of risk factors (obesity, physical inactivity, prolonged stress and smoking).

   (2) Injury prevention strategies.

   (3) Self-management strategies.

Obesity (Bariatrics)

1. **Medical problems associated with obesity.**

   a. Obesity is associated with many complications, including three of the leading causes of death: cardiovascular disease, diabetes mellitus and cancer. (See Table 7-1.)

   b. Other complications include: thromboembolic disorders, digestive tract disorders (reflux, gallstones), obstructive sleep apnea and pulmonary compromise with decreased gas exchange, vital capacity and expiratory volume.

   c. Obesity also increases the risk of hormone-related cancers, e.g., women: breast, cervical, endometrial and liver; men: rectal, prostate, colon.

2. **Physical problems associated with obesity.**

   a. Impaired functional mobility, ADL limitations, difficulty climbing stairs, difficulty walking.

   b. Increased risk for falls.

   c. Shortness of breath.

   d. Fatigue.

   e. Increased occurrence of back, hip and knee pain.

   f. Potential for skin breakdown and/or pressure ulcers, neuropathic ulcers and foot ulcerations.

   g. Knee osteoarthritis (OA).

   (1) Evidence supports an increased risk of knee OA in persons with obesity; there is not conclusive evidence of increased OA at other joints.

3. **Physical therapy interventions and considerations.**

   a. Gain "buy in" from individual for continued participation in activity modification.

   (1) Stress the overall health benefits of sticking with a consistent exercise program versus emphasizing weight loss.

CHAPTER 7

(a) Studies indicate that regular physical activity reduces cardiovascular morbidity for obese individuals even if they remain overweight.

(b) Studies indicate that in the obese individual more fat and less lean body tissue was lost when diet and exercise are combined.

(c) Studies show that exercise decreases visceral fat even if weight loss does not occur.

(d) Resistance exercise can increase lean body mass as well as improve ability to perform ADL.

(2) Assist the individual to identify potential barriers to a regular exercise program; develop strategies to mitigate.

(3) Seek input from individual regarding what type of aerobic and strengthening activity they would prefer to use; identify availability and incorporate into their program.

(4) Provide written program that includes pictures.

(5) Provide exercise flow sheet for tracking, monitoring and encouragement.

b. Potential complications during exercise.

(1) Increased risk for heat intolerance; carefully observe for signs of heat stroke or heat exhaustion.

(2) Angina pectoris or myocardial infarction.

(3) Excessive rise in blood pressure.

(4) Difficulty with blood sugar regulation.

(5) Hypohydration and reduced circulating blood volume.

(6) Joint problems: irritation of degenerative arthritis, ligamentous injuries.

(7) Excessive sweating; skin chafing.

c. Exercise prescription.

(1) Initial goal should be directed at regular compliance with a program that simply increases activity level and follows calorie intake recommendations.

(2) Include adequate warm up and stretching—avoid injury.

(3) Progressively increase intensity, frequency and duration.

(a) A simple program of incorporating walking in ADL activities can be sufficient to increase activity level in the beginning; e.g., walking to the bathroom versus doing bedside cares.

(b) Incorporate activities that are between 2 and 5 METs, e.g., standing, light house cleaning, wood working, walking at moderate speed, water aerobics, raking lawn, biking <10 mph.

(4) Consider foot wear—obesity affects foot mechanics; provide orthotic control and heel support to compensate for excessive pronation.

(5) Resistance exercises—begin by incorporating resistance exercise for duration (versus strength) to improve ability to perform work over time.

(a) Begin with resistance level of 30%–40% max resistance.

(b) Begin with one to two sets of 15–20 repetitions; include 3–10 exercises; progress to 30 minutes of resistance exercise.

(c) Perform resistance exercise on nonconsecutive days, 2–4 days/week, with ultimate goal 4 days/week.

(d) Resistance exercise with aerobic benefits: incorporate circuit style, low resistance and multiple repetitions and sets with rest breaks to gain benefit of resistance and aerobic exercise.

(6) Aerobic exercise.

(a) Intensity: begin aerobic activity at approximately 50% max heart rate. Instruct in self-monitoring using perceived exertion scale (RPE).

(b) Duration: begin with a goal of 20 minutes per day at the outset; this can be broken into 2- to 10-minute bouts that are incorporated into the daily routine and build to 60 minutes—again broken into 10- to 15-minute bouts of exercise.

(c) Frequency: slowly progress program to include exercise four to six times per week at aerobic capacities.

(7) Consider exercise position when exercising the patient who is unable to get out of bed. A semi-Fowler's (semi-sitting, 40–65 degrees) position is better than supine, as research shows most patients breathe better in this position.

(8) Decrease joint stress: choose stationary bike or pool program.

4. **Bariatric Equipment and Patient Management Options. Refer to Chapter 12.**

Thyroid Disorders

1. **Hypothyroidism: decreased activity of the thyroid gland with deficient thyroid secretion.**

a. Metabolic processes are slowed.

b. Etiology: decreased thyroid-releasing hormone secreted by the hypothalamus or by the pituitary gland; atrophy of the thyroid gland; chronic autoimmune thyroiditis (Hashimoto's disease); overdosage with antithyroid medication.

c. Symptoms include weight gain, mental and physical lethargy, dry skin and hair, low blood pressure, constipation, intolerance to cold and goiter.

d. If untreated, leads to myxedema (severe hypothyroidism) with symptoms of swelling of hands, feet, face. Can lead to coma and death.

e. Treatment: life-long thyroid replacement therapy.

f. **Red Flags:** Can result in exercise intolerance, weakness, apathy; exercise-induced myalgia; reduced cardiac output.

2. **Hyperthyroidism: hyperactivity of the thyroid gland.**
   a. Etiology unknown.
   b. Thyroid gland is typically enlarged and secretes greater than normal amounts of thyroid hormone (thyroxine), e.g., Graves' disease, thyroid storm, thyrotoxicosis.
   c. Metabolic processes are accelerated.
   d. Symptoms include nervousness, hyperreflexia, tremor, hunger, weight loss, fatigue, heat intolerance, palpitations, tachycardia and diarrhea.
   e. Treatment: antithyroid drugs.
   f. Radioactive iodine may also be prescribed or surgical ablation may be necessary.
   g. **Red Flags:** Can result in exercise intolerance; fatigue is associated with hypermetabolic state.

Adrenal Disorders

1. **Primary adrenal insufficiency (Addison's disease).**
   a. Partial or complete failure of adrenocortical function; results in decreased production of cortisol and aldosterone.
   b. Etiology: autoimmune processes, infection, neoplasm or hemorrhage.
   c. Signs and symptoms.
      (1) Increased bronze pigmentation of skin.
      (2) Weakness, decreased endurance.
      (3) Anorexia, dehydration, weight loss, gastrointestinal disturbances.
      (4) Anxiety, depression.
      (5) Decreased tolerance to cold.
      (6) Intolerance to stress.
   d. Medical interventions.
      (1) Replacement therapy: glucocorticoid, adrenal corticoids.
      (2) Adequate fluid intake, control of sodium and potassium.
      (3) Diet high in complex carbohydrates and protein.

2. **Secondary adrenal insufficiency: can result from prolonged steroid therapy (ACTH); rapid withdrawal of drugs; hypothalamic or pituitary tumors.**

3. **Cushing's syndrome: metabolic disorder resulting from chronic and excessive production of cortisol by the adrenal cortex or from drug toxicity (overadministration of glucocorticoids).**
   a. Etiology: most common cause is a pituitary tumor with increased secretion of ACTH.
   b. Signs and symptoms.
      (1) Decreased glucose tolerance.
      (2) Round "moon" face.
      (3) Obesity: rapidly developing fat pads on chest and abdomen; buffalo hump.
      (4) Decreased testosterone levels or decreased menstrual periods.
      (5) Muscular atrophy.
      (6) Edema.
      (7) Hypokalemia.
      (8) Emotional changes.
   c. Medical interventions.
      (1) Goal is to decrease excess ACTH; irradiation or surgical excision of pituitary tumor or control medication levels.
      (2) Monitor weight, electrolyte and fluid balance.

Psychiatric Conditions

States

1. **Anxiety: feelings of apprehension, worry, uneasiness; a normal reaction to tensions, conflicts or stress.**
   a. Degree of anxiety is related to degree of perceived threat and capacity to engage behaviors that can reduce anxiety.
   b. Anxiety can be constructive, stimulate an individual toward purposeful or neurotic (pathological) activity.
   c. Sympathetic responses (fight or flight) generally accompany anxiety; e.g., increased heart rate, dyspnea, hyperventilation, dry mouth, GI symptoms (nausea, vomiting, diarrhea), palpitations.

2. **Depression: altered mood characterized by morbid sadness, dejection, sense of melancholy. Can be a chronic, relapsing disorder.**
   a. **Red Flags:** Clinical manifestations.
      (1) Loss of interest in all usually pleasurable outlets, e.g., work, family.
      (2) Poor appetite, weight loss or weight gain.
      (3) Insomnia or hypersomnia, decreased energy.
      (4) Psychomotor imbalance: agitation or excessive fatigue; irritability.
      (5) Feelings of worthlessness, self-reproach, guilt, hopelessness.
      (6) Impaired concentration, ability to think.
      (7) Recurrent thoughts of suicide or death.

b. Management.
  (1) Treatment is pharmacological: tricyclic antidepressant drugs.
  ☞ **Red Flags:** Patients on these medications may exhibit disturbed balance, postural hypotension, falls and fractures, increased HR, dysrhythmias, ataxia, seizures.
  (2) Cognitive-therapy may help.
c. Physical therapy interventions.
  (1) Maintain a positive attitude, consistently demonstrate warmth and interest.
  (2) Acknowledge depression, provide hope.
  (3) Use positive reinforcement, build in successful treatment experiences.
  (4) Involve the patient in the treatment decisions.
  (5) Avoid excessive cheerfulness.
  (6) Take all suicide thoughts and acts seriously.

3. **Coping and adapting mechanisms: typically unconscious behaviors by which the individual resolves or conceals conflicts or anxieties.**
  a. Compensation: covering up a weakness by stressing a desirable or strong trait, e.g., a learning disabled child becomes an outstanding athlete.
  b. Denial: a refusal to recognize reality, e.g., refusal to acknowledge a fatal disease.
  c. Repression: refusal or inability to recall undesirable past thoughts or events.
  d. Displacement: the transferring of an emotion to a less dangerous substitute, e.g., yelling at your child instead of your boss.
  e. Reaction formation: a defensive reaction in which behavior is exactly opposite what is expected, e.g., a messy individual becomes neat.
  f. Projection: the attributing of your own undesirable behavior to another, e.g., "He made me do it."
  g. Rationalization: the justification of behaviors using reasons other than the real reason, e.g., presenting an attitude of not caring.
  h. Regression: resorting to an earlier, more immature pattern of functioning; e.g., in traumatic brain injury; common under high stress situations.

4. **General adaptation syndrome (GAS): total body coping/adaptation to a catastrophic event (illness, trauma).**
  a. Alarm stage, or "fight-or-flight" response: activation of the sympathetic system.
  b. Sustained resistance.
  c. Chronic resistance, exhaustion leading to stress-related illnesses.

Pathologies

1. **Anxiety disorders (anxiety neurosis): excessive anxiety not associated with realistically threatening specific situations; e.g., generalized anxiety.**
  a. Panic attacks: acute, intense anxiety or terror; may be uncontrollable, accompanied by sympathetic

signs, loss of mental control, sense of impending death.
  b. Phobias: excessive and unreasonable fear leads to avoidance behaviors, e.g., agoraphobia (fear of being alone or in public places).
  c. Obsessive-compulsive behavior: persistent anxiety is manifested by repetitive, stereotypic acts; behaviors interfere with social functioning; e.g., hand washing, counting and touching.

2. **Posttraumatic stress disorder (PTSD): exposure to a traumatic event produces a variety of stress-related symptoms.**
  a. PTSD symptoms.
    (1) Reexperiencing the traumatic event.
    (2) Psychic numbing with reduced responsiveness.
    (3) Detachment from the external world and survival guilt.
    (4) Exaggerated autonomic arousal, hyperalertness.
    (5) Disturbed sleeping.
    (6) Ongoing irritability.
    (7) Impaired memory and concentration.
  b. PTSD can be acute (symptoms last <3 months) or chronic (3 months or longer); onset can also be delayed.
  c. Symptoms should not be ignored. A mental health consultation is indicated.

3. **Psychosomatic disorders (somatoform disorders): physical signs or diseases that are related to emotional causes, e.g., psychosocial stress.**
  a. Characteristics.
    (1) Cannot be explained by identifiable disease process or underlying pathology.
    (2) Not under voluntary control; provides a means of coping with anxiety and stress.
    (3) Patient is frequently indifferent to symptoms.
  b. Types:
    (1) Conversion disorder (hysterical paralysis): loss or altered physical functioning representing psychosocial conflict or need, e.g., can result in paralysis, hemiplegia.
    (2) Hypochondria: abnormal or heightened concerns about health or body functions; false beliefs about suffering from some disease or condition.
  c. Management:
    (1) Physical symptoms are real: treat the patient as you would any other patient with similar symptoms.
    (2) Provide a supportive environment.
    (3) Identify primary gain (internal conflicts); assist patient in learning new, alternate methods of stress management.
    (4) Identify secondary gains (additional advantages, e.g., attention, sympathy); do not reinforce.
    (5) Provide encouragement and support for the total person.

4. **Schizophrenia: a group of disorders characterized by disruptions in thought patterns; of unknown etiology; a biochemical imbalance in the brain.**
   a. Symptoms:
      (1) Disordered thinking: fragmented thoughts, errors of logic, delusions, poor judgment, memory.
      (2) Disordered speech: may be coherent but unintelligible, or incoherent, mute.
      (3) Disordered perception: hallucinations and delusions.
      (4) Inappropriateness of affect: withdrawal of interest from other people and from the outside world; loss of self-identity, self-direction; disordered interpersonal relations.
      (5) Functional disturbances: inability to function in daily life, work.
      (6) Little insight in problems and behavior.
   b. Paranoia: a type of schizophrenic disorder characterized by feelings of extreme suspiciousness, persecution, grandiosity (feelings of power or great wealth), or jealousy; withdrawal of all emotional contact with others.
   c. Catatonia: a type of schizophrenic disorder characterized by mutism or stupor; unresponsiveness; catatonic posturing (remains fixed, unable to move or talk for extended periods).

5. **Bipolar disorder (manic-depressive illness): a disorder characterized by mood swings from depression to mania; a biochemical dysfunction.**
   a. Often intense outbursts, high energy and activity, excessive euphoria, decreased need for sleep, unrealistic beliefs, distractibility, poor judgment, denial.
   b. Followed by extreme depression (see depression symptoms).
   c. Treatment is pharmacological, e.g., lithium carbonate.

6. **Perseveration: the continued repetition of a movement, word, or expression, e.g., patient gets stuck and repeats the same activity over and over again; often accompanies traumatic brain injury or stroke.**

Grief Process

1. **The emotional process by which an individual deals with loss, e.g., of a significant loved one, body part or function, etc.**

2. **Characteristics.**
   a. Somatic symptoms: fatigue, sighing, hyperventilation, anorexia, insomnia, etc.
   b. Psychological symptoms: sorrow, discomfort, regret, guilt, anger, irritability, depression, etc.
   c. Resolution may take months or years.

3. **Stages.**
   a. Shock and disbelief, inability to comprehend loss.
   b. Increased awareness and anguish, crying or anger are common.

   c. Mourning.
   d. Resolution of loss.
   e. Idealization of lost person or function.

4. **Management.**
   a. Provide support and understanding of the grief process.
   b. Encourage expression of feelings, memories.
   c. Respect privacy, cultural or religious customs.

Death and Dying

1. **Physical symptoms: decreasing physical and mental functioning, gradual loss of consciousness.**

2. **Stages (Kubler-Ross).**
   a. Denial: patients insist they are fine, joke about themselves, are not motivated to participate in treatment.
      (1) Allow denial: denial is a protective compensatory mechanism necessary until such time as the patient is ready to face his/her illness.
      (2) Provide opportunities for patient to question, confront illness and impending death.
   b. Anger, resentment: patients may become disruptive, blame others.
      (1) Be supportive: allow patient to express anger, frustration, resentment.
      (2) Encourage focus on coping strategies.
   c. Bargaining: patients bargain for time to complete life tasks; turn to religion or other individuals; make promises in return for function.
      (1) Provide accurate information, honest, truthful answers.
   d. Depression: patients acknowledge impending death, withdraw from life; demonstrate an overwhelming sense of loss, low motivation.
      (1) Observe closely for suicide ideation.
      (2) Allay fears and anxieties, especially loneliness and isolation.
      (3) Assist in providing for comfort of the patient.
   e. Acceptance and preparation for death: acceptance of their condition; relate more to their family, make plans for the future.

3. **Management.**
   a. Support patient and family during each stage.
   b. Maintain hope without supporting unrealistic expectations.

Physical Therapy Goals, Outcomes and Interventions

1. **Motivating patients, managing the human side of rehabilitation**

2. **Establish boundaries of the professional relationship: identify problems, expectations, purpose, roles and responsibilities.**

3. Provide empathic understanding: the capacity to understand what your patient is experiencing from that patient's perspective.
   a. Recognize losses; allow opportunity to mourn "old self."
   b. Ask open-ended questions that reflect what the patient is feeling.
      (1) Empathetic response: "It sounds like you are worried and anxious about your pain and are trying your best."
      (2) Nonempathetic response: … "Don't worry about your pain," … "You're overreacting."
   c. Sympathy is not helpful or therapeutic; caregiver is closely affected by the patient's behaviors; e.g., therapist cries when the patient cries.

4. Set realistic, meaningful goals; involve the patient and family in the goal-setting process; self-determination is important.

5. Set realistic time frames for the rehabilitation program; recognize symptoms, stages of the grief process or death and dying and adjust accordingly.

6. Recognize and reinforce healthy, positive, socially appropriate behaviors; allow the patient to experience success.

7. Recognize secondary gains, unacceptable behaviors; do not reinforce these, e.g., malingering behaviors such as avoidance of work.

8. Provide an environment conducive to the patient's emotional state, learning and optimal function.
   a. Provide a message of hope tempered with realism.
   b. Keep patients informed.
   c. Lay adequate groundwork or preparation for expected changes or discharge.
   d. Help to re-establish personal dignity and self-worth; acknowledge whole person.

9. Help patients identify feelings, successful coping strategies, recognize successful conflict resolution and rehabilitation gains.
   a. Stress ability to overcome major obstacles.
   b. Stress that recovery is unique and highly individual.

Pediatric Physical Therapy

TIFFANY BOHM

Focus Areas for Content Review:
- Concepts of normal physical and motor development.
- Pathologies and conditions commonly seen in physical therapy that affect pediatric patients/clients.
- Physical therapy intervention strategies commonly utilized with pediatric clients including indications and contraindications, appropriate responses, and PTA response to adverse reaction.

- Tests and measures utilized with pediatric clients that provide information to guide the PTA in determining the child's ability to participate in and/or indication to discontinue intervention as well as to document the child's progress toward the established goals.
- Common goals/outcome expectations for children receiving physical therapy services.
- Psychosocial issues that are unique to the pediatric client and how to adjust interventions strategies to accommodate these issues.

The Typically Developing Child

Human development

1. The growth, change, evolution or maturation of an individual over time.

Learning/Developmental Theories

1. **Maturational: human behavior is innate and determined by a combination of genetic and biological factors.**

2. **Empirical: the environment provides the greatest influence on human development.**

3. **Behavioral.**
   a. Environmental reinforcement influences learned behavior.
   b. Behavior management.
      (1) Consistent or intermittent reinforcement can cause behaviors to be learned.
      (2) Ignoring behaviors can extinguish them.

4. **Social cognitive and sociocultural.**
   a. Social learning and reinforcement help a child develop new skills by building new behaviors and skills related to existing knowledge.
   b. Learning is accomplished through partnerships with more mature members of the learning community.

5. **Social maturational.**
   a. A child's readiness for learning particular skills is primarily biological, with modifications based on subsequent environmental experiences.
   b. Pattern of learning is sequential.
   c. The child will experience periods of equilibrium (mastery) and disequilibrium (lack of mastery).

Effect of Motor Control and Motor Learning on Development

1. **Motor control and motor learning are necessary for motor development to occur.**

2. **Refer to Chapter 3 for full explanation of motor control and motor learning.**

3. **Maturation.**
   a. Neural maturation determines motor development.
   b. Earliest movements, including reflexes, are determined by primitive neural structures.

Table 8-1 ➤ NORMAL REFLEXES & RESPONSES

Primitive Reflexes

REFLEX	STIMULUS	RESPONSE
Suck-swallow	Object touches roof of the mouth	• Sucking
Rooting	Stroke or brush on the cheek	• Turns head toward touch and open mouth
Flexor withdrawal	Noxious stimuli to sole of foot or palm of hand	• Flexion of knee or elbow to withdrawal from stimulus
Crossed extension	Noxious stimulus to sole of foot	• Flexion and then extension of contralateral leg
Traction response	Traction on upper extremities (as in pull-to-sit)	• Flexion of upper extremities with the appearance of "helping" into sitting position
Moro	Rapid neck extension	• Initially, arms abduct and extend followed quickly by arms flexing in as if grasping for parent and crying
Plantar grasp	Pressure on ball of the foot or toes	• Foot will dorsiflex and toes will curl
Positive support	Child is supported under the arms and feet bounce on a flat surface	• Extends legs for 20-30 seconds to support self in standing followed by flexion of legs and entering a sitting position
Stepping/Walking	Infant held upright (slightly tilted forward) with solid surface under feet	• Reciprocal stepping motion of legs
Galant	Stroke is made on the paravertebral area from neck to low back	• Lateral flexion of trunk towards the side being stroked with hips and legs moving toward side of stimulus
Asymmetric Tonic Neck Reflex (ATNR)	Head turned to one side	• Arm and leg on the face side extend, arm and leg on the skull side flex
Tonic Labyrinthine Reflex (TLR)	Supine or prone position	• In supine, trunk and extremities extend • In prone, trunk and extremities flex
Placing reaction (Proprioceptive placing)	Firm touch of dorsum of foot or hand on solid surface such as a table	• Flexion and subsequent extension of extremity resulting in hand or foot being place on surface (table)
Palmar grasp	Object placed in open hand	• Grasping of object
Babinski	Stroke to lateral plantar surface of foot	• Great toe extension and fanning of the other toes
Symmetric Tonic Neck Reflex (STNR)	Neck placed in flexion or extension	• When neck extends, arms extend and legs flex • When neck flexes, arms flex and legs extend

c. Mature movements are directed by advanced neural structures that differentiate complex movements.

4. Learning.
 a. Motor programs.
  (1) Intrinsic and automatic patterns of movement.
  (2) Can be modified to adapt to a situation based on sensory feedback and conditions.
 b. Generalization of skills occurs and child is able to use previously learned skills to decrease the time and effort necessary to learn a similar task.

5. Variables influencing development.
 a. Motivation.
 b. Muscle strength.
 c. Body weight.
 d. Level of arousal.
 e. Complexity and maturation of neural networks.
 f. Environmental forces.

Neonatal Development

1. Prematurity.
 a. Birth at less than 37 weeks of gestation.
 b. A fetus is considered viable at 22–23 weeks of gestation.

2. Reflexes.
 a. Basic unit of movement in the hierarchical theory of motor control.
 b. Involve the combination of a sensory stimulus and a motor response (Table 8-1).

3. Neonatal (primitive) reflexes.
 a. Normal for young infants and typically present at birth.
 b. Usually integrated in the first 9 months of life.
 ☞ **Red Flag**
  • Persistent, absent or asymmetrical reflexes usually indicate early brain damage and affect normal development (Table 8-2).

4. Postural control.
 a. The ability to maintain alignment of the body.
 b. Development.
  (1) Directional concepts.
   (a) Cephalocaudal: head control followed by upper extremity use followed by lower extremity use.
   (b) Proximal to distal: midline control must develop first to provide a stable base upon which the head and extremities may move.
   (c) General to specific: whole body movements develop before disassociation occurs.

Table 8-2 ➤ PRIMITIVE REFLEXES

REFLEX	AGE OF ONSET	AGE OF INTEGRATION	PROBLEMS IF REFLEX PERSISTS
Suck-swallow	28 weeks gestation	2–5 months	• Feeding • Releasing objects from mouth
Rooting	28 weeks gestation	3 months	• Oral motor development • Developing midline head control • Optical righting • Social interaction • Visual tracking
Flexor withdrawal	28 weeks gestation	1–2 months	• Standing and walking • Upper extremity functional activities
Crossed extension	28 weeks gestation	1–2 months	• Standing and walking
Traction response	28 weeks gestation	4–5 months	• Grading upper extremity response to traction
Moro	28 weeks gestation	4–6 months	• Sitting balance • Protective reactions in sitting • Eye-hand coordination • Visual tracking
Plantar grasp	28 weeks gestation	9 months	• Ability to stand with feet flat on a surface • Balance reactions and weight shift in standing
Positive support	35 weeks gestation	1–2 months	• Standing and walking • Balance reactions and weight shift in standing • *Can lead to plantar flexion contractures*
Stepping/Walking	Birth	2 months	• Balance and controlled ambulation when accommodating to uneven surfaces
Galant	Birth	3–6 months	• Development of sitting balance • *Can lead to scoliosis*
ATNR	Birth	4–6 months	• Feeding • Visual tracking • Bilateral hand use • Midline use of hands • Rolling • Development of crawling • *Can lead to muscular shortening and a variety of skeletal deformities (scoliosis, hip dislocation, etc.)*
TLR	Birth	4–6 months	• Initiating rolling • Propping on elbows with extended hips (in prone) • Flexing trunk and hips to sit from supine • Full body extension • Sitting and standing balance
Placing reaction (Proprioceptive placing)	Birth	6 months	• Organizing sensory input and motor output • Developing proprioception in extremities
Palmar grasp	Birth	9 months	• Voluntary grasp and release • Weightbearing on open hand • Crawling • Protective extension responses
Babinski	Birth	12 months	• Weightbearing on feet • Standing balance • Ambulation • *If present in a child over two years old, damage to the corticospinal tract may be present*
STNR	4–6 months	8–12 months	• Propping on arms in prone • Attaining and maintaining quadruped position • Reciprocal crawling • Sitting balance when head is moving • Using hands when looking at objects in sitting

Table 8-3 ➤ POSTURAL REACTIONS

Righting Reactions

REACTION	AGE OF ONSET	AGE OF INTEGRATION	BEHAVIOR ACHIEVED
Neonatal neck righting (neck on body: NOB)	Birth	4-6 months	• Rolling (log rolling and then segmental rolling)
Body righting on body (BOB)	4-6 months	5 years	
Optical righting	Birth-2 months	Persist	• Maintaining head in upright position (head control)
Labyrinthine righting			
Body righting on head (BOH)	4-6 months	5 years	
Landau	3-4 months	18-24 months	• Aligning head and body against gravity

Protective Responses

RESPONSE	AGE OF ONSET	AGE OF INTEGRATION	BEHAVIOR ACHIEVED
Parachute or Forward	5-6 months	Persist	• Protection in sitting
Lateral	7-8 months		
Posterior	9-10 months		
Stepping	15-18 months		• Protection against falling when standing or walking

Equilibrium and Tilting Responses

RESPONSE	AGE OF ONSET	AGE OF INTEGRATION	BEHAVIOR ACHIEVED
Prone	6 months	Persist	• Realigning the center of gravity in the base of support
Supine	7-8 months		
Sitting	7-8 months		
Quadruped	9-12 months		
Standing	12-24 months		

(d) Gross to fine: large muscle movements usually occur before small muscle movements.

(2) Kinesiological concepts (in order of development).

  (a) Physiological flexion: position in which babies are born.

  (b) Antigravity extension: active movements into extension occur first, as the extensors have been in a lengthened position and are prepared to move before flexors.

  (c) Antigravity flexion: as infant spends more time in supine, flexors are lengthened and strengthened by moving to overcome gravity.

  (d) Lateral flexion.

  (e) Rotation.

5. **Postural reactions.**

a. Assist child with orienting the world in an upright position.

b. Develop in infancy to early childhood.

c. Includes righting reactions, protective responses and equilibrium responses.

  (1) Righting reactions.

    (a) Responsible for orienting head and body in space.

    (b) Involve head and trunk movements.

  (2) Protective responses.

    (a) Utilized with rapid body displacement in response to an outside force.

    (b) Involve movement of extremities in the direction of displacement.

  (3) Equilibrium responses.

    (a) Utilized when slow changes occur between the center of gravity and base of support.

    (b) Degree of displacement determines the response used, beginning with movement of the head, then trunk and, if large enough, shoulder and/or hip abduction.

  ☞ **Red Flag**

    • Failure to develop postural reactions can pose a safety risk to the child (Table 8-3).

Developmental Milestones by Age and Domain (Table 8-4)

1. **During the first year, even months are typically the significant milestone months.**

a. Head control: 4 months.

b. Rolling: 6–8 months.

  (1) Log roll: 4–6 months.

  (2) Segmental roll: 6–8 months.

  (3) Rolling prone to supine usually occurs first, secondary to the developing antigravity extension first.

c. Sitting: 8 months.

d. Cruising: 10 months.

e. Walking: 12 months.

Table 8-4 ➤ DEVELOPMENTAL MILESTONES BY AGE AND DOMAIN

	GROSS MOTOR DEVELOPMENT	FINE MOTOR DEVELOPMENT
Birth to 1 month	• Physiological flexion • Head held to the side in prone • Full head lag in pull-to-sit	• Visually tracks objects to midline or beyond • Fisted hands
2–3 months	• Lifts head in prone 45-90 degrees • Can bear some weight through forearms in prone • Head to side in supine • Variable head lag in pull-to-sit • Head bobs in supported sitting • Hips in flexion in supported standing	• Hands begin to open more • Visually tracks objects 180 degrees • Reflexive palmar grasp
4–5 months	• Rolls prone to side or supine • Bears weight through forearms in prone • Rolls supine to side • Head steady in supported sitting • Scapular adduction with upper trunk extension in supported sitting • Bears most weight through flexed hips in supported standing	• Grasps toys • Ulnar-palmar grasp (Fingers opposing ulnar side of palm, thumb adducted and flexed) • Bilateral reaching with forearms pronated
6–7 months	• Rolls from supine to prone • Holds weight on one hand in prone to reach for toy • Holds weight on extended arms in prone • Lifts head in supine • Sits without support • Stands holding on • Bounces in standing	• Radial-palmar grasp (Rakes objects into palm with adducted thumb and flexed fingers) • Voluntary release to transfer objects between hands • Approaches objects unilaterally • Arm in neutral when approaching toy
8–9 months	• Gets into hands and knees position • Creeps on hands and knees • Moves from hands and knees to sitting • Sits without hand support for longer periods • Pulls-to-stand • Walks along furniture, "cruising" • Stands alone briefly	• Develops active supination in arms • Points and pokes with index finger • Takes objects out of containers • Develops more refined release of objects • Develops more variation in grasping including radial-digital grasp (thumb opposing side of index finger) • Radial-palmar grasp (Fingers raking object into palm) • Three-jaw-chuck grasp (First two fingers opposing thumb)
10–11 months	• Pulls to stand using half-kneel intermediate position • Stands without support for longer • Picks up object from floor while holding on • Bear walks on hands and feet • Walks with two hands held • Walks with one hand held • May walk a few steps without help	• Inferior pincer grasp (Thumb opposing ventral surface of index finger) • Fine pincer grasp (Tips of fingers oppose tip of thumb) • Puts objects into containers • Grasps crayon
12–15 months	• Walks alone • Walks backward and sideways • Bends over to look between legs • Creeps upstairs • Throws ball in sitting position • Runs–fast walks with wide-based gait	• Builds tower of two cubes • Marks paper with crayon • Uses neat pincer grasp
16–23 months	• Squats in play • Propels ride-on toys • Kicks ball in standing with minimum control • Throws ball in standing • Ascends and descends stairs with one hand held • Jumps off bottom step • Runs with more coordination	• Holds paper • Strings beads • Stacks six cubes • Imitates vertical and horizontal strokes with crayon on paper

(Continued on following page)

Table 8-4 ➤ continued

	GROSS MOTOR DEVELOPMENT	FINE MOTOR DEVELOPMENT
24–36 months	• Rides tricycle • Walks on tiptoe • Runs well • Catches large ball • Uses reciprocal gait pattern on stairs • Jumps with both feet • Hops on one foot • Cultural factors may influence development of movement skills (e.g., riding tricycle, ball play, hopping)	• Cuts with scissors • Builds tower using eight cubes • Opens and closes jar • Completes 3–4 piece puzzles • Folds clothes • Buttons clothes
3–4 years	• Throws ball overhand • Hops two to ten times on one foot • Stands on tiptoes • Walks on a line 10 feet • Runs fast and avoids obstacles • Jumps over 12 inch obstacles	• Copies a circle or cross • Draws a recognizable human figure with head and two extremities • Draws squares
5–8 years	• Skips on alternate feet • Gallops • Balances on one foot • Jumps with rhythm • Bounces large ball • Greater speed and control in running • Kicks ball with skill	• Hand preference is clear • Prints well • Starts to learn cursive writing • Able to fasten small buttons and hooks
9–12 years (pre-adolescent)	• More mature patterns of throwing and jumping • Able to run faster with more efficiency • Enjoys competitive games • Improved balance and coordination • Girls may develop pubescent body changes • Boys may develop preadolescent fat spurt	• Handwriting is well developed • Can do more skilled hand tasks such as those involved in art
13–18 years (adolescent)	• Rapid growth • Pubescent changes leading to increased size and strength; especially boys • Improved balance skills • Coordination • Endurance	• Greater dexterity developed for fine motor tasks • Develops skills in knitting, sewing, art, crafts, etc.
	SOCIAL DEVELOPMENT	LANGUAGE DEVELOPMENT
Birth to 1 month	• Eye contact • Molds body when held	• Monotonous cry to indicate needs
2–3 months	• Enjoys physical contact • Responds with smile	• Coos open vowel sounds like "aaa." • Laughs • Cries vary in pitch to communicate different emotions/needs • Vocalizes in response to conversation
4–5 months	• Socializes with strangers/others • Lifts arms to mother	• Reacts to music • Reacts to own name
6–7 months	• Recognizes mother visually • Anxious about strangers • Yells to get attention • Enjoys vigorous play • Anxious about separating from mother	• Waves bye-bye • Uses simple gestures • Babbles double consonants "baba" • Produces more consonant sounds when babbling
8–9 months	• Explores environment • Lets only mother meet needs • Enjoys social games	• Babbles single consonants • Uses "mama" or "dada" nonspecifically • Uses more mature pattern of inflection

Table 8-4 ➤ continued

	SOCIAL DEVELOPMENT	LANGUAGE DEVELOPMENT
10–11 months	• Tests parental reactions • Extends object to show	• Says "dada" and "mama" purposefully • Repeats sounds or gestures if laughed at • Babbles when alone • Language skills plateau while learning to walk
12–15 months	• Displays tantrum behaviors • Resists adult control • Easily distracted • Enjoys imitating adult behaviors	• Has one-to-three word vocabulary • Says "no" meaningfully • Uses words or approximations to express self • Uses exclamatory sentences ("uh-oh")
16–23 months	• Expresses affection • Plays alone for short time • Gets frustrated easily • Demonstrates parallel play • Interacts with peers	• Uses two-word sentences • Has a vocabulary of up to 50 words • Imitates sounds ("woof-woof") • Tries to sing songs • Uses own name
24–36 months	• Values own property ("Mine") • Talks loudly • Obeys simple rules • Has trouble with changes • May have tantrums • May develop fears of unfamiliar things such as animals or clowns	• Uses three to five word sentences • Uses expressive vocabulary of 50 to 200 words • Gives full name on request • Uses plurals and past tense • Frustrated if not understood • Recites nursery rhymes
3–4 years	• Plays cooperatively • Enjoys making friends • Enjoys helping with adult activities • Setting table • Needs praise and guidance from adults	• Has expressive vocabulary of up to 1000 words • Talks to self during play • Uses rhythmic language • Loves to talk • Learns entire songs
5–8 years	• Prefers to play with peers rather than adults • Learns to give and receive • Shares • Cares what other think of him/her	• Has vocabulary of 2000 to 4000 words • Uses tenses correctly • Uses pronouns correctly • Interested in new words • Recites songs and rhymes
9–12 years (pre-adolescent)	• Interested in organized sports • Enjoys group activities • Develops motivation and discipline to practice skills	• Increasing vocabulary and maturity of language skills • Improved self-expression
13–18 years (adolescent)	• Orientation changes away from family to peers • Self conscious • Usually interested in the opposite sex • More sophistication in social skills • Able to manage schedule	• Expressive skills in speaking and writing improve
	COGNITIVE DEVELOPMENT	ADAPTIVE DEVELOPMENT
Birth to 1 month	• Quiets when picked up • Consoles self by sucking	• Coordinates sucking, swallowing and breathing
2–3 months	• Looks for sound • Plays with own hands • Shows active interest in person for 1 minute	• Hands to mouth • Stays awake longer during day • Sleeps longer at night
4–5 months	• Looks for hidden voice • Plays for 2–3 minutes with one toy	• Eats pureed or strained foods • Naps 2–3 times per day
6–7 months	• Plays peek-a-boo • Plays with paper • Looks for familiar people when named • Shakes toys to hear sound	• Mouths solid food • Bites and chews toys • Feeds self a cracker • Very messy

(Continued on following page)

Table 8-4 ➤ continued

	COGNITIVE DEVELOPMENT	ADAPTIVE DEVELOPMENT
8–9 months	• Throws and drops objects • Enjoys looking at books • Stacks and unstacks ring toy	• Finger feeds self • Holds spoon • Chews using munching pattern • Up/down with jaw • Sleeps up to 14 hours at night
10–11 months	• Guides action toy manually • Dances	• Holds spoon • Helps with dressing
12–15 months	• Enjoys messy play including finger painting and feeding self • Helps to turn pages of books	• Brings spoon to mouth • Holds cup • Drinks with some spilling • Shows pattern of elimination behavior • Expresses discomfort with dirty diaper
16–23 months	• Names up to six body parts • Sorts objects • Puts things away • Understands personal pronouns • Turns pages one at a time	• Turns knob to open door • Feeds self with spoon • Some spilling • Helps with washing hands • Begins toilet training • Uses rotary movements to chew food
24–36 months	• Matches colors • Plays house • Loves being read to • Sorts shapes • Matches simple pictures • Matches pictures and objects • Engages in simple make-believe activities • Obeys two-part commands	• Recognizes common dangers • Uses spoon and fork • Uses napkin • Uses toilet consistently • Insists on doing things without help • Blows nose with help • Washes and dries hands • Dresses with help
3–4 years	• Identifies colors and shapes • Able to do at least a 30-piece puzzle • Identifies money • May confuse fantasy with reality	• Uses toilet without help • Uses eating utensils independently • Brushes teeth with supervision • May eliminate naps
5–8 years	• Learns to read • Learns addition and subtraction • Learns to write • Enjoys table games	• Learns to tie shoes • Can bathe independently • Washes hair with supervision • Takes role in household tasks • Can manage chores with supervision • Definite likes and dislikes with food • May have stomach aches related to school attendance
9–12 years (pre-adolescent)	• Increased attention span • Able to think more abstractly • Curious • Reads a variety of printed materials	• Independent in self-care activities • Learns to cook • Independent in simple household chores
13–18 years (adolescent)	• Formal thinking skills develop • Able to develop hypotheses, theories • Interests expand beyond self and local environment to world issues	• Learns to drive • Develops independence in most household tasks

2. Head control and sitting are the two most significant milestones.

Application Concept

Two significant developmental milestones:
  • Development of head control.
  • Ability to sit.

Posture and Gait

1. Postural flexibility.
  a. Infants under 1 year have normal physiological flexion.
  b. Younger children are usually more flexible than older children.

c. Girls exhibit more flexibility than boys at all ages.
d. During growth spurts children lose flexibility.
  (1) Bone to muscle length ratio changes.
  (2) Usually regain flexibility as muscles elongate to catch up to bone length.

2. **Typical pediatric posture and alignment.**
a. Birth–12 months.
  (1) Spine.
    (a) Changes from flexible rounded posture at birth to beginning lordosis in neck and lower spine.
    (b) Provides greater stability in the back and neck.
  (2) Lower extremities.
    (a) Change from physiological flexion to greater range in extension.
    (b) Transition from a more varus position of the hip and knee toward neutral position.
b. 1–6 years.
  (1) Spine develops greater lordosis in neck and low back.
  (2) Child learns to stand and walk (1–2 years).
    (a) Stands with a wide base of support and high guard position of the arms.
    (b) Hips decrease angle of anteversion.
  (3) Flexor tightness continues to decrease allowing full hip extension by 3–4 years.
  (4) Hips and knees develop greater valgus angles, sometimes having a "knock-kneed" appearance at age 3 years (maximum physiological genu valgum).
c. 6–12 years.
  (1) Boys lose flexibility throughout childhood.
  (2) Children continue to grow and to develop strength and coordination.
  (3) Major postural changes do not typically occur during this stage.
d. Adolescence.
  (1) Girls have slight genu valgum while boys have slight genu varum.
  (2) Final growth spurt occurs earlier in girls (8–14 years) than boys (11–16 years).
  (3) Full height and strength are achieved during adolescence.
  (4) Growth plates fuse in late adolescence to early 20s.

3. **Typical pediatric gait.**
a. Typically, developing children walk between the ages of 9–15 months.
b. Median age of gait achievement.
  (1) Stand independently by 10.5 months.
  (2) Take first steps by 11 months.
  (3) Walk independently by 11.5 months.
c. Prerequisite skills for standing.
  (1) Adequate body proportions.
  (2) Sufficient range of motion (ROM).
  (3) Adequate strength and motor control.
  (4) Coordination of visual, proprioceptive and vestibular systems for balance.
d. Standing.
  (1) Begin with bilateral upper extremity support and transition to unilateral support.
  (2) Initially stand using a wide base of support.
    (a) Hips in abduction, flexion and external rotation.
    (b) Upper extremities in abduction and external rotation for balance.
e. Early ambulation.
  (1) Cruising sideways using furniture for support emerges by 8–9 months.
  (2) Walking forward using support (hands held or holding a moving object) occurs by 9–10 months.
  (3) Characteristics.
    (a) Lower extremity positioning.
      • Wide base of support.
      • Excessive hip and knee flexion.
      • Full foot contact.
    (b) Gait deviations.
      • Short stride.
      • Longer stance phase.
      • Increased cadence.
      • Heel eversion in stance.
      • Relative footdrop in swing phase.
    (c) Electromyographic (EMG) studies show co-contraction of antagonistic muscle groups to promote stability.
  (4) Development of more mature gait pattern.
    (a) By 18 months:
      • Legs are closer together.
      • Cadence is slower.
      • Stride is longer.
    (b) By 2 years:
      • Consistent heel strike has emerged.
      • Center of gravity lowering allows for improved balance and stability.
      • Duration of the stance phase decreases as balance and coordination improve.
    (c) By 3 years:
      • More mature gait pattern is seen.
      • Joint angles in the hip and knee are similar to those of an adult.
      • Although continued heel eversion is seen in the stance phase, cocontraction of antagonists is more mature.
      • Balance and coordination have improved significantly by this point.
    (d) By 7 years, gait patterns can be assessed by adult standards.

Application Concepts

- Typical development requires the integration of a variety of intrinsic and extrinsic factors.
- Reflexes are the basis upon which a child develops and matures.
- Children require an extended period of practice and constant repetition to learn new skills.
- Although typical developmental stages and sequence are known, each child is different.
- Assessment of a child's early posture and gait should not be conducted using adult standards.

Physical Therapy Examination and Data Collection

Basic Assessments

1. **Strength.**
   a. Young children cannot cooperate with typical manual muscle tests.
   b. Usually assessed through observation and participation in play and functional skills.

2. **ROM.**
   a. Normal ROM changes through infancy, toddlerhood, childhood and adolescence.
   b. Growth spurts affect muscle length and, in turn, ROM.

3. **Developmental skills.**
   a. The *sequence* of developmental skills is similar for typically developing children.
   b. The *timing* of skill development is unique to each child within a normal range.

4. **Functional/adaptive skills.**
   a. Includes development of functional/adaptive skills such as dressing, eating and toileting.
   b. Dependent not only on individual maturation, but on environmental factors such as culture, parenting styles, environment and opportunities for practice.

Application Concepts

- The *sequence* of developmental skills is similar for the typically developing child.
- The *timing* of skill development is unique to each child within a normal range of time.

Screening Tests

1. **Usually administered by physicians or nurse practitioners.**

2. **Apgar (Named after physician Virginia Apgar).**
   a. Administered to newborn infants at 1 and 5 minutes after birth and again at 10 minutes if concerns are present.
   b. Measures heart rate, respiratory effort, muscle tone, reflex irritability and color.
   c. Each area has a score of 0, 1, or with a total score up to 10.
   d. Scores between 7 and 10 are considered normal.
   e. Low scores may indicate a lack of oxygen prior to or during birth.

3. **Denver Developmental Screening Test II (Denver II).**
   a. Screening tool most commonly used in pediatrician's offices during well-baby checks.
   b. Assesses the need for further developmental testing on children up to 6 years of age.
   c. Tests personal-social, fine motor, gross motor and language skills.

Standardized Developmental Tests Commonly Used by Therapists

1. **Neonatal Behavioral Assessment Scale (NBAS).**
   a. Used with typically developing infants from 37–48 weeks' gestational age.
   b. Assesses habituation, oral-motor, truncal, vestibular and social-interactive domains.

2. **Movement Assessment of Infants (MAI).**
   a. Used with infants birth to 12 months.
   b. Assesses muscle tone, reflexes, automatic reactions and volitional movement.

3. **Bayley Scales of Infant Development, 3rd edition (Bayley-III).**
   a. Used with children from birth to 42 months of age.
   b. Assesses adaptive, cognitive, language, motor and social-emotional development.

4. **Peabody Developmental Motor Scales, 2nd edition (PDMS-2).**
   a. Used with children from birth to 5 years of age.
   b. Measures gross and fine motor function.

Performance Scales Measuring Function and Outcomes of Therapy

1. **Gross Motor Function Measure, 2nd edition (GMFM-2).**
   a. Used for children with cerebral palsy and related disorders through acquisition of advanced gait activities.
   b. Measures gross motor skills including lying and rolling, sitting, crawling and kneeling, standing, walking, running and jumping.

2. **Functional Independence Measure for Children (WeeFIM).**
   a. For children between 6 months and 7 years for typically developing children; may be used up to age 21 for those with developmental disabilities.
   b. Measures self-care, mobility, locomotion, communication and cognitive skills.

3. **Pediatric Evaluation of Disability Inventory (PEDI).**
   a. Useful for children from 6 months to 7 years.
   b. Measures functional skills in the areas of self-care, mobility and social function, including notation of caregiver modifications.

Application Concepts

- While standard developmental timelines have been presented, it is important to remember development of such skills is dependent on both nature and nurture.
- Most assessments by the physical therapist or physical therapist assistant will take place while they are assessing the individual's completion of functional activities; standard manual muscle testing and goniometric techniques may be difficult to obtain accurately.
- A variety of assessments and performance scales are available based upon what information is desired.

Intervention

Overview

1. Most therapists achieve success by using an assortment of therapeutic techniques.

2. Several treatments used with adults with neurological disorders are also used with pediatric patients; see Chapter 3.

3. *Remember*: play is the work of children, so therapy has to be fun.

Intervention Approaches

1. **Neurodevelopmental treatment (NDT).**
   a. Developed by Karel and Berta Bobath.
   b. Normal movement sequences are facilitated and substitution/compensation is not permitted.
   c. Promote the use of involved body segments.
   d. Address innate postural and reflex responses to affect functional motor skills.
   e. Utilize sensory input to influence motor output.
   ☞ **Red Flag**
   - Substitution or compensation should not be permitted with NDT intervention.

2. **Sensorimotor integration (SI).**
   a. Developed by A. Jean Ayres.
   b. Attributes problems with learning, attention, behavior and visual perception to faulty integration of sensory input.
   c. Treatment focuses on providing systematic sensory input to help organize a child's motor output.

3. **Motor control approaches.**
   a. A number of approaches to therapy build on theories of motor control and motor learning.
   b. Refer to previous discussion and Chapter 3 regarding more information on motor control and motor learning.

Physical Therapy Tools for Working with Children

1. **Handling and environmental stimuli.**
   a. Use of sensory input to produce changes in motor output.
   b. Responses to sensory input can be affected by environment, health and emotions of child.
   c. For a child with low muscle tone, the goal is to increase motor output.
      (1) Handling techniques: tapping, brushing, vibrating, quick movements, deep pressure, spinning, swinging and bouncing.
      (2) Environmental stimuli: loud music, fast rhythms, loud voice, bright colors and changing activities frequently.

d. For a child with high muscle tone or dystonia, the goal is to decrease motor output.
   (1) Handling techniques: rocking, firm touch, rhythmic movements, slow movements, stroking, warm water and wrapping/swaddling.
   (2) Environmental stimuli: consistent sensory input, relaxing music, singing, quiet voice.
   ☞ **Red Flags**
      • It is essential the clinician correctly identify hypotonia or hypertonia.
      • Use of inhibition techniques with hypotonia or facilitation techniques with hypertonia can lead to undesired increases or decreases in tone, thereby decreasing the benefits of future therapeutic interventions provided during that session.

2. **Adaptive equipment.**
   a. Positioning for function.
      (1) Helps maintain alignment of trunk and limbs.
      (2) Prevents or minimizes contractures.
      (3) Promotes strengthening, balance and postural reflexes.
      (4) Facilitates functional skills.
      (5) Allows optimal mobility and participation in age-appropriate activities.
   b. Floor positioning and mobility devices.
      (1) Mat: allows free floor mobility and provides a safe, cushioned surface.
      (2) Wedge: allows a variety of positions for child to visually access environment, promotes weight bearing through extremities and facilitates postural reactions.
      (3) Sidelyer: gives child visual access to hands, keeps head in midline to decrease asymmetrical tonic neck reflex (ATNR) and allows flexion of hips and knees to decrease extensor tone.
      (4) Bolster: stimulates balance and postural reflexes and aids with development of dynamic postural control.
      (5) Ball: used to stimulate postural reflexes and to complete strengthening and coordination activities.
      (6) Scooter board: used to promote floor level mobility in prone, supine or quadruped position.
   c. Seated positioning and mobility devices.
      (1) Adapted chairs.
         (a) Allow access to typical environments (i.e., dining room table, classroom desks).
         (b) Provide child the needed support and stability that typical chairs do not have.
      (2) Adapted tricycle.
         (a) Foot pedals with straps.
         (b) Built-up handlebars.
         (c) Greater contour in seat.
         (d) Seat back: improves trunk alignment and provides greater stability in sitting.

Table 8-5 ➤ CHART ON WHEELCHAIR POSITIONING COMPONENTS

Head Support	Provides posterior, lateral or anterior support for head and for safety during transportation.
Lateral Trunk Supports	Provide postural support for upright positioning and for supporting scoliosis.
Lateral Hip Guides	Promotes neutral positioning of lower extremities, neutral position of the pelvis.
Medial Thigh Supports (Pommel)	Provides for neutral positioning of thighs. Not to be used as a weight bearing surface for groin to keep pelvis back in chair.
Foot Supports	Supports lower extremities, provides neutral positioning for lower extremities.
Lap Tray	Provides upper extremity positioning and support to assist with trunk extension. Provides a surface for upper extremity activities.
Pelvic Belt	Maintains pelvic positioning in chair. Provides a measure of safety to prevent falls out of the chair.
Chest Strap	Maintains trunk positioning and prevents falling forward. Used as a supplement to a posterior and lateral positioning aid.
Butterfly Strap	Provides a broad surface to promote anterior chest support for upright positioning.
Thigh Strap	Promotes pelvic alignment during seating. Supplements the pelvic belt.
Sub ASIS Bar	Promotes pelvic alignment while seated. Potential for skin breakdown if not fitted correctly. Could be viewed as a restraint.

      (3) Manual and power wheelchairs.
         (a) Benefits.
            • Allow custom positioning and mobility.
            • Can be used in multiple environments.
            • Allow independent mobility.
            • Available positioning components can be used in any wheelchair depending on specific postural needs of child (Table 8-5).
         (b) Stroller-type chairs: lighter than wheelchairs and usually foldable to provide portability.
         (c) Power scooters: less expensive than power wheelchairs but provide less trunk support and require greater balance and upper extremity skill to use.
   d. Standing positioning and mobility devices.
      (1) Benefits.
         (a) Child has standing level view of environment.
         (b) Weight bearing through long bones to decrease effects of osteoporosis.
         (c) Facilitate postural reflex mechanisms.
         (d) Allow use of arms and hands for functional tasks.
         (e) Dynamic standers can have wheels added to allow the child to move in a standing position through manual or powered propulsion.
      (2) Supine stander: provides posterior support for head control and encourages passive weight bearing with full posterior support.

(3) Prone stander: provides anterior support and stimulates postural activation to hold up head and upper trunk.

(4) Parapodium: allows child to move in a standing position at the same visual height as peers; can initially be used as a standing device and then child progresses to using it for pregait and gait activities.

(5) Anterior rolling walker: promotes upright posture, active weight bearing through lower extremities, strengthening, endurance and independent mobility skills.

(6) Posterior rolling walker: promotes trunk extension with more erect posture than an anterior walker, which may help decrease abnormal movements (i.e., poor reciprocal movement, lack of disassociation between lower extremities) during gait.

(7) Gait trainers: provide greater support through trunk and may attach hip-knee-ankle-foot orthosis (HKAFO) for lower extremity positioning.

(8) Axillary or forearm support crutches: require greater balance, trunk strength and postural control than walkers.

↪ **Red Flag**

• Adaptive equipment must be continually monitored for correct fit as the child grows in order to maximize its usefulness.

e. Orthoses.

(1) Benefits.

(a) Provide external support to maintain or correct alignment of extremities or trunk.

(b) Improve postural stability to allow greater mobility and functional skills.

(c) Reduce the effects of spasticity through alignment of joints and muscles.

(2) Submalleolar or University of California Biomechanics Laboratory (UCBL) shoe insert.

(a) Closely molded around the calcaneus to hold or prevent excessive calcaneal inversion or eversion.

(b) Helpful for children with foot posture problems.

(3) Supramalleolar orthosis (SMO).

(a) Provides support and alignment at the foot and medial/lateral ankle support.

(b) Provides added stability during standing and walking activities.

(4) Ankle foot orthosis (AFO).

(a) Maintains distal limb in optimal alignment and provides a stable base of support.

(b) Decreases the effects of abnormal muscle tone.

(c) Made of plaster or polypropylene and are bivalved, one piece, or articulating.

(d) May be useful for children with cerebral palsy, sacral levels of spina bifida, or general low muscle tone.

(5) Knee-ankle-foot orthosis (KAFO).

(a) Provides support and alignment of the foot, ankle and knee.

(b) Used for children who require greater external support because of significant weakness.

(6) HKAFO.

(a) Provides greater external stability for children with significant weakness at hips as well as knee and ankle.

(b) Allows standing and walking with assistive device.

(c) May be useful for children with high lumbar or low thoracic levels of spina bifida or spinal cord injury.

(7) Reciprocating gait orthosis (RGO).

(a) Allows children with significant weakness through lower extremities and trunk to walk with support.

(b) A body jacket with HKAFOs bilaterally and a cable system to facilitate reciprocal gait (2-point or 4-point gait pattern).

(c) May be useful for young children with T8-12 levels of spina bifida or traumatic spinal cord injury.

(8) Thoracic lumbar sacral orthosis (TLSO).

(a) Provides stability through the trunk to prevent or minimize spinal deformity and allow greater function.

(b) May be useful for children with no more than 40 degrees of scoliosis.

• Milwaukee orthosis (cervicothoracolumbosacral orthosis [CTLSO]) is used for all levels of scoliotic or kyphotic curves.

• Boston orthosis (thoracolumbosacral orthosis [TLSO]) is used with mid-thoracic or lower scoliosis curves.

↪ **Red Flags**

• Areas of redness that do not disappear within 20 minutes following removal of the orthotic device indicate a dangerous area of pressure.

• A trained individual should be consulted to adapt or refit the orthotic.

Application Concepts

• Play is the work of children and, therefore, it should be the basis for therapeutic interventions when working with pediatric patients.

• Many of the intervention approaches utilized with adult patients with neurological dysfunction can also be used with children presenting with neurological dysfunction.

• Adaptive equipment and orthoses should be used to increase function and facilitate quality of movement and body alignment.

• When selecting adaptive equipment, the needs of the family and their environment should be considered.

Conditions/Pathology/Diseases (CPD) with Intervention: Pediatric Orthopedic Disorders

Developmental Dysplasia of the Hip (DDH)

1. **Basic information.**
   a. A group of disorders involving poor alignment of the acetabulum and the head of the femur in the developing hip.
   b. Usually develops in the last trimester of pregnancy and may result from elevated levels of the female hormone relaxin, tight in utero positioning or breech positioning.
   c. Affects girls more than boys and left hip twice as often as the right hip.
   d. Exacerbated by swaddling and carrying infants with hips in extension and adduction.

2. **Clinical picture.**
   a. Nonambulatory child.
      (1) Asymmetrical hip abduction in flexion.
      (2) Asymmetrical groin or buttock skinfolds.
      (3) Pistoning of affected hip with manual traction.
      (4) Apparent femoral shortening on the affected side.
   b. Ambulatory child.
      (1) Trendelenburg's gait.
      (2) Decreased hip abduction.
      (3) Thigh pistoning.
      (4) Bilateral DDH presents with lordosis and swaying gait typical of a bilateral Trendelenburg.

3. **Medical intervention.**
   a. Bracing and splinting of hip in flexion and abduction.
      (1) Pavlik harness.
         (a) Typically used with infants under 9 months of age.
         (b) Allows active kicking to facilitate lower extremity strength and mobility and to decrease the complication of avascular necrosis of the hip.
      (2) Children over 9 months will need an abduction orthosis that allows walking.
   b. Traction and/or surgery (usually done after 18 months of age).
   ⇰**Red Flag**
      • Failure to correctly address the dysplasia can increase the risk of developing avascular necrosis of the hip.

4. **Physical therapy intervention.**
   a. Assessments.
      (1) Barlow's test: hip click felt when manually moving flexed hip from abduction to adduction.

   (2) Ortolani's test: hip click felt with passive movement of adducted and flexed hip into abduction with traction.
   b. Measuring and fitting brace.
   c. Parent education: brace application and positioning of hips in flexion and abduction.
   d. Direct intervention: strengthen, maintain or increase ROM and promote developmental skills.

Legg-Calvé-Perthes Disease (LCPD)

1. **Basic information.**
   a. Self-limiting degeneration of the femoral head due to a disturbance in blood supply.
   b. Due to genetic predisposition, trauma, anatomical variations or disorder of epiphyseal cartilage.
   c. Most commonly occurs in boys 4–7 years of age.
   d. Occurs less frequently in girls with onset at older ages and poorer rehabilitation potential.
   e. The younger the onset, the more positive the outcome.
   f. Approximately 20% occur bilaterally.

2. **Clinical picture.**
   a. 2- to 4-year progression of the disease with four stages.
      (1) Initial stage: failure of femoral head to grow due to decreased blood supply.
      (2) Fragmentation stage: fragmented epiphysis and revascularization of the femoral head.
      (3) Reossification stage: bone density returns to normal with changes in shape and structure of femoral head and neck.
      (4) Healed stage: femoral head and neck retain deformity from the repair process.
   b. Signs and symptoms.
      (1) Initial sign is a limp with ambulation, typically a Trendelenburg gait.
      (2) Mild pain in groin, medial knee or thigh.
      (3) Decreased ROM most noticeable in hip abduction and internal rotation.
      (4) Thigh, calf or buttock atrophy from disuse.
      (5) Limb length discrepancy.

3. **Medical intervention.**
   a. Some physicians recommend no treatment, allowing condition to heal on its own.
   b. Most physicians advocate treatment.
      (1) Observation and monitoring course of disease via radiographs.

(2) Avoid participation in contact sports in favor of non–weight-bearing exercise such as swimming.

(3) If condition is more vigorous, avoid weight-bearing with use of crutches.

(4) For advanced condition, splinting in abduction and internal rotation or surgery to contain the femoral head in the acetabulum may be necessary.

⚐ Red Flag
- Failure to follow the necessary precautions can slow the recovery process.

4. **Physical therapy intervention.**
   a. Ongoing assessment of ROM, strength and functional skills.
   b. Patient and family education: gait training, ROM, strengthening exercises, transfers and functional skills training.
   c. Consultation with school staff to encourage and support inclusion and mobility.

Slipped Capital Femoral Epiphysis (SCFE)

1. **Basic information.**
   a. Hip deformity related to slippage of the femoral epiphysis.
   b. May result from a genetic predisposition or hormonal influences leading to weak growth plates.
   c. Occurs in children who are tall, with delayed skeletal maturity, obese, near the onset of puberty (9–16 years of age).
   d. More common in boys than girls and children of African American or Polynesian ethnicity.
   e. Bilateral slips may occur in 25%–30% of cases.

2. **Clinical picture.**
   a. Onset.
      (1) Chronic slip: most common with a gradual onset and progression of symptoms for 3 weeks or more.
      (2) Acute slip: sudden onset of severe pain and is usually precipitated by trauma.
      (3) Acute-on-chronic slip: gradual symptoms that build up over a period of time and a traumatic episode cause an onset of severe symptoms.
   b. Grades of slippage.
      (1) Preslip: mild changes in the x-ray including a widened growth plate.
      (2) Grade 1 (mild slip): femoral head slipped $<1/3$ the width of the femoral neck.
      (3) Grade 2 (moderate slip): femoral head slipped $1/3–1/2$ the width of the femoral neck.
      (4) Grade 3 (severe slip): femoral head slipped $>1/2$ the width of the femoral neck.
   c. Signs/symptoms.
      (1) Intermittent limp and pain in groin, buttock, knee or thigh.
      (2) Antalgic and/or Trendelenburg's gait.

(3) Leg held in external rotation and hip flexion is accompanied by external rotation.

(4) Limitations of hip internal rotation, abduction and sometimes flexion.

3. **Medical intervention.**
   a. With early changes but no slip, conservative measures may help avoid surgery until skeletal maturity is reached.
      (1) Vigilant monitoring by radiograph.
      (2) Non–weight-bearing using crutches.
      (3) Weight loss.
      (4) Forbidding athletics.
   b. Surgery is usually required to pin the hip and prevent further slippage in mild or moderate cases.
   c. Varus osteotomy may be required to change the angle of the femoral neck to shaft for more severe cases.

⚐ Red Flag
- When early changes are apparent but no slip exists, conservative measures must be followed. This allows surgery to be withheld until skeletal maturity and likely decreases the number of surgeries the child will require.

4. **Physical therapy intervention.**
   a. Aim to minimize or reduce slippage, maintain hip ROM and function and prevent or minimize degenerative changes in later years.
   b. Order adaptive equipment (crutches, wheelchair).
   c. Patient and family education: home exercise program for strength and ROM, proper use of adaptive equipment and transfers, mobility and/or gait training.
   d. Home evaluation for accessibility.
   e. Consultation with school staff regarding mobility issues.

Juvenile Rheumatoid Arthritis (JRA)

1. **Basic information.**
   a. Group of disorders characterized by inflammation of connective tissue including joints and other systems.
   b. Occurs in children under 16 years of age where arthritis is present for 6 weeks or more.
   c. Cause is unknown but may be a genetic predisposition or due to a viral or bacterial infection triggering an autoimmune response.

2. **Clinical picture.**
   a. Classification.
      (1) Oligoarticular or pauciarticular.
         (a) Characterized by arthritis in fewer than five joints.
         (b) Affected joints usually have asymmetrical distribution.
      (2) Polyarticular.
         (a) Characterized by arthritis in five or more joints.

(b) Affected joints have a symmetrical distribution.

(c) Slow onset with gradual joint pain developing or acute onset with low-grade fever.

(3) Systemic

(a) Characterized by acute onset with high spiking fevers, rash on trunk and proximal extremities and possible organ inflammation (pericardium, heart, lungs).

(b) Causes joint destruction and potential disability.

b. Signs/symptoms.

(1) Joint pain, swelling and stiffness.

(2) Decreased ROM in affected joints.

(3) Myalgia (muscle pain).

3. Medical intervention.

a. Pharmaceutical management.

(1) Aspirin and nonsteroidal anti-inflammatory drugs (NSAIDS) (e.g., ibuprofen, naproxen and indomethacin).

(2) Slow-acting antirheumatic drugs (SAARDS) (e.g., gold salts, hydroxychloroquine and penicillamine).

(3) Corticosteroids (e.g., prednisone).

(4) Immunosuppressive and cytotoxic agents (e.g., cyclosporine, methotrexate).

b. Surgical management.

(1) Synovectomy.

(2) Soft tissue release.

(3) Osteotomy or epiphyseodesis (joint fusion).

(4) Total joint replacement.

4. Physical therapy intervention.

a. Splinting to maintain joint ROM.

b. Stretching to maintain soft tissue flexibility.

c. Modalities for pain control.

d. Activities to improve strength and endurance.

e. Patient and family education.

(1) Avoidance of joint trauma, especially during inflammation flares.

(2) Facilitating appropriate developmental skills for age and ability.

(3) Instruction, assistance and adaptations for functional skills such as mobility and self-help skills.

⚑ **Red Flag**

• Failure to identify disease flares and make the necessary accommodations in intervention approach can ultimately lead to a more rapid onset of joint damage.

Osteogenesis Imperfecta (OI)

1. Basic information.

a. Abnormality in the collagen gene causing problems with the amount and quality of collagen in the body.

b. Equal likelihood in boys and girls with a genetic predisposition.

2. Clinical picture.

a. Characterized by fragile bones that break easily and often for no apparent reason.

b. Other common symptoms: dental problems, scoliosis, kyphosis, short stature and hearing loss.

c. Four types.

(1) Type I: most common, usually have triangular-shaped face, thin, smooth skin and hearing loss beginning in teens or 20s.

(2) Type II: most severe form with newborns often suffering fractures before birth and dying shortly after birth.

(3) Type III: least common, involves progressive deformity of the long bones, skull and spine resulting in very small stature, dental and hearing problems, barrel-shaped rib cage and respiratory compromise secondary to severe kyphoscoliosis.

(4) Type IV: relatively rare, presents with loose, easily overstretched joints, dental problems and mild short stature.

3. Medical intervention.

a. Orthotic devices such as splints, lower extremity orthotics or body jackets for protection, to allow weight bearing and to prevent deformity.

b. Assurance of adequate calcium intake.

c. Assess for and treat fractures.

4. Physical therapy intervention.

a. Aim to minimize fractures through joint protection, maximize activity and weight bearing for bone and muscle strength and facilitate maximum functional skills.

b. Active exercise for strengthening with positioning and stretching to maintain ROM.

⚑ **Red Flag**

• Passive stretching is not recommended due to risk of fracture or joint subluxation.

c. Assistive devices such as walkers, crutches or wheelchairs to improve mobility.

d. For some children with type IV, weight training with a very low amount of weight can be indicated.

e. Low-impact endurance activities such as swimming and walking.

f. Parent education including supporting child at the head and trunk region, not at long bones and rolling child during diaper changes not lifting at the ankles.

Arthrogryposis Multiplex Congenita

1. Basic information.

a. Nonprogressive neuromuscular disorder causing multiple joint contractures at birth.

b. Etiology is usually unknown but may result from lack of fetal movement, trauma or insult during 1st trimester of pregnancy, maternal history of fevers during pregnancy, or maternal multiple sclerosis, myasthenia gravis or myotonic dystrophy.

2. **Clinical picture.**
   a. Variability in clinical picture usually includes severe joint contractures and absence of muscle development.
      (1) Contractures with severity increasing distally.
      (2) Joint dislocation at hips or knees.
      (3) Thin subcutaneous tissue.
      (4) Absence or decreased size of muscle groups.
   b. Typically affected body parts in order of prevalence.
      (1) Foot: clubfoot.
      (2) Hip: flexion or abduction and external rotation deformities.
      (3) Wrist: flexion, ulnar deviation.
      (4) Knee: extension or flexion.
      (5) Elbow: extension or flexion.
      (6) Shoulder: internal rotation and extension or flexion.
   c. Children with distal involvement have a good prognosis for being community ambulators while children with systemic joint involvement may be household ambulators or use wheelchairs.

3. **Medical intervention.**
   a. Lower and upper extremity splints and orthotic devices.
   b. Body jackets and other braces to prevent formation of scoliosis.
   ➤ **Red Flag**
      • Development of scoliosis can lead to decreased lung capacities.
   c. Surgical intervention.
      (1) Clubfoot surgery may be deferred until the child is ready to stand.
      (2) Hip dislocation.
         (a) If one hip is dislocated, surgery is done to prevent pelvic obliquity and scoliosis.
         (b) If bilateral dislocation, surgical intervention may be withheld because painless dislocated hips are better than stiff located hips.
      (3) Knee flexion contractures: usually addressed when child is ambulatory, involving hamstring lengthening or posterior capsulotomy of knee joint.
      (4) Knee extension contractures: quadriceps lengthening is performed when knee position interferes with sitting or ambulation.
      (5) Scoliosis may be managed via surgical fusion.

4. **Physical therapy intervention.**
   a. Strengthening of neck, trunk and extremity muscles using developmental activities (i.e., prone on elbows, sitting, rolling, kneeling and standing).
   b. Functional mobility training: rolling, crawling/creeping, ambulation and/or power wheelchair training.
   c. Use of assistive devices: cane, walker, gait trainer, adapted stroller or wheelchair.
   d. Parent instruction in daily stretching and positioning to maintain and increase ROM.

Pediatric Fractures

1. **Basic information.**
   a. Multiple causes: trauma, child abuse, motor vehicle accident and genetics.
   b. Fracture patterns are different than adults due to bones that are more flexible, more porous and less dense than adult bones.
   c. Children's periosteum is thicker than adults, leading to better blood supply and faster rate of healing (2–4 weeks).
   d. Active epiphyseal plates are affected in 30% of pediatric fractures.

2. **Clinical picture.**
   a. Common fracture sites include distal radius, tibial shaft, clavicle and elbow.
   b. Signs and symptoms: redness, swelling, pain, heat, muscle spasm, deformity and nonuse of extremity.
   c. Types of fractures.
      (1) Buckle fracture (torus fracture): compression of long bone on one side.
      (2) Greenstick fracture: compression on one side of long bone with distraction on other side.
      (3) Bending fracture (plastic deformation): bending of long bone in the direction of force.
      (4) Epiphyseal fracture: fracture involving the epiphyseal plate.
      (5) Spiral fracture: caused by twisting force on long bone.

3. **Medical intervention involves splinting or casting and analgesics for pain control.**

4. **Physical therapy intervention includes instructing patient and family in use of assistive device and providing strengthening, balance and endurance exercises.**

Foot and Ankle Deformities

1. **Basic information: causes of congenital deformity include in utero positioning, neuromuscular disorders and genetic disorders.**

2. **Clinical picture.**
   a. Classification.
      (1) Metatarsus adductus: metatarsals deviated medially.

(2) Talipes equinovarus (clubfoot): adduction of forefoot, varus position of hindfoot and equinus at ankle.

(3) Calcaneovalgus: foot dorsiflexion, eversion or valgus of hindfoot and abduction of metatarsals.

b. Signs/symptoms: visual deformity, gait disturbances and delays in development of gross motor and mobility skills.

3. **Medical intervention involves casting and, if not successful, surgery to fuse the ankle joint in a functional position.**

4. **Physical therapy intervention.**

a. Stretching to counter deformity and supplement splinting or bracing.

⚑ **Red Flag**
   - It is essential to stretch the gastrocnemius/soleus muscles while avoiding breakdown of the mid-foot ligaments.

b. Serial casting.
   (1) Splints or casts are applied to counter the deformity (e.g., for clubfoot).
   (2) The cast is applied in the direction of forefoot abduction, hindfoot valgus and ankle dorsiflexion.
   (3) Casts are changed every 1–2 weeks for several months until bones have remodeled.

c. Gait training.

d. Promote normal developmental skills through play.

e. Sensory input.
   (1) Casted limbs may need sensory stimulation during periods of time out of the cast.
   (2) Sensory stimulation includes rubbing with textured material, water and sand play, massage and weight bearing.

⚑ **Red Flag**
   - Failure to provide the necessary sensory stimulation can lead to difficulties with ambulation if the child is not able to tolerate sensory input on the soles of the feet.

Brachial Plexus Injury

1. **Basic information.**

a. Damage to all or some of the nerve roots from C5 through T1.

b. Commonly caused by a traction or compression injury.

c. Degree of injury.

(1) Avulsion: nerve is torn from the spinal cord.

(2) Rupture: nerve sheath or nerve fibers are torn, but not at the spinal attachment.

(3) Neuroma: nerve was torn and healed, but scar tissue prevents nerve conduction to the tissues.

(4) Neuropraxia or stretch: most common type of injury when nerve is damaged but not torn.

2. **Clinical picture (See Musculoskeletal chapter).**

3. **Medical intervention.**

a. Surgery may be necessary to repair avulsion injuries.

b. With onset of spasticity, oral muscle relaxers or Botox may be used.

4. **Physical therapy intervention.**

a. Initial positioning.
   (1) Infant swaddled with arm across upper abdomen.
   (2) Arm across the body (shoulder adduction and internal rotation).
   (3) Utilized for 1–2 weeks to allow nerve to rest and recover.

b. After initial recovery.
   (1) Gentle ROM to prevent contractures.
   (2) Facilitate awareness of involved extremity.
   (3) Facilitate motor output through sensory inputs (i.e., stroking, approximation).
   (4) Facilitate muscle activity via hand-over-hand activities and weight bearing.

c. As child grows, teach strategies to accomplish age-appropriate tasks and introduce assistive devices to increase functional skills.

Application Concepts

- A number of the pediatric orthopedic conditions utilize non–weight bearing, aquatic exercise and other conservative approaches to decrease the risk of further damage.
- It is important to address the child's mobility and assistive device needs with the educational staff to ensure appropriate inclusion in the academic environment.
- Once medical restrictions are lifted, therapeutic intervention should focus on facilitating achievement of developmental mobility and other age-appropriate skills.
- Positioning plays a very important part in prevention of further deformity and increasing the child's rehabilitation potential.

Conditions/Pathology/Diseases (CPD) with Intervention: Pediatric Neurological and Genetic Disorders

Cerebral Palsy (CP)

1. **Basic information.**
   a. Insult to the brain during development, at birth or within the first few years resulting in permanent, nonprogressive damage.
   b. Etiology.
      (1) Prenatal causes: maternal infections, diabetes, malnutrition, seizures or radiation exposure.
      (2) Perinatal causes: prematurity, low birth weight, multiple births, prolapsed umbilical cord, intraventricular hemorrhage and asphyxia.
      (3) Postnatal causes: infection (meningitis, encephalitis), asphyxia, traumatic brain injury (TBI) (falls, shaken baby syndrome), stroke, near drowning and brain tumor.

2. **Clinical picture.**
   a. Distribution of motor involvement.
      (1) Diplegia.
         (a) Both legs affected while trunk and arms may be affected to a lesser degree.
         (b) Typical standing posture.
            • Hip flexion, adduction and internal rotation.
            • Knee flexion.
            • Ankle plantar flexion.
         (c) Typical gait.
            • Poor disassociation between legs, noted trunk rotation and high guard positioning of arms for balance.
            • May use wheelchair, walker or crutches.
      (2) Hemiplegia.
         (a) One arm and leg on the same side affected.
         (b) Typical standing posture.
            • Shoulder adduction and internal rotation.
            • Elbow and wrist flexion.
            • Hip internal rotation.
            • Knee extension.
            • Ankle plantar flexion.
         (c) Typical gait.
            • Asymmetrical gait with circumduction of lower extremity.
            • May use cane or crutch for balance.
      (3) Quadriplegia/tetraplegia.
         (a) All four extremities and trunk involved.
         (b) With greater levels of trunk involvement the child may demonstrate head involvement.
   b. Classification of muscle tone.
      (1) Hypotonia (floppy, rag doll or low tone).

         (a) Muscle tone lower than normal, usually throughout the body.
         (b) Characteristics.
            • Excessive ROM.
            • Weak deep tendon reflexes and primitive reflexes.
            • Child is usually overweight due to deficient energy output.
            • Impaired speech due to poor oral motor control.
            • Gait characterized by wide base of support, short stride length and poor balance.
         (c) Physical therapy interventions specific to children with hypotonia.
            • Support all limbs to prevent injury.
            • Use care to prevent hyperextension at elbows and knees.
            • Use vigorous passive and active movement to stimulate increased muscle output.
            • Promote active weightbearing to stimulate postural reflexes.
      (2) Hypertonia (tight, spastic, stiff, or rigid).
         (a) Muscle tone higher than normal with location determined by area of motor cortex involved.
         (b) Characteristics.
            • ROM of motion may be limited.
            • Common contractures: hip adduction, internal rotation and flexion; knee flexion; ankle plantar flexion.
            • Hyperreflexive deep tendon reflexes.
            • Persistence of primitive reflexes (asymmetrical neck reflex (ATNR), symmetrical neck reflex (STNR), tonic labyrinthine reflex (TLR) limiting the development of normal movements.
            • Child usually thin due to excessive energy output.
            • Speech usually impaired due to poor oral motor control.
            • Gait characterized by poor muscle control and decreased balance with variations related to the distribution of muscle tone.
         (c) Physical therapy interventions specific to children with hypertonia.
            • Position hips and knees in greater than 90 degrees of flexion to inhibit strong reflexive extension.
            • Use midline symmetrical positioning to inhibit abnormal reflexes.

- Use gentle, rhythmic movement to encourage controlled movement.
- Promote active weight bearing with aligned limbs and trunk to allow optimal independence in motor skills.

(3) Athetosis or dystonia.
  - (a) Poor stability in midline resulting from a lesion in the basal ganglia or cerebellum.
  - (b) Identified by writhing movements, fluctuating tone and constantly moving between end ranges.
  - (c) Characteristics.
    - Distribution throughout body, including face.
    - ROM usually normal but may be excessive due to constant movement throughout range.
    - Hyperreflexive deep tendon reflexes.
    - Hypotonia in infancy changes to athetosis as child matures.
    - Persistence of primitive reflexes (ATNR, STNR, TLR) limiting the development of normal movements.
    - Child usually thin due to excessive energy output.
    - Speech usually impaired due to poor oral motor control.
    - Many children are unable to obtain enough stability to stand and walk; those who do have excessive movements and poor balance and likely require a walker, crutches or wheelchair for mobility.
  - (d) Physical therapy interventions specific to children with athetosis.
    - Encourage midline, symmetrical posture to minimize effects of abnormal reflexes.
    - Use gentle, rhythmic movements to encourage controlled motor output.
    - Allow abnormal movements if they contribute to functional skills.
    - Encourage child to problem solve motor difficulties.

(4) Ataxia.
  - (a) Results from a lesion in the cerebellum.
  - (b) Identified by wide base of support and high guard position of the upper extremities during gait, poor balance, tremors, low postural tone and poor visual tracking.
  - (c) Characteristics.
    - Distribution throughout body.
    - Poor balance.
    - ROM usually normal or excessive due to low tone.
    - Hyporeflexivity of deep tendon reflexes.
    - Weak primitive reflexes.
  - (d) Physical therapy interventions specific to a child with ataxia.

- Encourage midline, symmetrical posture for maximum function.
- Provide sensory input (tactile, proprioceptive, auditory, visual) to help the child orient in space.
- Weighted vest or belts to increase proprioceptive feedback and improve balance.
- Use aids to assist with balance (e.g., weighted walker, crutches and canes).

(5) Mixed.
  - (a) More than one type of muscle tone.
  - (b) Hypertonicity and athetosis is the most common form of mixed CP.

c. Classification based on severity.
  (1) Mild: independent functional skills including feeding and walking, develop at least some language skills.
  (2) Moderate: independent mobility (crawling or walking with support), need assistance for some functional skills such as feeding, may develop a few words of language.
  (3) Severe: needs help for most functional tasks including mobility and feeding, does not develop language skills.

d. Related problems.
  (1) Mental retardation (50%–75%).
  (2) Visual impairment (50%).
  (3) Speech/language deficits or delays and oral-motor problems (50%).
  (4) Seizures (30%).
  (5) Hearing impairment (10%).
  (6) Visual-motor and perceptual disorders.
  (7) Behavior disorders.
  (8) Orthopedic disorders: joint contracture, hip subluxation or dislocation, scoliosis, kyphosis, or lordosis, tibial torsion and clubfoot.

⚑ **Red Flag**
  - It is essential to be aware of related problems children present with in order to safely provide intervention, including seizure and oral-motor problems.

3. **Medical intervention.**
  a. Medications.
    (1) Seizures: Tegretol, Dilantin, Depakote, phenobarbital, Clonazepam.
    (2) Spasticity.
      (a) Botulinum toxin A (Botox) injections.
        - Prevents release of acetylcholine at the neuromuscular junction.
        - Lasts 1–4 months.
        - Common muscles of injection: gastrocnemius/soleus, hamstrings, hip flexors and hip adductors.
      (b) Baclofen.
        - Decreases excitatory input into alpha motor neurons.

- May be given orally or by intrathecal injection (through lumbar puncture or catheter).
  - **Red Flags**
    - Children who have Botox injections must be given extensive therapy to stretch tight agonist muscles and strengthen the antagonist muscles.
    - Following administration of any muscle relaxant, loss of spasticity may present difficulty with previously acquired functional mobility skills and ambulation.
  b. Surgical procedures.
    (1) Dorsal rhizotomy: cutting of dorsal nerve rootlets supplying the affected muscles to decrease spasticity and increase function.
    (2) Z-plasty: release of a muscle or tendon to reverse contractures.

4. **Physical therapy intervention.**
  a. Intervention is individualized, working as a team with the child and family in setting goals.
  b. Positioning and adapted equipment.
    (1) Benefits.
      (a) Allow visual access to the environment.
      (b) Facilitate functional use of extremities.
      (c) Encourage mobility.
      (d) May allow standing when otherwise impossible.
        - Improves weight bearing through long bones.
        - Improves visceral function (bowel and bladder elimination, respiratory function, venous return).
        - Decreases risk of developing lower extremity flexion contractures.
    (2) Good positioning.
      (a) Symmetrical posture.
      (b) Aligned trunk, pelvis and extremities.
      (c) Head in midline to minimize persistent primitive reflexes.
      (d) Hips and knees at 90 degrees when sitting.
      - **Red Flag**
        - It is imperative to utilize proper positioning to increase functioning and to avoid further limitations of the child.
    (3) Special considerations.
      (a) If strong extensor tone is present, hips and knees can be positioned in more than 90 degrees.
      (b) Posterior tilt-in-space wheelchair can be used if gravity needed to help keep trunk and head aligned in upright position.
      (c) Prompts can be used and reduced as child improves stability and mobility skills.

      (d) Serial casting may be necessary to obtain optimal positioning for use of equipment.
    (4) Examples: corner seat, molded seat, sidelyer, wheelchair with appropriate supports and prone or supine stander.
  c. Orthoses.
  d. Dynamic positioning supports.
  e. Optimizing functional skills.
    (1) Handling: elongate shortened muscle groups, facilitate dynamic movement, inhibit primitive reflexes and facilitate optimal muscle tone.
    (2) Promote weight bearing.
    (3) Provide postural challenges to improve balance, muscle tone and strength.
    (4) Utilize principles of motor learning to help a child learn new skills.

Traumatic Brain Injury (TBI)

1. **For full discussion, refer to Chapter 3.**

2. **Special considerations of TBI in the pediatric patient.**
  a. For children, length of time of unconsciousness (coma) is a predictor of outcome.
  b. Behavioral scales that assess a child's recovery
    (1) Pediatric Glasgow Coma Scale.
      (a) Same areas of assessment and scoring as with Adult Glasgow Coma Scale.
      (b) Indicators given for both infant and pediatric patients.
    (2) Glasgow Coma Scale.
    (3) Rancho Los Amigos scale.
  c. Educate family members and caregivers to provide sensory stimulation and, when appropriate, facilitate return of functional mobility.

Spina Bifida

1. **Basic information.**
  a. Group of congenital malformations of the spine, including the vertebrae and the spinal cord.
  b. Caused by a genetic predisposition, maternal deficiency of folic acid and maternal exposure to alcohol or valproic acid during the first 4 weeks of pregnancy.

2. **Clinical picture.**
  a. Classification.
    (1) Occulta (not visible).
      (a) Results from incomplete fusion of the posterior vertebral arch with no protrusion of neurological or superficial tissues.
      (b) May be indicated by a hair tuft, fat pad, dimple or sinus at base of spine.
      (c) No disability usually results from this disorder.

(2) Acculta or cystica (visible).
  (a) Meningocele.
   • Cerebrospinal fluid and superficial tissue protrudes from the spine in a sac at the level of lesion but neurological tissue is rarely involved.
   • If disability is present, impaired bowel and bladder function and foot weakness are most likely.
  (b) Myelomeningocele.
   • Meninges and parts of the spinal cord protrude from the abnormally formed spine in a sac at the level of lesion.
   • Disability includes paralysis and loss of sensation below the level of the lesion.
   • Extent of disability depends on level of lesion and scope of neurological involvement.
 b. Signs/symptoms.
  (1) Meningitis may result due to infection of exposed tissue if lesion is not closed soon after birth.
  (2) Hydrocephalus.
   (a) Increased accumulation of cerebrospinal fluid within the ventricles of the brain occurs in 60%–90% of children with myelomeningocele.
   (b) Treated with a ventriculoperitoneal shunt.
    • Shunt precautions.
     * Avoid placing pressure on the shunt.
     * Avoid stretching the neck.
     * Do not place child in Trendelen burg's position.
    ⚑ **Red Flag**
     • The clinician must be aware of the signs of shunt malfunction: irritability, vomiting, fontanel bulging, lethargy, headache and changes in behavior, coordination or seizure activity.
  (3) Arnold-Chiari malformation, type II.
   (a) Common in children with myelomeningocele.
   (b) Brainstem and cerebellum protrude into the spinal canal through the foramen magnum.
   (c) Can result in compression of spinal cord with resulting symptoms.
    • Dysphagia.
    • Feeding difficulties.
    • Trouble breathing.
    • Choking.
    • Arm stiffness.
  (4) Tethered cord.
   (a) Congenital anomaly or scarring/adhesion of the spinal cord tissue to overlying dura or skin.

   (b) May result in increased neurological problems as child grows and traction of spinal nerves results in damage to the nerves.
   ⚑ **Red Flag**
    • Older children who demonstrate a rapid decline in function or increase in and development of new symptoms may be experiencing a tethered cord and further medical evaluation is warranted.
  (5) Orthopedic deformities from lack of movement in utero.
   (a) Clubfeet.
   (b) Bowed long bones.
   (c) Hip flexion contractures.
   (d) Dislocated hips.
   (e) Scoliosis or kyphosis.
  (6) Additional complications.
   (a) Obesity.
   (b) Osteoporosis.
   (c) Incontinence of bowel and bladder (with lesion at or above S2).
   (d) Skin breakdown due to lack of sensation.
   (e) Learning problems.
   (f) Visual-perceptual problems.
   (g) Seizures.
   (h) Developmental delays.
   (i) Latex allergy.
   ⚑ **Red Flag**
    • Latex allergy can range from a rash to severe pulmonary crisis. Inspect all items that will come in contact with the child for the presence of latex. Common items include medical gloves, balloon, rubber toys, adhesive tape and pacifiers.
  (7) Level of disability (Table 8-6).

3. **Physical therapy intervention.**
 a. Family education.
  (1) Positioning to prevent/minimize joint deformities, especially hip, knee and ankle flexion contractures.
  (2) Handling to support flaccid lower limbs and reduce risk of fracture due to osteoporosis.
  (3) Activities to promote development.
  (4) Use of assistive devices to promote optimal development in all areas.
  (5) Awareness of potential shunt malfunction.
 b. Maximize functional skills.
  (1) Strengthening through play.
  (2) Stretching tight joints and muscles.
  (3) Fit and teach use of appropriate assistive devices to promote normal developmental activities.
  (4) Fit and teach use of proper orthotic devices.
  (5) Facilitation of functional motor development.

Table 8-6 ➤ LEVEL OF FUNCTIONAL SKILLS FOR MYELOMENINGOCELE

LEVEL OF LESION	INNERVATED MUSCLES	FUNCTIONAL PROGNOSIS	ASSISTIVE DEVICES
Thoracic	Neck, upper limbs, shoulder girdle, trunk muscles.	No lower limb movements. Trunk muscles may be weak. Arms may be weak due to lack of trunk stability. Will use wheelchair for most mobility. No bowel or bladder control.	Power wheelchair, manual wheelchair, reciprocating gait orthosis, standing frame, and body jacket for spinal stability.
High lumbar (L1-2)	As above, plus hip flexors.	Weak hip flexion. May develop dislocated hips. May ambulate short distances with assistive devices. No bowel and bladder control. At risk for hip flexion contractures.	Power wheelchair, manual wheelchair, reciprocating gait orthosis, standing frame, HKAFO, rollator walker, forearm crutches.
Mid lumbar (L3-4)	As above, plus hip adductors, knee extensors and flexors, may have some ankle dorsiflexion (L4).	No sensation in lower legs or feet. Walks short distance with aids while young. No bowel or bladder control.	KAFO, AFO, walker, forearm crutches, wheelchair for longer distances.
Low lumbar (L4-5)	As above plus weak hip extension and abduction, weak plantar flexion against gravity with eversion.	Sensation impaired in lower legs and feet. Can walk without orthoses, but needs aids due to fatigue. Can ride a bicycle, no bowel and bladder control.	AFO, crutches.
Sacral	As above plus increased strength in ankle plantar flexion and dorsiflexion, more control of intrinsic foot muscles.	Sensation impaired in feet. Good hip strength and function. Can walk without support. Bowel and bladder control may be impaired.	AFO

Down's Syndrome (Trisomy 21)

1. **Basic information.**
   a. Results from malformation of the 21st chromosome.
   b. Types.
      (1) Nondisjunction.
         (a) Extra chromosome present on the 21st pair.
         (b) Over 90% of individuals with Down's syndrome have this type.
      (2) Translocation.
         (a) Third copy of the 21st chromosome is attached to another pair of chromosomes.
         (b) In 25% of cases it results from one or both parents being carriers.
      (3) Mosaic.
         (a) Some cells in the body exhibit normal chromosomes and others exhibit abnormal chromosomes in the 21st pair.
         (b) Degree of disability is dependent on the percent of cells exhibiting abnormal chromosomes.
   c. Increasing maternal and, in a small percentage, paternal age has been linked to increased incidence of Down's syndrome.

2. **Clinical picture.**
   a. Characteristic features.
      (1) Upward slant to eyes.
      (2) Small ears and mouth with protruding tongue.
      (3) Palmar crease on feet or hands.
      (4) Microcephaly with flattened occiput.
      (5) Short stature (average height is under 5 feet).
   b. Hypotonia leading to decreased strength and joint hypermobility.

   c. Congenital heart defects.
   d. Visual and hearing deficits.
   e. Mental retardation.
   f. Speech and articulation disorders.
   g. Feeding difficulties, especially in the early years.
   h. Developmental delays in all areas, including delayed postural reactions and motor development.
   i. Other related problems.
      (1) Hypothyroidism.
      (2) Vertebral instability at the atlantoaxial (C1-2) joint.
         (a) Acute or gradual spinal cord injury, especially with a sudden incident of hyperflexion.
         (b) Important to identify as early symptoms as these indicate a medical emergency.
            • Weakness and loss of functional skills, including ambulation.
            • Change in deep tendon reflexes and sensation.

   ➢ **Red Flag**
      • If a screening radiograph demonstrates instability, activities to avoid include diving, tumbling, headstands, contact sports and any other activities that could cause a hyperflexion injury to the neck.

3. **Physical therapy intervention.**
   a. Facilitate gross motor skill development.
      (1) Encourage postural control and movement.
      (2) Promote activities that facilitate increasing strength, motor control and gross and fine motor development.
   b. Support oral-motor skills: facilitate lip closure and inhibit tongue protrusion.
   c. Patient and family education.

Duchenne Muscular Dystrophy (Pseudohypertrophic Muscular Dystrophy)

1. Basic information.

a. Most common form of congenital, degenerative sex-linked disease of muscle tissue.

b. Almost all affected are boys.

c. Lack of dystrophin increases muscle cell membrane permeability: calcium infiltrates cells and muscle tissue breaks down.

2. Clinical picture.

a. Progressive muscle weaknesses from proximal to distal muscles.

  (1) Gower's sign.

    (a) Child pushes up from the floor on his hands, walking hands up legs to stand.

    (b) Due to weak knee and hip extensors.

    (c) Typically occurs by 4 to 7 years of age.

  (2) Waddling gait and falls are typical.

b. Pseudohypertrophic muscles: muscles appear hypertrophied as fat and connective tissue replace muscle tissue in calves, deltoids, quadriceps and tongue.

c. Contractures: result from significant muscle imbalances, most commonly in heel cords, tensor fascia latae, hip flexors and hamstrings.

d. Lumbar lordosis, thoracic kyphosis and scoliosis.

e. Cardiac muscle myopathy.

f. Mild to moderate intellectual impairment becomes evident as child gets older.

g. Progression:

  (1) Age 3–5: weakness, tripping, Gower's sign.

  (2) Age 6–8: gait deviations (toe walking, wide base of support), lordosis, unable to ascend stairs, poor endurance.

  (3) Age 9–11: walks with braces or may lose ambulation skills.

  (4) Age 12–14: loss of ambulation skills, increased obesity, development of spinal deformities, increasing contractures at hips, knees and elbows.

  (5) Age 15–17: increased respiratory compromise may lead to assisted ventilation, dependent in most ADLs.

  (6) Young adulthood: increased dependence, death in early 20s due to increasing respiratory compromise.

3. Physical therapy intervention.

a. Work with family, child and team of providers to determine how to best support child as functional skills diminish.

b. Maintain range of motion via positioning, splinting and stretching.

c. Maintain ambulation and standing skills.

d. Utilize assistive devices: braces, crutches, standing frames and dynamic standers.

e. Maintain functional skills, including communication and mobility, by utilizing power wheelchairs and augmentative and alternative communication devices.

f. Maintain cardiorespiratory function and strength via spontaneous, active motion through normal recreation and ADL.

☞ Red Flag

• The clinician should avoid strengthening exercises in order to preserve muscle tissue. Aquatic therapy may be a good alternative as it can build strength and endurance while not increasing rate of tissue breakdown.

Pervasive Developmental Disorder (PDD)

1. Basic information.

a. Spectrum of neurobiological disorders related to specific abnormalities in brain function, of which autism is the most common.

b. Causes of autism are largely unknown but some genetic factors have been identified.

c. Other common disorders in the PDD spectrum.

  (1) Rett's syndrome: onset 6–18 months, only in girls, with severe apraxia, seizures, lack of speech and hand flapping.

  (2) Asperger's disorder: milder form of autism with social isolation, eccentric behavior and differences in speech inflection and patterns.

  (3) PDD-NOS (not otherwise specified): marked impairment of social interaction, communication and stereotyped behavior patterns but does not meet the full definition for a diagnosis of autism.

  (4) Childhood disintegrative disorder: period of at least 2 years of typical development followed by loss of previously acquired skills occurring before the age of 10.

2. Clinical picture of autism.

a. Symptoms usually become apparent between 2 and 3 years of age.

b. Impairments in communication.

  (1) Delays or abnormalities in expressive and receptive language skills.

  (2) Nonverbal communication.

  (3) Echolalic (immediate, involuntary repetition of words heard from another person) speech.

  (4) Flat and monotonous, or high pitched and loud voice.

c. Impairments in socialization.

  (1) Difficulty maintaining eye contact.

  (2) Do not understand gestures and social cues.

  (3) Prefer to be alone.

d. Impairments in imagination.

  (1) Prefer predictable events and objects.

    (2) Play with objects in stereotypical ways rather than imaginative (spinning car wheels instead of making car "drive").

  e. Abnormal relationships to objects and events.

    (1) Routine is essential and changes to routine can lead to behavior issues.

    (2) Difficulty with new situations, objects, people.

    (3) Stereotypical mannerisms and behaviors (hand flapping, head banging, rocking).

  f. May have abnormalities in muscle tone (usually low), decreased strength, poor balance, clumsiness and delays in gross motor skills.

  g. Difficult behaviors including temper tantrums and social withdrawal.

3. Physical therapy considerations.

  a. Use familiar objects and routines.

  b. Prepare the child for changes in routine.

  c. Follow behavioral protocols.

  d. Speak clearly and keep instructions simple.

  e. Encourage eye contact with child during communication.

  f. Structure environment to teach appropriate social skills with peers.

  g. Use daily activities to increase strength and functional skills (e.g., climbing stairs, running on the playground).

  ▷ **Red Flag**

    • Each child will likely follow a different behavior plan. The clinician must know the guidelines of the plan and follow it every day in order to help the child develop appropriate behaviors.

    • Consistency in approach and daily schedule is necessary.

Mental Retardation/Developmental Disability/Developmental Delay

1. Basic information.

  a. Mental retardation: subaverage intellectual functioning that manifests before age 18.

  b. Developmental disability: manifests before age 22 and likely continues through life.

  c. Developmental delay: usually diagnosed in children less than 3 years of age; can be used with children as old as 9 years in order to qualify for special education under the Individuals with Disabilities Education Act (IDEA).

2. Clinical picture.

  a. Mental retardation is decreased intellectual functioning with concurrent limitations in two or more adaptive skill areas: communication, self-care, home living, social skills, community use, self-direction, health and safety, functional academics, leisure and work.

  b. Developmental disability substantially limits functioning in three or more areas: self-care, receptive and expressive language, learning, mobility, self-direction, capacity for independent living, economic self-sufficiency; requires individualized interdisciplinary services for extended duration.

  c. Developmental delay.

    (1) Delay in one or more of the following areas: gross motor skills, fine motor skills, language skills and social skills.

    (2) May result in later diagnosis of developmental disability or resolve with intervention or maturation.

3. Physical therapy intervention.

  a. Services utilized are dependent on strengths and needs of the child and family.

  b. Common goals of intervention: gait, strength, endurance, flexibility, balance and motor planning.

  c. Treatment focuses on play to increase strength, endurance and functional activities.

  d. Utilize orthoses, adaptive equipment and assistive technology.

  e. Work with the child as part of a team that includes the child and family.

Sickle Cell Anemia

1. Basic information: autosomal recessive genetic trait found in people of African or Mediterranean descent.

2. Clinical picture.

  a. Abnormally shaped red blood cells cause health impairments.

    (1) Sickled cells cannot pass through small capillaries and cause blockages resulting in poor oxygen supply to some tissues.

    (2) Cells break down faster than normal, causing jaundice.

    (3) Lack of adequate red blood cells causes anemia.

  b. Symptoms (vary with each child).

    (1) Fatigue due to anemia.

    (2) Organ enlargement, necrosis, scarring and pain due to occluded blood vessels in highly vascularized organs such as spleen, liver, bones and kidneys.

    (3) Stroke.

    (4) Skin ulcers.

3. Physical therapy intervention.

  a. Dependent on needs of the child and must occur as part of a team effort.

  b. Encourage general exercise to maintain strength and endurance.

  c. Strengthening exercises to address orthopedic needs.

  d. Intervention considerations.

(1) Developmental therapy for children with motor delays due to pain, fatigue, multiple surgeries or stroke.

(2) Orthopedic intervention for children with fractures due to osteoporosis.

(3) Wound care (including debridement) for children with skin ulcers.

Application Concepts

- Contracture formation is present in a variety of the congenital pediatric disorders. While not totally preventable, the PTA can play a major role in limiting contractures by providing appropriate patient and family education on positioning and stretching.
- Persistence of primitive reflexes (ATNR, STNR, TLR) often limits the development of normal movements. The PTA should work to decrease the influence of these reflexes prior to implementing functional activity training.
- Physical therapy will often focus on increasing functional mobility and independence in the school and home environments. The PTA should remember this when working with the patient and family to determine goals and therapeutic activities.
- Since many of these disorders have a genetic component or are related to a maternal issue during pregnancy, the PTA should be prepared to face family members taking or placing blame for the child's condition. Additionally, many family members will be going through the grieving process in the early stages following diagnosis. If not comfortable dealing with these issues, the PTA should consult with a social worker.

Special Considerations when Working with the Pediatric Population

Team Members

1. **Family.**
   a. Family is the primary context for the child and, as such, PTs and PTAs must collaborate with family members as full members of any team servicing a child.
   b. Family members are constant in a child's life, whereas medical and educational personnel change.

2. **Teamwork.**
   a. Intradisciplinary: involves collaborating with colleagues in the same discipline about a particular child or problem.
   b. Multidisciplinary: many disciplines work with the same child, each writing separate reports and developing discipline-specific goals and treatment activities.
   c. Interdisciplinary: many disciplines work with the same child and collaborate with each other in some aspects of care, including assessment, report writing, planning goals and providing intervention.
   d. Transdisciplinary: requiring "role release" between disciplines it is most likely to occur in early intervention settings where multiple service providers would be inefficient, intrusive and confusing to the child and family.

Environments of Care

1. **Medical systems.**
   a. Usually address acute and chronic health issues.
   b. Settings include hospitals, rehabilitation centers, outpatient clinics.
   c. May assist a child and family with the transition to community care systems such as early intervention programs and schools.

2. **Educational systems.**
   a. Usually address educational and vocational issues.
   b. Settings include early intervention programs, schools and vocational programs.
   c. Services for children are tailored to the system of care that is providing the service and therefore may vary according to the setting.

Legislation Guiding the Provision of Services

1. **IDEA.**
   a. Initially authorized in 1975 as the Education for All Handicapped Children's Act (Public Law 94-142) and most recently reauthorized in 2004 (Public Law 108-446).
   b. A federal program overseen by the states and implemented at the district level.

c. Part C provides services for children birth to three years of age and their families.
    (1) Includes public awareness, child find activities (identification of children in need of services) and service to eligible children.
    (2) Providers deliver services that are family directed and occur in natural environments whenever possible.
    (3) An Individualized Family Service Plan (IFSP) is developed by providers and the child's family to address the needs of the child and the family.
d. Part B provides services for individuals between 3 and 21 years of age.
    (1) Services are child-centered and mandated to support the individual's educational (not medical) needs.
    (2) FAPE: all children are guaranteed a *free, appropriate, public education.*
    (3) LRE: educational services must be provided in the *least restrictive environment.*
    (4) IEP: an Individualized Educational Plan is devised for each child.
        (a) Developed by all individuals working with the child, including classroom staff and parents.
        (b) Includes present levels of performance, goals and objectives, services to be provided and evaluation criteria.
    (5) Special education is provided to meet the unique and individual needs of the child.
    (6) Related services, including physical therapy, are provided when necessary to allow the child to benefit from the special education services provided.

(7) Vocational programs.
    (a) Schools are required to have transition plans in place in the IEP by the time a child is 16 years of age.
    (b) Adult vocational service systems may be part of this plan.
    (c) Children must be eligible to receive services.

2. **The Rehabilitation Act of 1973, Section 504.**
    a. Civil rights legislation that addresses the rights of all children with disabilities, whether or not they qualify for special education.
    b. Includes appropriate accommodations, educational and related services needed by the child.

3. **The Americans with Disabilities Act (ADA).**
    a. Legislation passed in 1990 that addresses civil rights for all Americans with disabilities, including children.

Application Concepts

- Play is what children are about and, in turn, should be the focus of pediatric therapy.
- Multidisciplinary teams are the most beneficial when working with children and families but take a great deal of trust and coordination on the part of the team members.
- All children, regardless of ability or disability, have the right to receive an education that is appropriate for their level of functioning.
- While many parents will desire services, all related services (including physical therapy) can only be provided in the school district when they are limiting the child's ability to benefit from their special education.

Geriatric Physical Therapy

SUSAN B. O'SULLIVAN

Focus Areas for Content Review:

- Anatomy and physiology changes that occur due to the normal aging process.
- Pathologies and injuries common to geriatric patient's/client's seen in physical therapy.
- Physical therapy intervention strategies commonly utilized with older adult clients including indications and contraindications, appropriate responses, and PTA response to adverse reaction.

- Tests and measures utilized with older adult clients that provide information to guide the PTA in determining the patient's ability to participate in and/or indication to discontinue intervention as well as to document the patient's progress toward the established goals.
- Common goals/outcome expectations for older adults receiving physical therapy services.
- Psychosocial issues that are unique to older adults and how to adjust interventions strategies to accommodate these issues.

Definitions and Theories of Aging

Aging

1. General Concepts and Definitions

2. Aging: the progressive and cumulative physiological, biological and functional changes in the body systems. A complex and variable process from individual to individual; common to all members of a given species; evidenced by a decline in homeostatic efficiency; increasing probability that reaction to injury will not be diminished or unsuccessful.

3. Gerontology: the scientific study of the factors impacting the normal aging process and the effects of aging.

4. Geriatrics: the branch of medicine concerned with the illnesses of old age and their care.

5. Life span: maximum survival potential, the inherent natural life of the species.

6. Life expectancy: the number of years of life expectation from year of birth.
   a. 77.7 years in United States, 2006.
   b. Women live 6.6 years longer than men.

7. Senescence: last stages of adulthood through death.

8. Categories of elderly: young elderly ages 65–74 (60% of elderly population); old elderly ages 75–84; old, old elderly or frail elderly: ages >85.

9. Ageism: discrimination and prejudice leveled against individuals on the basis of their age.

Theories of Aging

Many theories on aging exist. They can be grouped into the following categories.

1. Developmental – Genetic theories.
   a. Concepts include: aging is intrinsic in the organism; there are preprogrammed biological changes of tissues and cells that lead to aging; there are limits in the number of cell divisions that can be performed; cell damage results from free radicals, poor nutrition or hydration.

2. Nongenetic theories.
   Concepts include: environmental factors damage DNA; genetic mutation or changes in genes occur over time;

accumulation of cross-linked proteins damage tissues and cells.

3. **New theories of aging.**

a. Includes theories related to sleep and sleep pattern changes, imbalances and changes at the hormonal and cellular levels and genetic influences.

Demographics and Socioeconomic Costs

Demographics, Mortality and Morbidity

1. **Persons over 65 represent a rapidly growing segment of the population; by year 2030, it is expected that there will be over 69 million (21% of total population) elderly Americans.**
   a. Elderly women outnumber elderly men.
   b. Minority populations are projected to represent 25% of those aged 65+ by year 2030.

2. **Projections demonstrate those aged 85 and older will make up one-quarter of the elderly population by the year 2050.**

3. **Reasons for increased life expectancy, aging of the population.**
   a. Advances in healthcare include improved infectious disease control.
   b. Advances in infant/child care resulting in decreased mortality rates.
   c. Improvements in nutrition and sanitation.

4. **Leading causes of death (mortality) in persons over 65, in order of frequency.**
   a. Coronary heart disease (CHD), accounts for 31% of deaths.
   b. Cancer, accounts for 20% of deaths.
   c. Cerebrovascular disease (stroke).
   d. Chronic obstructive pulmonary disease (COPD).
   e. Pneumonia/flu.

5. **Leading causes of disability/chronic conditions (morbidity) in persons over 65, in order of frequency.**
   a. Arthritis, 49%.
   b. Hypertension, 37%.
   c. Hearing impairments, 32%.
   d. Heart impairments, 30%.
   e. Cataracts and chronic sinusitis, 17% each.
   f. Orthopedic impairments, 16%.
   g. Diabetes and visual impairments, 9% each.
   h. Tinnitus and varicose veins, 8% each.
   i. Most older persons (60%–80%) report having one or more chronic conditions.

Socioeconomic Factors

1. **Most elderly Americans live on fixed incomes.**

2. **About half of older persons have completed high school.**

3. **Noninstitutionalized elderly: most live in family setting.**

4. **Institutionalized elderly: about 5% of persons over 65 reside in nursing homes; percentage increases dramatically with age (22% of persons over 85).**

5. **Older persons account for:**
   a. 12% of population and 36% of total healthcare expenditures.
   b. 33% of all hospital stays and 44% of all hospital days of care.

Patient Care Concepts

Principles of Geriatric Rehabilitation

1. **Recognize variability of older adults.**
   a. Uniqueness of the individual.
   b. Developmental issues unique to the elderly.

2. **Focus on careful and accurate clinical assessments to identify remediable problems.**

a. Determined by physical therapist at time of initial evaluation.
b. Ongoing assessment by physical therapist assistant.
   (1) Determine capacity for safe function.
   (2) Determine effects of inactivity versus activity.
   (3) Determine effects of normal aging versus disease pathologies.

3. Focus on functional goals.
   a. Determine priorities, remediable problems.
   b. Implement plan of care in conjunction with patient/caregiver.

4. Promote optimal health.
   a. Focus on increasing health conducive behaviors, prevention of disability.
   b. Minimize and compensate for health-related losses and impairments of aging.

5. Recognize that research supports factors beyond genetics that contribute to quality of life.
   a. Psychosocial factors: e.g., perceptions of health, balance between abilities and challenges, relationships, social support, external resources, personal attitude.
   b. Maximize patient involvement in goal setting and treatment planning.
   c. Maximize patient autonomy: e.g., assistive devices, environmental modification.
   d. Be sensitive to cultural and ethnicity issues.
   e. Enhance coping skills: seek/provide resources for social networking.
   f. Maximize patient active role in rehabilitation process, recognize functional abilities.

6. Holism: consider the whole patient; integrate all facets of an individual's life; determine social support systems, effects of social isolation; determine effects of losses; determine effects of depression, dementia.

7. Recognize demands for continuity of care, interactions in a complex healthcare delivery system.
   a. Advocate for needed services.
   b. Provide effective documentation.

Ethical and Legal Issues

1. Professional practice affirms patient rights and dignity (professional ethical standards, American Physical Therapy Association [APTA] Code of Ethics).

2. Informed consent.
   a. Respect for personal autonomy.
      (1) Competent patients have the right to refuse treatment; e.g., do not resuscitate (DNR) orders.
   b. Legal right to self-determination.
      (1) Information must be provided to patient that outlines:
         (a) The nature and purpose of treatment.
         (b) Treatment alternatives.
         (c) Risks and consequences of treatment.
         (d) Likelihood of success or failure of treatment.
   c. Consent must be obtained from a legal guardian if the individual is judged incompetent.
      (1) Older adults with fluctuating mental abilities must be carefully evaluated for periods of lucidity.
      (2) Documentation with a mental status exam is essential.

3. Advance Care Medical Directive (Living Will) established by federal Patient Self-Determination Act of 1990.
   a. Healthcare proxy (durable power of attorney)
      (1) Identifies a valid agent who is granted the authority to make healthcare decisions for an individual should that individual become incapacitated.
   b. Requirements.
      (1) Regulated by individual states; specific requirements vary by state.
      (2) Must be in writing.
         (a) Signed by principal; witnessed by two adults.
      (3) Empowers healthcare agent.
         (a) Includes specific guidelines as to which treatment options will be allowed, which will not; e.g., artificial life support, feeding tubes.
      (4) Defines conditions/scope of agent's authority.

Physiological Changes and Adaptations Associated with Aging

Cellular Changes

1. Total number of cells decreases with age.
   a. Cells are less organized in function and have more variation.

2. Aging interferes with apoptosis (the preprogrammed cell death that does not release harmful substances into surrounding tissues).
   a. Apoptosis slowed; programmed cell death does not occur, leads to cancers such as leukemia. Cancer cells do not die but rather they invade surrounding healthy tissue.
   b. Apoptosis accelerated, killing healthy good cells, leads to tissue damage and disorders such as Parkinson's, Alzheimer's and Huntington's diseases.

Cartilage

1. **Cartilage: relies on blood flow from adjacent bones and movement of synovial fluid for nutrients.**
   a. Normally thins with age; degenerative changes are not reversible; decreased hydration and increasing fibrous growth around bony prominences can contribute to stiffness at joints.
   b. Cellular changes in the matrix of cartilage decreases the ability of cartilage to maintain hydration and nutrition.
   c. Regular weight-bearing exercise is critical to maintain hyaline cartilage; with inactivity, hyaline cartilage is converted to fibrocartilage.
   d. Compressive forces followed by release are necessary for movement of nutrients and waste products into and out of cartilage.

2. **Red Flag: Intervention implications.**
   a. Activity that reinforces alternate compressive (weight bearing) and relaxing forces can help maintain health of cartilage.
   b. Maintenance of strength around joints can help decrease joint stress.

Muscular System

1. **Changes in muscle may be due more to decreased activity levels and disuse than directly from the aging process.**
   a. Some loss of strength and muscle mass is part of the normal aging process (sarcopenia); decreased activity levels can lead to weakness resulting in increased prevalence of falls; dietary changes such as decreased intake of energy and protein can negatively affect muscle loss.
   b. Muscular endurance: muscles fatigue more readily due to decreased muscle tissue oxidative capacity and decreased peripheral blood flow.
   c. Muscle strength: will be less than that of a younger person; however, it can be increased and maintained in the elderly; girth measurements are not a reliable measure of improved strength in the elderly.
      (1) Strength peaks at age 30 and remains relatively constant until age 50, after which there is accelerating loss of strength (15%–20% per decade) in the sixth to seventh decade and increases to 30% per decade after that in the nonexercising adult.
   d. Muscle power: significant declines due to losses in speed of contraction secondary to changes in nerve conduction and synaptic transmission.

2. **Intervention implications.**
   a. Muscle strength can be increased and maintained in the aging individual.

   b. Norms for muscle strength testing will be less than that of a younger individual and are best judged on ability to perform functional and recreational activities rather than on strength testing.
   c. Girth measurements are not reliable measures of improved strength (see section 1.b above).

Skeletal System

1. **Normal aging results in bone mass and density loss; decreasing levels of activated vitamin D$_3$ circulating in blood stream causes less calcium to be absorbed; imbalance in osteoblast (bone building) and osteoclast (bone breakdown) activity; osteoclast activity is stronger and leads to bone loss.**
   a. Women who are postmenopausal have decreased estrogen levels which influence parathyroid hormone and calcitonin to increase bone reabsorption.
   b. Other contributing factors to bone loss can include: hyperthyroidism, steroid therapy, decreased progesterone.
   c. Peak bone mass is gained in the late teens and twenties, bone loss begins after that; between ages 45 and 70, bone mass decreases (women by about 25%; men by 15%); decreases another 5% by age 90; with aging, calcium absorption diminishes.
      (1) Loss of calcium, bone strength, especially trabecular bone (age-related trabecular bone loss starts at age 35, cortical bone loss starts around age 40).
   d. Postural changes: forward head, increased kyphosis of the thoracic spine, flattening of lumbar lordosis, hip and knee flexion contractures secondary to increased sitting.

2. **Intervention implications.**
   a. Weight-bearing exercise can help maintain and improve bone strength.
   b. Muscle cocontractions and progressive resistive exercise has been shown to improve bone strength.
   c. **Red Flag:** Persons with weaker bones are more prone to fracture; fall risk assessment should be performed.

Body Fat Composition

1. **Body fat increases in mid life (women until late 60s; men until late 50s) and then decreases; women's body fat decreases more slowly.**

2. **Body fat distribution changes: moves from under skin to deeper areas of body; women tend to store fat in their lower body (hips, thighs) and men tend to store it in the abdomen.**

Neurological System

1. Age-related changes.

a. Atrophy of nerve cells in cerebral cortex: overall loss of cerebral mass/brain weight of 6%–11% between ages of 20 and 90; accelerating loss after age 70.

b. Changes in brain morphology.

  (1) Generalized cell loss in cerebral cortex: especially frontal and temporal lobes' association areas (prefrontal cortex, visual).

  (2) Presence of lipofuscins, senile or neuritic plaques and neurofibrillary tangles (NFTs): significant accumulations associated with pathology; e.g., Alzheimer's dementia.

  (3) More selective cell loss in basal ganglia (substantia nigra and putamen), cerebellum, hippocampus, locus ceruleus; brainstem minimally affected.

c. Decreased cerebral blood flow and energy metabolism.

d. Changes in synaptic transmission.

  (1) Decreased synthesis and metabolism, as well as delay in impulse conduction and synaptic transmission of major neurotransmitters: e.g. serotonin, catecholamines and dopamine. (Dopamine loss is associated with Parkinson's disease).

  (2) Slowing of many neural processes, especially in polysynaptic pathways.

e. Changes in spinal cord/peripheral nerves.

  (1) Neuronal loss and atrophy: 30%–50% loss of anterior horn cells, 30% loss of posterior roots (sensory fibers) by age 90.

  (2) Loss of motoneurons results in increase in size of remaining motor units (development of macromotor units).

  (3) Loss of sympathetic fibers may account for: diminished autonomic stability, increased incidence of postural hypotension in older adults.

f. Age-related tremors (essential tremors [ETs]).

  (1) Occur as an isolated symptom, particularly in hands, head and voice.

  (2) Characterized as postural or kinetic, rarely resting.

  (3) Benign, slowly progressive; in late stages may limit function.

  (4) Exaggerated by movement and emotion.

2. Movement implications.

a. Effects on movement.

  (1) Overall speed and coordination are decreased; increased difficulties with fine motor control.

  (2) Slowed recruitment of motoneurons contributes to loss of strength.

  (3) Both reaction time and movement time are increased.

  (4) Older adults are affected by the speed/accuracy trade-off.

    (a) The simpler the movement, the less the change.

    (b) More complicated movements require more preparation, longer reaction and movement times.

    (c) Faster movements decrease accuracy, increase errors.

  (5) Older adults typically shift in motor control processing from open to closed loop; e.g., demonstrate increased reliance on visual feedback for movement.

  (6) Demonstrate increased cautionary behaviors; an indirect effect of decreased capacity.

b. General slowing of neural processing: learning and memory may be affected.

c. Problems in homeostatic regulation: stressors (heat, cold, excess exercise) can be harmful, even life threatening.

3. Medical management.

a. Correction of medical problems.

b. Improve health: diet, smoking cessation.

4. Intervention, implications and compensatory strategies.

a. Increase levels of physical activity: encourages neuronal branching, slows rate of neural decline, improves cerebral circulation.

b. Provide effective strategies to improve motor learning and control.

  (1) Allow for increased reaction and movement times: will improve motivation, accuracy of movements.

  (2) Allow for limitations of memory: avoid long sequences of movements.

  (3) Allow for increased cautionary behaviors: provide adequate explanation and/or demonstration when teaching new movement skills.

  (4) Stress familiar, well-learned skills: incorporate repetitive movements.

Application Concepts

• Allow additional reaction time: overall movements and reaction times become slower; there may be decreased functional mobility and movement limitations; movements may be stiffer, fewer automatic movements.

• Approach tissue-stretching activities carefully: connective tissues become more dense and stiff and less elastic; increased risk for strains/strains/tears; increased tendency for fibrinous adhesions and contractures.

• Recognize normal gait changes: slower cadence, shorter steps, wider base of support, increased double-support phase (safety, compensate for

balance disturbance), decreased trunk rotation and arm swing; less steady gait.
- Provide strength training: significant increases in strength can be achieved through isometric and progressive resistive programs; higher intensity training (70%–80% max) produces changes more quickly and more predictably than moderate-intensity programs (both, however, are successful). Decreases in muscle function are typically more related to decreased levels in activity than to the aging process itself.

Sensory Systems

1. **Vision.**
   a. Aging changes: there is a general decline in visual acuity; gradual prior to sixth decade, more rapid decline between ages 60 and 90; visual loss may be as much as 80% by age 90. Changes can include.
      (1) Presbyopia: visual loss in middle and older ages characterized by inability to focus properly and blurred image; due to loss of accommodation, elasticity of lens.
      (2) Decreased reaction time to adapt to changes of dark and light; reduced ability to quickly change focus from far to near.
      (3) Increased sensitivity to light and glare.
      (4) Loss of color discrimination, especially for blues and greens.
      (5) Decreased pupillary responses; size of resting pupil increases.
      (6) Decreased sensitivity of corneal reflex; less sensitive to eye injury or infection.
      (7) Oculomotor responses diminished: restricted upward gaze; reduced pursuit eye movements; ptosis may develop.
   b. Additional vision loss with pathology.
      (1) Cataracts: opacity; clouding of lens due to changes in lens proteins; results in gradual loss of vision: central first, then peripheral; increased problems with glare; general darkening of vision: loss of acuity, distortion.
      (2) Glaucoma: increased intraocular pressure, with degeneration of optic disc; atrophy of optic nerve; results in early loss of peripheral vision (tunnel vision), progressing to total blindness.
      (3) Senile macular degeneration: loss of central vision associated with age-related degeneration of the macula compromised by decreased blood supply or abnormal growth of blood vessels under the retina; initially patients retain peripheral vision, may progress to total blindness.
      (4) Diabetic retinopathy: damage to retinal capillaries, growth of abnormal blood vessels and hemorrhage leads to retinal scarring and finally

retinal detachment; central vision impairment; complete blindness is rare.
      (5) CVA, homonymous hemianopsia: loss of one-half visual field in each eye (nasal half of one eye and temporal half of other eye); produces an inability to receive information from right or left side; corresponds to side of sensorimotor deficit.
      (6) Medications: impaired or fuzzy vision may result with antihistamines, tranquilizers, antidepressants, steroids.
   c. Intervention, implications and compensatory strategies.
      (1) Assess for visual deficits: acuity, peripheral vision, light and dark adaptation, depth perception, diplopia.
      (2) Be sure individual is wearing glasses if applicable.
      (3) Allow extra time for visual discrimination and response.
      (4) Work in adequate light, reduce glare; avoid abrupt changes in light, light to dark.
      (5) Decreased peripheral vision may limit social interactions, physical function: stand directly in front of patient at eye level when communicating with patient.
      (6) Assist in color discrimination: use warm colors (yellow, orange, red) for identification and color coding.
      (7) Provide other sensory cues when vision is limited: e.g., verbal descriptions to new environments, touching to communicate you are listening.
      (8) Provide safety education; reduce fall risk.
      (9) Report all findings to physical therapist for appropriate changes to plan of care warranted.

2. **Hearing.**
   a. Aging changes: occur as early as fourth decade; affects a significant number of elderly (23% of individuals aged 65–74 have hearing impairments and 40% over age 75 have hearing loss; rate of loss in men is twice the rate of women; also starts earlier).
      (1) Outer ear: build-up of cerumen (ear wax) may result in conductive hearing loss; common in older men.
      (2) Middle ear: minimal degenerative changes of bony joints.
      (3) Inner ear: significant changes in sound sensitivity, understanding of speech and maintenance of equilibrium may result with degeneration and atrophy of cochlea and vestibular structures, loss of neurons.
   b. Types of hearing loss.
      (1) Conductive: mechanical hearing loss from damage to external auditory canal, tympanic membrane or middle ear ossicles; results in hearing

loss (all frequencies); tinnitus (ringing in the ears) may be present.

   (2) Sensorineural: central or neural hearing loss from multiple factors; e.g., noise damage, trauma, disease, drugs, arteriosclerosis.

   (3) Presbycusis: sensorineural hearing loss associated with middle and older ages; characterized by bilateral hearing loss, especially at high frequencies at first, then all frequencies; poor auditory discrimination and comprehension, especially with background noise; tinnitus.

c. Additional hearing loss with pathology.

   (1) Otosclerosis: immobility of stapes results in profound conductive hearing loss.

   (2) Paget's disease.

   (3) Hypothyroidism.

d. Intervention, implications and compensatory strategies.

   (1) Determine if patient/client uses hearing aids; check for proper functioning.

   (2) Minimize auditory distractions: work in quiet environment.

   (3) Speak slowly and clearly, face patient/client.

   (4) Use nonverbal communication to reinforce your message: e.g., gesture, demonstration.

   (5) Orient person to topics of conversation that cannot be heard to reduce paranoia, isolation.

3. Vestibular/balance control.

a. Aging changes: vestibular system functions to monitor head position and detect movements of the head. Degenerative changes in otoconia of utricle and saccule; vestibular ocular reflex (VOR) gain decreases; begins at age 30, accelerating decline at ages 55–60 resulting in diminished vestibular sensation.

   (1) Diminished acuity, delayed reaction times, longer response times.

   (2) Reduced function of VOR; affects retinal image stability with head movements, produces blurred vision.

   (3) Altered sensory organization: older adults more dependent upon somatosensory inputs for balance.

   ⚑ (4) **Red Flag:** Less able to resolve sensory conflicts when presented with inappropriate visual or proprioceptive inputs due to vestibular losses.

   (5) Postural response patterns for balance are disorganized: characterized by diminished ankle torque, increased hip torque, increased postural sway.

b. Additional loss of vestibular sensitivity with pathology.

   (1) Ménière's disease: episodic attacks characterized by tinnitus, dizziness, a sensation of fullness or pressure in the ears; may also experience sensorineural hearing loss.

   (2) Benign paroxysmal positional vertigo (BPPV): brief episodes of vertigo (less than 1 minute) associated with position change; the result of degeneration of the utricular otoconia that settle on the cupula of the posterior semicircular canal; common in older adults.

   (3) Medications: antihypertensives (postural hypotension), anticonvulsants, tranquilizers, sleeping pills, aspirin, nonsteroidal anti-inflammatory drugs (NSAIDs).

   (4) Cerebrovascular disease: vertebrobasilar artery insufficiency (transient ischemic attack [TIAs], strokes), cerebellar artery stroke, lateral medullary stroke.

   (5) Cerebellar dysfunction: hemorrhage, tumors (acoustic neuroma, meningioma); degenerative disease of brainstem and cerebellum; progressive supranuclear palsy.

   (6) Migraine.

   (7) Cardiac disease.

c. Intervention, implications and compensatory strategies.

   ⚑ (1) **Red Flag:** Increased incidence of falls in older adults.

   (2) See section on falls and instability (VI.B).

4. Somatosensory.

a. Aging changes: decline in sensitivity to touch, temperature and vibration due to decline in sensibility of peripheral sensory receptors Meissner's corpuscles (touch, texture receptors), pacinian's corpuscles (pressure, vibration receptors) and Krause's corpuscles (temperature receptors).

   (1) Lower extremities may be more affected than upper.

   (2) Proprioceptive losses: increased thresholds in vibratory sensibility, beginning around age 50; greater in lower extremities than upper extremities; greater in distal extremities than proximal.

   (3) Loss of joint receptor sensitivity; losses in lower extremities; cervical joints may contribute to loss of balance.

   (4) Cutaneous pain thresholds increased: greater changes in upper body areas (upper extremities, face) than for lower extremities.

b. Additional loss of sensation with pathology.

   (1) Diabetes, peripheral neuropathy, cerebrovascular accident (CVA), central sensory losses, peripheral vascular disease, peripheral ischemia.

c. Intervention, implications and compensatory strategies.

   (1) Allow extra time for responses with increased thresholds.

   (2) Use touch to communicate: maximize physical contact; e.g., rubbing, stroking.

   (3) Highlight or enhance naturally occurring intrinsic feedback during movements: e.g., stretch, tapping.

CHAPTER 9

(4) Provide augmented feedback through appropriate sensory channels: e.g., walking on carpeted surfaces may be easier than on smooth floor.

(5) Teach compensatory strategies to prevent injury to anesthetic limbs, falls.

(6) Provide assistive devices as needed for fall prevention.

(7) Utilize biofeedback devices as appropriate (e.g., limb load monitor).

5. **Taste and smell.**
   a. Changes: gradual decrease in taste sensitivity; decreased smell sensitivity.
   b. Additional loss of sensation with:
      (1) Smoking.
      (2) Chronic allergies, respiratory infections.
      (3) Wearing dentures.
      (4) CVA, involvement of hypoglossal nerve.
   c. Clinical implications/compensatory strategies:
      (1) Decreased taste, enjoyment of food leads to poor diet and nutrition.
      (2) Older adults frequently increase use of taste enhancers: e.g., salt or sugar.
      (3) Decreased home safety: e.g., gas leaks, smoke.

Cognitive Changes

1. **Age-related changes.**
   a. No uniform decline in intellectual abilities throughout adulthood.
      (1) Changes do not typically show up until mid 60s; significant declines affecting everyday life do not show up until early 80s.
      (2) Most significant decline in measures of intelligence occurs in the years immediately preceding death (termed terminal drop).
   b. Tasks involving perceptual speed: show early declines (by age 39); require longer times to complete tasks.
   c. Numeric ability (tests of adding, subtracting and multiplying): abilities peak in mid 40s; well maintained until 60s.
   d. Verbal ability: abilities peak at age 30; well maintained until 60s.
   e. Memory: impairments are typically noted in short-term memory; long-term memory retained; most difficulty noted with novel or new learning conditions; use of memory tools, e.g., notes, reminder calls, beneficial.
   f. Learning: the ability to learn is not lost; new learning may take longer. Affected by increased cautiousness, anxiety, fast pace, interference from prior learning.

2. **Medical management.**
   a. Improve health.
      (1) Correction of medical problems: imbalances between oxygen supply and demand to central nervous system (CNS); e.g., cardiovascular disease, hypertension, diabetes, hypothyroidism.
      (2) Pharmacological changes: drug reevaluation; decreased use of multiple drugs; monitor closely for drug toxicity; reduction in chronic use of tobacco and alcohol; correction of nutritional deficiencies.

3. **Intervention, implications and compensatory strategies.**
   a. Use context-based strategies (e.g., practice stair climbing, perform many transfers in same situation) versus memorization (young adults); stress relationship, importance for function; decrease pace as appropriate, incorporate repetition; use memory tools.
   b. Increase physical activity.
   c. Increase mental activity.
      (1) Keep mentally engaged ("Use it or lose it"); e.g., chess, crossword puzzles, high level of reading, math games/puzzles.
      (2) Encourage engaged lifestyle: socially active; e.g., clubs, travel, work.
      (3) Cognitive training activities.
   d. Auditory processing may be decreased; provide written instructions.
   e. Provide stimulating, "enriching" environment; avoid environmental dislocation: e.g., hospitalization or institutionalization may produce disorientation and agitation in some elderly.
   f. Reduction of stress: counseling and family support.

Application Concepts

- Compensate for possible vestibular changes and balance difficulties.
- Provide additional time for responses with new learning.
- Use repetition.
- Use and encourage use of memory tools.
- Provide additional feedback: walking surface, touch, etc.
- Provide written instructions.
- Speak slowly, clearly, enunciating clearly, use appropriate volume for individual's abilities.
- Ensure well-lighted treatment and home environments; minimize glare.
- Limit moving from well-lighted to dark areas quickly.
- Use visual markers, warm colors (yellows, oranges and reds).

Cardiovascular System

1. **Age-related changes.**
   a. Changes more due to inactivity and disease than aging; no significant alteration in the work capacity of the heart.

b. Degenerative changes: slight increased heart size; mild increased thickness of ventricular wall; mild thickening of endocardium and valves (due to increased tissue density, cross-linking); nodular thickening at atrioventricular valves (due to repeated mechanical stress).

c. Heart rate (HR): resting HR and cardiac output show minimal changes; max HR decreases; HR response typically not affected at sub-max levels.
   (1) Rate at which HR peaks is increased: can lead to lower cardiac output and stroke volume, creating increased possibility of orthostatic hypotension.
   (2) Exercise response: aging heart will increase cardiac output by increasing stroke volume to meet demands.

d. Decline in neurohumoral control: baroreceptors less responsive to position changes; can lead to orthostatic hypotension.

e. Changes in conduction system: loss of pace maker cells in sinoatrial node (SA) node.

f. Changes in blood vessels: arteries thicken, less distensible; slowed exchange capillary walls; increased peripheral resistance.

g. Resting blood pressure rises: systolic greater than diastolic.

h. Decreased blood volume, hemopoietic activity of bone.

i. Increased blood coagulability.

2. **Implications for intervention.**
   a. Changes at rest are minor: resting heart rate and cardiac output relatively unchanged; resting blood pressures increase.
   b. Cardiovascular responses to exercise: blunted, decrease in heart rate acceleration, decrease maximal oxygen uptake and heart rate, reduced exercise capacity, increased recovery time.
   c. Decreased stroke volume due to decreased myocardial contractility.
   d. Maximum heart rate declines with age (HRmax = 220 – age).
   e. Cardiac output decreases 1% per year after age 20; due to decreased heart rate and stroke volume.
   f. Orthostatic hypotension: common problem in elderly due to reduced baroreceptor sensitivity and vascular elasticity.
   g. Increased fatigue; anemia common in elderly.
   h. Systolic ejection murmur common in elderly.
   i. Possible electrocardiographic (ECG) changes: loss of normal sinus rhythm; longer PR and QT intervals; wider QRS; increased arrhythmias.

Application Concepts
- Avoid quick changes to position—secondary to increased potential for orthostatic hypotension.

- Avoid exercise following a moderate meal.
- Maximum heart rate is decreased in elderly.
- Healthy life styles help decrease effects of aging.

Pulmonary System

1. **Age-related changes.**
   a. Chest wall stiffness, changes in spinal curvature and declining strength of intercostal muscles results in increased work of breathing.
   b. Loss of lung elastic recoil, decreased lung compliance.
   c. Changes in lung parenchyma: alveoli enlarge, become thinner; fewer capillaries for delivery of blood; less effective oxygen uptake.
   d. Changes in pulmonary blood vessels: thicken, less distensible.
   e. Decline in lung capacity: residual volume increases (amount of air remaining in lungs after maximum expiration), vital capacity (volume of air that can be forcibly exhaled) decreases.
   f. Forced expiratory volume (airflow) decreases.
   g. Altered pulmonary gas exchange: oxygen tension falls with age, at a rate of 4 mm Hg/decade; PaO_2 at age 70 is 75 versus 90 at age 20.
   h. Blunted ventilatory responses of chemoreceptors in response to respiratory acidosis: decreased homeostatic responses.
   i. Blunted defense/immune responses: decreased ciliary action to clear secretions, decreased secretory immunoglobulins, alveolar phagocytic function.

2. **Implications for intervention.**
   a. Respiratory responses to exercise: similar to younger adult at low and moderate intensities; at higher intensities, responses include increased ventilatory cost of work, greater blood acidosis, increased likelihood of breathlessness, increased perceived exertion.
   b. Clinical signs of hypoxia are blunted; changes in mentation and affect may provide important cues.
   c. Cough mechanism is impaired.
   d. Gag reflex is decreased; increased risk of aspiration.
   e. Recovery from respiratory illness prolonged in the elderly.
   f. Significant changes in function with chronic smoking, exposure to environmental toxic inhalants.

3. **Intervention, implications and compensatory strategies.**
   a. Complete cardiopulmonary assessment by the physical therapist prior to commencing an exercise program is essential in older adults due the high incidence of cardiopulmonary pathologies.
      (1) Selection of appropriate exercise tolerance testing protocol (ETT) is important.

(2) Absence of standardized test batteries and norms for elderly.

(3) Many elderly cannot tolerate maximal testing; submaximal testing commonly used.

b. Individualized exercise prescription essential.

(1) Choice of training program is based on fitness level, presence or absence of cardiovascular disease, musculoskeletal limitations, individual's goals and interests.

(2) Prescriptive elements (frequency, intensity, duration and mode) are the same as for younger adults; developed by the physical therapist.

(3) Walking, chair and floor exercises, modified strength/flexibility calisthenics well-tolerated by most elderly.

(4) Consider pool programs (exercises, walking and swimming) for aging adults with bone and joint impairments.

(5) Consider multiple modes of exercise (circuit training) on alternate days to reduce likelihood of muscle injury, joint overuse, pain, fatigue.

c. Aerobic training programs can significantly improve cardiopulmonary function in the elderly. Benefits of aerobic training programs:

(1) Decreased heart rate at a given submaximal power output.

(2) Improved maximal oxygen uptake (VO_2max).

(3) Greater improvements in peripheral adaptation, muscle oxidative capacity than central changes; major difference from training effects in younger adults.

(4) Improved recovery heart rates.

(5) Decreased systolic blood pressure; may produce a small decrease in diastolic blood pressure.

(6) Increased maximum ventilatory capacity: vital capacity.

(7) Reduced breathlessness, lowers perceived exertion.

(8) Psychological gains: improved sense of well-being, self-image.

(9) Improved functional capacity.

d. Improve overall daily activity levels for independent living.

(1) Lack of exercise is an important risk factor in the development of cardiopulmonary diseases.

(2) Lack of exercise contributes to problems of immobility and disability in the elderly.

Application Concepts

- Monitor exercise response carefully using a variety of tools (observation of patient verbal responses, rate of perceived exertion; blood pressure (BP) and HR changes may be blunted by medication.
- Changes in rib cage excursion and postural changes can also diminish respiration.

- There will be a prolonged recovery time following exertion—lengthen cool-down phase of aerobic activity.

Integumentary System

1. Changes in skin composition.
   a. Dermis thins with loss of elastin.
   b. Decreased vascularity; vascular fragility results in easy bruising.
   c. Decreased sebaceous activity and decline in hydration.
   d. Appearance: skin appears dry, wrinkled, yellowed, inelastic, aging spots appear (clusters of melanocyte pigmentation); increased with exposure to sun.
   e. General thinning and graying of hair due to vascular insufficiency and decreased melanin production.
   f. Nails grow more slowly, become brittle and thick.

2. Loss of effectiveness as protective barrier.
   a. Skin grows and heals more slowly; less able to resist injury and infection.
   b. Inflammatory response is weakened.
   c. Decreased sensitivity to touch, perception of pain and temperature; increased risk for injury from concentrated pressures or excess temperatures.
   d. Decreased sweat production with loss of sweat glands results in decreased temperature regulation and homeostasis.

Gastrointestinal System

1. Decreased salivation, taste and smell along with inadequate chewing (tooth loss, poorly fitting dentures); poor swallowing reflex may lead to poor dietary intake, nutritional deficiencies.

2. Esophagus: reduced motility and control of lower esophageal sphincter.
   a. Lower esophageal sphincter hesitant to relax may result in feeling of fullness at substernal area; lower esophageal sphincter weakens which may result in acid reflux and heartburn.

3. Stomach: reduced motility, delayed gastric emptying; decreased digestive enzymes and hydrochloric acid; decreased digestion and absorption of nutrients; indigestion common.

4. Liver: decreased blood flow; diminished capacity to regenerate cells; changes in medication metabolism.

5. Small intestine: generally maintains ability to absorb nutrients; however, reduced blood supply can hinder absorption; changes in metabolism and absorption of lactose, calcium and iron.

a. **Red Flag:** Decrease in calcium necessitates increased calcium intakes.

6. Large intestine: decreased motility, decreased mobility and dehydration can all lead to constipation; can be offset with increased activity and fiber intake.

Hepatic, Renal and Genitourinary Systems

1. Renal system: loss of kidney mass and total weight with nephron (filtering unit) atrophy, decreased renal blood flow (by as much as 10% per decade), decreased filtration.
   a. Blood urea rises.
   b. Decreased excretory and reabsorptive capacities.
   c. Reduced hormonal response (vasopressin): leads to impaired ability to conserve salt and contribute to increased risk for dehydration.

2. Pancreas: beta cells possess decreased ability to increase insulin production in response to increases in blood glucose levels.

3. Bladder: muscle weakness; decreased capacity causing urinary frequency; difficulty with emptying causing increased retention; increased incidence of urinary tract infections due to reflux of urine into ureters.
   a. Urinary incontinence common: affects over 10 million adults; over half of nursing home residents and one-third of community dwelling elders; affects older women with pelvic floor weakness and older men with bladder or prostate disease.
   b. Inadequate hydration: causes concentrated urine which irritates the lining of bladder wall, which causes involuntary contractions and leakage.

Endocrine System

1. Insulin (secreted by pancreas): muscle cells may become less responsive to insulin; after age 50, normal fasting blood glucose levels rise 6–14 milligrams per deciliter every 10 years.

2. Adrenal glands: aldosterone (important in regulating electrolyte and fluid balance) levels decrease; can cause problems with orthostatic hypotension.

Application Concepts

- Monitor skin condition and protect as needed.
- Diminished capacity to regulate body temperature; control environment, advise dressing in layers.
- Encourage water consumption.
- Encourage intake of high fiber foods.
- Encourage maintenance of or increased activity levels.
- Encourage attention to intake of dietary minerals.

Pathological Conditions Associated with the Aging Adult

Musculoskeletal System

1. Osteoporosis: disease process that results in reduction of bone mass; a failure of bone formation (osteoblast activity) to keep pace with bone reabsorption and destruction (osteoclast activity).
   a. World Health Organization (WHO) diagnostic criteria (Table 9-1).
      (1) Osteopenia (systemic, evenly distributed, decrease in bone loss): defined by bone mineral density (BMD) between 1.0 and 2.5 standard deviations (SDs) below the young normal mean reference population.
      (2) Osteoporosis: defined by BMD at the hip or spine that is ≤2.5 SDs below the young normal mean reference population.
      (3) Severely osteoporotic: defined as BMD ≤2.5 SDs below the young normal mean reference population plus one or more fragility fractures.
   b. Etiological factors.
      (1) Hormonal deficiency associated with menopause and hypogonadism: loss of estrogens or androgens.
      (2) Nutritional deficiency: inadequate calcium, impaired absorption of calcium; excessive alcohol, caffeine consumption.
      (3) Decreased physical activity: inadequate mechanical loading.
      (4) Diseases that affect bone loss: hyperthyroidism, diabetes, hyperparathyroidism, rheumatic disease (lupus), celiac disease, gastric bypass, pancreatic disease, multiple myeloma, sickle cell disease, end-stage renal disease, Paget's disease, cancer and chemotherapeutic drugs.
      (5) Medications that affect bone loss: corticosteroids, thyroid hormone, anticonvulsants, catabolic drugs, some estrogen antagonists, chemotherapy.

Table 9-1 ➤ BONE MINERAL DENSITY AND TREATMENT RECOMMENDATIONS

CATEGORY	TREATMENT RECOMMENDATIONS
WHO (World Health Organization) Criteria for Bone Mineral Density	
Normal	
BMD <1 SD below young normal mean distribution.	Weight-bearing exercise
*Presents average or below average risk of fracture	Trunk extension activities and exercise
	Resistance exercise
Osteopenia	
BMD 1.0–2.5 SD below young normal mean distribution	Weight-bearing exercise
*Presents increased risk for fracture	Trunk extension activities and exercise
	Functional activities
	Resistance exercise
	Postural/balance training
	Safety education/fall prevention
Osteoporosis	
BMD >2.5 SD below young normal mean distribution	Same as above—also add:
* Presents significantly increased risk of fracture	Deep breathing exercise
Severe Osteoporosis	
BMD >2.5 SD below young normal mean distribution + one or more fragility fractures	Same as above—also add:
*Presents extremely high risk for fracture	Environmental modification
	Incorporation of protective clothing

BMD, bone mineral density; SD, standard deviation

(6) Additional risk factors: family history, white/Asian race, early menopause, thin/small build, smoking.

c. Characteristics.
  (1) Estimated 10 million Americans with osteoporosis; will affect about one in two women.
  (2) Bone loss is about 1% per year (starting for women at ages 30–35, for men ages 50–55); accelerating loss in postmenopausal women, approximately 5% per year for 3–5 years.
  (3) Structural weakening of bone.
  (4) Decreased ability to support loads.
  (5) High risk of fractures.
  (6) Trabecular bone more involved than cortical bone.
    (a) Common areas affected: vertebral column, femoral neck, distal radius/wrist, humerus.
    (b) Potential for deformity: feet—hammer toes, bunions lead to antalgic gait; postural kyphosis, forward head position; hip and knee flexion contractures.

d. Assessment.
  (1) Medical tests: BMD testing; x-rays for known or suspected fractures.
  (2) Physical therapist examination will include: physical activity/fall history, history, physical exam, nutritional history.

  (3) Physical therapist assistant ongoing assessments.
    (a) Assess dizziness: may use Dizziness Handicap Inventory.
    (b) Sensory integrity: vision, hearing, somatosensory, vestibular, sensory integration.
    (c) Motor function: strength, endurance, motor control.
    (d) Range of motion (ROM)/flexibility.
    (e) Postural hypotension.
    (f) Gait and balance assessment.

e. Medical management.
  (1) Medical therapy: initiated with BMD T-scores ≤–2.5 at femoral neck or spine (obtained by dual-energy x-ray absorptiometry [DXA]) or individuals >50 years with low bone mass (T-score between 1.0 and 2.5, osteopenia). Current Food and Drug Administration (FDA)–approved pharmacological options include medications (Table 9-2).
  (2) Promote health; provide counseling on risk of osteoporosis and related fractures, health behaviors.
    (a) Daily calcium intake, individuals age 50 or older: 1200 mg per day.
    (b) Daily vitamin D intake, individuals age 50 or older: 800–1000 IU per day.
    (c) Diet: low in salt, avoid excess protein: inhibits body's ability to absorb calcium.
    (d) Avoid tobacco smoking and excessive alcohol intake.

f. Intervention, implications and compensatory strategies.
  (1) Promote maintenance of bone mass by including regular weight-bearing exercise:
    (a) Walking (30 min/day); stair-climbing; use of weight belts to increase loading.
    (b) Muscle strengthening (resistance exercises) reduces risk of falls and fractures.
  (2) Postural/balance training.
    (a) Postural reeducation, postural exercises to reduce kyphosis, forward head position.
    (b) Flexibility exercises.
    (c) Functional balance exercise: e.g., chair rises, standing/kitchen sink exercises (e.g., toe raises, unilateral stance, hip extension, hip abduction, partial squats).
    (d) Tai chi.
    (e) Gait training.
  (3) Safety education/fall prevention.
    (a) Advise patients to avoid forward bending and exercises with trunk flexion, especially in combination with twisting.
    (b) Avoid long-term bed rest.
    (c) Proper shoes: flat shoes enhance balance abilities (no heels).
    (d) Assistive devices to decrease fall risk: cane, walker as needed.

Table 9-2 ➤ COMMONLY PRESCRIBED MEDICATIONS AND ASSOCIATED PRECAUTIONS*

MEDICATION**	PRESCRIBED FOR	SIDE EFFECTS	INTERACTIONS	PHYSICAL THERAPY CONSIDERATIONS
Medications used for Bone Disorders				
alendronate (Fosamax) calcitonin (Miacalcin, Calcimar) raloxifene (Evista)	Bone disorders (e.g.: osteoporosis and Paget's disease)	Constipation Indigestion Diarrhea Abdominal pain Deterioration (osteonecrosis) of the jaw Muscle cramps Headaches Calcitonin: nasal spray can cause irritation in nose (e.g., sores, dryness, itching, bleeding). Injectable can cause: stomach pain, diarrhea, nausea or vomiting, flushing (face, ears, hands, feet), loss of appetite	Can cause increases in abdominal distress if combined with use of aspirin Calcium or antacids taken with medication can interfere with uptake of medication Calcium intake should be monitored by MD Calcitonin: may interfere with other meds taken for Paget's disease Calcium intake should be monitored by MD Raloxifene: may affect blood clotting (an increased risk of blood clots with this medication); individuals on warfarin (Coumadin) Calcium intake should be monitored by MD as levels could become too high	Alendronate: patient should take the medication on an empty stomach, should not lie down within 30 minutes of taking the medication; increased chance of irritation of esophagus Raloxifene: monitor carefully for bruising. Ensure the patient is getting blood test for clotting times (prothrombin time, international ratio)
Medications Used to Treat Inflammatory Disorders				
Nonsteroidal Anti-inflammatory Drugs (NSAIDs) aspirin ibuprofen (Motrin, Advil) naproxen (Aleve, Naprosyn)	Inflammatory conditions and pain Rheumatoid arthritis Osteoarthritis	Stomach and gastrointestinal irritation Can cause symptoms of dizziness, fatigue, dyspnea, tinnitus, headache		
COX-2 inhibitors Celecoxib (off the market: Vioxx)	Inflammatory conditions and pain Rheumatoid arthritis	Produce less stomach and gastrointestinal irritation than NSAIDs; however, increased risk for potential heart problems Liver dysfunction, contributes to declining kidney function. Fluid accumulation mimicking congestive heart failure	When taken with anticoagulants, aspirin, corticosteroids or SSRIs may cause increased risk of stomach bleeding Effectiveness of ACE inhibitors or diuretics may be decreased by this medication	
Corticosteroid Injections	Arthritis inflammation and other painful inflammatory conditions	Weakens tissues, especially with repeated use		Be cautious of weakened tissues and cartilage in the case of multiple injections
Disease-Modifying Anti-rheumatic Drugs (DMARDs) Gold Therapy Compounds	Rheumatoid arthritis		Modifies the immune system response to the inflammatory process and stops or slow its progress	
Steroids methylprednisolone (Medrol) Prednisone	Rheumatoid arthritis	Significant weakening of tendon, muscle, and bone can occur May weaken the immune system	Prednisone may increase or decrease effects of anticoagulant medications	Clinician should pay careful attention to posture, monitor for changes that may reflect weakening of the spine or other support structures

*Medications used in the medical management of diseases and conditions are included in the licensure exam. PTAs should be familiar with categories of medications and their indications for use. PTAs should also be acutely aware of potential effects on tolerance to physical therapy intervention.

**Generic drug names appear first followed by brand names in parenthesis; brand names may be trademarked or registered.

(Continued on following page)

Table 9-2 ➤ continued

MEDICATION**	PRESCRIBED FOR	SIDE EFFECTS	INTERACTIONS	PHYSICAL THERAPY CONSIDERATIONS
Medications Used to Treat Ischemic Conditions of the Heart				
Cholesterol-Lowering Medications Lovastatin, colestipol (Colestid), fluvastatin (Lescol), pravastatin (Pravachol), atorvastatin ((Lipitor), cholestyramine (Questran), fenofibrate (Antara, Fenoglide, Lipofen), gemfibrozil (Lopid), rosuvastatin calcium (Crestor)	Hyperlipidemia Atherosclerosis Ischemic heart disease	Nausea, fatigue, diarrhea, weakness, myalgia, myositis		
Fish Oil (Lovaza)	Hyperlipidemia, fish oil helps to lower triglyceride levels; may help decrease risk of heart disease, may help lower blood pressure	May cause belching, bad breath, loose stools, heartburn, nausea, rash, nosebleeds May reduce immune system activity	May lower blood pressure in persons who are taking blood pressure lowering medications May cause slow blood clotting; potential for increased bruising or bleeding, especially if combined with medications such as aspirin, naproxen, ibuprofen, warfarin May increase symptoms of depression	Monitor for hypotension
Beta-Blockers atenolol (Tenormin) Carvedilol (Coreg) metoprolol (Lopressor) propranolol (Inderal)	Atherosclerosis Ischemic heart disease Angina pectoris • Slows heart rate and decreases the force needed to contract the heart muscle • Decreases blood pressure and myocardial oxygen demand	Nausea, fatigue, slow pulse, weakness, increased blood glucose levels, nightmares, depression, asthmatic attacks, sexual dysfunction		Use RPE scale to monitor patient tolerance to exercise • Blood pressure and heart rate are not good indicators of the work being done as they are being artificially controlled by the medication
Calcium Channel Blockers nifedipine (Procardia) verapamil (Calan, Verelan) Nicardipine (Cardene) diltiazem (Cardizem)	Atherosclerosis Ischemic heart Disease Angina pectoris • Medications cause vasodilation of the coronary arteries, lowers blood pressure, and can suppress some arrhythmias	Hypotension, postural hypotension, dizziness, headache, fluid retention - peripheral edema, palpitations, flushes		Be aware of possibility of postural hypotension. Warrants MD notification Use RPE scale to monitor patient tolerance to exercise • Blood pressure and heart rate are not good indicators of the work being done as they are being artificially controlled by the medication
aspirin	Atherosclerosis Ischemic heart disease • Decreases the risk of a blood clot forming in the coronary arteries			
Nitrates (Vasodilators) nitroglycerine (Nitrostat, Nitro-Bid)	Atherosclerosis Ischemic heart disease Angina pectoris • Act to cause vasodilation of coronary arteries	Nausea, vomiting, tachycardia, transient headache, hypotension, weakness, flush on face and neck		Orthostatic hypotension and tachycardia warrant notification of MD and PT

Table 9-2 ➤ continued

MEDICATION**	PRESCRIBED FOR	SIDE EFFECTS	INTERACTIONS	PHYSICAL THERAPY CONSIDERATIONS
Medications Used to Treat Congestive Conditions of the Heart				
Diuretics hydrochlorothiazide (HydroDIURIL, Aquazide H) spironolactone (Aldactone) furosemide (Lasix) bumetanide (Bumex)	Congestive heart conditions • Work to increase excretion of sodium and water thus decrease amount of fluid in the body	Potential electrolyte imbalances, muscle cramps, weakness, joint pains, drowsiness, dehydration, gout, nausea, blood glucose abnormalities		Dizziness and lightheadedness warrants notification of the MD and PT
Digitalis Compounds digoxin (Lanoxin, Digitek)	Congestive Heart Conditions • Increases force of the heart's contractions • Slows heart rate to allow chambers to fill completely	Nausea, vomiting, diarrhea, confusion, loss of appetite, heartbeat irregularities		
Ace Inhibitors (Angiotensin-Converting Enzyme Inhibitors) enalapril maleate (Vasotec) ramipril (Altace) Captopril (Capoten) lisinopril (Prinivil, Zestril)	Congestive Heart Conditions • Decreases how hard the heart has to work to pump blood through the heart by decreasing pressure in vessels of heart • Prevents constrictions of blood vessels and retention of sodium and fluid	Persistent dry cough, weakness, headache, palpitations, swelling of feet or abdomen, dizziness, fainting, numbness or tingling of hands, feet or lips	May cause congenital defects if taken during the first trimester of pregnancy	May cause postural hypotension Swelling of feet or abdomen, dizziness, or fainting warrant notification of MD
Beta-blockers atenolol (Tenormin) carvedilol (Coreg) metoprolol (Lopressor, Toprol-XL) propranolol (Inderal)	Congestive Heart Conditions • Reduces the output of blood and heart rate by counteracting a hormone called norepinephrine • Relaxes blood vessels of the heart muscle by blocking sympathetic conduction of B-receptors on the SA node and myocardial cells; reduces force of contraction and decreases heart rate	Nausea, fatigue, slow pulse, weakness, increased blood glucose levels, nightmares, depression, asthmatic attacks, sexual dysfunction		Dizziness warrants contacting MD and PT Can cause postural hypotension
Medications Used to Treat Arrhythmias of the Heart				
Digitalis Drugs digoxin Antiarrhythmics quinidine (Cardioquin) Procainamide HCl (Procanbid, Procan Sr)	Atrial Fibrillation • Work to slow or alter the electrical conduction patterns of the heart • Increases heart muscle's ability to contract and pump correctly	Nausea, palpitations, vomiting, insomnia, dizziness, symptoms of CHF, shortness of breath, swollen ankles, coughing up blood		If symptoms of CHF develop immediately contact MD, supervising PT and document
Medications used to Treat Cognitive Disorders				
Tricyclics amitriptyline (Elavil)	Depression • Meds work on chemical imbalances in brain	Dry mouth or eyes, weight gain, drowsiness, constipation, nausea, sweating		Tricyclic antidepressants can cause postural hypotension
nortriptyline (Pamelor, Aventyl HCl) Desipramine (Norpramin) *Serotonin and Norepinephrine Reuptake Inhibitors (SNRIs)* venlafaxine (Effexor, Effexor XR) duloxetine HCl (Cymbalta) *Selective Serotonin Reuptake Inhibitors (SSRIs)* fluoxetine (Prozac, Sarafem) paroxetine (Paxil) escitalopram (Lexapro) sertraline (Zoloft) citalopram (Celexa)	• SSRIs increase brain serotonin levels	SSRIs: symptoms that will likely diminish: anxiety, restlessness, increased sleepiness, heartburn; symptoms that may not resolve unless SSRI is stopped - sexual problems		

(Continued on following page)

Table 9-2 ➤ continued

MEDICATION**	PRESCRIBED FOR	SIDE EFFECTS	INTERACTIONS	PHYSICAL THERAPY CONSIDERATIONS
Symptom Modifying Medications Levodopa (Sinemet, Stalevo) Dopamine Agonists COMT Inhibitors Selegiline (Eldepryl, Zelapar)	Parkinson's disease • Body works to turn levodopa into dopamine • Dopamine agonists increase effect of levodopa • COMT inhibitors block the enzyme that breaks down levodopa; prolong its effect when taken at same time • Selegiline agents prevent breakdown of dopamine	Mental confusion, hallucinations, abnormal movements, restlessness, heart rhythm disturbances, insomnia, mouth sores, constipation, back pain, nausea and vomiting Note: dopamine agonists can increase the side effects of levodopa	Narcotic painkillers, antidepressants, decongestants, alcohol, foods high in tyramine (aged meats, aged cheese, sausage, herring, and more)	Levodopa may cause postural hypotension With selegiline agents, notify MD immediately if any of the following occur: lightheadedness, restlessness, irritability, twitching or muscle movement, painful or difficult urination
Anticholinergic	Parkinson's disease • Works to decrease tremors	Dry mouth, constipation, urine retention, blurred vision In elderly patients, can cause confusion and hallucinations		
Acetyl cholinesterase inhibitors donepezil (Aricept) rivastigmine (Exelon) Galantamine (Razadyne) memantine (Namenda)	Alzheimer's disease • Increases the availability of acetylcholine • Namenda may regulate glutamate through its action on the NMDA receptors in the brain			

ACE, angiotensin-converting enzyme; CHF, congestive heart failure; COMT, catecholamine *O*-methyl transferase; NMDA, *N*-methyl-D-aspartate; RPE, rate of perceived exertion; SSRIs, selective serotonin reuptake inhibitors.

(e) Fracture prevention: counseling on safe activities; avoid sudden forceful movements, twisting, standing, bending over, lifting, supine sit-ups.

(f) Include home assessment for fall risk.

2. **Paget's disease (osteitis deformans): progressive metabolic bone disease: characterized by increased bone resorption and excessive, unorganized new bone formation (new bone lacks structural stability of normal bone); eventual replacement of bone marrow with vascular fibrous tissue.**

   a. Affects both men and women with slight increased prevalence in men; often familial.

   b. Etiology: often inherited in an autosomal dominant pattern; genetic basis not well understood.

   c. Musculoskeletal manifestations: primarily affects axial skeleton; lesions occur in multiple sites in the spine, pelvis, femur, tibia as well as the skull; can cause pathological fractures; affected bones change shape and size.

   d. Clinical presentation/symptoms: pain; if periosteum is irritated pain may be described as "deep, boring"; pain is likely worse at night; pain is reduced (not eliminated) with activity; fatigue; lightheadedness; general stiffness; headache and muscular aches.

   (1) Active disease process can cause increased release of calcium (due to overactive osteoclasts)

in the blood to cause hypercalcemia state; results in fatigue, weakness, loss of appetite, abdominal pain, constipation.

   (2) Clinical findings: increased kyphosis, bowing of femurs or tibias; waddling gait due to femoral neck causing coxa vara; pain from altered mechanical stresses if joint deformities exist.

   e. Medical management and tests.

   (1) Diagnostics: may take years; often made incidentally through radiographic or laboratory tests looking for other pathology; laboratory tests assessing alkaline phosphatase levels; bone scan.

   (2) Treatment: bone resorption inhibitors oral alendronate or risedronate (nitrogen-containing bisphosphonates); treatment can induce remission of the disease process; pain control through use of non-steroidal anti-inflammatory; surgical intervention in cases of potential compromise to vital structures or if severe degenerative joint exists (see Table 9-2).

   f. Physical therapy screening: difficult to diagnose. Physical therapist must be aware of symptomatic complaints: vague diffuse headache; hearing loss; tinnitus; incontinence; diplopia; swallowing difficulties.

   g. Intervention, implications and compensatory strategies.

(1) Physical therapy: encourage regular cardiovascular and strengthening activity; postural exercises; weight-bearing exercise; strengthening exercises to help maintain joint alignment; coordination and balance exercises; maintenance of ROM.

➢ (2) **Red Flag:** Avoid high-impact activities such as jogging, running and jumping (particularly in cases of spinal involvement); avoid forward bending and twisting exercises.

3. **Fractures.**
   a. High risk of fractures in the elderly associated with low bone density and multiple risk factors: e.g., age, comorbid diseases, dementia, psychotropic medications.
   b. Hip fracture: common orthopedic problem of older adults.
      (1) Mortality rate 20%, associated with complications.
      (2) About 50% will not resume their premorbid level of function; e.g., walk independently.
      (3) May result in dependency; continued institutionalization occurs in as many as one-third of hip fracture patients.
      (4) Majority of hip fractures are treated surgically; 95% are femoral neck or intertrochanteric fractures; remaining 5% are subtrochanteric fractures.
      (5) Intensive interdisciplinary rehabilitation program with early mobilization may improve outcome.
      (6) Treatment protocols are based on the type of fracture and surgical procedure used; internal fixation versus prosthetic replacement.
   c. Vertebral compression fractures.
      (1) Usually occur in lower thoracic, lumbar regions (T8-L3).
      (2) Typically result from routine activity: bending, lifting, rising from chair.
      (3) Chief complaints: immediate, severe local spinal pain, increased with trunk flexion.
      (4) Lead to shortening of spine, progressive loss of height; spinal deformity (kyphosis); can progress to respiratory compromise.
      (5) Intervention, implications and compensatory strategies.
         (a) Acute phase: horizontal bed rest; out of bed 10 minutes every hour; isometric extension exercises in bed.
         (b) Emphasis on extension postures (sleeping, sitting, standing) and exercises; avoid flexion activities; postural training.
         (c) Modalities for relief of pain.
         (d) Safety education/modify environment.
         (e) Decrease vertebral loading; use soft-soled shoes.

         (f) Surgical repair: kyphoplasty or vertebroplasty can be performed for individuals with painful vertebral fractures.
      ➢ (6) **Red Flag:** Use caution when patient/client is taking pain medications that can cause disorientation or sedation that can result in falls.
   d. Stress fractures: fine, hairline fracture (insufficiency fracture) without soft tissue injury.
      (1) In elderly, common in pelvis, proximal tibia, distal fibula, metatarsal shafts, foot.
      (2) May be unsuspected source of pain.
      (3) Observe for signs of local tenderness and swelling; e.g., postexercise.
      (4) Interventions, goals and outcomes as established by the physical therapist.
         (a) Rest.
         (b) Correction of exercise excesses or faulty exercise program.
         (c) Reduction of vertical loading; e.g., soft-soled shoes.
   e. Upper extremity fractures: humeral head, Colles' fractures.
   f. For discussion of fracture assessment and management, see chapter 2 on Musculoskeletal Physical Therapy.
   g. Clinical implications of fracture management in the aging adult.
      (1) Fractures heal more slowly.
      (2) Older adults are prone to complications: pneumonia, decubitus ulcers, mental status complications with hospitalization.
      (3) Rehabilitation may be complicated or prolonged by lack of support systems, comorbid conditions, decreased vision, poor balance.

4. **Degenerative arthritis/osteoarthritis (OA): a noninflammatory progressive, degenerative process affecting articular cartilage of synovial joints; eventually produces bony remodeling and overgrowth (spurs, lipping); eventual synovial and capsular thickening and joint effusion; typically affects weight-bearing joints such as hips, knees, the cervical and lumbar spine, the distal interphalangeal joints of fingers and the carpometacarpal joint of the thumb.**
   a. Risk factors: genetic link especially in hands, hips, smaller incidence in knees; obesity; weak quadriceps muscle; joint impact; repetitive impact and twisting (e.g., sports activities); occupational activities involving kneeling and squatting with heavy lifting.
   b. Clinical manifestations.
      (1) Tissue degradation: thinning and splitting of cartilage; decreased ability to withstand stress of use; eventual exposure of subchondral bone.
      (2) Characterized by: pain, swelling and stiffness, worse early morning (usually <30 minutes); increased pain with weight-bearing and strenuous activity; muscle spasm; loss of ROM and

mobility; bony deformity, crepitus; muscle weakness secondary to disuse.

   (3) Bony deformities.

     (a) Herberden's nodes: enlargement of distal interphalangeal joints of fingers.

     (b) Bouchard's nodes: enlargement of proximal interphalangeal joints.

  c. Medical management: NSAIDs, corticosteroid injections, topical analgesics, joint replacements (see Table 9-2).

  d. Intervention, implications and compensatory strategies.

    (1) Reduction of pain and muscle spasm; modalities, relaxation training.

    (2) Interventions.

     (a) Maintain or improve ROM: stretch muscle; manage joint restrictions with joint play and mobilization techniques.

     (b) Correct muscle imbalances; strengthening exercises to promote neuromuscular control of joint; improve balance and ambulation.

     (c) Balance training exercises—tai chi.

     (d) Aerobic conditioning: low-impact (walking, biking, swimming) and low-moderate or high-intensity aerobic conditioning programs.

     (e) Aquatic programs; e.g., pool walking, Arthritis Foundation program, produces beneficial effects similar to aerobic conditioning, enhances ease of movement.

    (3) Patient education and empowerment.

     (a) Teach patients about disease, taking an active role in care, symptom management.

     (b) Teach joint protection, safe exercise for strength and muscle performance, ROM and endurance.

    (4) Provide assistive devices for ambulation and activities of daily living; e.g., canes, walkers, shoe inserts, reachers.

    (5) Promote healthy lifestyle: weight reduction to relieve stress on joints.

- Evidence supports aerobic conditioning and strengthening exercise programs can help to decrease joint symptoms, decrease disability, decrease pain and improve overall sense of well-being.
- Evidence supports hip joint mobilizations to improve arthrokinematics which can have a greater clinical effect on muscle function and joint motion than active exercise alone.

---

5. Rheumatoid arthritis (RA): diffuse connective tissue disease resulting in inflammation of synovial membrane, release of proteolytic enzymes that perpetuate inflammation and joint damage; inflammatory changes in tendon sheaths (tenosynovitis); pannus formation (granulation tissue) covers and erodes articular cartilage, bone, ligaments and the joint capsule.

  a. Affects approximately 10 in 1000 people; affects women two to four times more often than men at all ages.

  b. Characterized by: systemic manifestations; e.g., morning stiffness more pronounced and lasting longer than with OA; symmetrical, bilateral joint involvement; joint erythema and swelling; elevated serum rheumatoid factor; periods of exacerbation and remission; eventual rheumatoid nodules and joint malalignment.

    (1) Joints commonly affected.

     (a) Cervical spine: atlantoaxial joint, mid-cervical region; involvement at C1-2 can be life threatening (transverse ligament rupture leading to odontoid encroachment on foramen magnum).

     (b) Costovertebral joints, spinal facet joints, sacroiliac joint: ankylosing spondylitis of one or more vertebrae of the spine.

     (c) Shoulders: glenohumeral, sternoclavicular or acromioclavicular joints.

     (d) Elbows, wrists and hands.

    (2) Joint deformities.

     (a) Swan neck deformity: proximal interphalangeal (PIP) hyperextension with distal interphalangeal (DIP) flexion.

     (b) Boutonniere deformity: DIP extension with PIP flexion.

     (c) Thumb deformities: termed types I–III; affect all joints.

     (d) Foot deformities: splayed foot with weakening of the transverse arch from synovitis; hallux valgus and bunions may exist; hammer toes—volar subluxation of metatarsophalangeal joints combined with flexion of the PIP and hyperextension of the DIP joints; claw toes—volar subluxation of metatarsal head with flexion of the PIP and DIP joints.

    (3) Muscle involvement: atrophy may be seen; unknown if result of disuse or other unknown mechanism. In long-standing disease, atrophy of intrinsic hand musculature and quadriceps may be observed.

    (4) Tendon involvement: inflammation of synovial lining of tendon sheaths leading to tenosynovitis.

  c. Medical management.

    (1) Laboratory testing: for elevated erythrocyte sedimentation rate (ESR) or C-reactive protein (CRP), elevated rates are indicative of active inflammation; laboratory testing for rheumatoid factor (RF) does not confirm or rule out diagnosis of RA. Complete blood count (CBC), red blood cells often decreased, white blood cell

count typically normal, thrombocytosis (high platelet count) not uncommon.

(2) Synovial fluid analysis: enhances differential diagnosis; will be cloudy, less viscous and will clot; increase in fluid; presence of crystals can confirm diagnosis of gout.

(3) Radiographic imaging: PT or MD will review for joint alignment, bone density and condition of joint surface, cartilaginous spacing, soft tissue swelling evidence.

(4) Medications: NSAIDS and disease-modifying antirheumatic drugs (DMARDS) including biological response modifiers (BRMs) and corticosteroids (see Table 9-2).

(5) Surgical management: selectively chosen for appropriate individuals.

   (a) Soft tissue surgeries: synovectomy, soft tissue release, tendon transfer.

   (b) Bone and joint surgeries: osteotomy, arthroplasty, arthrodesis.

d. Intervention, implications and compensatory strategies.

(1) Decrease pain: modalities (use caution with cold applications due to Raynaud's phenomenon with RA); gentle massage, relaxation techniques.

(2) Increase or maintain ROM sufficient for functional activities: active or passive ROM within pain limits; manual techniques, grades I and II oscillations, teach self ROM; implement appropriate neurological stretching techniques (**Red Flag:** Do not stretch swollen joints.); avoid exercise-induced pain that lasts greater than an hour following treatment.

(3) Joint protection: use orthoses or splints to support joints when appropriate, specially designed shoes to decrease forces through foot.

(4) Resistance exercises: include isometric exercise (submaximal effort); use concentric and eccentric muscle contractions; do not cause pain with resistance.

(5) Establish regular exercise and physical activity routine: include endurance; crucial to long-term quality of life.

(6) Promote independence in activities of daily living (ADL).

(7) Gait: improve safety, improve efficiency of pattern.

(8) Teach joint protection principles (see Table 9-3).

Evidence supports that patients with medically controlled RA respond favorably to carefully supervised exercise programs. Benefits of exercise program include improved function and muscle strength, decreased number of clinically active joints and decreased disease activity. Long-term adherence to these programs can lead to improved aerobic capacity, improved strength and functional ability, improved psychological well-being.

Table 9-3 ➤ JOINT PROTECTION PRINCIPLES RHEUMATOID ARTHRITIS

- Respect fatigue: alternate activities; stop activity when fatigue begins to develop.
- Conserve energy: work or exercise in short episodes, several times/day rather than long episodes; balance work and rest activities.
- Work postures: avoid performing work/exercise in deforming positions; avoid prolonged positions—change every 20–30 minutes throughout day.
- Avoid pain: decrease activity level, or omit, if pain persists following activity that lasts >1 hour.
- Maintain joint alignment: use appropriate adaptive equipment to decrease joint forces and workload.

Neurological Disorders and Diseases

1. **Stroke (CVA): sudden, focal neurologic deficit resulting from ischemic or hemorrhagic lesions in the brain.**

a. Stroke is the most common cause of serious long-term disability in United States.

(1) Incidence of stroke increases dramatically with age; most strokes (43%) occur in persons over the age of 74; incidence doubles with every decade of life after age 55; women have 20% less chance of stroke than men.

b. Risk factors.

(1) Modifiable risk factors: hypertension (BP above 160/95 mm Hg); lowering diastolic BP by 5–6 mm Hg decreases risk of stroke by up to 40%.

(2) Nonmodifiable risk factors: age, race, sex.

c. Medical diagnosis and management.

(1) Doppler ultrasound studies of blood flow through arteries; neuroimaging (CT, computed tomography; MRI, magnetic resonance imaging; DWI, diffusion-weighted [magnetic resonance] imaging; PET, positron emission tomography).

(2) Treatment.

   (a) Embolic stroke: maintaining cerebral perfusion, maintain appropriate blood pressure levels through diuretics, beta-blockers or angiotensin-converting enzymes; control edema through use of water restriction or agents that increase serum osmolarity.

   (b) Ischemic stroke: thrombolytic and antithrombotic agents; emergent care includes use of recombinant tissue plasminogen activator (tissue plasminogen activator activates plasmin which, in turn, actively digests fibrin strands and aids in dissolving thrombosis or clots); when administered within 3 hours of initial stroke, tissue plasminogen activator results in a 30% greater chance of recovery.

   (c) Intracerebral hemorrhage: reduction of elevated blood pressures through rapid-acting antihypertensive medications; control edema; hyperventilation and diuretics (mannitol) to move fluid from the intracranial compartment can be used; however, it has rebound effects and can worsen the condition; surgical draining most appropriate for cerebellar hemorrhage.

(d) Subarachnoid hemorrhage: consists of management of secondary complications of rebleeding, vasospasm, hydrocephalus, hyponatremia and seizures; increase fluids; avoid antihypertensive drugs.

d. Clinical signs, symptoms and interventions: see chapter 3 on Neuromuscular Physical Therapy.

e. Functional impairments: impaired functional mobility skills; impaired gait; impaired postural control and balance; impaired function in basic ACL, self-care.

f. For additional discussion, see chapter 3 on Neuromuscular Physical Therapy.

2. **Parkinson's disease.**

a. Degenerative, chronic, progressive disease of nervous system resulting in loss of midbrain dopamine neurons; characterized by rigidity, tremor, bradykinesia (slow movements) and postural instability.

(1) Parkinsonism and Parkinson's disease (PD) affects >800,000 adults in the United States.

(2) Clinical signs and symptoms: rigidity, bradykinesia, resting tremor, impaired movement initiation and impaired reflexive or automatic movements. See chapter 3 on Neuromuscular Physical Therapy for further information.

(3) Functional impairments.

(a) Impaired functional mobility skills; e.g., problems with initiating movements and freezing episodes, slowed movements.

(b) Impaired gait: shuffling gait, festinating (an abnormal and involuntary increase in the speed of walking), loss of arm swing and reciprocal trunk movements.

(c) Impaired postural control and balance; e.g., flexed or stooped posture, impaired balance reactions.

(d) Impaired speech and oro-motor control.

(e) Bradykinesia of hands; impaired handwriting, dressing, self-care.

b. Medical diagnosis and management.

(1) Diagnosis: assessment of the triad of tremor, rigidity and akinesia coupled with asymmetry of symptoms and presence of resting tremor and good response to levodopa can best differentiate PD from parkinsonism from other causes. Functional brain imaging is also sensitive to changes in brain metabolism and receptor binding.

(2) Medical treatment: drug administration to treat symptoms; patients develop tolerance for med-

ications with resultant increases in doses and decreased time frame for relief of symptoms; common medications: levodopa, carbidopa, catechol-O-methyl (COMT); dopamine agonists (bromocriptine), anticholinergic drugs to improve motor functions (see Table 9-2).

c. For additional discussion, see chapter 3 on Neuromuscular Physical Therapy.

3. **Implications for intervention for neurological rehabilitation in the aging adult.**

a. Older adults are prone to complications/indirect impairments: e.g., contracture and deformity, decubitus ulcers, mental status complications.

b. Rehabilitation may be complicated or prolonged by lack of support systems, comorbid conditions, decreased sensorimotor function, poor balance.

c. With irreversible neurologic disease, it is important to address the impairments and functional limitations responsive to interventions; overall focus should be on improved function and safety.

d. Compensatory treatment strategies should be utilized when impairments cannot be remediated; strategies can include environmental modifications, assistive devices, use of home health aides.

Cognitive Disorders

1. **Delirium: fluctuating attention state causing temporary confusion and loss of mental function, disorientation to place and time; an acute disorder, potentially reversible (Table 9-4).**

a. Etiology: drug toxicity and/or systemic illness, oxygen deprivation to brain; environmental changes and sensory deprivation: e.g., recent hospitalization, institutionalization.

b. Characteristics.

(1) Acute onset, often at night; fluctuating course with lucid intervals; worse at night.

(2) Duration; hours to weeks.

(3) May be hypo- or hyperalert, distractible; fluctuates over course of day.

(4) Orientation and memory impaired; difficulty with concentration; easily distracted.

(5) Illusions/hallucinations, periods of agitation.

(6) Memory deficits: immediate and recent.

(7) Disorganized thinking, incoherent speech.

(8) Sleep/wake cycles always disrupted; sundowning (increased agitation late in day and early evening) may be present.

c. Treatment principles.

(1) Environment: keep calm and quiet environment; low-level lighting without shadows; exposure to natural light; keep familiar objects near by; having familiar individuals involved is beneficial.

Table 9-4 ➤ DIFFERENTIAL DIAGNOSIS: ORGANIC BRAIN SYNDROMES

	MULTI-INFARCT DEMENTIA	SENILE DEMENTIA ALZHEIMER'S TYPE (SDAT)	PRESENILE DEMENTIA ALZHEIMER'S TYPE (PDAT)
Age of Onset	55–70	60+	40–60
Gender Distribution	M:W = 3:1	M:W = 2:3	M:W = 2:3
Duration	varies: days>years	varies: months>years; mean survival 7–11 yr.	rapid mean survival 4 years
Mode of Onset	sudden	gradual	less gradual than SDAT
Course	intermittent step-wise	slowly or rapidly progressive	rapidly progressive
Prognosis	varies	poor: mod. or severe cases	very poor
Outcome	death from CVA, CAD, or infection	death from general system failure, infection	
Hereditary Precipitating Factors	atherosclerosis some familial tendency	multifactorial: age genetic: chromosome 21 abnormality; APOE4 gene; traumatic brain injury, Down Syndrome	
Neuropathology	small or large areas of infarction secondary gliosis, senile plaques not common	neuronal degeneration, neurofibrillary tangles, amyloid deposits, senile plaques, decreased cholinergic neuronal activity	
Clinical Signs of Brain Damage	diffuse or focal, areas of preserved function	diffuse, generalized	diffuse, generalized, more severe than SDAT
Impairment of Higher Cortical Functions	isolated impairments, focal signs, episodes of confusion with lucid intervals, some insight	progressive dementia, progressive disorientation, memory loss, impaired cognition, judgment, abstract thinking, visuospatial deficits, apraxia, delusions, hallucinations; late stages: disorders of sleep, eating, sexual behavior, no insight	
Affect	emotional lability, anxious, depressed	variable: depressed anxious, paranoid, hostile, restlessness, agitation, wandering, "sundowning" late: apathy personality changes: egocentricity, impulsivity, irritability, inappropriate social behaviors	
Neuromuscular	focal signs: may see hemiparesis, hemisensory loss	occasional tremors, generalized weakness, unsteady gait, increased tone: rigid postures, decreased postural reflexes, increased fall risk, repetitive behaviors	
Seizures	yes	rare	occasional
Medical	TIAs, CVA, hypertension, headaches	infections, contractures, fractures, decubitus ulcers, urinary and fecal incontinence	

(2) Physical therapy implications: include reorientation activities; use clear explanations; ensure that patient has eyeglasses and hearing aids in place if appropriate.

☞(3) **Red Flag:** avoid restraining individual.

2. Dementia: loss of intellectual functions and memory causing dysfunction in daily living (see Table 9-4).
   a. Incidence: estimated that between 1.5 and 2.3 million persons are suffering moderate to severe dementia in the United States; prevalence increases with age.
   b. Criteria for dementia.
      (1) Deterioration of intellectual functions: impoverished thinking; impaired judgment; disorientation, confusion, impaired social functioning.
      (2) Disturbances in higher cortical functions: language (aphasia); motor skills (apraxia); perception (agnosia).
      (3) Memory impairment; recent and remote.
      (4) Personality changes: alteration or accentuation of premorbid traits; behavioral changes.
      (5) Alertness (consciousness) usually normal.
      (6) Sleep often fragmented.
   c. Reversible dementias: 10%–20% of dementias; multiple causes.
      (1) Drugs: sedatives, hypnotics, antianxiety agents, antidepressants, antiarrhythmics, antihypertensives, anticonvulsants, antipsychotics, drugs with anticholinergic side effects.
      (2) Nutritional disorders: B_6 deficiency, thiamine deficiency, B_{12} deficiency/pernicious anemia, folate deficiency.
      (3) Metabolic disorders: hyper/hypothyroidism, hypercalcemia, hyper/hyponatremia, hypoglycemia, kidney or liver failure, Cushing's syndrome, Addison's disease, hypopituitarism, carcinoma.
      (4) Psychiatric disorders: depression, anxiety, psychosis.
      (5) Toxins: air pollution, alcohol.
   d. Primary degenerative dementia, Alzheimer's type, 50%–70% of dementias.

(1) Third costliest disease in United States.; fourth leading cause of death.

(2) Etiology unknown: evidence of chromosomal abnormalities; predisposing factors: family history, Down's syndrome, traumatic brain injury, aluminum toxicity.

(3) Pathophysiology.

    (a) Generalized atrophy of brain with decreased synthesis of neurotransmitters, diffuse ventricular dilation.

    (b) Histopathological changes: neurofibrillary tangles; neuritic senile plaques, build-up of beta-amyloid protein.

(4) Types (see Table 9-4).

(5) Characteristics.

    (a) Dementia: insidious onset with generally progressive deteriorating course; irreversible; mean survival time post-diagnosis is 4 years.

    (b) May have periods of agitation, restlessness, wandering.

    (c) Sundowning syndrome: confusion and agitation increases in late afternoon.

e. Multi-infarct dementias (MIDs), 20%–25% of dementias.

(1) Etiology: large and small vascular infarcts in both gray and white matter of brain, producing loss of brain function.

(2) Characteristics.

    (a) Sudden onset rather than insidious: stepwise progression.

    (b) Spotty and patchy distribution of deficits: areas of preserved ability along with impairments.

    (c) Focal neurological signs and symptoms: e.g., gait and balance abnormalities, weakness, exaggerated deep tendon reflexes (DTRs).

    (d) Emotional liability common.

    (e) Associated with history of stroke, cardiovascular disease, hypertension.

f. Other types of dementias.

(1) Parkinson's disease: dementia is sometimes found in late stages of the disease.

(2) Alcohol-related; chronic alcoholism with prolonged nutritional (B_1) deficiency; e.g., Korsakoff's psychosis.

g. Examination: performed by physical therapist on evaluation. The physical therapist assistant should be aware of information gathered at initial evaluation and assess for changes throughout treatment sessions and throughout the episode of care.

(1) History: determine onset of symptoms, progression, triggering events; common problems, social history.

(2) Examine cognitive functions: orientation, attention, calculation, recall, language. Standardized test: Mini-Mental State Exam (MMSE); score of

<24 of a possible 30 is indicative of mental decline/dementia.

(3) Examine for impairments in higher cortical functions; inability to communicate, perceptual dysfunction.

(4) Examine for behavioral changes: restless, agitated, distracted, paranoid, wandering, inappropriate social behaviors, repetitive behaviors.

(5) Examine self-care: ability to carry out ADL; e.g., limitations in grooming and hygiene, continence.

(6) Examine motor abilities: dyspraxia, gait and balance instability.

(7) Examine environment for safety, optimal function.

h. Interventions, implications and compensatory strategies.

(1) Environment.

    (a) Provide safe environment: prevent falls, injury or further dysfunction, safety from wandering, utilize safety monitoring devices as needed (e.g., alarm device).

    (b) Provide soothing environment with reduced environmental distractions; reduces agitation, increases attention.

(2) Support individual's remaining function.

    (a) Approach the patient in a friendly, supportive manner; model calm behavior.

    (b) Use consistent, simple commands; speak slowly.

    (c) Use nonverbal communication: sensory cues, gesture, demonstration.

    (d) Provide reorienting information: use prompts, wall calendars, daily schedules, memory aids whenever possible.

    (e) Avoid stressful tasks, emphasize familiar, well-learned skills; provide redirection.

    (f) Approach learning in a simple, repetitious way; proceed slowly, provide adequate rest time.

    (g) Provide mental stimulation; utilize simple, well-liked activities, games.

(3) Provide regular physical activity: safe walking program, balance activities for fall prevention, activities to promote body awareness and sensory stimulation.

(4) Participate in restraint reduction program.

(5) Educate/support family, caregivers.

(6) Present a realistic, consistent team approach to management.

3. Depression: a disorder characterized by depressed mood and lack of interest or pleasure in all activities and associated symptoms for a period of at least 2 weeks.

a. Incidence.

(1) Up to 20% of community-dwelling and institutionalized elderly have depressive symptoms or major depression.

b. Assess for predisposing factors performed by physical therapist.
   (1) Family history, prior episodes of depression.
   (2) Illness, drug side effects; hormonal.
   (3) Chronic condition; loss of physical functions, pain (e.g., stroke).
   (4) Sensory deprivation (loss of vision or hearing).
   (5) History of losses: death of family and friends, job, income, independence.
   (6) Social isolation, lack of family support.
   (7) Psychological losses; memory, intellectual functions.
c. Assess for associated depressive symptoms.
   (1) Nutritional problems: significant weight loss or weight gain, dehydration.
   (2) Sleep disturbances: insomnia or hypersomnia.
   (3) Psychomotor changes: inactivity with resultant functional impairments, weakness, agitation.
   (4) Fatigue or loss of energy.
   (5) Feelings of worthlessness, low self-esteem, guilt.
   (6) Inability to concentrate, slowed thinking, impaired memory, indecisiveness.
   (7) Withdrawal from family and friends; self-neglect.
   (8) Recurrent thoughts of death, suicidal ideation, document and immediately report all threats of suicide to nursing and physical therapist.
   (9) Decline in cognitive function (i.e., document with MMSE).
   (10) Standardized test: Geriatric Depression Scale; 30-item yes/no scale; score >8 indicates depression.
d. Medical treatment: pharmacotherapy widely used; psychotherapy; electroconvulsive shock therapy (ECT); may be used if drug treatment is unsuccessful or contraindicated (see Table 9-2).
e. Interventions, implications and compensatory strategies.
   (1) Avoid excessive cheerfulness; provide support and encouragement.
   (2) Assist patient in adjustment process to losses, coping strategies.
   (3) Encourage activities, exercise program; aerobic training is associated with increased feelings of well-being.
   (4) Assist in improving/maintaining independence; emphasize mastery by patient, achievement of short-term goals rather than long-term goals.

Cardiovascular System Disorders and Diseases

1. **Hypertension: pressures in excess of 160/95 mm Hg; can be classified according to type (systolic or diastolic).**

(a) Significant risk factors associated with cardiovascular disease.
   (1) Stroke.
   (2) Renal failure.
   (3) Death.
(b) Treatment to lower blood pressure significantly decreases risk of these complications.
   (1) Medication.
   (2) Lifestyle modifications; i.e., increasing activity level.
   (3) Dietary changes.

2. **Coronary artery disease (CAD)/ischemic heart disease: affects an estimated 12 million persons in the United States; although death rates from CAD have decreased, there has not been a decline in the incidence of CAD.**

3. **Angina pectoris: angina pain not always a consistent indicator of ischemia in elderly; shortness of breath, ECG ST segment depression may be more reliable indicators.**

4. **Acute myocardial infarction (MI).**
   a. Clinical presentation: occur more frequently in the morning hours; may vary from younger adult, may present with sudden dyspnea, acute confusion, syncope; silent attacks may occur (painless, asymptomatic) in adults >75 years of age; more common among nonwhites, smokers and adults with diabetes.
   b. Clinical course often more complicated in the elderly; mortality rates twice that of younger adults.

5. **Congestive heart failure.**

6. **Conduction system diseases; pacemaker dysfunction results in low cardiac output.**

7. **Peripheral vascular disease.**

8. **See chapter 4 on Cardiovascular Physical Therapy for discussion of these diseases.**

Pulmonary Disorders and Diseases

1. **Chronic bronchitis.**

2. **Chronic obstructive pulmonary disease (COPD).**

3. **Asthma.**

4. **Pneumonia.**
   a. Initial symptoms may vary: instead of high fever, productive cough may see altered mental status, tachypnea and dehydration.

5. **Lung cancer.**

6. **See chapter 5 on Pulmonary Physical Therapy for a discussion of these diseases.**

Integumentary Disorders and Diseases

1. Pressure ulcers (decubitus ulcers).
   a. Characteristics:
      (1) Risk factors: immobility and inactivity, sensory impairment, cognitive deficits, decreased circulation, poor nutritional status, incontinence and moisture.
      (2) Common over bony prominences: ischial tuberosities, sacrum, greater trochanter, heels, ankles, elbows, scapulae.
      (3) If not treated promptly, can progress to damage of deep structures.

      (4) Potentially fatal in frail elderly and chronically ill.
   b. Intervention, clinical signs and symptoms refer to the Integumentary chapter.

Metabolic Pathologies

1. Diabetes mellitus.
   a. Aging is associated with deteriorating glucose tolerance; type II diabetes affects as many as 10%–20% of individuals over age of 60.
   b. Associated with obesity and sedentary lifestyle.
   c. Intervention, clinical signs and symptoms and examination. Refer to chapter 7 on Other Systems for discussion.

Common Problem Areas for Aging Adults

Immobility-Disability

1. Impaired mobility and disability can result from a host of diseases and problems.

2. Limitations in function increase with age; includes difficulty with personal care activities and home management activities.

3. Immobility can result in additional problems.
   a. Immobility can lead to complications in almost every major organ system: e.g., pressure sores, contractures, bone loss, muscular atrophy, deconditioning.
   b. Metabolic changes can include: negative nitrogen and calcium balance, impaired glucose tolerance, decreased plasma volume, altered drug pharmacokinetics.
   c. Psychological changes can include loss of positive self-image, depression.
   d. Behavioral changes can include; confusion, dementia secondary to sensory deprivation, egocentricity.
   e. Loss of independence and dependency.

4. Physical therapist examination to identify source of immobility or disability.

5. Interventions, goals and outcomes.
   a. Establishment of a supportive relationship and promote self-determination of goals.
   b. Focus on optimal function, gradual progression of physical daily activities.
   c. Prevent further complications or injury.
   d. A team approach of health professionals to address all aspects of the patient's problems; patient participation in decision making.

Falls and Instability

1. Falls and fall injury are a major public health concern for the elderly.
   a. Each year approximately 30% of persons over the age of 65 fall.
   b. Falls often result in soft tissue injuries and fractures; are a factor in 40% of admissions to nursing homes.
   c. Falls result in: increased caution and fear of falling, loss of confidence to function independently, reduced motivation and levels of activity, increased risk of recurrent falls.

2. Fall etiology: most falls are multifactorial, the result of multiple intrinsic and extrinsic factors and their cumulative effects on mobility; e.g., disease states, age-related changes.
   a. Intrinsic/physiological factors.
      (1) Age: incidence of falls increases with age.
      (2) Sensory changes.
         (a) Reduced vision, hearing, cutaneous proprioceptive, vestibular function.
         (b) Altered sensory organization for balance, reduced resolution of sensory conflict situations, increased dependence on support surface somatosensory inputs.
      (3) Musculoskeletal changes: weakness; decreased ROM; altered postural synergies.
      (4) Neuromotor changes: dizziness, vertigo common.
         (a) Timing and control problems: impaired reaction and movement times, slowed onset.
      (5) Cardiovascular changes: orthostatic hypotension; hyperventilation, coughing, arrhythmias.

(6) Drugs.
   (a) Strong evidence linking psychotropic agents.
   (b) Some evidence linking certain cardiovascular agents, especially those that cause peripheral vasodilation.
   (c) Conflicting evidence linking analgesics, hypoglycemics.
b. Intrinsic/psychosocial factors.
  (1) Mental status/cognitive impairment.
  (2) Depression.
  (3) Denial of aging.
  (4) Fear of falling, associated with self-imposed activity restriction.
  (5) Relocation.
c. Extrinsic/environmental factors.
  (1) Setting: three times as many falls for institutionalized or hospitalized elderly than for community dwelling.
  (2) Consider ground surfaces, lighting, doors/doorways, stairs.

(3) At home most falls occur in bedroom (42%), bathroom (34%).
d. Activity-related risk factors.
  (1) Most falls occur during normal daily activity: getting up from bed/chair, turning head/body, bending, walking, climbing/descending stairs.
  (2) Some falls are caused by improper use of assistive device: walker, cane, wheelchair.

3. Fall prevention.
a. Examination, performed by PT.
  (1) Accurate fall history: location, activity, time, symptoms, previous falls.
  (2) Physical examination of patient: cognitive, sensory, neuromuscular, cardiopulmonary.
  (3) Standardized tests and measures for functional balance and instability (see Table 9-5).
b. Identify fall risk; determine all intrinsic and/or extrinsic factors.

Table 9-5 ➤ FUNCTIONAL BALANCE TESTS

TEST	DESCRIPTION	REFERENCE VALUES
Performance-Oriented Mobility Assessment (POMA, Tinetti)	Examines balance (balance subtest, nine items including sitting, sit-to-stand, standing, standing feet together, turn 360 degrees, sternal nudge, stand on one leg, tandem stand, reaching up, bending over, stand-to-sit, timed rising) and walking (gait subtest, eight items including gait initiation, path, turning timed walk, step over obstacles)	Maximum score is 28; patients who score <19 are at high risk for falls; patients who score 19–24 are at moderate risk
Berg Balance Scale	Examines functional balance (14 items) including sitting unsupported, sit-to-stand, stand-to-sit, transfers; in standing: EO to EC, feet together, forward reach, pick object off floor, head turns, turning 360 degrees, stepping up, tandem stand, stand on one leg	Maximum score is 56; patients who score <45 are at high risk for falls; with scores 54–46, a 1-point drop is associated with a 6%–8% increase in fall risk
Timed Up and Go (TUG)	Examines functional balance during rise from a chair, walk 3 m, turn, and return to chair. Performance on the Get Up & Go test (GUG) is untimed	Normal intact adults can perform the test in (10 seconds; 11–20 seconds is considered normal for frail elderly or disabled patients; patients who take >20 seconds are at increased risk for falls; patients who take >30 seconds are at high risk
Functional Reach (FR)	Examines maximal distance a person can reach forward beyond arm's length while maintaining a fixed position in standing (single item test)	Forward reach norms: above average >12.2 inches, below average <5.6 inches; a forward reach of <10 is indicative of increased fall risk
Multidirectional Reach Test (MDRT)	Examines maximal distance a person can reach forward, backward, and lateral to right and left	Backward: above average >7.6 inches, below average <1.6 inches; lateral: above average >9.4 inches, below average <3.8 inches
Short Physical Performance Battery (SPPB)	Includes repeated chair stands (sit-to-stand rises), semitandem, tandem, and side-by-side stands as well as a timed 8 ft (2.44 meter) walk	Tests are scored in terms of time to complete: 5 sit-to-stands, 10 sec in each of the standing conditions and 8 ft walk. An ordinal score is given for each section. Summary ordinal score: 0 (worst performance) to 12 (best performance).
Dynamic Gait Index (DGI)	Examines dynamic gait (eight items) including changes in gait speed, head turns, pivot turns, obstacles, and stairs	Normal intact adults received a score of 21 ± 3; patients with history of falls received a mean score of 11 ± 4
Balance Efficacy Scale (BES)	Examines level of self-confidence when performing functional tasks encountered in daily life; 18 questions are scored from 0%–100% confidence; activities include getting out of chair, walking up and down flight of 10 stairs, getting out of bed, getting into and out of tub or shower, removing items from cupboard, walking on uneven ground, standing on one leg	Total score is divided by 18 to yield mean BES score; scores <50 indicate low confidence

c. Interventions, goals and outcomes as established by physical therapist. Followed up by the physical therapist assistant.
 (1) Eliminate or minimize all fall risk factors; stabilize disease states, medications.
 (2) Improve functional mobility.
 (3) Provide exercise to increase strength, flexibility.
 (4) Provide sensory compensation strategies.
 (5) Balance and gait training.
 (6) Functional training.
  (a) Focus on sit-to-stand transitions, turning, walking, stairs.
  (b) Modify ADL; provide assistive devices, adaptive equipment as appropriate.
  (c) Allow adequate time for activities; instruct in gradual position changes.
 (7) Safety education.
  (a) Identify risks.
  (b) Provide instructions in writing.
  (c) Communicate with family and caregivers.
 (8) Modify environment to reduce falls and instability.
  (a) Use environmental checklist.
  (b) Ensure adequate lighting.
  (c) Use contrasting colors to delineate hazardous areas.
  (d) Simplify environment, reduce clutter.
d. When the patient falls:
 (1) Do not attempt to lift patient by yourself: get help, provide first aid and call emergency services if necessary.
 (2) Check for dizziness that may have preceded the fall.
 (3) Provide reassurance.
 (4) Contact supervising physical therapist.
 (5) Solicit witnesses of fall event.
 (6) Document event.

Medication Errors

1. Scope of the problem.
 a. Most elderly (60%–85%) utilize prescription drugs to address a chronic medical problem.
 b. One-third have three or more medical problems requiring multiple medications and complex dosage schedules.
 c. Average older person takes between four and seven prescription drugs each day.
  (1) Also, an additional 3.2 over-the-counter drugs.
 d. Adverse drug reactions are associated with:
  (1) Hospital admissions.
  (2) High incidence of falls/hip fracture: e.g., effects of psychotropic agents.
  (3) Motor vehicle accidents.

2. Older adults are at increased risk for drug toxicity.

 a. Factors include age-related changes in pharmacokinetics.
  (1) Alterations in drug absorption, distribution to tissues, oxidative metabolism.
  (2) Altered sensitivity to the effects of drugs.
   (a) Increased with certain drugs (e.g., narcotic analgesics, benzodiazepines).
   (b) Decreased with certain drugs (e.g., drugs mediated by beta-adrenergic receptors, isoproterenol, propranolol).
  (3) Alterations in excretion associated with a decline in hepatic and renal function: decreased clearance in certain drugs (e.g., digoxin, lithium).
  (4) Drugs may interfere with brain function, cause confusion (e.g., psychoactive drugs, sedatives, hypnotics, antidepressants, anticonvulsants, antiparkinsonism agents).
  (5) Older adults have less homeostatic reserve (e.g., more susceptible to orthostatic hypotension with vasodilating drugs due to dampened compensatory baroreceptor response).
  (6) Drug-processing effects: multiple drugs compete for binding sites.
   (a) Drug-to-drug interactions (e.g., levadopa combined with monoamine oxidase inhibitors [MAOIs] may result in hypertensive response).
   (b) Most drugs exert more than one specific action in the body (polypharmacological effects: e.g., prednisone prescribed for anti-inflammatory action may benefit arthritic symptoms but will aggravate a coexisting diabetic state (augments blood glucose levels).
 b. Physicians may prescribe medications that are inappropriate for use with some elderly persons: e.g., those causing hypotension or dizziness.
 c. Most patients are not knowledgeable about drug actions, drug side effects.
 d. Drug-food interactions can interfere with effectiveness of medications (e.g., efficacy of levadopa is compromised if ingested too soon before or after a high-protein meal); potential vitamin/drug interactions.
 e. Polypharmacy phenomena: multiple drug prescriptions.
  (1) Exacerbated by elderly who visit multiple physicians, use different pharmacies.
  (2) Lack of integrated care; e.g., computerized system of drug monitoring.
 f. Health status influences/socioeconomic factors.
  (1) Older adults have a high rate of medication dosage errors: associated with memory impairment, visual impairments, uncoordination, low literacy.
  (2) Financial issues: due to high costs and/or fixed incomes the elderly may skip dosages or stop taking medications.

g. Common adverse effects.
  (1) Confusion/dementia (e.g., tranquilizers, barbiturates, digitalis, antihypertensives, anticholinergic drugs, analgesics, antiparkinsonians, diuretics, beta-blockers).
  (2) Sedation/immobility (e.g., psychotropic drugs, narcotic analgesics).
  (3) Weakness (e.g., antihypertensives, vasodilators, digitalis, diuretics, oral hypoglycemics).
  (4) Postural hypotension (e.g., antihypertensives, diuretics, tricyclic antidepressants, tranquilizers, nitrates, narcotic analgesics).
  (5) Depression (e.g., antihypertensives, anti-inflammatory, antimycobacterial, antiparkinsonians, diuretics, sedative-hypnotics, vasodilators).
  (6) Drug-induced movement disorders.
    (a) Dyskinesias: involuntary, stereotypic and repetitive movements (e.g., lip smacking, hand movements) associated with long-term use of neuroleptic drugs and anticholinergic drugs, levadopa.
    (b) Akathisia (motor restlessness) associated with antipsychotic drugs.
    (c) Essential tremor associated with tricyclic antidepressants, adrenergic drugs.
    (d) Parkinsonism: associated with antipsychotics, sympatholytics.
  (7) Incontinence: caused by or exacerbated by a variety of drugs (e.g., barbiturates, benzodiazapines, antipsychotic drugs, anticholinergic drugs).

3. **Interventions, goals and outcomes.**
  a. Assess in adequate monitoring of drug therapy.
    (1) Recognize drug-related side effects.
      (a) Adverse reactions to drugs.
      (b) Potential drug interactions in the elderly.
    (2) Carefully document patient responses to medications, exercise and activity.
  b. Assist in patient and family drug education/compliance; e.g., understanding of purpose of drugs, dosage, potential side effects.
  c. Encourage centralization of medications through one pharmacy.
  d. Assist in simplification of drug regimen and instructions.
    (1) Administration of drugs (e.g., daily pill box, drug calendar).
    (2) Check to see if patient is taking medications on schedule.
    (3) Time doses in conjunction with daily routine.
  e. Coordinate physical therapy with drug schedule/optimal dose; e.g. exercise during peak dose with individual on Parkinson's medications.
  f. Recognize potentially harmful interaction effects: modalities that cause vasodilatation in combination with vasodilating drugs.

Nutritional Deficiency

1. **Many older adults have primary nutritional problems.**
  a. Nutritional problems in elderly are linked to health status and poverty rather than to age itself.
    (1) Chronic diseases alter the overall needs for nutrients/energy demands, the abilities to take in and utilize nutrients and overall activity levels; e.g., Alzheimer's disease, CVA, diabetes.
    (2) Limited, fixed incomes severely limit food choices and availability.
  b. Both undernourishment and obesity exist in the elderly and contribute to decreased levels of vitality and fitness.
  c. Contributing factors to poor dietary intake.
    (1) Decreased sense of taste and smell.
    (2) Poor teeth or poorly fitting dentures.
    (3) Reduced gastrointestinal function: decreased saliva, gastromucosal atrophy, reduced intestinal mobility, reflux.
    (4) Loss of interest in foods.
    (5) Lack of social support, socialization during meals.
    (6) Lack of mobility: inability to get to grocery store, shop; inability to prepare foods.
  d. There is an age-related slowing in basal metabolic rate and a decline in total caloric intake. Most of the decline is associated with a concurrent reduction in physical activity.
  e. Dehydration is common in the elderly, resulting in fluid and electrolyte disturbances.
    (1) Thirst sensation is diminished.
    (2) May be physically unable to acquire/maintain fluids.
    (3) Environmental heat stresses may be life threatening.
  f. Diets are often deficient in nutrients, especially vitamins A and C, B_{12}, thiamine, protein, iron, calcium/vitamin D, folic acid, zinc.
  g. Increased use of taste enhancers, e.g., salt and sugar or alcohol, influences nutritional intake.
  h. Drug/dietary interactions influence nutritional intake (e.g., reserpine, digoxin, antitumor agents, excessive use of antacids).

2. **Assessment, performed by physical therapist. Ongoing assessment by the physical therapist assistant.**
  a. Dietary history: patterns of eating, types of foods.
  b. Psychosocial: mental status, desire to eat/depression, social isolation.
  c. Body composition: weight/height measures; skin fold measurements (triceps/subscapular skin fold thickness); upper arm circumference.
  d. Sensory function: taste and smell.
  e. Dental and periodontal disease, fit of dentures.

f. Ability to feed self: mastication, swallowing, hand/mouth control, posture, physical weakness, fatigue.

g. Integumentary: skin condition, edema.

h. Compliance to special diets.

i. Functional assessment: basic ADL, feeding, overall exercise/activity levels.

3. Interventions, goals and outcomes.

a. Assist in monitoring adequate nutritional intake.

b. Assist in health promotion.

(1) Maintain adequate nutritional support.

(a) Nutritional consults as necessary.

(b) Nutritional educational programs.

(c) Assistance in grocery shopping, meal preparation; e.g., recommendations for home health aides.

(d) Elderly food programs: home delivered/"meals on wheels"; congregate meals/senior center daily meal programs; federal food stamp programs.

(2) Maintain physical function, adequate activity levels.

Therapeutic Exercise Foundations

THOMAS BIANCO
SUSAN B. O'SULLIVAN

Focus Areas for Content Review:
- Principles of exercise physiology.
- Application of therapeutic exercise strategies to address patient goals/outcomes.
- Contraindications for therapeutic exercise strategies.

Strength Training

Concepts of Muscle Function and Strength

1. **Strength is the force output of a contracting muscle and is directly related to the amount of tension a contracting muscle can produce.**

2. **Contractile elements of muscle.**
   a. Muscles are composed of fibers, which are made up of myofibrils. Myofibrils are composed of sarcomeres that are connected in series. The overlapping cross bridges of actin and myosin make up a sarcomere.
   b. When a muscle contracts, the actin-myosin filaments slide together and the muscle shortens. The cross bridges slide apart when the muscle relaxes and returns to its resting length.

3. **Motor unit nerve supply to the muscle.**
   a. Slow-twitch (ST) fibers (type I).
      (1) Slow contraction speed.
      (2) Low force (tension) production.
      (3) Highly resistant to fatigue.
   b. Fast-twitch (FT) fibers (type IIa).
      (1) Fast contraction speed.
      (2) Fatigue resistant.
      (3) Characteristics can be influenced by the type of training.
   c. Fast-twitch (FT) fibers (type IIb).
      (1) Fast contraction speed.

   (2) High-force production.
   (3) Susceptible to quick fatigue.
   d. Hereditary influences and fiber type distribution.
      (1) The percentage of either FT or ST fibers in the body is determined by genetics. This ratio cannot be changed via normal exercise.
      (2) Specific training can modify metabolic characteristics of all fiber types: e.g., high-intensity, anaerobic strength training will stimulate optimal FT adaptation.
   e. Order of fiber type recruitment.
      (1) Recruitment order depends upon type of activity, force required, movement pattern and position of the body.
      (2) ST motor units have the lowest functional thresholds and are recruited during lighter, slower efforts such as low-intensity, long-duration endurance activities.
      (3) Higher forces with greater velocity cause the activation of more powerful, higher threshold FT motor units.
      (4) Order of recruitment is ST, followed by FT IIa and finally followed by FT IIb motor units.

4. **Length-tension.**
   a. As the muscle shortens or lengthens through the available ROM, the tension it produces varies.

251

Table 10-1 ➤ RESISTANCE TRAINING SPECIFICITY CHART

RELATIVE LOADING	OUTCOME	% 1 RM	REPETITION RANGE	# OF SETS	REST BETWEEN SETS
Light	Muscular Endurance	<70	12 20	1 3	20 30 seconds
Moderate	Hypertrophy and Strength	70 80	8 12	1 6	30 120 seconds
Heavy	Maximum Strength	80 100	1 8	1 5+	2 5 minutes

Maximum tension is generated at some midpoint in the ROM; less tension is developed in either shortened or lengthened ROM.

b. The weight lifted or lowered cannot exceed that which the muscle is able to control at its weakest point in the ROM.

c. When a muscle is stretched beyond the resting length, there is a mechanical disruption of the cross bridges as the microfilaments slide apart and the sarcomeres lengthen. Releasing the stretch allows the sarcomeres to return to their resting length. This change in ratio of length to tension is called *elasticity*.

d. Once released, a muscle stretched into the elastic range will contract and produce a force or tension as the muscle returns to its original length.

Adaptations to Strength Training

1. **Muscle.**
   a. Hypertrophy is an increase in muscle size as a result of resistance training and can be observed after at least 6–8 weeks of training.
   b. Remodeling: individual muscle fibers are enlarged, contain more actin and myosin and have more, larger myofibrils; sarcomeres are increased.
   c. An increase in motor unit recruitment and synchronization of firing facilitates contraction and maximizes force production.
   d. The average person has a ratio of 50% fast to ST motor units. Performing workloads of low intensity will challenge half of the body's muscle mass. High-intensity exercises for shorter durations (less than 20 repetitions) are needed to train the highly adaptable FT IIa fibers.
   e. Disuse atrophy occurs when a muscle loses both size and strength from lack of use or when a limb is immobilized.
   f. Cross-section area of a muscle highly correlates with strength gains. The larger the muscle, the greater the strength of that muscle.

2. **Positive changes in impairments. Improvement in:**
   a. Strength.
   b. Bone mass.
   c. Body composition: fat to lean body composition.
   d. Weight control and weight maintenance; decreased risk of adult-onset diabetes.
   e. Reaction time.

f. Metabolism, calorie burning during and after exercise.
g. Cardiovascular status: reduction in resting blood pressure.
h. Immunologic function.

3. **Positive changes in function and quality of life.**
   a. Improved balance and coordination.
   b. Improved gait and functional mobility.
   c. Improved activities of daily living.
   d. Improved job/recreational/athletic performance.
   e. Improved sense of well-being, posture and self image.

Guidelines to Develop Strength (see Table 10-1)

1. **Overload principle:** To increase strength, the muscle must be loaded or challenged beyond its current force capability. Higher levels of tension will cause hypertrophy and recruitment of muscle fibers. This level will change with each adaptation.

2. **Specificity of training** refers to adaptations in the metabolic and physiological systems of the body depending on the type of overload imposed. Specific modes of exercise elicit specific adaptations, creating specific training effects.

3. **Reversibility:** benefits of training are not sustained unless muscles are continuously challenged. Detraining effects include decreased muscle recruitment and muscle fiber atrophy.

4. **Metabolic effects of strength training.**
   a. Muscle contraction to about 60% of its force-generating capacity causes a blockage of blood flow to the working muscle. This is a result of increased intramuscular pressure. The energy source for this level of muscle contraction is mainly anaerobic and does not improve with aerobic conditioning.
   b. Strength training of specific muscles has a brief activation period and uses a relatively small muscle mass, producing less cardiovascular metabolic demand than vigorous walking, running, swimming, etc.
   c. Rhythmic activities increase blood flow to exercising muscles via a contraction and relaxation "milking action." The primary energy source is aerobic.
   d. Circuit training (cross training) with high repetitions and low weights incorporates all modes of training

and provides more general conditioning to improve body composition, muscular strength and some cardiovascular fitness.

5. Common errors associated with resistance or strength training.
   a. Valsalva's maneuver: forcible exhalation with the glottis, nose and mouth closed while contraction is being held. This maneuver increases intrathoracic pressure, slows HR, decreases return of blood to the heart, increases venous pressure and cardiac work.
   b. Inadequate rest after vigorous exercise. Three to 4 minutes are needed to return the muscle to 90%–95% of preexercise capacity. Most rapid recovery occurs in the first minute.
   c. Increasing exercise progression too quickly (intensity, duration, frequency) can overwork muscles and cause injuries.
   d. Substitute motions occur from too much resistance, incorrect stabilization and when muscles are weak from fatigue, paralysis or pain.

Exercises to Improve Strength and Range

1. Manual resistance is a type of active exercise in which another person provides resistance.
   a. Advantages.
      (1) Useful in the early stages of an exercise program when the muscle is weak. The therapist can judge the capability of muscle to safely meet demands of exercise.
      (2) Can be modified for a painful arc in the joint range of motion (ROM).
      (3) Safe resistance exercise when the joint movement needs to be carefully controlled and the resistance is mild to moderate.
      (4) Can be easily changed to include diagonal or functional patterns of movement, (e.g., proprioceptive neuromuscular facilitation [PNF]) or appropriate facilitation techniques (e.g., quick stretch) (Table 10-2).
         (a) Extremity as well as trunk PNF patterns can be used to facilitate strength, motor recruitment and ROM.
   b. Disadvantages.
      (1) The amount of resistance cannot be measured quantitatively.
      (2) It may be difficult to maintain the same resistance during the full joint ROM and to consistently repeat the same resistance.
      (3) The amount of resistance is limited by the strength of the clinician or caregiver.

2. Mechanical resistance is a type of active exercise in which resistance is applied through the use of equipment or mechanical apparatus.

Table 10-2 ➤ PROPRIOCEPTIVE NEUROMUSCULAR FACILITATION PATTERNS

DIAGONAL PATTERN	JOINT POSITION AND/OR MOTION
UPPER EXTREMITY	
D1 Flexion	Begin in: glenohumeral medial rotation, abduction and extension
	Move to: lateral rotation, adduction and flexion
	D1 Extension: is the opposite
D2 Flexion	Begin in: glenohumeral medial rotation, adduction and extension
	Move to: lateral rotation, abduction and flexion
	D2 Extension: is the opposite
LOWER EXTREMITY	
D1 Flexion	Begin in: medial rotation, abduction and extension
	Move to: lateral rotation, adduction and flexion
	D2 Extension: is the opposite
D2 Flexion	Begin in: lateral rotation, adduction and extension
	Move to: medial rotation, abduction and flexion
	D2 Extension: is the opposite
HEAD AND TRUNK DIAGONAL PATTERNS	
Chopping	Sitting or Supine: upper trunk flexion with rotation and upper extremity D1 extension—facilitates rolling to prone position
Lower Trunk Rotation	Supine trunk flexion with rotation to right or left, knees flexing
Lower Extremity D1 Pattern	D1 flexion helps rolling in any direction

   a. Advantages.
      (1) The amount of resistance can be measured quantitatively and increased over time.
      (2) Can be used when amounts of resistance are greater than the clinician can apply manually.
   b. Disadvantages.
      (1) Not easily modified to exercise in diagonal or functional patterns.
      (2) May not be safe if resistance needs to be carefully controlled or maintained at low levels.

3. Goals and indications for resistance exercise.
   a. Increase strength as a muscle group that lifts, lowers or controls heavy loads for relatively low number of repetitions.
   b. Increase muscular endurance by performing low-intensity repetitive exercise over a prolonged period of time.
   c. Improve muscular performance related to strength and speed of movement.

4. Precautions.
   a. Local muscle fatigue is a normal response of the muscle from repeated dynamic or static contractions

over a period of time. Fatigue is due to depleted energy stores, insufficient oxygen and build-up of lactic acid. It is characterized by a decline in peak torque and increased muscle pain with occasional spasm and decreased AROM.

b. General muscular fatigue affects the whole body after prolonged activities such as walking or jogging, usually due to low blood sugar, decreased glycogen stores in muscle and liver, depletion of potassium.

c. Fatigue may be associated with specific clinical diseases: e.g., multiple sclerosis, cardiac disease, peripheral vascular dysfunction and pulmonary diseases. These patients fatigue more rapidly and require longer rest periods.

d. Overwork or overtraining causes temporary or permanent loss of strength as a result of exercise. In normal individuals, fatigue causes discomfort so overtraining and muscle weakness do not usually occur. Patients with lower motor neuron disease who participate in vigorous resistance exercise programs can have a deterioration of strength: e.g., postpolio syndrome. Overwork can be avoided with slow progression of the exercise intensity, duration and progression.

e. Osteoporosis makes the bone unable to withstand normal stresses and highly susceptible to pathological fracture. It may develop as a result of prolonged immobilization, bed rest, the inability to bear weight on an extremity and as a result of a nutritional or hormonal factor.

f. Acute muscle soreness develops during or directly after strenuous anaerobic exercise performed to the point of fatigue. Decreased blood flow and reduced oxygen (ischemia) creates a temporary build up of lactic acid and potassium. A cool-down period of low intensity exercise can facilitate the return of oxygen to the muscle and reduce the soreness.

g. Delayed-onset muscle soreness (DOMS) can begin 12–24 hours after vigorous exercise or muscular overexertion. It peaks 24–48 hours after exercise. Muscle tenderness and stiffness can last up to 5–7 days. Usually, it is greater after muscle lengthening or eccentric exercise. Severity of soreness can be lessened by gradually increasing intensity and duration of exercises.

5. **Contraindications.**

a. Inflammation: resistance exercises can increase swelling and cause damage to muscles or joints.

b. Pain: severe joint or muscle pain during exercise or for more than 24 hours after exercise requires an elimination or reduction of the exercise.

6. **Types of resistance exercise.**

a. Isometric exercise is static and occurs when a muscle contracts without a length change. Resistance is variable and accommodating. Contractions should be held for at least 6 seconds to obtain adaptive changes in the muscle.

(1) Strengthening of muscles is developed at a point in the ROM, not over the entire length of the muscle.

(2) This type of resistance exercise can increase blood pressure and should be used cautiously with the patient with a cardiac condition.

(3) Monitor for potential Valsalva's maneuver.

b. Isotonic exercise is dynamic and can have a constant (free weights) or a variable (machine) load as the muscle lengthens or shortens through the available ROM. Speed can be variable for this type of exercise.

(1) Weight-lifting machines have an oval-shaped cam or wheel that mimics the length-tension curve of the muscle: e.g., Nautilus or Cybex. These machines vary the resistance as the muscle goes through the ROM, providing resistance that the muscle can safely complete at various points of the ROM.

(2) Free weights do not vary the resistance through the ROM of a muscle. The weakest point along the length-tension curve of each muscle limits the amount of weight lifted.

(3) Weight-lifting machines are safer than free weights and used early in a resistance exercise or rehabilitation program.

c. Isokinetic exercise is dynamic and has a speed control for muscle shortening and lengthening. Resistance is accommodating and variable.

(1) Peak torque, the maximum force generated through the ROM, is inversely related to angular velocity, the speed the body segment moves through its ROM: i.e., increasing angular velocity decreases peak torque production.

(2) Concentric or eccentric resistance exercise can be performed on isokinetic equipment.

(3) Isokinetic exercise provides maximum resistance at all points in the ROM as the muscle contracts.

(4) During isokinetic testing, the weight of a body segment creates a torque output around the joint: e.g., the lower leg around the knee joint in sitting knee flexion. This gravity-produced torque adds to the force generated by the muscle when it contracts and gives a higher torque output than is actually created by the muscle. The higher value can affect the testing values of the muscle group and which muscle group needs to be strengthened. Software can correct for the effects of gravity.

d. Eccentric (lengthening) versus concentric (shortening).

(1) Maximum eccentric contraction produces more force than maximal concentric contraction.

(2) Resistance training performed concentrically improves concentric muscle strength and eccentric training improves eccentric muscle strength (specificity of training).

(3) Eccentric contractions occur in a wide variety of functional activities such as lowering the body against gravity: e.g., sitting down or descending stairs.

(4) Eccentric contractions provide a source of shock absorption during closed-chain functional activities.

(5) Eccentric contractions consume less oxygen and fewer energy stores than concentric contractions against similar loads.

7. ROM.

a. Short-arc exercise: resistance exercise performed through a limited ROM, e.g., initial exercise after knee surgery (anterior cruciate repair), painful full ROM.

b. Full arc exercise: resistance exercise performed through full ROM.

8. Open-versus closed-chain exercises.

a. Open-chain exercise occurs when the distal segment (hand or foot) moves freely in space: e.g., when an arm lifts or lowers a hand-held weight.

b. Resistance exercises usually are open chain, which may be the only option if weight bearing is contraindicated.

c. Open-chain exercise does not adequately prepare a patient for functional weight-bearing activities.

d. Closed-chain exercise occurs as the body moves over a fixed distal segment: e.g., stair climbing or squatting activities.

e. Closed-chain exercise loads muscles, bones, joints and noncontractile soft tissues such as ligaments, tendons and joint capsules.

f. Mechanoreceptors are stimulated by closed-chain exercises adding to joint stability, balance, coordination and agility in functional weight-bearing postures.

Specific Exercise Regimens

1. Progressive resistive exercise (PRE) uses the repetition maximum (RM) or the greatest amount of weight a muscle can move through the ROM a specific number of times (e.g., DeLorme, well-known physician who developed this exercise protocol, used 10 RM as baseline). Three sets of 10 repetitions are completed with brief rests (1–2 minutes) between sets. Progression (DeLorme): exercise begins with 10 repetitions at 50% RM, followed by 10 repetitions at 75% RM and finally 10 repetitions at 100% RM.

2. Circuit weight training is a sequence of exercises for total-body conditioning. A rest period of usually 30 seconds to 1 minute is taken between each exercise. Exercises can be done with free weights or weight-training machines.

3. Plyometric training, or stretch-shortening activity, is an isotonic exercise that combines speed, strength and functional activities. Used in later stages of rehabilitation to achieve a high level of performance: e.g., jumping off of a platform and then up onto the platform at a rapid pace to improve vertical jumping abilities.

4. Brief repetitive isometric exercise occurs with up to 20 maximum contractions held for 5–6 seconds and performed daily. A 20-second rest after each contraction is recommended to prevent increases in blood pressure. Strength gains occur in 6 weeks.

Endurance Training

Training Strategies to Develop Muscular Endurance

1. Muscular endurance is the ability of an isolated muscle group to perform repeated contractions over time.

2. Muscular endurance is improved by performing low-load resistance exercise for many repetitions. Exercise programs that increase strength also increase muscular endurance.

3. Muscular endurance programs are indicated after injuries to joints and soft tissues. Dynamic exercises at a high number of repetitions against light resistance are more comfortable and create less joint irritation than heavy resistance exercises.

4. Early in a strength-training program, high repetitions and low-load exercises cause less muscle soreness and reduce the risk of muscle injury.

Training Strategies to Develop Cardiovascular Endurance

1. Cardiovascular endurance is the ability to perform large muscle dynamic exercise, such as walking, swimming and/or biking, for long periods of time.

2. Overload principle is used to enhance physiological improvement and bring about a training change. Specific exercise overload must be applied.
   a. Training adaptation occurs by exercising at a level above normal.
   b. The appropriate overload for each person can be achieved by manipulating combinations of training frequency, intensity and duration.

3. Specificity principle refers to adaptations in the metabolic and physiological systems depending on the type of overload imposed.
   a. Specific exercise elicits specific adaptations creating specific training effects: e.g., swim training will increase cardiovascular conditioning only when tested in swimming. There is no crossover for conditioning from swimming to running.

4. Individual differences principle: training benefits are optimized when programs are planned to meet the individual needs and capacities of the participants.

5. Reversibility principle: detraining occurs rapidly, after only 2 weeks, when a person stops exercising. Beneficial effects of exercise training are transient and reversible.

6. FITT equation: includes factors that affect training: frequency, intensity, time and type. Intensity is interrelated with both duration (time) and frequency.
   a. Frequency is the number of exercise sessions per week. If training at a lower intensity, then more frequent exercise is indicated.
      (1) If the intensity is constant, the benefit from two versus four or three versus five times per week is the same.
      (2) For weight loss, 5–7 days per week increases the caloric expenditure more than 2 days per week.
      (3) Less than 2 days per week does not produce adequate changes in aerobic capacity or body composition.
   b. Intensity (overload) is the primary way to improve cardiovascular endurance.
      (1) Relative intensity for an individual is calculated as a percentage of the maximum function: e.g., maximum oxygen consumption (Vo_2max) or maximum heart rate (HRmax).
      (2) The Vo_2max or HRmax can be measured directly or indirectly based on different methods: e.g., 3-minute step, 12-minute run or 1-mile walk test.
      (3) HR max can be estimated using 220 minus the age of the individual. Training level or target heart rate (THR) can be established at 70% of maximum to increase aerobic capacity.
      (4) The Karvonen formula is used to predict heart rate reserve (HRR) or HR max minus the resting heart rate (RHR) and correlates directly to Vo_2max. THR = (HRmax – RHR) × % of desired training intensity + RHR.
      (5) Rating of perceived exertion (RPE) can be used to evaluate training at submaximal evels. A cardiorespiratory training effect can be achieved at a rating of "somewhat hard" or "hard" (13–16 on the original Borg scale of 6–19). An appropriate level of training should result in conversational exercise or "talk test": moderate exercise that is not too strenuous and can improve endurance.
   c. Duration (time).
      (1) Duration is increased when intensity is limited, e.g., by initial fitness level. Improvements in aerobic capacity, therefore, depend on increasing exercise duration and frequency; e.g., 3–5 minutes per day produces training effects in poorly conditioned individuals, whereas 20–30 minutes, three to five per week is optimal for conditioned people.
      (2) Multiple sessions of short durations are also indicated when intensity is limited by environmental conditions, such as heat and humidity or by medical conditions, such as intermittent claudication or congestive heart failure.
      (3) Obese individuals should exercise at longer durations and lower intensities. At this exercise level, the person can speak without gasping and does not have muscle ache or burn from lactic acid accumulation.
      (4) Obesity increases the mechanical work of the heart and can lead to cardiac and left ventricular dysfunction.
   d. Type of exercise needed to increase cardiovascular endurance should involve large muscle groups activated in rhythmic aerobic nature. Specificity of training should be considered.
   e. Refer to Chapter 4.

Training Strategies to Develop Pulmonary Endurance

1. Pulmonary endurance is related to the ventilation of the lungs and oxygen consumption.

2. Ventilation is the process of air exchange in the lungs. The volume of air breathed each minute or minute ventilation (Ve) is 6 liters. Ve = breathing rate × tidal volume. In maximum exercise, increases in breathing

rate and depth may produce ventilation as high as 200 liters per minute.

3. Energy is produced aerobically as oxygen is supplied to exercising muscles. Oxygen consumption rises rapidly during the first minutes of exercise then levels off as the aerobic metabolism supplies the energy required by the working muscles (steady state).

4. The more fit a person is, the more capable their respiratory system is of delivering oxygen to sustain aerobic energy production at increasingly higher levels of intensity.
   a. Obesity can impair pulmonary function because of the added effort to move the chest wall.

5. In severe pulmonary disease, the cost of breathing can reach 40% of the total exercise oxygen consumption. This would decrease the oxygen available to the exercising nonrespiratory muscles and limit exercise capabilities. Obesity can significantly increase the level of impairments.

6. Exercise-induced asthma (EIA) can occur when the normal initial bronchodilatation is followed by bronchoconstriction. The reduction in airflow from airway obstruction affects the ability of the lungs to provide oxygen to exercising muscles.
   a. EIA is an acute, reversible airway obstruction that develops 5–15 minutes after strenuous exercise when a person does not breathe through the nose, which warms and humidifies the air.
   b. When a person mouth breathes, the air is cold and dry, contributing to the bronchoconstriction.
   c. Lowering the intensity level and allowing the person to breathe through the nose can allow prolonged aerobic exercise to continue.
   d. The problem is rare in activities that require only short bursts of activity, such as baseball, and is more likely to occur in endurance activities, such as soccer.
   e. When exercising in humid versus dry environments, the exercise-induced asthmatic response is considerably reduced. Refer to Chapter 5.

Aerobic Training

1. Aerobic training (cardiorespiratory endurance training) can result in higher fitness levels for healthy individuals, slow the decrease in functional capacity in the elderly and recondition those that have been ill or have chronic disease.

2. Positive effects of aerobic training on the cardiovascular and respiratory systems.
   a. Improve breathing volumes and increased Vo_2max.
   b. Increase heart weight and volume; cardiac hypertrophy is normal with long-term aerobic training.
   c. Increase total hemoglobin and oxygen delivery capacity.
   d. Decrease resting and submaximal exercise heart rates. Can be utilized to measure improvements from aerobic training.
   e. Increase cardiac output and stroke volume.
   f. Improve distribution of blood to working muscles and enhance capacity of trained muscles to extract and use oxygen.
   g. Reduce resting blood pressure.

3. Continuous training at a submaximal energy requirement can be prolonged for 20–60 minutes without exhausting the oxygen transport system.
   a. Work rate is increased progressively as training improvements are achieved; overload can be accomplished by increasing the exercise duration.
   b. In healthy individuals, continuous training is the most effective way to improve endurance.

4. Circuit training uses a series of exercise activities that are repeated several times.
   a. Several exercise modes can be utilized involving large and small muscle groups both statically and dynamically.
   b. Circuit training improves endurance and strength by stressing the aerobic and anaerobic energy systems.

5. Interval training includes an exercise period followed by a prescribed rest interval. It is perceived to be less demanding than continuous training and tends to improve strength and power more than endurance.
   a. The relief interval can be passive or active; its duration ranges from a few seconds to several minutes. Active or work recovery involves doing the exercise at a reduced level. During the relief period, a portion of the ATP and oxygen used by the muscles during the work period is replenished by the aerobic system.
   b. The longer the work interval, the more the aerobic system is stressed and the duration of the rest period is not important.
   c. In a short work interval, a work-recovery ratio of 1:1 to 1:5 is appropriate to stress the aerobic system. A ratio of rest interval 1:1/2 work interval allows exercise to begin before recovery is complete. This stresses the aerobic system.
   d. With appropriate spacing of work-relief intervals, a significant amount of high-intensity work can be achieved. The total amount of work completed with interval training is greater than the amount of work accomplished with continuous training.

6. Warm-up and cool-down periods: each exercise session includes a 5–15 minute warm-up and a 5–15 minute cool-down period.
   a. The warm-up period prevents the heart and circulatory system from being suddenly taxed. It includes

a. low-intensity cardiorespiratory activities and flexibility exercises.

b. The cool-down period also consists of exercising at a lower intensity. It reduces abrupt physiological alterations that can occur with sudden cessation of strenuous exercise: e.g., venous pooling in the lower extremities which causes decreased venous return to the heart.

c. Longer warm-up and cool-down periods may be needed for deconditioned or older individuals.

Common Errors Associated with Muscular, Cardiovascular and Pulmonary Endurance Training

1. Lack of exercise tolerance testing (ETT) before the exercise prescription is determined could result in a training program set too high or too low for that particular individual.

2. Starting out at too high a level can overly stress the cardiorespiratory and muscular systems and potentially cause injuries.

3. Increasing intensity too fast can create a problem for an individual during endurance training.

4. Exercising at too intense a level can use the anaerobic energy system, not aerobic system; this increases strength and power, not endurance.

5. Insufficient warm-up or cool-down results in inadequate cardiorespiratory and muscular adaptation; there is inadequate time to prepare for or recover from higher intense activity.

6. Inconsistent training frequency, duration, or intensity does not properly stress or overload the aerobic system to create training effects.

Exercise at High Altitude

1. At altitudes of 6,000 feet (2,000 m) or higher there can be a noticeable drop in performance of aerobic activities.

2. The partial pressure of oxygen is reduced resulting in poor oxygenation of hemoglobin.

3. This hypoxia at altitude can result in immediate compensatory hyperventilation (stimulation of the baroreceptors) and increased heart rate.

4. Reduction in CO_2 from hyperventilation results in more alkaline body fluids.

5. Adjustments or acclimatization to higher altitude.
   a. Takes 2 weeks at 2,300 m and an additional week for every additional 600 m in altitude.

b. There is a decrease in plasma volume (concentrating red blood cells) and an increase in total red blood cells and hemoglobin improving oxygenation.

c. Changes in local circulation may facilitate oxygen transport.

d. Adjustments do not fully compensate for altitude. Maximum V_{O_2} is decreased 2% for every 300 m above 1,500 m. Thus, there is a drop in performance for endurance activities.

e. Training at altitude does not provide any improvement in sea-level performance.

6. The air in mountainous regions tends to be cool and dry. Body fluids can be rapidly lost through evaporation and result in dehydration.
   a. Ensure adequate hydration for those exercising or engaged in sport at altitude.

Exercise in Hot Weather

1. When exercising in the heat, muscles require oxygen to produce energy.

2. To decrease metabolic heat, blood is shunted to the periphery; thus, working muscles are deprived of needed oxygen.

3. Core temperature increases and sweating increases. Fluids must be continually replaced or core temperatures can rise to dangerous levels.

4. Hot, humid environments diminish the evaporative cooling component even with profuse sweating. Excess fluid loss can compromise cardiovascular function.

5. Fluid replacement.
   a. Maintain plasma volume.
   b. Colder fluids are emptied from the stomach more rapidly than room temperature fluids.
   c. Concentrated carbohydrate drinks impair gastric emptying and slow fluid replacement.
   d. Glucose-polymer drinks do not impair physiological functioning. They may also resupply lost electrolytes.

6. Repeated heat stress results in acclimatization in about 10 days of exposure.
   a. Exercise capacity is increased.
   b. Cardiac output is better regulated.
   c. Sweating is more efficient.
   d. Acclimatization to heat stress does not seriously deteriorate with age.

7. Men and women can adapt equally well to heat even though the mechanisms of thermoregulation differ slightly. The menstrual cycle is not a factor.

8. Obesity is a major consideration when exercising in the heat.

a. Excess fat slows conduction of heat to the periphery.

b. Excess fat increases the metabolic cost of activity.

9. **The addition of sports gear (e.g., football pads, helmets) coupled with a hot, humid environment and activity can compromise thermoregulation.**

a. This can potentially end in fatal results, especially with the person who is obese.

Exercise Recommendations for Individuals with Obesity (see Chapter 7)

Mobility and Flexibility Training

Flexibility

1. **Flexibility refers to the ability to move a joint through an unrestricted, pain-free ROM; the musculotendinous unit elongates as the body segment moves through the ROM.**

2. **Dynamic flexibility refers to the active ROM of a joint and is dependent upon the amount of tissue resistance met during active movement.**

3. **Passive flexibility is the degree to which a joint can be passively moved through the available ROM and is dependent upon the extensibility of the muscle and connective tissue around the joint.**

Stretching

1. **Stretching involves any therapeutic technique that lengthens shortened soft tissue structures and increases ROM.**

2. **Type of stretching is determined by the type of force applied, the intensity of stretch and duration of stretch to contractile and noncontractile tissues.**

   a. Manual passive stretching takes the structures beyond the free ROM to elongate tissues beyond their resting length.

      (1) The stretch force is applied for at least 15–30 seconds and repeated several times during a session.

      (2) Manual stretching is considered a short duration stretch, maintained statically for less time than mechanical stretching.

      (3) Intensity and duration depend on patient tolerance and therapist strength and endurance.

      (4) Low-intensity manual stretch, applied as long as possible, is better tolerated and results in optimal improvement in tissue length with minimal risk of injury to any weakened tissue.

   b. Ballistic stretching is a high-intensity very short-duration "bouncing" stretch. By contracting the opposite muscle group, the patient uses body weight and momentum to elongate the tight muscle.

      (1) It is considered unsafe because of poor control and the potential of rupturing weakened tissues. It should not be performed after an injury or surgery.

      (2) Ballistic stretch facilitates the stretch reflex, causing an increase in tension in the muscle that is being stretched. It is contraindicated in spastic muscles.

   c. Prolonged mechanical stretching is a low intensity external force (5–15 lb to 10% of body weight) applied over a prolonged period by positioning a patient with weighted pulley and traction systems. Dynamic splints or serial casts may also be used.

      (1) Prolonged stretch may be maintained for 20–30 minutes or as long as several hours.

      (2) Dynamic splints are applied for 8–10 hours to increase ROM.

      (3) Low-intensity prolonged mechanical stretching has been shown to be more effective than manual passive stretching with long-standing flexion contractures.

   d. Active stretching occurs when voluntary, unassisted movement by the patient provides the stretch force to a joint. It requires strength and muscular contraction of the prime mover to actively stretch the antagonist muscle group.

      (1) The force is controlled by the patient and is considered low intensity (to tolerance). The risk of tissue injury is low.

      (2) Duration is equal to passive manual stretching or about 15–30 seconds and is limited by prime mover muscular endurance.

   e. Active inhibition (facilitated stretching) refers to techniques in which the patient reflexively relaxes the muscle to be elongated prior to or during the stretching technique; e.g., proprioceptive neuromuscular facilitation (PNF).

      (1) Hold-relax (HR): is a relaxation technique usually performed at the point of limited ROM in the agonist pattern; an isometric contraction of

the range-limiting antagonist is performed against slowly increasing resistance, followed by voluntary relaxation and passive movement by the therapist into the newly gained range of the agonist pattern. The muscle relaxes as a result of autogenic inhibition possibly from the Golgi tendon organ (GTO) firing and decreasing muscular tension.

(2) Hold-relax-active contraction (HRAC): following hold-relax technique, active contraction into the newly gained range of the agonist pattern is performed. The muscle is further relaxed through the inhibitory effects of reciprocal inhibition.

(3) Contract-relax-active contraction (CRAC): a relaxation technique usually performed at a point of limited ROM in the agonist pattern; isotonic movement in rotation is performed followed by an isometric hold of the range-limiting muscles in the antagonist pattern against slowly increasing resistance, voluntary relaxation and active movement into the new range of the agonist pattern.

(4) Indications for active inhibition techniques include limitations in ROM caused by muscle tightness or muscle spasm. CR techniques may be more painful, especially if muscle cocontraction is present.

3. Contractile tissue.
   a. A muscle that is lengthened over a prolonged period of time will have an increase in the number of sarcomeres in series. The muscle will adjust its length over time.
   b. A muscle immobilized in a shortened position will have a decrease in the number of sarcomeres and an increase in connective tissue.
   c. The sarcomere adaptation is transient. A muscle allowed to resume its normal length will produce or absorb sarcomeres (lengthen or shorten).

4. Neurophysiological properties of contractile tissue.
   a. The muscle spindle monitors the velocity and length changes in muscle.
   b. A quick stretch to a muscle stimulates the alpha motoneurons and facilitates muscle contraction via the monosynaptic stretch reflex. This can increase tension in a muscle to be lengthened.
   c. The GTO inhibits contraction of the muscle. When excessive tension develops, the GTO fires, inhibiting alpha motoneuron activity and decreasing tension in the muscle.
   d. Slow stretching especially applied at end range causes the GTO to fire and inhibit the muscle (autogenic inhibition), allowing the muscle to lengthen (stretch-protection reflex).

5. Noncontractile connective tissue, including ligaments, tendons, joint capsules, fasciae and skin, can affect joint flexibility and requires remodeling to increase length.
   a. Low-magnitude loads over long periods increase the deformation of noncontractile tissue, allowing a gradual rearrangement of collagen bonds (remodeling). This type of stretch is better tolerated by the patient.
   b. Fifteen or twenty minutes of low-intensity sustained stretch, repeated on 5 consecutive days, can cause a change in the length of muscles and connective tissue.
   c. Intensive stretching is usually not done every day in order to allow time for healing. Without healing time, a breakdown of tissue will occur, as in overuse syndromes and stress fractures.
   d. With aging, collagen loses its elasticity and tissue blood supply is decreased, reducing healing capability. Stretching in older adults should be performed cautiously.

6. Overstretch is a stretch well beyond the normal joint ROM resulting in hypermobility. If the supporting structures of a joint are insufficient and weak, they cannot hold a joint in a stable, functional position during functional activities. This is known as stretch weakness.

7. Contracture is the adaptive shortening of muscle or other soft tissues that cross a joint; contracture results in decreased ROM.
   a. Myotatic contracture (pertaining to muscle) involves a musculotendinous unit that has adaptively shortened with loss of ROM. Usually occurs without specific tissue pathology and in two-joint muscles such as the hamstrings, rectus femoris or gastrocnemius. It can typically be resolved in a short time with gentle stretching exercises and active inhibition techniques.
   b. Adhesions can occur if tissue is immobilized in a shortened position for extended periods of time, resulting in a loss of mobility.
   c. Scar tissue adhesions develop in response to injury and the inflammatory response. Initially, new fibers develop in a disorganized pattern and will restrict motion unless remodeled along lines of stress: e.g., the patient with burns.
   d. Irreversible contracture is a permanent loss of soft tissue extensibility that cannot be released by nonsurgical treatment. It occurs when normal soft tissue is replaced by an excessive amount of nonextensible tissue such as bone or fibrotic tissue.

Relaxation of Muscles

1. Local relaxation techniques can assist in the lengthening of contractile and noncontractile tissue.

2. Heat increases the extensibility of the shortened tissues. Warm muscles relax and lengthen more easily,

reducing the discomfort of stretching. Connective tissue stretches with less force and shorter duration.

   a. The GTO sensitivity is increased which makes it more likely to fire and inhibit muscle tension.

   b. Low-intensity active exercise performed prior to stretching will increase circulation to soft tissue and warm the tissues to be stretched.

   c. Heat without stretching has little or no effect on long-term improvement in muscle flexibility. The combination of heat and stretching produces greater long-term gains in tissue length than stretching alone.

3. Massage increases local circulation to the muscle and reduces muscle spasm and stiffness.

4. Biofeedback helps the patient reduce the amount of tension in a muscle and improves flexibility while decreasing pain. Increased level of feedback signals (auditory, visual) assists the patient in recognizing tense muscles.

Common Errors Associated with Mobility and Flexibility Training

1. Passively forcing a joint beyond its normal ROM.

2. Aggressively stretching a patient with a newly united fracture or osteoporosis may result in fracture.

3. Using high-intensity, short-duration stretching procedures on muscles and connective tissues that have been immobilized over a long time or recovering from injury or surgery.

4. Stretching muscles around joints without using strengthening exercises to develop an appropriate balance between flexibility and strength.

5. Overstretching of weak muscles, especially postural muscles that support the body against gravity.

Postural Stability Training

Stability (Static Postural Control)

1. Refers to the synergistic coordination of the neuromuscular system enabling an individual to maintain a stable position in an antigravity, weight-bearing position.

2. Stability control involves prolonged holding; it is an endurance function.

Dynamic Stabilization, Controlled Mobility

1. Proximal segments and trunk provide a stable base for functional movements.

   a. An individual maintains postural stability of the trunk while weight shifting.

   b. Distal segments are fixed while proximal segments are moving.

   c. Movement normally occurs through increments of range (small range to large range).

2. Patients with hyperkinetic movement disorders (e.g., ataxia) need to be progressed from large-range to small-range movements and finally to holding steady (stability control).

Dynamic Stabilization, Static-Dynamic Control

1. An individual maintains postural stability of the trunk during dynamic extremity movements (e.g., reaching, kicking a ball).

2. Strength, endurance, flexibility and coordination are needed for static and dynamic stabilization.

Guidelines to Develop Postural Stability

1. It is important to consider exercise protocols that effectively challenge core muscle groups and create adequate stability to perform functional activities. Stability requires the recruitment of tonic, slow-twitch muscle fibers for sustained periods of time.

2. Start training by teaching safe spinal ROM in a variety of basic postures. Teach chin tucking with axial extension of the cervical spine and pelvic tilting with ROM of the lumbar spine.

3. Incorporate procedures to retrain kinesthetic awareness of postural position. Teach the neutral pelvis position first to ensure a stable base.

a. Emphasis is placed on strength and endurance of back multifidi and oblique abdominals rather than erector spinae.

b. Focus on patient awareness of normal alignment of the spine and pelvis feel of the muscles contracting to maintain that position while exercising.

c. Visual, verbal and proprioceptive cues (e.g., resistance of elastic bands or light manual resistance) can be used to improve postural awareness.

4. To safely develop strength and endurance in the stabilizing muscles, practice maintained holding in a variety of postures. The higher the center-of-mass and smaller the base-of-support, the greater the degree of postural challenge: e.g., sitting versus standing.

5. Movements of the extremities challenge the trunk and neck stabilization; functional position must be maintained as movements are carried out.

6. Resistance can be applied to the trunk or to the moving extremities; functional position must be maintained as the resistance is increased.

7. Alternating isometric contractions between antagonists can enhance stabilizing contractions and develop postural control; e.g., PNF techniques of alternating isometrics (AI) and rhythmic stabilization (RS).

a. Alternating isometrics (AI): isometric holding is facilitated first on one side of the joint, followed by alternate holding of the antagonist muscle groups. May be applied in a variety of directions; i.e. anterior-posterior, mediallateral, diagonal.

b. Rhythmic stabilization (RS): simultaneous isometric contractions of both agonist and antagonist patterns performed without relaxation using careful grading of resistance; results in cocontraction of opposing muscle groups; RS emphasizes rotational stability control.

8. During early training, emphasize muscles needed for trunk support in the upright posture, for performing basic body mechanics and for upper extremity lifting.

9. Teach control of functional positions while moving from one position to another. This is called transitional stabilization and requires graded contractions and adjustments between the trunk flexors and extensors. Consider moving out of a posture (eccentric control) before moving into a posture (concentric control).

10. Introduce simple patterns of motion that develop safe body mechanics and movement.

11. Closed-chain tasks are good choices to enhance postural stabilization (e.g., partial squats and controlled lunges); add arm motions and weights as tolerated.

12. More complex patterns of movement (e.g., rotation and diagonal motions) can be added (e.g., PNF trunk patterns of chop/reverse chop or lift/reverse lift.) Postures can be progressed to add difficulty; e.g., supine to sitting to standing.

13. Incorporate stretching into the postural exercise program. Adequate flexibility is necessary for postural muscles to hold body parts in proper alignment.

Common Errors Associated with Postural Stability Training

1. Inadequate stretching of tight muscles (e.g., tight hip flexors that hold the pelvis in an anterior pelvic tilt or tight hamstrings that hold the pelvis in a posterior tilt); both prevent a stable postural base (neutral pelvis and spine position).

2. Inadequate control of core muscles could place excessive stress on proximal structures during functional activities: e.g., the vertebrae and discs of the spine during sitting.

3. Progressing too quickly or starting at too high a functional level for the patient to maintain postural stability.

4. Exercising past the point of fatigue; this is determined by the inability of the trunk or neck muscles to stabilize the spine in its functional position.

5. Attempting to force a patient into a general neutral position, instead of finding the proper and safe position for each individual.

Stability Ball Training (also known as Swiss Ball, Physio Ball, or Therapy Ball)

1. Benefits/uses.

a. Promotes balance; provides an unstable base of support, requiring continuous adjustments in balance. Moving the feet and/or the ball changes the base of support and challenges balance. Allows safe practice of falling.

b. Works muscles in functional, synergistic patterns.

(1) Recruits and retrains core muscles (deep spinal and abdominal muscles).

(2) Promotes postural relearning: e.g., neutral position in sitting, cervical or trunk rotation.

(3) Enhances coordination, movement combinations: e.g., arm and leg bilateral symmetrical, bilateral asymmetrical movements, four-limb Mexican hat dance.

c. Heightens proprioception and sensory perception, awareness of the body moving in space.

d. Improves ROM, allows safe stretching: e.g., total body extension or flexion, upper or lower extremity stretches.

e. Allows relaxation training: e.g., gentle bouncing combined with deep breathing. Gentle rocking can be used to decrease tone in hypertonic patient.

f. Allows a safe, dynamic cardiovascular workout: e.g., dynamic bouncing with extremity movements.

g. Increases strength. Can be combined with resistance training (e.g., lifting the ball with arms or legs; using hand weights or resistive bands while on ball) or closed chain exercises (e.g., partial squats using the ball).

h. Has been used to replace chairs in schools; improves posture and concentration, calms hyperactive children.

2. Advantages: light, portable, durable and inexpensive.

3. Determining appropriate ball size.
   a. Sitting on ball with feet flat, the ball height should place the hips and knees at 90-degree angles.
   b. Supine with ball under knees, the ball height should equal the distance between the greater trochanter and the knee.
   c. Quadruped, the ball height should equal the distance between the shoulder and the wrist.

4. Firmness/inflation.
   a. Ball should be comfortable and have some bounce.
   b. A firm ball moves more quickly.
   c. A soft ball moves more slowly; may make patient feel safer, more secure.
   d. Surface affects movement of the ball: quicker on hard surface, slower on mat or soft surface.

5. Precautions.
   a. Obese individuals, exceeding ball weight limits.
   b. Avoid sharp belt buckles, zippers when over the ball; check surface for sharp objects.
   c. Lack of foot traction, feet slipping: use bare feet, rubber-soled shoes, or yoga sticky mat.
   d. Requires adequate space around exercising individual.
   e. Watch for sensory overload: sympathetic signs (e.g., children, adults with traumatic brain injury).
   f. Increased pain with mobility exercises and degenerative joint disease.
   g. Muscle fatigue.

6. Contraindications.
   a. Dizziness or nausea.
   b. Extreme anxiety or fear of being on the ball.

Coordination and Balance Training

Goals and Outcomes

1. Motor function (motor control and learning) is improved.

2. Postural control, biomechanical alignment and symmetrical weight distribution are improved.

3. Strength, power and endurance necessary for movement control and balance are improved.

4. Sensory control and integration of sensory systems (somatosensory, visual and vestibular) necessary for movement control and balance are improved.

5. Performance, independence and safety are improved in transfers, gait and locomotion.

6. Performance, independence and safety are improved in basic activities of daily living (BADL) and instrumental activities of daily living (IADL).

7. Aerobic capacity and endurance are improved.

8. Self-management of symptoms is improved.

Training Strategies to Improve Coordination and Balance

1. Motor learning strategies are important to assist the CNS in adaptation for movement control.
   a. Learning requires repetition. Practice schedules should be carefully organized. Initial practice may feel threatening to patient: e.g., patient may feel in danger of losing control or balance. Progression should be gradual; the therapist should ensure patient confidence and safety, continuing motivation.
   b. Sensory cues are used to enhance motor performance.
   c. Feedback should stress knowledge of results (KR). Attention is drawn to the success of the outcome. It is important to establish a reference of correctness during early, cognitive learning.
   d. Feedback should address knowledge of performance (KP). Attention is drawn to missing elements, how to recruit, correct responses and sequence responses.
   e. Feedback schedules: feedback given frequently (after every trial) improves initial performance. Feedback given less frequently (summed after a given number of trials or fading with decreasing frequency) improves retention of skills.

f. A variety of activities and environments should be used to promote adaptability and generalizability of skills. Practice is from a closed (fixed) environment to open variable environments.

g. Patient decision-making skills are promoted.

2. **Remedial strategies focus is on use of involved body segments (e.g., affected extremities in the patient with stroke).**

a. Control is first developed in isolated movements and progressed to more complex movements. Developmental postures/activities can be used to isolate body segments and focus on specific body skills; e.g., weight shifts to improve hip control are practiced first in kneeling before standing.

b. Control is first achieved in holding (stability) before moving in a posture (stability-dynamic control) and skill level function (e.g., gait).

c. Specific techniques can be used to remediate impairments (weakness, incoordination and adaptive shortening, abnormal tone): e.g., tapping to improve responses of a weak quadriceps in standing.

d. As quality of movement improves, speed of movement and control are increased.

e. Active responses and active learning should be promoted; progression is to unassisted or unfacilitated movements as soon as possible.

3. **Compensatory strategies are utilized as appropriate to promote safety and early resumption of functional skills: e.g., the patient with delayed or absent recovery, multiple comorbidities. Compensatory training may lead to learned nonuse of impaired extremities and delay recovery in those patients with recovery potential; e.g., the patient with stroke.**

a. Safety is improved by substitution: intact segments (sound limbs) for impaired segments; cognitive control for impaired motor control; e.g., the patient with ataxia.

b. Safety is improved by altering postural strategies; e.g., widening the base of support (BOS) and lowering the center of mass (COM).

c. Safety is improved by use of appropriate assistive devices and shoes: e.g., weighted walker, athletic shoe.

d. Safety is improved through environmental adaptations: e.g., handrails, adequate lighting and removal of throw rugs, contrast tape on stairs.

Interventions to Improve Coordination

1. **Functional training.**

a. Initial focus is on postural stability activities: e.g., holding.

(1) A number of different weight-bearing postures can be used: e.g., prone-on-elbows, sitting, quadruped, kneeling, plantigrade and standing.

Progression is to gradually decrease BOS while raising height of COM.

(2) Specific exercise techniques to enhance stability include alternating isometrics (AI) and rhythmic stabilization (RS).

(3) Use slow-reversal-hold (SRH) through decreasing ROM with ataxic movements.

b. Progress to controlled mobility activities: weight shifting through decrements (decreasing) of ROM progressing to stability (steady holding); moving in and out of postures (movement transitions).

(1) Specific exercise techniques include slow reversals (SR), SRH, guided movements.

(2) PNF patterns can be utilized to enhance synergistic control and reciprocal action of muscles; techniques of SR or SRH can be used to modulate timing and force output.

c. Aquatic exercises: water increases proprioceptive loading, slows down ataxic movements, provides buoyancy and light resistance.

d. Stabilization devices (e.g., air splints, soft neck collars) stabilize body segments and eliminate unwanted movement.

e. Environment: patients with ataxia do better in a low-stimulus environment, which allows better utilization of cognitive strategies.

2. **Sensory training.**

a. Patients with proprioceptive losses.

(1) Visual compensation strategies: e.g., Frenkel's exercises in which position is varied from supine to sitting to standing; movements are guided visually.

(2) Light weights: wrist cuffs, ankle cuffs, weighted walkers, elastic resistance bands to increase proprioceptive loading.

b. Patients with visual losses benefit from cognitive training strategies along with environmental adaptations and assistive devices.

Interventions to Improve Balance

1. **Exercises to improve ROM, strength and synergistic responses in order to withstand challenges to balance. Key activities include:**

a. "Kitchen sink exercises": heel-cord stretches, heel-rises, toe-offs, partial wall squats, single-leg activities (side kicks, back kicks), marching in place, look-arounds (head and trunk rotation), hip circles. Progression from bilateral upper extremity (UE) touch-down support to unilateral UE support to no UE support.

b. Postural awareness training: focus on control of body position, centering the center of mass (COM) within the limits of stability (LOS).

   c. Weight shifts (postural sway): training of ankle strategies, hip strategies. Can include postural sway biofeedback (e.g., Balance Master).

   d. Training of change-of-support strategies: stepping strategies (forward, backward, sideward, crossed-step); UE reaching and protective extension.

2. **Functional training activities.**

   a. Sit-to-stand (STS) and sit-down (SIT) activities. Practice moving body mass forward over BOS, extending lower extremities (LEs) and raising body mass over feet and reverse. Focus on balance control while pivoting body mass over feet.

   b. Floor-to-standing rises. Practice rising from floor to standing in the event of a fall: e.g., side sit to quadruped to kneeling to half-kneeling to standing transitions.

   c. Gait activities: practice walking forward, backward, sideward; slow to fast; normal BOS to narrowed BOS; wide turns to the right and left; 360-degree turns; head turns right and left; crossed-step walking and braiding; over and around obstacles.

   d. Elevation activities: practice step-ups, lateral step-ups, stair climbing and ramps.

   e. Dual-task training. In standing or walking, practice simultaneous UE activities (e.g., bouncing a ball, catching or throwing a ball); in standing, practice LE activities (e.g., kicking a ball, tracing letters with one foot).

   f. Community activities: Practice walking in open (variable) environments; pushing or pulling doors, car transfers, grocery shopping, etc.

   g. Practice anticipatory timing activities: e.g., getting on/off elevator, escalator.

3. **Disturbed balance activities including manual perturbations, moveable BOS devices (stability ball, wobble board, split foam roller, dense foam).**

   a. Therapist-initiated manual perturbations (sitting, standing); carefully grade force of perturbations, range and speed of movements.

   b. Stability ball training. Practice sitting, active weight shifts (e.g., pelvic clock), UE movements (e.g., arm circles, reaching), LE movements (e.g., stepping, marching), trunk movements (e.g., head and trunk turns).

   c. Wobble board/equilibrium boards. Practice both self-initiated and therapist-initiated shifts in sitting or standing. Gradually increase range and speed of shifts.

4. **Sensory training.**

   a. Visual changes. Practice standing and walking eyes open (EO) to eyes closed (EC); full lighting to reduced lighting.

   b. Somatosensory changes. Practice standing and walking on tile floor to carpet (low pile to high); dense foam, outside terrain.

   c. Vestibular changes. Practice standing and walking and moving head side-to-side, up-and-down; on a moving surface (e.g., escalator, elevator, bus).

   d. Introduce sensory conflict situations (e.g., standing on foam cushion with eyes closed).

5. **Safety education/fall prevention.**

   a. Assist patient in identification of fall risk factors; e.g., effect of medications, postural hypotension.

   b. Lifestyle counseling: assist the patient in recognizing unsafe activities, harmful effects of a sedentary lifestyle.

   c. Refer to section on Falls and Instability, Chapter 9, VI, B.

Interventions to Improve Aerobic Capacity and Endurance

1. Treadmill walking: focus on velocity control, progression is from slow to fast. Safety harness can be worn to provide partial body-weight support (BWS) if patient is unstable: e.g., the patient with ataxia or stroke. Incline and distance can also be modified.

2. Ergometers. Pace pedaling on a cycle ergometer; progression is from slow to fast. Resistance and distance can also be modified. Can include both LE and UE training.

3. Strength training.

   a. Active/active assistive exercise.

   b. Manual resistance; PNF patterns can be used to promote synergistic control, improve timing using techniques of slow reversals or slow reversal hold.

   c. Weights, pulleys, hydraulics, elastic resistance bands, mechanical or electromechanical devices.

4. Stretching exercises.

Teach Activity Pacing and Energy Conservation Strategies as Appropriate

1. The patient with ataxia has increased energy expenditure and can experience debilitating fatigue.

Relaxation Training

Relaxation

1. **Relaxation refers to a conscious effort to relieve excess tension in muscles.**
   a. Excess muscle tension can cause pain, which leads to muscle spasm, which in turn produces more pain. To break the pain/spasm cycle, patients must learn to relax tense muscles.
   b. Excess tension in tissues can result from maintaining a constant posture or sustaining muscle contractions for a period of time. Abnormal shortening or lengthening of muscles and ligaments is termed postural stress syndrome (PSS).
   c. Habituation of compensatory movement patterns that contribute to the persistence of pain is termed movement adaptation syndrome (MAS).

2. **Awareness of prolonged muscle tension is accompanied by techniques designed to promote relaxation, improve circulation and maintain flexibility.**

Training Strategies to Promote Relaxation

1. **Start with the patient in a comfortable resting position with all body parts well supported.**

2. **Jacobson's progressive relaxation technique includes a systematic distal to proximal progression of conscious contraction and relaxation of musculature.**
   a. A period of reflex relaxation follows active contraction of muscle. The stronger the contraction, the greater the relaxation.
   b. Breathing control: deep breathing is coupled with the progressive relaxation to further promote relaxation. In diaphragmatic breathing, the patient breathes in slowly and deeply through the nose, allowing the abdomen to relax and expand and then relaxes and allows the air to be expired through the relaxed open mouth.

3. **Cognitive strategies/guided imagery: the patient is instructed to focus on relaxing the body, visualizing calmness and relaxation.**
   a. The patient focuses on letting go of all muscular effort, letting tension melt away.
   b. The patient focuses on a relaxing environment or pleasant images to promote relaxation: e.g., lying on a tropical beach in the warm sunshine.

4. **Active ROM: AROM can be used to reduce tension by moving body segments slowly.**

5. **The technique of rhythmic rotation (RRo) involves slow, passive, rotational movements of the limbs or trunk and can be very effective in relieving muscular tension and spasticity: e.g., hook-lying (lying on your back with hips and knees partially bent) with both lower extremities on a Swiss ball, gently rocking the knees on the ball from side-to-side.**

6. **Slow vestibular stimulation: slow vestibular stimulation applied with gentle rocking techniques can also be used to enhance relaxation; e.g., gentle rocking of the infant with colic.**

7. **Biofeedback training can be an effective modality to promote relaxation: e.g., training to reduce the level of tension in the frontalis muscle.**

8. **Stress management/lifestyle adaptation techniques.**
   a. Careful identification and evaluation of life stressors, e.g., Life Events Scale, Holmes-Rahe Social Readjustment Scale, the Hassles Scale, is critical in developing an appropriate plan of care to reduce chronic stress. Stress-control techniques include both cognitive and physical strategies.
   b. Life style modification reduces frequency of high-stress situations and events. It is important to ensure adequate rest and activity and adequate nutrition.
   c. Enhance coping skills: ensure the patient maintains some level of control and decision making.
   d. Maximize effective use of social support systems.

Common Errors Associated with Relaxation Training

1. **Lack of awareness of the effects of the environment on an individual. Failure to have the patient in a low-stress environment and comfortably positioned.**

2. **Lack of awareness of stress factors affecting the patient. Failure to evaluate stressors carefully and incorporate stress-management techniques.**

3. **When using progressive relaxation techniques, progressing too fast from one body segment to another: e.g. distal to proximal body parts. Failure to combine slow deep breaths with each contraction and relaxation.**

4. **Lack of effective training of kinesthetic awareness. Patients do not recognize when their muscles are tense. They perceive the tense muscle as normal, not needing any relaxation intervention.**

CHAPTER 10

Aquatic Exercise

Goals and Outcomes

1. Motor function and motor learning are enhanced.

2. ROM and flexibility are improved.

3. Postural control, biomechanical alignment and symmetrical weight distribution are improved.

4. Strength, power and endurance are improved.

5. Sensory control and integration of sensory systems (somatosensory, visual and vestibular) are improved.

6. Performance, independence and safety in balance, gait and locomotion are improved.

7. Aerobic capacity and endurance are improved.

8. Relaxation, reduction of pain and decreased muscle spasm are enhanced.

Strategies

1. Immersion in pools or tanks is used to facilitate exercise. Water buoyancy, buoyant devices and various depths of immersion decrease body weight and enhance movement; similar movements on land may be more difficult or impossible to perform.

2. Allows greater freedom and range of movement than is permitted in whirlpools or Hubbard tanks.

3. Pools or tanks with a walking track, with or without a treadmill, are used to enhance gait and endurance.

Physics Related to Aquatic Exercise

1. Buoyancy: the upward force of the water on an immersed or partially immersed body or body part. It is equal to the weight of the water that it displaces (Archimedes' principle). This creates an apparent decrease in the weight and joint unloading of an immersed body part, thereby allowing easier movement in water.

2. Cohesion: the tendency of water molecules to adhere to each other. The resistance encountered while moving through water is due to cohesion; some force is needed to separate water molecules.

3. Density: the mass per unit volume of a substance. The density of water is proportional to its depth; deeper water must support the water above it.

4. Hydrostatic pressure: the circumferential water pressure exerted on an immersed body part. A pressure gradient is established between the surface water and deeper water due to the increase in water density at deeper levels.
   a. Pascal's law states that the pressure exerted on an immersed body part is equal on all surfaces.
   b. Increased pressure counteracts effusion and edema and enhances peripheral blood flow.

5. Turbulence: movement of a body part through water creates circular motion of the water (eddy current) near the surface of the part producing frictional drag.
   a. As speed of movement increases, greater resistance is encountered.
   b. Moving through turbulent water creates greater resistance as compared to calm water.
   c. Use of equipment (e.g., paddle or boot) increases resistance and drag as the patient moves through water.

Thermodynamics

1. Water temperature affects body temperature and performance.

2. Water temperature is determined by specific needs of patient and intervention goals.
   a. Cooler temperatures are used for higher intensity exercise.
   b. Warmer temperatures are used to enhance mobility and flexibility: e.g., patients with arthritis.
   c. Ambient air temperature should be close to water temperature (e.g., within 3°C).

3. There is decreased heat dissipation through sweating with immersion.

4. At temperatures >37°C patients will have increased cardiovascular demands at rest and during exercise.

5. At temperatures <25°C patients will have difficulty maintaining core temperature.

Special Equipment

1. Buoyancy assistance devices: inflatable cervical collar, flotation rings, buoyancy belt or vest, kick board.

2. Buoyant dumbbells (swimmers') are used for upright or horizontal support.

3. Webbed gloves and hand paddles are used to increase resistance to upper extremity movement.

4. Fins and boots are used to increase resistance to LE movement.

Exercise Applications

1. Movement horizontal to or upward toward the water surface (active assistive exercise) is made easier due to the buoyancy of water. A flotation device may be needed to support very weak patients.

2. Movement downward into the water is more difficult because of the buoyancy of water.
   a. A flotation device or hand-held paddle can be used to increase the resistance.
   b. A paddle turned to slice through the water decreases the resistance.

3. Resistance exercise can be controlled by the speed of the movement.
   a. Resistance is increased with increased velocity of movement due to the cohesion and turbulence of the water.
   b. Slower movements meet less resistance.
   c. Ataxic movements are slowed and more controlled against the resistance of water.

4. Stretching exercises can be assisted by the buoyancy of water.

5. The amount of weight bearing on the lower extremities is determined by the height of the water/level of immersion (buoyancy) relative to the upright patient.
   a. The greater the water depth, the less the weight/loading on extremities.
   b. Can be used for partial weight bearing (PWB) gait training.

6. Lower extremity reciprocal movements are enhanced by use of a kick board and using kicking movements.

7. Aerobic conditioning is enhanced with deep water walking or running, high step marching. Progression is to reduced water levels to land walking/running.
   a. Immersed equipment (e.g., cycle ergometer, treadmill or upper body ergometer) can be used to enhance conditioning.
   b. Swimming is an excellent aerobic training activity.
   c. Regular monitoring of exercise responses (e.g., heart rate, ratings of perceived exertion) is required.

8. Treatment time varies with the type of activity, patient tolerance and level of skill.

Contraindications

1. Bowel or bladder incontinence.

2. Severe kidney disease.

3. Severe epilepsy.

4. Severe cardiac or respiratory dysfunction: e.g., cardiac failure, unstable angina, severely reduced vital capacity, unstable blood pressure.

5. Severe peripheral vascular disease.

6. Large open wounds, skin infections, colostomy.

7. Bleeding or hemorrhage.

8. Water and airborne infections: e.g., influenza, GI infections.

Precautions

1. Fear of water, inability to swim.

2. Ataxic patients with postural instability.

3. Patients with heat intolerance: e.g., patients with multiple sclerosis.

4. Use waterproof dressings on small open wounds and intravenous lines.

Therapeutic Modalities

KAREN E. RYAN

Focus Areas for Content Review:

- Physics principles that underlie therapeutic modalities utilized in physical therapy interventions.
- Physiological effects of various physical modalities.

- Application of therapeutic modalities including indications, contraindications, safety considerations and procedures of application.
- Tests and Measures indicating patient ability to participate in and/or indication to discontinue intervention as well as to document the patient's progress toward the established goals.

Superficial Thermotherapy

Physics Related to Heat Transmission

1. Conduction: heat transfer from a warmer object to a cooler object through direct molecular interaction of objects in physical contact. Conductive modalities: hot packs, cold packs, paraffin.

2. Convection: heat transfer by movement of air or fluid from a warmer area to a cooler area or moving past a cooler body part. Convective modalities: whirlpool, Hubbard tank, fluidotherapy.

3. Radiation: transfer of heat from a warmer object to a cooler object through the transmission of electromagnetic energy without heating an intervening medium. Infrared waves absorbed by cooler body. Radiation modality: infrared lamp.

Physiological Effects of General Heat Application

1. Large areas of the body surface area exposed to heat modality, e.g., whirlpool (hip and knee immersed) and Hubbard tank (lower extremities and trunk immersed) (Table 11-1).

Table 11-1 ➤ PHYSIOLOGICAL EFFECTS OF GENERAL HEAT APPLICATION

INCREASED	DECREASED
Cardiac output	Blood pressure
Metabolic rate	Muscle activity (sedentary effect)
Pulse rate	Blood to internal organs
Respiratory rate	Stroke volume
Vasodilation	

Physiological Effects of Small Surface Area Heat Application

1. Heat modality applied to discrete area of body, e.g., low back, hamstring, neck.

2. Body tissue responses to superficial heat.
   a. Skin temperature rises rapidly and exhibits greatest temperature change.
   b. Subcutaneous tissue temperature rises less rapidly and exhibits smaller change.
   c. Muscle and joint show least temperature change, if any, depending on size of structure.

3. Physiological effects on body systems and structures to small surface area heat modalities are listed in Tables 11-2 and 11-3.

Table 11-2 ➤ INCREASED PHYSIOLOGICAL RESPONSES OF BODY SYSTEMS AND STRUCTURES TO LOCAL HEAT APPLICATION

SYSTEM/STRUCTURE	MECHANISM
Blood flow	Dilation of arteries and arterioles
Capillary permeability	Increase in capillary pressure
Elasticity of nonelastic tissues	Increased extensibility of collagen tissue
Metabolism	For every 10°C increase in tissue temperature there is a two- to threefold increase rate of cellular oxidation (Van't Hoff's law)
Vasodilation	Activation of axon reflex and spinal cord reflex, release of vasoactive agents (bradykinin, histamine, prostaglandin)
Edema	Increased capillary permeability

Table 11-3 ➤ DECREASED PHYSIOLOGICAL RESPONSES OF BODY SYSTEMS AND STRUCTURES TO LOCAL HEAT APPLICATION

SYSTEM/STRUCTURE	MECHANISM
Joint stiffness	Increased extensibility of collagen tissue and decreased viscosity
Muscle strength	Decreased function of glycolytic process
Muscle spasm	Decreased firing of II afferents of muscle spindle and increased firing of Ib Golgi tendon organ fibers reduces alpha motor neuron activity and thus decreases tonic extrafusal activity
Pain	Presynaptic inhibition of A delta and C fibers via activation of A beta fibers (gate theory), disruption of pain-spasm cycle

Goals and Indications for Superficial Thermotherapy

1. Pain modulation: increase connective tissue extensibility; reduce or eliminate soft tissue inflammation and swelling; accelerate the rate of tissue healing; reduce or eliminate soft tissue and joint restriction and muscle spasm.

2. Preparation for electrical stimulation: massage, passive and active exercise.

Precautions for Use of Superficial Thermotherapy

1. Cardiac insufficiency: edema, impaired circulation, impaired thermal regulation, metal in treatment site and open wounds.

Contraindications to the Use of Superficial Thermotherapy

1. Acute and early subacute traumatic and inflammatory conditions, decreased circulation, decreased sensation, deep vein thrombophlebitis, impaired cognitive function, malignant tumors, tendency toward hemorrhage or edema, age (very young and very old patients). Additional contraindications relative to specific modality listed separately.

General Treatment Preparation for Thermotherapy and Cryotherapy

1. The application of physical agents must be performed by a qualified physical therapist or personnel supervised by a physical therapist (physical therapist assistant, affiliating physical therapist or physical therapist assistant student). The treatment and expected sensations must be explained to the patient.

2. Place patient in comfortable position.

3. Expose treatment area and drape patient properly.

4. Inspect skin and check temperature sensation prior to treatment.

5. If patient has good cognitive function, a call bell or other signaling device can be given to patient to alert personnel of any untoward effects of treatment. Check patient frequently during initial treatment. A patient with impaired cognitive function, such as Alzheimer's disease, senility or mental retardation, should be checked frequently (every five minutes) during treatment.

6. Dry and inspect skin at conclusion of treatment.

7. Specific procedures for each physical agent listed separately.

Superficial Thermotherapy Agents

Hydrocollator Pack (Hot Pack)

1. Description: a canvas pack of varying size filled with silica gel which is heated by immersing in water heated between 165°–170°F.
   a. Mechanism of energy transfer: conduction.

2. Indications for superficial thermotherapy.
   a. Joint stiffness.
   b. Musculoskeletal pain.
   c. Muscle spasm.
   d. Preparation for electrical stimulation and massage.
   e. Preparation for passive stretching/exercise or active exercise.
   f. Subacute conditions.
   g. Chronic conditions
   h. Traumatic conditions.
   i. Inflammatory conditions.

3. Contraindications for superficial thermotherapy.
   a. Acute and subacute traumatic and inflammatory conditions.
   b. Impaired circulation.
   c. Impaired sensation.
   d. Deep vein thrombophlebitis.
   e. Impaired cognitive function.
   f. Malignant tumors.
   g. Potential of hemorrhage or edema.
   h. Pediatric or frail elderly patients (precaution).

4. Method of application.
   a. Properly position and drape patient.
   b. Visually inspect the area to be treated.
      (1) Assess the patient's ability to report sensory changes.
   c. The area should be clear of jewelry and clothing.
   d. Check pack for ruptures.
   e. Place pack in terry cloth cover (equal to 4 layers) and place one folded towel between commercial cover and patient.
      (1) Place 8–12 layers between patient and hot pack.
   f. Cover the pack to minimize heat loss.
   g. If patient must lie on pack, use additional towels and pillows to support patient.
   h. Secure pack to patient with towels, sandbags or straps if indicated.
   i. Check skin during treatment.
   j. Monitor initial response to treatment during first 5–10 minutes by asking patient for feedback and visually inspecting skin.
   k. Treatment time is generally 20–30 minutes.

Hydrotherapy (Whirlpool and Hubbard Tank)

1. Description: partial or total immersion baths in which water is agitated and mixed with air and directed at or around a specific area.
   a. Mechanism of energy transfer: convection.

2. Physics.
   a. Specific heat is the heat-absorbing capacity of water. The specific heat of water is about four times that of air.
      (1) The body is able to deal with extremes of heat through perspiration (vaporization).
      (2) As more of the body is submerged in the water, less body surface area is available to perspire.
         (a) Temperatures of the hydrotherapy tank need to decrease as more of body is submerged.
   b. Hydrostatic pressure is the circumferential water pressure exerted on an immersed body part.
      (1) This pressure can have a positive effect on edema in the area treated; however, it may not be sufficient to overcome the dependent position during treatment.
   c. Buoyancy is the upward force of the water on an immersed or partially immersed body or body part, which is equal to the weight of the water that is displaced (Archimedes' Principle).

3. Indications for hydrotherapy.
   a. Wound care and debridement.
   b. Status post–hip fracture.
   c. Postsurgical conditions of the hip, knee, ankle, hand or elbow.
   d. Subacute and chronic musculoskeletal conditions of the neck, shoulder, back or hip.
   e. Rheumatoid arthritis.

4. Contraindications for hydrotherapy.
   a. Refer to contraindications for hydrocollator packs.
   b. Precautions:
      (1) Avoid overutilization with wound care.
         (a) Clean wounds.
         (b) Primarily closed.
         (c) Reepithelializing or granulating tissue.
      (2) Chronic wounds with >50% adherent black eschar.
         (a) Wounds with nonlocalized infection.
         (b) Tissues with cellulitis.
      (3) Split-thickness skin grafts before 3–5 days.
         (a) Full-thickness skin grafts before 7–10 days.

(4) Patient tolerance for treatment.
    (a) Systemic factors, allergy or sensitivity to additives need to be considered.

5. Method of application.
  a. Clean the tank following outlined procedures.
    (1) Use an approved disinfectant, in approved manner, for appropriate length of time.
    (2) Thoroughly rinse the disinfectant prior to filling the tank for patient use.
  b. Fill tank with water to appropriate level and temperature.
    (1) Whirlpool liners may be used.
      (a) Wounds, burns, or for patients with blood-borne pathogens (HIV or hepatitis).
    (2) 103°–110°F general extremity whirlpool.
    (3) 100°F Hubbard tank (full-body immersion).
    (4) 95°–100°F if the patient has peripheral vascular disease.
    (5) 92°–96°F if open wounds are present.
    (6) 88°F with multiple sclerosis.
  c. Add disinfectant if open wounds are present. Bactericidal additives most frequently used.
    (1) Povidone-iodine 4 parts per million.
    (2) Sodium hypochlorite (bleach) 200 parts per million.
    (3) Chloramine-T, 100–200 parts per million.
  d. Standard precautions (gowns, goggles, masks and gloves) should be applied in infected environment and if splashing is suspected.
    (1) Refer to Table 8-1 for details.
  e. Assist patient in immersing body or body part into tank.
    (1) With Hubbard tank use stretcher or pneumatic lift.
    (2) Lower to waterline to allow patient to get accustomed to water temperature before immersing completely.
    (3) Keep patient's head elevated.
      (a) Secure head end of stretcher to bracket in tank.
      (b) Remove the hoist when stretcher is resting on bottom of tank.
    (4) Use towels to pad any pressure points to minimize compression on tank edges.
    (5) Adjust agitator for desired effect.
      (a) Position, force, direction, depth, aeration.
    (6) Monitor patient's response and tolerance to treatment.
    (7) At termination of treatment, assist patient from tank.
    (8) Dry and inspect skin.

6. Treatment time.
  a. 20 minutes.
    (1) Up to 30 minutes if other therapeutic procedures are being performed.

7. General cleaning procedures.
  a. Procedures may vary in different settings.
  b. After draining water from the tank, rinse the entire tank including the openings in the agitator and all the drains.
  c. Wipe all areas that were in contact with water with a clean towel.
  d. Wash/scrub the inside of the tank.
    (1) Outside of the agitator.
    (2) The drains with a disinfectant diluted in warm water.
  e. Wash/scrub the agitator thermometers and all equipment used in the treatment.
    (1) Allow disinfectant to stand for at least one minute.
  f. Place the agitator in a bucket of disinfectant/water mixture covering all openings with the solution.
  g. Turn on agitator for about 20–30 seconds.
  h. Turn off motor and remove agitator from bucket.
  i. Rinse entire tank and all equipment until all residue is removed.
    (1) When treating a patient with burns or with wounds.
      (a) Refill the tank with hot water and disinfectant.
      (b) Let stand for 5 minutes before rinsing with clean water.
  j. Rinse the tank a second time with hot water (110°–115°F) to speed drying.
  k. Wipe inside and outside of the tank with a clean towel.

8. Electrical safety.
  a. Safety precautions must be taken with any modality that potentially exposes the patient to electrical hazard from a faulty electrical connection.
    (1) A ground fault circuit interrupter should be installed at the circuit breaker or receptacle of all whirlpool and Hubbard tanks.
      (a) The electrical circuit is broken if the current is diverted to the patient who is grounded rather than to a grounded modality.
    (2) All whirlpool turbines, tanks and motors including motors on lifts should be checked for broken or frayed connections.

Fluidotherapy is no longer tested on the NPTE

Paraffin Bath

1. Description: the therapeutic application of a mixture of paraffin and mineral oil to a body part. The paraffin bath is a double-walled, thermostatically controlled unit.

a. The low specific heat of the paraffin mixture (6:1 or 7:1 ratio of paraffin wax and mineral oil) allows the patient to tolerate the higher temperatures (125°–127°F).
b. Paraffin/mineral oil melts between 118°F and 130°F.
c. Mechanism of energy transfer: conduction.

2. **Indications for paraffin bath.**
   a. Most often used on smaller irregularly shaped areas such as wrists hands or feet for painful joints due to arthritis or other inflammatory conditions in the subacute or chronic phase.
   b. Joint stiffness.

3. **Contraindications for paraffin bath.**
   a. Allergic rash.
   b. Open wounds.
   c. Recent scars or sutures.
   d. Skin infection.

4. **Method of application.**
   a. Treatment temperature ranges 125°–127°F.
   b. Assess patient's sensation and heat tolerance.
   c. Inform patient of what to expect during treatment and to report abnormal sensations.
   d. Instruct patient not to touch sides or bottom of the unit.
   e. Inspect skin for infection or open areas.
   f. Wash area to be treated; dry thoroughly.
   g. Remove or cover jewelry with several layers of gauze.
   h. Dip and remove part 6–12 times.
   i. Wrap part in plastic and several layers of toweling. Secure with tape or rubber bands.
   j. Position patient comfortably.

5. **Treatment time: 15–20 minutes.**

Contrast Bath

1. **Description: alternating immersion of body part in a hot and cold water bath to produce a vascular exercise through active vasodilatation and vasoconstriction of the blood vessels.**
   a. Mechanism of energy transfer: conduction.

2. **Indications for contrast bath.**
   a. Any condition requiring stimulation of peripheral circulation in limbs.
   b. Peripheral vascular disease.
   c. Sprains.
   d. Strains.
   e. Trauma (after first few hours).
   f. Persistent edema.

3. **Contraindications for contrast bath.**
   a. Advanced arteriosclerosis.
   b. Arterial insufficiency.
   c. Loss of sensation to heat or cold.

4. **Method of application.**
   a. Treatment begins in hot water (100°–110°F) for 6–10 minutes.
   b. Transfer body part to cold water (55°–65°F) for 1 minute.
   c. Transfer to hot water for 4 minutes.
   d. Continue sequence of 4:1 ending in hot water.
      (1) Hot/cold ratios may be modified depending on patient's tolerance.
   e. Ending in cold water may benefit treatment of edema.
   f. During the initial treatment, patient's tolerance may be optimal by beginning at the lower end of the hot range and the higher end of the cold range.

5. **Treatment time: 20–30 minutes.**

Nonimmersion Irrigation Device

1. **Small, hand-held electric water pump that produces a water jet to create a shearing force to loosen tissue debris. Some devices produce a pulsed lavage and include suction to remove debris.**

2. **Procedure.**
   a. Treatment should take place in an enclosed area.
   b. Face and eye protection, gloves and waterproof gown are required.
   c. Sterile, warm saline is used. Antimicrobials may be added.
   d. Select appropriate treatment pressure, usually 4–8 psi. Pressure may be increased in presence of large amounts of necrotic tissue or tough eschar. Pressure should be decreased with bleeding, near a major vessel or if a patient complains of pain.
   e. Treatment time is usually 5–15 minutes, once a day. Wound size and amount of necrotic tissue may increase treatment parameters.

Aquatic Therapy

1. **A form of hydrotherapy used primarily for weight-bearing activities, active exercise or horizontal floating activities. Swimming pools or Hubbard tanks with or without walking troughs and treadmill units are used.**

2. **Principles.**
   a. Movement horizontal to or upward toward the water surface (active assistive exercise) is made easier by the buoyancy of the water. A flotation device may be used as well.
   b. Movement downward is more difficult. A flotation device would increase resistance.
   c. Increasing speed of movement increases resistance because of turbulence and cohesion of water. Use of hand-held paddles held width-wise will increase

resistance. Streamlining can be achieved by turning the paddle and slicing through the water.

d. Amount of weight-bearing can be determined by the water depth. The greater the depth, the less the load on the extremities because of buoyancy.

e. Water temperature is 92°–98°F.

f. Treatment time varies with patient tolerance.

g. Open wounds and skin infections must be covered.

h. Goals are to improve standing balance; partial weight-bearing ambulation; aerobic exercise; improve range of motion (ROM); increase muscle strength via active assistive, active or resistive exercise.

i. Contraindications are incontinence, urinary tract infections, severe epilepsy, unprotected open wounds, unstable blood pressure or severe cardiopulmonary dysfunction.

Superficial Cryotherapy Techniques

Physics Related to Cryotherapy Energy Transmission, the removal of heat via conduction or evaporation

1. Conduction: transfer of heat from a warmer object to a cooler object through direct molecular interaction of objects in physical contact. Conductive modalities: cold pack, ice pack, ice massage, cold bath.

2. Evaporation (heat of vaporization): highly volatile liquids that evaporate rapidly on contact with warm object. Evaporative modality: vapocoolant sprays (Fluori-Methane).

Physiological Effects of Large Surface Area (General) Cold Application (Table 11-4)

Physiological Effects of Small Surface Area (Local) Cold Application

1. Effects of cold application on body tissues:
   a. Skin temperature falls rapidly and exhibits greatest temperature change.
   b. Subcutaneous temperature falls less rapidly and displays smaller temperature change.
   c. Muscle and joint show least temperature changes, requiring longer cold exposure.

2. Vasoconstriction of skin capillaries resulting in blanching of skin in center of contact area and hyperemia due to histamine reaction around the edge of contact area in normal tissue.

3. Cold-induced vasodilation: cyclic vasoconstriction and vasodilation following prolonged cold exposure (>15 minutes). Occurs mostly in hands, feet and face where arteriovenous anastomoses are found. Called the "hunting" reaction. Recent studies have questioned the clinical significance of this reaction.

4. Physiological effects on body systems and structures to small (local) surface area cold modalities (Tables 11-5 and 11-6).

5. Adverse physiological effects of cold due to hypersensitivity.

Table 11-4 ➤ PHYSIOLOGICAL EFFECTS OF GENERAL COLD APPLICATION

DECREASED	INCREASED
Metabolic rate	Blood flow to internal organs
Pulse rate	Cardiac output
Respiratory rate	Stroke volume
Venous blood pressure	Arterial blood pressure. Shivering (occurs when core temperature drops)

Table 11-5 ➤ DECREASED PHYSIOLOGICAL RESPONSES OF BODY SYSTEMS AND STRUCTURES TO LOCAL COLD APPLICATION

SYSTEM/STRUCTURE	MECHANISM
Blood flow	Sympathetic adrenergic activity produces vasoconstriction of arteries, arterioles and venules
Capillary permeability	Decreased fluids into interstitial tissue
Elasticity of nonelastic tissues	Decreased extensibility of collagen tissue
Metabolism	Decreased rate of cellular oxidation
Muscle spasm	Decreased firing of II afferents of muscle spindle, increased firing of Ib Golgi tendon organ fibers reduces alpha motor neuron activity and thus decreases tonic extrafusal activity
Muscle strength	Decreased blood flow, increase in viscous properties of muscle (long duration: >5–10 min)
Spasticity	Decrease in muscle spindle discharge (afferents: primary, secondary), decreased gamma motor neuron activity
Vasoactive agents	Decreased blood flow

Table 11-6 ➤ INCREASED PHYSIOLOGICAL RESPONSES OF BODY SYSTEMS AND STRUCTURES TO LOCAL COLD APPLICATION

SYSTEM/STRUCTURE	MECHANISM
Joint stiffness	Decreased extensibility of collagen tissue and increased tissue viscosity
Pain threshold	Inhibition of A delta and C fibers via activaton of A-beta fibers (gate theory), interruption of pain-spasm cycle, decreased sensory and motor conduction, synaptic transmission slowed or blocked.
Increased blood viscosity	Decreased blood flow in small vessels facilitates red blood cells adhering to one another and vessel wall impeding blood flow.
Muscle strength	Facilitation of alpha motor neuron (short duration: 1–5 min)

a. Cold urticaria: erythema of the skin with wheal formation associated with severe itching due to histamine reaction.
b. Facial flush, puffiness of eyelids, respiratory problems and, in severe cases, anaphylaxis (decreased blood pressure, increased heart rate) with syncope are also related to histamine release.

Goals and Indications for Cryotherapy

1. Modulate pain: reduce or eliminate soft tissue inflammation or swelling, reduce muscle spasm, reduce spasticity.

Precautions

1. Hypertension, impaired temperature sensation, open wound, over superficial nerve, very old or young.

Contraindications to Use of Cryotherapy

1. Cold hypersensitivity (urticaria), cold intolerance, cryoglobulinemia, peripheral vascular disease, impaired temperature sensation, Raynaud's disease.

Cryotherapy (Cold) Agents

Cold Packs

1. Description: commercial packs containing semigelled substance covered in durable plastic.
   a. Available in various sizes and stored in freezer units.
   b. Remains cold for up to 10 minutes after removal from the freezer unit.
   c. Advantage: can conform to irregular surfaces of the body.
   d. Mechanism of energy transfer: conduction.

2. Indications for cold packs.
   a. Acute and chronic traumatic and inflammatory conditions.
   b. Edema.
   c. Muscle spasm.
   d. Musculoskeletal pain.
   e. Thermal burns.

3. Contraindications for cold packs.
   a. Impaired circulation.
   b. Impaired sensation.
   c. Peripheral vascular disease.
   d. Prolonged application over superficial nerves.
   e. Raynaud's disease.
   f. Sensitivity or allergic reaction to cold.

4. Method of application.
   a. Cold packs are maintained at 0°–10°F.
   b. Keep patient warm throughout treatment.
   c. Dampen towel with warm water.
      (1) Wring out excess water.
      (2) Fold in half and place cold pack on towel.
   d. Place on area to be treated and cover with dry towel.
   e. Secure pack to the patient.

5. Treatment time: 10–20 minutes.

Ice Massage

1. Description: ice applied directly to the treatment area.
   a. Ice cylinder formed by freezing water in paper or Styrofoam cup.
      (1) A tongue depressor or popsicle stick can be placed in water before freezing for ease of handling.
   b. Mechanism of energy transfer: conduction.

2. Indications and contraindications for ice massage.
   a. Refer to cold pack section.

3. Method of application.
   a. Remove ice from container.
      (1) Wrap ice in towel or hold onto stick.

b. Apply ice massage to area no larger than 4 × 6 inches in slow (2 inches/sec) overlapping circles or overlapping longitudinal strokes.
   (1) If treating large area, divide into smaller areas.
c. Avoid bony areas or superficial nerves (e.g., peroneal/fibular).
d. Use towel to dab melting ice.
e. Treat until anesthesia is achieved.
f. Monitor skin during application.
   (1) Vasoconstriction of capillaries results in blanching (whitening) of skin in center of contact area and hyperemia (reddening) around edge of contact area (in normal tissue).
      (a) This is a histamine reaction.
   (2) The patient will experience the following sensations, typically in this order: cold, burning, aching, numbness.

4. **Treatment time varies.**
   a. Typically 5–10 minutes until analgesia is achieved.

Vapocoolant Spray

1. Description: a nontoxic, nonflammable liquid, which produces rapid cooling via evaporation when sprayed on skin.

a. Mechanism of energy transfer: evaporation.

2. **Indications for vapocoolant spray.**
   a. Myofascial referred pain.
   b. Muscle spasms.
   c. Desensitize trigger points.

3. **Contraindications for vapocoolant spray.**
   a. Refer to cold pack section.

4. **Method of application.**
   a. Hold nozzle down 18–24 inches from treatment area.
   b. Spray at a 30-degree angle and "sweep" spray over area at 4 inches per second.
   c. Apply over entire treatment area, starting at pain site and moving to the area of referred pain.
   d. Allow liquid to completely evaporate before sweep spraying again.
   e. Caution.
      (1) Do not frost the skin.
   f. Passively stretch muscle before and during application.
   g. Instruct patient to perform active exercise after spraying.

5. **Treatment time: 10–15 minutes.**

Deep Thermotherapy (Deep Heating Agents)

Short-Wave Diathermy (SWD)

1. **Description.**
   a. Uses an alternating current with a frequency of oscillations of a million or more per second.
   b. No longer covered on PTA examination.

Microwave Diathermy (MWD)

1. **Description.**
   a. Method of applying electromagnetic energy via conversion through a director (treatment applicator).
   b. No longer covered on PTA examination.

Ultrasound

1. Description: high-frequency acoustical energy source delivered through a sound head applied directly to the tissue being treated.
   a. Applicator contains a piezoelectric crystal (transducer).

   (1) The transducer converts electrical energy into acoustical energy via reverse piezoelectric effect (conversion).
   b. Frequency range: 0.8–3.0 MHz.

2. **Method of application.**
   a. A coupling gel is used for effective sound wave transmission.
   b. Can also be used under water to treat irregular body parts such as the ankle or wrist.
      (1) Immersion technique.
   c. Transducer size.
      (1) Transducers come in a variety of sizes—from 1 cm² to 10 cm²; 5 cm² is the most common.
      (2) Transducer size should be selected relative to the size of the treatment area (1 cm² = wrist; 5 cm² = shoulder, leg).
   d. The depth of penetration is generally 3–5 cm; based on frequency of delivery.
      (1) Use 3 MHz for superficial tissues, due to greater scatter (attenuation) of sound waves in superficial tissues.
      (2) Use 1 MHz for deeper tissues, due to less scatter in superficial tissues allowing for more energy penetration to deeper tissues.

e. Mode of application.
(1) Continuous mode results in greater heating of the tissues; use for chronic or noninflammatory conditions.
(2) Pulsed mode results in intermittent delivery of ultrasound (US) energy, thus decreasing overall heating; use for acute or inflammatory conditions; 20% duty cycle most common.
f. Direct contact (transducer/skin interface).
(1) Description: moving sound head in contact with relatively flat body part (e.g., lumbar area). Sound head in contact with body-part at all times.
g. Indirect contact.
(1) Description: water immersion or fluid-filled balloon, condom or surgical glove. Used with irregular body parts.

3. Indications for ultrasound.
a. Open wounds.
b. Neuromas.
c. Periarticular conditions.
d. Joint contractures.
e. Musculoskeletal pain.
f. Muscle spasm.
g. Subacute and chronic traumatic and inflammatory conditions.

4. Contraindications for ultrasound.
a. Acute inflammatory joint pathologies.
b. Healing fractures.
c. Thrombophlebitis.
d. Use of radium or radioactive isotopes.
e. Do not apply over vital organs, epiphysis of growing bones, eye, heart, cervical ganglia, carotid sinuses, reproductive organs, spinal cord, close to or directly over cardiac pacemakers, close to or directly over pregnant uterus.

5. Precautions for ultrasound.
a. Metal implants in field.
b. Osteoporosis.
c. Plastic implants.
d. Primary repair of tendons, ligaments or scar tissue.

6. Method of application.
a. Select method of application.
(1) Direct contact (moving technique).
(a) Apply generous amount of gel to skin for effective sound wave transmission.
(b) Place sound head at right angle to skin surface.
(c) Move sound head slowly (1.5 inches/sec) in overlapping circles or longitudinal strokes, keeping sound head in contact with skin.
(d) With sound head moving and in firm contact, turn up intensity to desired level.
(e) Treatment intensities: 0.1–3.0 watt/cm².
• Lower intensities recommended for acute conditions or on thin tissues.
• Higher intensities recommended for chronic conditions and thicker/deeper tissues.
(f) Watch for periosteal pain.
• Occurs when intensity is too high.
• Occurs if sound head movement is slowed.
• If this occurs, stop and readjust intensity.
(2) Indirect contact (immersion).
(a) Fill container (plastic is preferred) with water high enough to cover treatment area.
(b) Place part in water.
(c) Place sound head in water, keeping it 1 inch from body part at right angle.
(d) Move sound head slowly (1.5 inches/sec) as in direct contact.
(e) Turn up intensity to desired level.
• Refer to direct contact-moving technique.
(f) Wipe off any air bubbles that may form on the sound head or body part during treatment.
(3) Fluid-filled bag technique.
(a) Place bag around sound head, squeezing out fluid until all air is removed and sound head is immersed in water.
(b) Apply coupling agent to skin and place bag over treatment area.
(c) Move sound head slowly (1.5 inches/sec) within bag, maintaining a right angle to body part.
• Do not slide bag on skin.
(d) Turn up intensity to desired level.
• Refer to direct contact-moving technique.

Phonophoresis

1. Description: the use of ultrasound to administer medications through the skin into deeper tissues.
(1) Analgesics: lidocaine.
(2) Anti-inflammatory drugs: dexamethasone.

2. Indications for phonophoresis.
a. Subacute and chronic musculoskeletal conditions.

3. Contraindications for phonophoresis.
a. Refer to ultrasound.
b. Allergy to medication.

4. Method of application.
a. Method of application: same as direct contact method.
(1) The medicinal agent is used as or part of the coupling medium.
b. Treatment intensity is 1–2 watt/cm².
(1) Lower intensity and longer treatment time is more effective in driving medications into tissue.
c. Treatment time.
(1) 5–10 minutes.

Radiant Energy Agents

Infrared

1. No longer covered on the PTA examination.

Ultraviolet

1. No longer covered on the PTA examination.

Electrical Stimulation

Characteristics

1. Wave forms (Figure 11-1).
   a. Monophasic (direct or galvanic current).
      (1) A unidirectional flow of charged particles.
   b. Biphasic wave (alternating current).
      (1) A bidirectional flow of charged particles.
   c. Polyphasic wave.
      (1) A biphasic current modified to produce three or more phases in a single pulse.

2. Description.
   a. Used in physical therapy to treat dysfunction, typically pain or muscle weakness.
   b. The outcomes and methods of application are varied dependent upon type of modality or current used.
   c. Generic forms of current.
      (1) Direct current (DC).
      (2) Alternating current (AC).
      (3) Pulsatile (pulsed) current.

General Indications for Electrical Stimulation

1. Pain modulation.
   a. Activation of gate mechanisms (gate theory) for pain management.
   b. Gate theory.
      (1) Noxious (or painful) stimuli are transmitted to the spinal cord by descending pathways from the brain using the (small) C and A-delta fibers.
      (2) Nonpainful stimuli are transmitted by the (large) A-beta fibers believed to block the pain signal.
      (3) A-delta fibers conduct impulses faster than the C fibers.
         (a) A-delta fibers.
            • Produce short duration, sharp, well-localized sensations.
         (b) C fibers.
            • Produce longer lasting, poorly localized dull pain.
         (c) All fiber types are located in the dorsal root ganglia at various levels of the spinal cord.
            • Transmitted by axonal processes to specific areas of the spinal cord.
         (d) Within the dorsal horn of the spinal cord is substantia gelatinosa believed to be where T (transmission) cells are and where the basis for the gate control theory arises.
         (e) C and A-delta nerve impulses excite the T cells.
            • Receive a combination of both excitatory and inhibitory influences.
            • May significantly affect the final pain experience.
      (4) Melzack and Wall (authors of the gate control theory) proposed that descending control from the

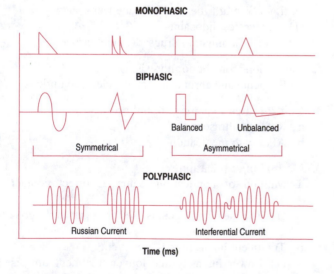

MONOPHASIC

BIPHASIC

Balanced   Unbalanced

Symmetrical   Asymmetrical

POLYPHASIC

Russian Current   Interferential Current

Time (ms)

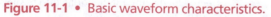

Figure 11-1 • Basic waveform characteristics.

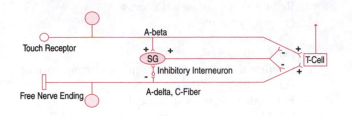

Figure 11-2 • Schematic of gate control theory (Melzack and Wall).

brainstem and cortex strongly influence the excitability of the transmission cells and that "psychological factors (e.g., past experience, attention and emotion) influence pain response and perception by acting on the gate control system."

(5) The gate control theory suggests that sensory information traveling on small fibers (A-delta and C) open the gate while information traveling on large fibers (A-beta) closes the gate.

    (a) See Figure 11-2.

2. General muscle stimulation.

a. Unipolar/monopolar placement.

    (1) One single or multiple (bifurcated) active electrodes placed over treatment area.

b. The larger (dispersive) electrode is placed ipsilaterally away from the treatment area.

c. The space between the active and dispersive electrodes should be at least the diameter of the active electrode.

d. The greater the distance between electrodes, the less risk of skin irritation and unwanted stimulation of adjacent muscles.

e. Vigilant inspection of skin is very important with long-term use.

f. Secure electrodes to body part.

g. Settings.

    (1) Frequency.

    (2) Waveform.

    (3) Modulation rate.

        (a) Refer below for desired treatment outcome.

3. Muscle strengthening.

a. Amplitude (intensity) until muscle response (contraction) is observed.

    (1) Intensity should be enough to produce >grade 3 muscle contraction.

    (2) The current should be continuous with slow ramp-up time.

b. Duty cycle.

    (1) 1:3 on:off cycle or greater will minimize muscle fatigue.

c. 10–25 muscle contractions recommended to obtain treatment outcome.

4. Muscle spasm (fatigue).

a. Continuous or interrupted mode of current.

b. Intensity sufficient to produce a twitch muscle contraction.

5. Muscle reeducation.

a. Training muscles to respond appropriately to volitional effort.

b. Parameters and procedures are similar to muscle strengthening techniques.

c. Stimulation for multiple sets of singular or multiple repetitions.

    (1) Used in conjunction with functional activity.

d. Provides proprioceptive feedback.

e. Assist in coordinated muscle movement.

f. Treatment sessions 10–30 minutes, dependent on patient tolerance.

6. Other general conditions for electrical stimulation.

a. Wound healing.

    (1) Pulsed currents (monophasic, biphasic, polyphasic) with interrupted modulations.

        (a) Improves circulation via the muscle pump to improve tissue nutrition and accelerates metabolic waste disposal.

        (b) Alters chemical balance of tissues to facilitate healing.

b. Increase or maintain joint range of motion.

    (1) Mechanical stretching of connective tissue and muscles associated with a joint.

        (a) Utilized when muscle strength is deficient.

        (b) Neuromuscular dysfunction (e.g., spasticity) prevents adequate joint movement.

    (2) Decreases pain to encourage joint motion.

    (3) Decreases edema if significant obstruction to motion.

c. Delivery of medications through skin (iontophoresis).

d. Assists in the management of scoliosis.

General Contraindications for Electrical Stimulation

1. Healing fractures.

a. Some patients have used electrical stimulation devices prescribed by their surgeons as part of their recovery. These are called bone stimulators.

2. Over superficial metal implants.

3. In areas of active bleeding.

4. Distal to or adjacent to an area of thrombophlebitis or phlebothrombosis.

5. Malignancies in the area.

a. Some exception occurs when treatment is palliative only for pain management. Physician script is recommended.

6. Pregnancy.
   a. If treatment is to be applied to the abdominal area.

7. Patients with cardiac pacemaker, cardiac arrhythmias, conduction disturbances.

8. Over pharyngeal or laryngeal muscles.

9. Patients with active tuberculosis.

10. Over carotid sinuses.

Precautions for Electrical Stimulation

1. Use electrical stimulation cautiously in the presence of obesity.

2. Use precaution in applying electrical stimulation to areas of absent or decreased sensation.

3. Severe edema.

4. Electrical stimulation can exacerbate eczema, psoriasis, acne, dermatitis. It may also spread infection.

5. Patients with diabetes or thin, fragile skin can be at risk of breakdown from electrodes.

6. Patients with peripheral neuropathies may not achieve muscle contraction if maintaining intensity at a comfortable/safe level.

7. Denervated muscles will only respond to direct current.

8. Be aware of presence of any metal devices (internal or external).
   a. Electrodes should be positioned with the metal well outside the pathway of the current.

9. Caution is needed with diminished cognition or with patients who have difficulty understanding instructions or giving feedback.

10. Stimulation to patients with spinal cord injury may contribute to the risk of autonomic dysreflexia.

11. Do not use electrical modality when.
    a. There is evidence of broken or frayed wires.
    b. The unit is not connected to a ground fault circuit interrupter; refer to whirlpool section for details.

General Method of Application

1. General muscle stimulation procedures.
   a. Explain procedure, sensation to expect and treatment effects to patient.
   b. Position patient comfortably, with treatment area properly exposed and supported.
   c. Assess skin condition and sensation.
   d. Reduce skin resistance if necessary.
      (1) Apply hot pack.
      (2) Alcohol.
      (3) Gentle abrasion.
   e. Confirm that all controls are in the starting position before turning on the modality.
   f. Electrode placement sites are determined.
      (1) May be predetermined by supervising PT.
   g. Treatment area is cleaned.
   h. Electrodes are prepared and secured.
   i. Preset parameters are adjusted.
      (1) Frequency.
      (2) Pulse/phase duration.
      (3) Delivery mode.
         (a) Continuous or interrupted.
      (4) On-off time.
      (5) Ramp.
      (6) Choice of polarity.
      (7) Treatment timer.

2. Electrode selection.
   a. Two electrodes (leads) are required to complete the current circuit.
      (1) When two or four electrodes of the same size are used, all are considered active; typical for pain management.
      (2) Bipolar set-up. When two electrodes are used and one is larger (two times) than the other, the smaller electrode is considered the active electrode and the larger the dispersive; typical for neuromuscular electrical stimulation (NMES).
   b. Current density (the amount of current concentrated under the electrode) is relative to the electrode size.
      (1) A given current intensity passing through the smaller active electrode produces high current density and thus a stronger stimulation.
      (2) The same current is perceived as less intense under the larger dispersive electrode because of the lesser current density.
   c. Electrode size should be relative to the size of the treatment site.
      (1) Large electrodes in a small treatment area (e.g., forearm) could result in current overflowing to surrounding muscles producing undesired effects.
      (2) Conversely, small electrodes applied to a large muscle (i.e., quadriceps) could result in high current density under the electrodes, making stimulation uncomfortable for the patient.
      (3) The active electrode is usually placed over the treatment site (motor point), to produce a stimulation effect.
      (4) The dispersive electrode may be placed on the treatment site or at a remote site.
   d. Refer to electrode placement section.

3. Electrode preparation.
   a. Metal plate/sponges.
      (1) Saturate sponge with water.

(2) Remove excess water so sponge is not dripping wet.

b. Carbonized rubber.

  (1) Place a small amount of gel in the center of the electrode.

  (2) Spread gel to cover the entire surface.

c. Pregelled electrode.

  (1) Remove protective cover.

  (2) Place a small amount of gel (metal mesh/foil electrode) or water (Karaya electrode) on the electrode.

4. **Electrode placement.**

a. Refer to general muscle stimulation section.

5. **Delivery.**

a. Increase amplitude to stimulation level but always within patient's tolerance.

b. Ask patient what he or she feels and where the sensation is felt.

c. Adjust any parameters as indicated.

d. Stay with patient for several minutes.

  (1) To monitor reaction and tolerance.

  (2) To adjust amplitude as needed.

e. Continue to monitor patient periodically throughout treatment.

6. **Completion.**

a. Turn amplitude to zero.

b. Remove electrodes.

c. Turn unit off.

d. Inspect treatment area.

e. Note all variables set for treatment and document.

f. Unplug unit from wall outlet.

7. **Documentation.**

a. Include patient's problem.

b. Outcome desired.

c. Intervention given.

d. Skin status.

e. Electrode type, size, placement and number.

f. Commercial stimulation unit used.

g. Electrical parameters of treatment.

h. Treatment time.

i. Patient response.

j. Remember: the written note should assure consistent replication of the treatment.

Transcutaneous Electrical Nerve Stimulation (TENS)

Description

1. Transcutaneous electrical nerve stimulation is designed to provide afferent stimulation for pain management.

2. Is typically delivered via a portable, battery operated stimulator.

Physiological Effects of TENS

1. Pain modulation through activation of central inhibition of pain transmission.

a. Gate control theory.

b. Large-diameter A—beta fibers activate inhibitory interneurons, producing inhibition of the smaller pain-transmitting fibers (A-delta, C fibers).

2. Pain modulation through descending pathways creating endogenous opiate (Figure 11-3).

a. Noxious stimuli generate endorphin production from the pituitary gland.

b. Endogenous opiate-rich nuclei, periaqueductal gray matter (PAG) in the midbrain and thalamus are also activated by strong stimuli.

c. Neurotransmitters from the PAG facilitate the cells of the nucleus raphe magnus (NRM), and reticularis gigantocellularis (RGC).

d. Efferents from these nuclei travel through the dorsal lateral funiculus to terminate on the enkephalinergic

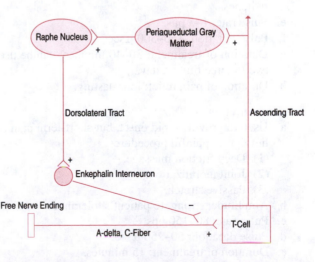

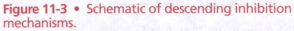

Figure 11-3 • Schematic of descending inhibition mechanisms.

interneurons in the spinal cord to presynaptically inhibit the release of substance P from the A-delta and C fibers.

Electrical Stimulation Characteristics of TENS

1. **Waveform.**
   a. Typically, asymmetrical biphasic with a zero net direct current component.
   b. Other variations, including pulsed monophasic current, have been used.

2. **Modulations: continuous or burst.**

Method of Application

1. **Conventional (high rate) TENS.**
   a. Most common mode of TENS.
   b. Can be applied during acute or chronic phase of pain.
   c. Modulation of pain via the activation of the gate theory.
   d. Onset of pain relief is relatively fast.
   e. Amplitude: comfortable tingling sensation; no muscle response.
   f. Pulse rate: 50–80 pps.
   g. Pulse duration: 50–100 μsec.
   h. Duration of treatment: 20–60 minutes; can be used several times throughout the day.
   i. Duration of pain relief: temporary.

2. **Acupuncture-like (strong low rate) TENS.**
   a. Can be applied during chronic phase of pain.
   b. Produces analgesia through stimulation-evoked production of endogenous opiates.
   c. Onset of pain relief may be as long as 20–30 minutes.
   d. Amplitude: strong but comfortable rhythmic muscle twitches.
   e. Pulse rate: 1–5 pps.
   f. Pulse duration: 150–300 μsec.
   g. Duration of treatment: 30–40 minutes; can be used two to three times a day.
   h. Duration of pain relief: long-lasting.

3. **Brief, intense TENS.**
   a. Used to provide rapid onset, but short-term pain relief during painful procedures.
      (1) Deep friction massage.
      (2) Joint mobilization.
      (3) Passive stretch.
   b. Amplitude: strong, to patient's tolerance.
   c. Pulse rate: 80–150 pps.
   d. Pulse duration: 50–250 μsec.
   e. Duration of treatment: 15 minutes.
   f. Duration of pain relief: temporary.

4. **Burst mode (pulse trains) TENS.**
   a. Combines both high- and low-rate TENS.
   b. Stimulation of endogenous opiates but with more comfortable current than low-rate TENS.
   c. Onset of pain relief similar (analgesia) to low-rate TENS.
   d. Amplitude: comfortable, intermittent paresthesia.
   e. Pulse rate: 50–100 pps delivered in packets or bursts of 1–4 pps.
   f. Pulse duration: 50–200 μsec.
   g. Duration of treatment: 20–30 minutes.
   h. Duration of pain relief: long-lasting.

5. **Hyperstimulation (point stimulation) TENS.**
   a. Use of a small probe to locate and noxiously stimulate acupuncture or trigger points.
   b. Multiple sites can be stimulated per treatment.
   c. Onset of pain relief is similar to acupuncture-like TENS.
   d. Amplitude: strong, within patient's tolerance.
   e. Pulse rate: 1–5 pps.
   f. Pulse duration: 150–300 μsec.
   g. Duration of treatment: 15–30 second increments.
   h. Duration of pain relief: long-lasting.

6. **Modulation mode TENS.**
   a. Method of modulating the parameters of the above-listed TENS modes for preventing neural or perceptual adaptation due to constant electrical stimulation.
   b. Frequencies, intensities or pulse durations can be altered by ten or more percent one or two times per second.

Electrode Placement

1. **Several options should be considered.**
   a. Acupuncture site.
   b. Dermatome distribution of involved nerve.
   c. Over painful site.
   d. Proximal or distal to the pain site.
   e. Segmentally related myotomes.
   f. Trigger points.

Indications

1. **Acute and chronic pain.**

Contraindications

1. **Patients with demand-type pacemakers or over the chest of a patient with cardiac disease.**

2. **TENS should not be applied in these areas/conditions.**
   a. Over the eyes.
   b. Laryngeal or pharyngeal muscles.
   c. Head and neck of patients following cerebral vascular accident.
   d. Patients who suffer from epilepsy.

3. **TENS should not be applied to mucosal membranes.**

Functional Electrical Stimulation (FES)

Description

1. Usually portable units that are designed to be worn by patients.
   a. Enhance the voluntary contraction of innervated muscles.
   b. Decrease disuse atrophy.
   c. Improve impaired ROM.
   d. Re-educate muscles.
   e. Decrease muscle spasm.
   f. Manage spasticity management.

2. FES is also called functional neuromuscular stimulation.

3. This section will describe FES as a supplement or alternative to the use of orthotic devices.

Dorsiflexion Assist in Gait Training

1. Patients with hemiplegia sometimes exhibit paralyzed dorsiflexor and evertor muscles.

2. FES uses.
   a. Foot drop.
   b. Facilitates dorsiflexors and evertors during swing phase.

3. Electrical stimulation characteristics.
   a. Electrode placement.
      (1) Bipolar.
      (2) Active electrode placed over motor point (peroneal nerve near head of fibula or anterior tibialis muscle).
   b. Treatment parameters.
      (1) Amplitude: tetanic muscle contraction sufficient to decrease plantar flexion.
      (2) Pulse rate: 30–300 pps.
      (3) Pulse duration: 80–100 msec.
      (4) Treatment mode.
         (a) Heel switch contains pressure-sensitive contact.
            • Stops stimulation during stance phase.
            • Activates stimulation during swing phase.
         (b) Hand switch also allows the assistant to control stimulation during gait.

Other Gait-Assisted Protocol Considerations

1. Placement of electrodes on appropriate muscles.
   a. Plantar flexors during push-off.

b. Hamstrings during late swing phase.
c. Quadriceps and/or gluteus during stance phase.

2. Electrical stimulation characteristics.
   a. Similar to dorsiflexion protocol.

3. Method of application.
   a. Similar to dorsiflexion protocol except for electrode placement.

Idiopathic Scoliosis Management

1. Lateral curve of the spine commonly found in children.

2. FES considerations.
   a. The patient needs to be compliant and cooperative.
   b. The patient needs to demonstrate a progressive and idiopathic curve.
      (1) The curve needs to measure 20–45 degrees.

3. Electrical stimulation characteristics.
   a. Wave form: rectangular constant current.
   b. Pulse duration: 225 μsec.
   c. Modulation: interrupted.

4. Method of application.
   a. Electrode placement.
      (1) Bipolar.
      (2) Midaxillary line on the convexity of the curve.
      (3) Superior and inferior to the rib attached to the vertebra attached to the apex of the spine.
   b. Treatment parameters.
      (1) Amplitude: tetanic muscle contraction to patient's tolerance.
      (2) Pulse rate: 25 pps.
      (3) Duration of treatment.
         (a) Up to 8 hours.
         (b) On:off ratio 1:1 (6 sec:6 sec).

Shoulder Subluxation

1. Patients with a cerebrovascular accident (CVA) may initially exhibit weakness or flaccid paralysis of the muscles supporting the glenohumeral joint, especially the supraspinatus and the posterior deltoid musculature.

2. The force of gravity acting on the unsupported upper extremity tends to stretch the ligaments surrounding the glenohumeral joint.
   a. Result is severe pain and decreased upper extremity function.

3. Electrical stimulation characteristics of FES:
   a. Waveform: asymmetrical biphasic square.
   b. Modulation: continuous.

4. Method of application.
   a. Electrode placement.
      (1) Bipolar.
      (2) Electrodes on the supraspinatus and posterior deltoid musculature.

   b. Treatment parameters.
      (1) Amplitude: tetanic muscle contraction to the patient's tolerance.
      (2) Pulse rate: 25–50 pps.
      (3) Duration of treatment.
         (a) 15–30 minutes.
         (b) Three times daily up to 6–8 hours.
         (c) On/off ratio 1:3 (2 sec:6 sec) progressing to 12:1 (24 sec: 2 sec).

Iontophoresis

Description

1. The method of transferring medicinal agents through the skin or mucous membrane for therapeutic benefit by continuous direct current.

Physics

1. Like charges repel like charges.

Ion Transfer

1. Opposing charges of medicine and current are the basis for ions transferred into the tissues.

2. Duration of treatment, current density and concentration of ions in the solution determine effect of treatment.

Electrical Characteristics of Iontophoresis

1. Waveform: monophasic.

2. Modulation: continuous.

Method of Application

1. Clean and inspect skin.

2. Position patient and support area to be treated.

3. Select appropriate size electrode and apply the ion (medication) to the electrode (active).

4. Place active electrode on the treatment area and attach appropriate lead wire.
   a. Active electrode lead should be the same polarity as ion prescribed.

   b. Dispersive electrode is twice the size of the active electrode and opposite charge of ion.
      (1) Placed either proximally or distally to the treatment site.
      (2) Completes the circuit.

5. The space between the active and dispersive electrodes should be at least the diameter of the active electrode.
   a. Some commercial electrode sets have a fixed distance that limits the spacing between electrodes.

6. Determine dose.
   a. The physical therapist will determine the ion and current dose. Typical treatment dose is 40 mA per minute. Thus, 1mA for 40 minutes equals 40 mA-minute dosage.

7. Turn the intensity up slowly, to increase patient tolerance.
   a. Note that lower intensities result in longer treatment times. May also help to decrease chance of poor tissue reaction (burn, blister).

8. Ask the patient how current feels; discontinue and check tissue if patient complains of pain.

9. Monitor skin following treatment. Report adverse reactions.

General Indications

1. See Table 11-7.

Contraindications for Iontophoresis

1. Refer to general contraindications for electrical stimulation.

2. Impaired skin sensation.

Table 11-7 ➤ INDICATIONS FOR THE USE OF IONTOPHORESIS AND IONS COMMONLY USED

INDICATIONS	ION	POLARITY	SOURCE
Analgesia	Lidocaine, Xylocaine	Positive	Lidocaine, Xylocaine
	Salicylate	Negative	Sodium salicylate
Calcium deposits	Acetate	Negative	Acetic acid
Dermal ulcers	Zinc	Positive	Zinc oxide
Edema reduction	Hyaluronidase	Positive	Wyadase
Fungal infections	Copper	Positive	Copper sulfate
Hyperhidrosis	Water	Positive/negative	Tap water
Muscle spasm	Calcium	Positive	Calcium chloride
	Magnesium	Positive	Magnesium sulfate
Musculoskeletal inflammatory conditions	Dexamethasone	Negative	
	Hydrocortisone	Positive	

3. Allergy or sensitivity to therapeutic agent or direct current.

4. Denuded area or recent scar.

5. Cuts.

6. Bruises.

7. Broken skin.

8. Metal in or near treatment area.

High-Voltage Galvanic Stimulation (Twin-Spiked Monophasic): High-Voltage Pulsed Current

Description

1. High-voltage pulsed current (HVPC).
   a. Typically, monophasic twin-peaked pulses of short duration.

Physics

1. The skin offers high resistance to the flow of low-voltage current.

2. Passage of HVPC decreases the skin resistance due to the current flowing toward the skin capacitors rather than the skin resistors.
   a. Thermal effects are insignificant (little resistance to current).

Characteristics of HVPC

1. Waveform: paired monophasic with instantaneous rise and exponential fall of current.

2. Modulations: continuous, surged and interrupted.

Procedural interventions for high voltage galvanic stimulation

1. Muscle stimulation protocol.
   a. Refer to General Procedure section.

2. Wound healing parameters.
   a. Amplitude: comfortable tingling sensation, paresthesia, no muscle response.
   b. Pulse rate: 80–100 pps.
   c. Pulse duration: 20–100 μsec.
   d. Duration of treatment: 0–60 minutes.

3. Method of application.
   a. Inspect wound area.
   b. Position patient and support treatment area.
   c. Clean and debride wound site.
      (1) Pack with sterile saline-soaked gauze.
   d. Place active electrode over gauze.
   e. For bactericidal effect.
      (1) The active electrode should have negative polarity.
      (2) For a culture-free wound, the active electrode should be positive.
   f. The dispersive electrode is placed proximally to the wound site.

g. Turn up intensity slowly to selected level.

h. At conclusion of treatment, turn intensity down slowly to zero.

Indications

1. Refer to general stimulation indications.

Contraindications

1. Refer to general stimulation contraindications section.

Electromyographic (EMG) Biofeedback

Description

1. **Electronic instrument used to measure motor unit action potentials (MUAP) that are generated by active muscles.**

   a. Signals are detected, amplified and converted into audiovisual signals that are used to reinforce voluntary control of muscles.

   b. The use of EMG biofeedback in clinical practice by the physical therapist assistant is usually restricted to surface, not needle electrodes.

Procedural Interventions for EMG Biofeedback

1. **Electrode selection.**

   a. Electrode selection is dependent on the size of the muscle or muscle group being measured.

2. **Electrode placement.**

   a. Bipolar technique.

      (1) Two active electrodes (one positive and one negative) and a single reference ground electrode.

         (a) The reference electrode may be placed between or adjacent to active electrodes.

         (b) This arrangement minimizes or eliminates extraneous electrical activity (noise or crosstalk).

   b. Active electrodes are placed on or near motor point of targeted muscle or muscle groups.

   c. Active electrodes are usually placed parallel to muscle fibers.

      (1) About 15 cm apart.

      (2) The reference electrode is placed near the treatment area.

   d. Active electrodes placed close together.

      (1) Minimize cross-talk.

      (2) Yield small signals.

      (3) Provide more precise signal.

   e. Active electrodes placed further apart.

      (1) Yield large signals.

      (2) Detection from more than one muscle.

   f. Treatment setting should be quiet for optimal patient concentration.

   g. Prepare skin to allow for optimal recording.

      (1) Same as electrical stimulation.

   h. Apply conductive gel.

   i. Secure electrodes to the area to be treated.

Specific Procedural Interventions for EMG Biofeedback

1. **Technique to increase muscle activity.**

   a. Weak muscles.

      (1) Begin with electrodes widely spaced and with the biofeedback unit set for high sensitivity (to increase detection of signal).

      (2) For a single weak muscle.

         (a) Begin with electrodes close together or if a more precise signal is desired.

   b. Instruct patient to attempt an isometric contraction (holding for 6–10 seconds).

      (1) Produce an audiovisual signal.

   c. As the patient's motor recruitment ability improves, decrease the sensitivity of the signal.

   d. Use facilitation techniques to encourage response of muscle if necessary.

      (1) Tapping.

      (2) Cross-facilitation.

      (3) Vibration.

   e. Progress from simple to more complex functional movements as patient gains motor control.

   f. Treatment time: 5–10 minutes to 30 minutes or more, depending on patient's tolerance.

   g. At conclusion of session: clean patient's skin and clean or dispose of electrodes.

2. **Technique for decreasing muscle activity (muscle relaxation).**

a. Begin with electrodes spaced close together and with the biofeedback instrument sensitivity set to low.
   (1) Minimizes cross-talk.
b. Instruct the patient to relax and try to lower the audiovisual signal.
   (1) Relaxation techniques can be used.
c. Progress from low- to high-sensitivity settings as the patient gains ability to relax muscles and perform functional activities.
d. Treatment time: 5–10 minutes to 30 minutes, depending on patient's tolerance.
e. At end of session: clean patient's skin and clean or dispose of electrodes.

Criteria for Patient Selection for Biofeedback Training

1. Good vision.
2. Good hearing.
3. Good communication abilities.
4. Good comprehension skills.
5. Ability to follow simple commands.
6. Good motor planning skills.
7. No profound sensory or proprioceptive deficits.

Continuous Passive Motion (CPM)

Description

1. Uninterrupted passive motion of a joint delivered through a controlled range of motion. A mechanical device provides the continuous movement for extended period of time.

Physiological Effects (Table 11-8)

Procedural Interventions for Continuous Passive Motion

1. Should be applied immediately postoperatively.
2. Rate of motion set at one cycle per 1 or 2 minutes.

3. If applied to the knee, the ROM may be 20–40 degrees of flexion initially.
   a. Increase it by 5–10 degrees as patient can tolerate until optimal range is reached.
4. Treatment time: as little as 1 hour sessions, three times a day to 24 hours continuously.
5. Patient's limb can/should be removed periodically to allow for active or active-assistive exercises as well as activities of daily living (ADL) training.
6. Treatment duration: 1–3 weeks or until therapeutic outcomes are attained.

Indications for Continuous Passive Motion

1. Postimmobilization fracture.
2. Tendon or ligament repair.
3. Total knee replacement.
4. Total hip replacement.

Contraindications for Continuous Passive Motion

1. Discontinue treatment if patient experiences.
   a. Increased inflammation.
   b. Increased edema or pain.
2. Always inform the PT immediately.

Table 11-8 ➤ PHYSIOLOGICAL EFFECTS OF CONTINUOUS PASSIVE MOVEMENT

INCREASED	DECREASED
1. Synovial fluid lubrication of the joint	1. Contractures
2. Circulation	2. Postoperative pain
3. Improvement of wound, articular cartilage, ligament and tendon healing	3. Adhesions
4. Acceleration rate of intra articular effusion cartilage healing and regeneration	4. Edema and joint
5. Nutrition to articular cartilage and periarticular tissues	

Tilt Table

Description

1. A mechanical or electrical table designed to elevate a patient from horizontal (0 degrees) to vertical (90 degrees) position in a controlled incremental manner.
   a. There are usually three straps attached to the table to stabilize the patient securely.
      (1) At the upper thorax.
      (2) The pelvis and the knees.
      (3) With a standing platform at the feet.

Physiological Effects of Tilt Table

1. Stimulation of postural reflexes to counteract orthostatic hypotension.
2. Facilitates postural drainage.
3. Provides a gradual loading response to one or both lower extremities.

Method of Application

1. Position the patient supine on the table.
2. To counteract venous pooling.
   a. Abdominal binder.
   b. Thigh-high elastic stockings.
   c. Ace bandages wrapped around the lower extremities.
3. Secure the three straps firmly to adequately stabilize the patient on the table.
4. Elevate the table gradually in increments.
   a. 30 degrees.
   b. 45 degrees.
   c. 60 degrees.
   d. 80 degrees.
   e. 90 degrees.
   f. To patient's tolerance.
5. Maintain new position for 30–60 minutes or to patient's tolerance.

6. Monitor the patient at each increment of elevation and while at new elevation to assure patient's tolerance to the positional change.
   a. Blood pressure.
   b. Heart rate.
   c. Respiratory rate.
7. Watch for cyanotic lips or nail beds as they may indicate compromised circulation.
8. Treatment time varies with patient condition and tolerance.

Indications for Tilt Table

1. Prolonged bed rest.
2. Immobilization.
3. Spinal cord injury.
4. Head injury.
5. Pulmonary congestion.
6. Difficulty with maintaining limited weight-bearing through lower extremities.

Contraindications for Tilt Table

1. Any condition that is irritated by an upright or semi-upright position.

Precautions for Tilt Table

1. Orthostatic hypotension.
   a. The table is elevated gradually, to allow the body to accommodate to positional changes while decreasing the risk of blood pressure dropping.
2. Postural hypotension.
   a. Decrease in blood pressure that occurs with positional changes from horizontal to vertical.
   b. Occurs frequently with spinal cord injuries.
   c. Ace wrapping and/or compressive stockings, as well as an abdominal binder, in conjunction with the tilt table, will minimize the effects.

Soft Tissue Massage

Description

1. Manipulation of soft tissue by the hands.

Physiological Effects of Soft Tissue Massage

1. Increased venous and lymphatic flow.

2. Stretching and loosening of scar tissue.

3. Edema reduction.

4. Sedation.

5. Muscle relaxation.

6. Pain reduction.

Selected Massage Techniques

1. Stroking (effleurage).
   a. Gliding movements of hands over the surface of the skin.
      (1) Superficial stroking is light contact.
      (2) Deep stroking is heavy pressure.
      (3) Used initially and at conclusion of treatment session.
      (4) Mold hand around body part and move distally to proximally.
      (5) Stroking is utilized to move the clinician's hand from one body part to another and between other strokes.

2. Kneading (petrissage).
   a. Grasping and lifting tissue.
      (1) The milking effect aids in loosening adhesions and increasing venous return.
      (2) Lift and wring tissue using one or both hands, fingers or thumb and first finger.
      (3) Stroke direction is distal to proximal along extremity to increase venous return.

3. Friction.
   a. Compression of tissue using small circular or long stroking movements with the palmar surface of hand or fingertips.
      (1) Pressure may be light initially.
         (a) Progresses to heavy.
         (b) Moves superficial tissue over deeper tissue.
      (2) Heavy compression over soft tissue will stretch scars and loosen adhesions.

      (3) Pressure gradually increases to patient's tolerance as the technique moves up, down or around treatment area.
      (4) Pressure should never be abruptly released.
      (5) Cross-fiber friction uses deep strokes across the muscle fibers rather than along longitudinal axis of the fibers.

4. Tapping (tapotement).
   a. Rapid striking with the palmar surface of the hands and/or fingers, cupped hand (clapping or percussion), or the ulnar edge of the hand and fingers (hacking) in an alternating manner.
      (1) Tapping is used when stimulation is desired.
      (2) Cupping is used at the chest to mobilize secretions during postural drainage sessions.

5. Vibration.
   a. Shaking of tissue using short, rapid quivering motions with both hands on the body part.
   b. Often used in conjunction with cupping during postural drainage to loosen adherent secretions.

Method of Application

1. Position the patient in a comfortable, relaxed position.
   a. Place body part in a gravity-eliminated position or in a gravity-assisted position (depending upon treatment desired).

2. Body part is exposed and supported.
   a. No clothing to restrict circulation.

3. Begin with light effleurage and progress to deep effleurage to warm the tissues, then to kneading or friction technique depending upon treatment goals identified.

4. Massage should begin at proximal section of an extremity, or centrally on the trunk (to clear the area).
   a. Move distally or peripherally.
   b. Return to the proximal section.

5. All stroke movements are directed distal to proximal, especially in the case of edema; on the trunk, movements begin centrally.

6. Complete treatment with effleurage strokes, moving from deep to superficial technique.

7. Treatment time varies with condition, tissue response and patient tolerance.

Indications for Soft Tissue Massage

1. Subacute and chronic pain.

2. Muscle spasm.

3. Superficial scar formation.
    a. From trauma or burns.

4. Edema.

5. Postural drainage.

Contraindications for Soft Tissue Massage

1. Acute inflammation in area.

2. Acute febrile condition.

3. Severe atherosclerosis.

4. Severe varicose veins.

5. Phlebitis.

6. Areas of recent surgery.

7. Thrombophlebitis.

8. Cardiac arrhythmia.

9. Malignancy.

10. Hypersensitivity.

11. Severe rheumatoid arthritis.

12. Hemorrhage in area.

13. Edema secondary to kidney dysfunction, heart failure and venous insufficiency.

Mechanical Spinal Traction

Description

1. A distraction force applied to the spine to separate or attempt to separate vertebral bodies and elongate spinal structure.
    a. Force can be applied in an intermittent or sustained (continuous) manner.

General Treatment Outcomes for Mechanical Spinal Traction

1. Reduction of radicular signs and symptoms associated with disc protrusion, lateral stenosis, degenerative disc disease.

2. Reduction in muscle guarding/spasm.

3. Reduction in joint pain.

4. Increasing range of motion.

5. Use of traction in the treatment of skeletal fractures is not a part of this chapter.

Cervical Traction

1. In current practice the occipital halter is commonly used.
    a. It has no mandibular strap and pulls exclusively from the occiput.

2. Cervical traction can be applied in sitting or supine position.
    a. Supine has been shown to be more effective.

Method of Application

1. The angle of pull will vary depending upon the target area.
    a. Approximately 0–5 degrees of cervical flexion to increase intervertebral space at C1-5.
    b. Up to 25–30 degrees of cervical flexion to increase intervertebral space at C5-7.
    c. Zero degrees of cervical flexion is advised for disc dysfunction.
    d. Otherwise, the neck should be positioned in and maintained at 20–30 degrees of flexion with use of a pillow.

2. Traction force should be applied at the occipital region.

3. If pain is reported, the treatment should be stopped and the halter readjusted.

4. Treatment force.
    a. 10–15 pounds to effect disc protrusion, elongation of soft tissue, muscle spasm.
    b. 20–30 pounds to achieve joint distraction.

5. Treatment time.
    a. 5–10 minutes for acute conditions and herniated disk.
    b. 15–30 minutes for other conditions.

6. Cycle time.
   a. Dependent on condition and treatment outcome.
   b. Facet problems seem to respond better to shorter but equal on/off times.
   c. Disks seem to respond to longer on/off times with approximately a 3:1 ratio or sustained traction.

7. **The patient's response to the traction treatment is crucial.**
   a. If the patient complains of increased pain after the treatment session, the amount of traction force/time applied should not be increased.
      (1) The physical therapist must be notified.

Indications for Mechanical Spinal Traction

1. **Degenerative disc.**

2. **Discogenic pain.**

3. **Herniated nucleus pulposus (disc protrusion).**

4. **Joint disease.**

5. **Joint stiffness (hypomobility).**

6. **Meniscoid-blocking muscle spasm.**

7. **Nerve root impingement.**

8. **Subacute or chronic joint pain.**

Contraindications for Mechanical Spinal Traction

1. **Impaired cognitive function.**

2. **Spinal tumors.**

3. **Spinal infections.**

4. **Spondylolisthesis.**

5. **Rheumatoid arthritis.**

6. **Osteoporosis.**

7. **Vascular compromise.**

8. **Pediatric or elderly patients.**

Precautions for Mechanical Spinal Traction

1. **Acute inflammation aggravated by traction.**

2. **Acute sprains and strains.**

3. **Claustrophobia.**

4. **Hiatal hernia.**

5. **Joint instability.**

6. **Pregnancy.**

7. **TMJ problems if using a chin strap.**

Lumbar Traction

1. Description.
   a. A programmable traction machine is most frequently used in current practice because of its versatility.
   b. A split table minimizes friction between the body and table.
   c. Lumbar traction is usually applied in supine with pillows under the knees.
      (1) The prone position is often used in the case of a posteriorly herniated lumbar disc.
   d. The top edge of the pelvic harness is above the iliac crest.
      (1) The inferior margin of the thoracic harness is slightly below the lower ribs.
   e. The thoracic harness provides countertraction to pull on the pelvis.

Method of Application

1. Position of the hips and knees will vary depending on the treatment area being targeted. Hip flexion to approximately:
   a. 45–60 degrees will provide laxity at the L5-S1 level.
   b. 60–75 degrees will provide laxity at the L4-5 level.
   c. 75–90 degrees will provide laxity at the L3-4 level.

2. Treatment force.
   a. Acute phase 25–45 pounds.
   b. Disk protrusion, spasm; elongation of soft tissues 25% of body weight.
   c. Joint distraction 50 pounds or 50% of body weight.
   d. Poundage needed to overcome the frictional forces of the lower body (when not using a split table) is one-fourth the patient's body weight.

3. Optimal traction force varies depending on resources.
   a. Ranging from 300 pounds to one-fourth the body weight.
   b. Maximum tolerance of T11-12 disks is reported to be 440 pounds; estimates for the lumbar spine are much greater.

4. Treatment time depends on desired outcome.
   a. 5–10 minutes for herniated disc.
   b. 10–30 minutes for other conditions.

5. Cycle time.
   a. Intermittent traction allows for greater traction forces.
      (1) Facet problems respond better to shorter and equal on/off times.
         (a) 10 seconds on/10 seconds off.
      (2) Herniated disc problems respond to longer on/off times with approximately 3:1 ratios with sustained pulls.
         (a) 60 seconds on/20 seconds off.

Intermittent Compression

Description

1. Pneumatic pump that applies external pressure to an extremity through inflatable sleeves of various sizes to fit upper or lower extremities (ankle, ankle and lower leg or full extremity).
   a. The sleeves are attached to a pump by a rubber tube.
   b. Sleeves are designed to allow either uniform compression on the extremity (single compartment) or sequential pressure on the extremity (multiple compartments).
   c. The pressure is greater distally and decreases proximally.
   d. Cold can be applied simultaneously with intermittent compression when a coolant (50°–77°F) is pumped through the inflatable sleeve.

Physiological Effects of Intermittent Compression

1. External pressure on the extremity increases the pressure in the interstitial fluids, forcing fluids to move into the lymphatic and venous systems.

2. Reduces the fluid volume in the extremity.

3. Normalizes tissue texture and increases comfort.

Method of Application

1. Check.
   a. Blood pressure.
      (1) Treatment pressures approximate to or greater than the diastolic pressure should encourage movement of the lymph and reabsorption of edema.
      (2) Maximum pressure should not exceed the systolic pressure; this may exceed the arterial system's ability to withstand the pressure and be uncomfortable for the patient.
   b. Heart rate.
   c. The affected extremity's circumferential measurement.

2. Place patient in a comfortable position.
   a. Affected extremity elevated approximately 45 degrees (above the heart) and abducted 20–70 degrees.

3. Remove all jewelry and apply stockinet over extremity; smooth out all wrinkles.
   a. Cover any open areas with gauze or appropriate covering.

4. Place sleeve over extremity and attach rubber tubing to sleeve and compression unit.

5. Adjust the inflation and deflation ratio to approximately 3:1 for reduction of edema, venous stasis.
   a. Generally 80–100 seconds on and 25–50 seconds off.
   b. For residual limb shaping use a 4:1 ratio, 40–60 seconds on and 10–15 seconds off.

6. Turn power on and slowly increase pressure to desired level.

7. Treatment time is dependent on the patient's tolerance.
   a. Minimum daily treatment times.
      (1) Lymphedema: 2 hours to two 3-hour sessions.
      (2) Traumatic edema: 2 hours.
      (3) Venous ulcers: 2.0–2.5 hours, three times a week.
      (4) Residual edema: 1- to 3-hour sessions totaling 4 hours of total treatment.
   b. Some conditions may require shorter treatment times initially.

Special Considerations for Intermittent Compression

1. The patient's blood pressure determines the setting.
   a. Some manufacturers recommend that the setting never exceed the patient's diastolic blood pressure.
   b. Others advise that the pressure can fall between the diastolic and systolic pressure since the unit's pressure is only on for a short period.
   c. The PT usually determines the settings following the guidelines identified in section C.1 above.

2. Numbness, tingling, pulse or pain should not be felt during the treatment.

3. At the end of the treatment session.
   a. Turn off the unit.
   b. Remove the sleeve and stockinet.
   c. Assess the skin.

4. Usually an elastic bandage or compression stocking is placed on the limb to retain the reduction before a dependent position is allowed.

CHAPTER 11

Indications for Intermittent Compression

1. Chronic edema.

2. Lymphedema (postmastectomy).

3. Stasis ulcer.

4. Traumatic edema.

5. Venous insufficiency.

6. Amputation.

Contraindications for Intermittent Compression

1. Acute inflammation.

2. Acute deep venous thrombosis.

3. Arterial insufficiency.

4. Acute pulmonary edema.

5. Cancer.

6. Diminished skin sensation.

7. Kidney or cardiac insufficiency.

8. Hypertension.

9. Cognitive dysfunction.

10. Obstructed lymph channels.

11. Infection in the area to be treated.

12. Pediatric or elderly frail patients.

Documentation

1. The documentation should assure consistent replication of the intervention given.

2. Document each episode of intervention.

3. Document patient/client self-report as appropriate.

4. Document specific intervention provided.
   a. Frequency.
   b. Intensity.
   c. Duration, as appropriate.
   d. Area of intervention, as appropriate.

5. Document patient/client response to the intervention.

6. Document all communication between the PTA and the supervising PT.

7. As with all documentation, only use medically approved abbreviations or symbols.

APPENDIX 11-1

Conversion formula for Celsius (centigrade) to Fahrenheit and vice versa

1. You may need to convert from Celsius to Fahrenheit or vice versa.
   a. Conversion formulas:
      (1) Celsius to Fahrenheit: $9/5\ C + 32 = F$.
      (2) $C \times 9$ divided by $5 + 32 = F$.
      (3) Fahrenheit to Celsius: $5/9\ F - -32 = C$.
      (4) $F \times 5$ divided by $9 - 32 = C$.

The authors wish to acknowledge the contributions of Lisa J. Ford, PTA, AS, to previous editions of this chapter.

chapter 12

Gait, Functional Training, Equipment and Devices

SUSAN B. O'SULLIVAN

Focus Areas for Content Review:
- Mechanics and pathomechanics of gait.
- Physical therapy interventions and strategies to address gait and mobility deficits including indications, contraindications, equipment and environmental considerations.

- Standard wheelchair components and specialized features. Seating and positioning strategies and wheelchair training strategies.
- Prosthetic and orthotic devices components, training in safe and efficient use and care of the device.

Gait

Phases of Gait

1. **The gait cycle is broken down into two phases: stance and swing, each referring to a single limb.**
   a. *Stance phase* refers to the time the limb remains on the ground; it represents approximately 60% of the gait cycle.
      (1) "Double stance" refers to the period of time during the stance phase when portions of both feet are in contact with the ground: during this time the weight is being shifted from one limb to the next. This does not exist with running.
   b. *Swing phase* refers to the time the limb remains in the air; it represents approximately 40% of the gait cycle.

2. **The phases of gait can be described using two different sets of terminology, Traditional (T) and Rancho Los Amigos (RLA); both are used clinically so it is recommended that readers be familiar with both (Table 12-1).**
   a. *Traditional terminology* refers to lengths of time in the gait cycle.
   b. *Rancho Los Amigos* (RLA) refers to points in time during the gait cycle.

Stance Phase

1. **Heel strike (T): the instant the heel of the stance limb contacts the ground at the beginning of the stance phase. Initial contact (RLA): The instant the foot of the leading limb comes in contact with the ground. This is the beginning of the stance phase.**
   a. Muscle activation patterns (Table 12-2): Hip muscles (gluteus maximus, hamstrings and adductor magnus) contract isometrically to stabilize the hip; knee extensors (quadriceps) contract eccentrically to control a small amount of knee flexion for shock absorption; ankle dorsiflexors (tibialis anterior, extensor hallucis longus, extensor digitorum longus) act eccentrically to oppose the plantar flexion moment, thus controlling the foot to avoid foot slap.

2. **Foot flat (T): plantar surface of the foot of the stance limb makes contact with ground; occurs immediately after heel strike. Loading response (RLA): the gait cycle's period of double support occurs immediately after initial contact until the opposite leg leaves the ground. The time between the initial contact and the beginning of swing phase for the other limb.**
   a. Muscle activation patterns (see Table 12-2): Hip extensors (gluteus maximus, hamstrings) contract isometrically to stabilize the hip; knee extensors

Table 12-1 ➤ GAIT TERMINOLOGY

TRADITIONAL TERMINOLOGY		RANCHO LOS AMIGOS TERMINOLOGY	
TERM	**DEFINITION**	**TERM**	**DEFINITION**
Stance Phase = Approximately 60% of Gait Cycle			
Heel Strike	Beginning of stance phase, heel contacts ground.	Initial Contact	Beginning of stance phase, heel or other part of foot contacts the ground.
Foot Flat	Occurs following heel strike. Plantar surface of foot touches ground. Loading response of limb.	Loading Response	Beginning of double-support phase of stance, from initial contact until the opposite extremity leaves the ground.
Midstance	Full body weight is taken over the stance limb.	Midstance	Beginning of single-support phase of stance when opposite limb leaves the ground and full body weight is taken over stance limb.
Heel-Off	Occurs following midstance; heel of this limb leaves the ground.	Terminal Stance	Last period of single-limb support, begins when heel rises and ends when the contralateral limb makes contact with the ground.
Toe-Off	The last portion of stance phase, follows heel-off when only the toe of the stance limb is in contact with the ground.	Preswing	The second period of double-support from initial contact of opposite limb to lift off of the support limb.
Swing Phase = approximately 40% of Gait Cycle			
Acceleration	First portion of swing phase, from toe-off until mid swing.	Initial Swing	First portion of swing phase from toe off of the contralateral limb until maximum knee flexion of this extremity.
Mid Swing	Mid portion of swing when this extremity moves directly under the body.	Mid Swing	Begins with maximum knee flexion of this limb and ends when the tibia is perpendicular to the ground.
Deceleration	Starts immediately after mid swing when limb is slowing down and knee is extending in preparation for heel strike.	Terminal Swing	Begins when the tibia is perpendicular to the floor and ends when the foot touches the ground.

(quadriceps) contract eccentrically to control the knee; ankle plantar flexor (gastrocnemius, soleus) muscles contract eccentrically to control forward tibial motion.

3. **Midstance (T): the point at which full body weight is taken on the leading limb as the opposite limb leaves the ground. Midstance (RLA): the opposite limb leaves the ground; body weight is taken and advanced over and ahead of the support limb. This is a period of single-limb support.**
   a. Muscle activation patterns (see Table 12-2): Hip, knee and ankle extensors are active through stance to oppose antigravity forces/stabilize the limb; hip extensors control forward motion of trunk; hip abductors stabilize the pelvis during unilateral stance.

4. **Heel off (T): occurs after midstance as the heel of the leading leg leaves the ground. Terminal stance (RLA): the last period of single limb support that begins when the heel rises and ends when the other limb makes contact with the ground.**
   a. Muscle activation patterns: peak activity of plantar flexors occurs just after heel-off to push off and generates forward propulsion of the body.

5. **Toe-off (T): the last portion of the stance phase follows heel-off when only the toe of the stance limb is in contact with the ground. Preswing (RLA): the second period of double support from initial contact of the opposite limb to lift off of the support limb.**

   a. Muscle activation patterns (see Table 12-2): Hip and knee flexors contract concentrically to assist with elevation of the limb, the hip and knee extensors may contribute to forward propulsion of the body with a brief burst of activity; ankle plantarflexors (gastrocnemius, soleus) contract concentrically to assist with forward propulsion of the limb.

Swing Phase

1. **Acceleration (T): first portion of swing phase from toe off until midswing. Initial swing (RLA): first portion of the swing phase from toe off of the contralateral limb until maximum knee flexion of the same extremity.**
   a. Muscle activation patterns (see Table 12-2): hip flexors (iliopsoas) act concentrically to assist with forward motion of the hip; knee extensors (quadriceps) are active early in the phase to assist with swing, by mid swing the extensors are silent as forward momentum carries the limb; ankle dorsiflexors act concentrically to clear the toe of the advancing limb.

2. **Midswing (T): mid portion of swing when the referenced extremity moves directly under the body. Midswing (RLA): begins with maximum knee flexion and ends when the tibia is perpendicular to the ground.**

Table 12-2 ➤ MUSCLE ACTIVITY DURING GAIT AND THE RESULT OF WEAKNESS

PORTION OF GAIT	MUSCLE ACTIVITY	RESULT OF WEAKNESS	POSSIBLE COMPENSATION
Heel strike to foot flat	HIP: erector spinae, gluteus maximus, hamstrings.	Excessive hip flexion and anterior pelvis tilt	Forceful trunk extension and backward leaning to prevent excessive hip flexion.
	KNEE: quadriceps contract initially to hold knee in extension (loading response), then eccentrically to control knee flexion. Gastrocnemius (late in phase) begins contraction.	Quadriceps: excessive knee flexion. Gastrocnemius: excessive knee flexion.	Trunk lurches forward or external rotation of extremity to lock knee into extension.
	ANKLE & FOOT: pretibial group works eccentrically to control plantar flexion.	Foot slap	Lack of heel strike at initial contact resulting in foot placed flat on floor or toes-first gait.
Foot flat through midstance	HIP: gluteus maximus works to oppose hip flexion.	Excessive hip flexion and anterior pelvic tilt.	Trunk extension initially to prevent excessive hip flexion.
	KNEE: quadriceps contract in early phase to extend knee, then no activity is required; gastrocnemius and soleus eccentric contraction. Hamstrings: work to prevent genu recurvatum.	Quadriceps: excessive knee flexion. Hamstrings: knee hyperextension.	Plantar flexion at ankle so that foot flat occurs instead of heel strike; eliminates excessive flexion moment of the knee. This occurs early in midstance – no compensation is needed in later part of phase.
	ANKLE & FOOT: gastrocnemius and soleus act eccentrically to control forward advance of tibia	Excessive dorsiflexion and uncontrolled forward motion of the tibia.	Ankle may be maintained in plantar flexion to avoid excessive dorsiflexion.
Midstance to heel-off	HIP: extensors in early phase to maintain stability.	Pelvis drop on swing limb, decreased ability to clear limb.	Lateral trunk shift over weak (stance) limb.
	Hip abductors (gluteus medius) work concentrically to control lateral pelvis tilt during swing of opposite limb.		
	KNEE: gastrocnemius and soleus work eccentrically to control advance of the tibia.	Gastrocnemius: excessive dorsiflexion and uncontrolled forward motion of the tibia resulting in knee snapping into extension at late phase.	Loss of heel rise at the ankle resulting in dropping of pelvis on this side during pre-swing activities.
	ANKLE & FOOT: Tibialis posterior isometric	Tibialis posterior: controls amount of pronation.	Gastrocnemius: ankle may be maintained in plantar flexion to avoid excessive dorsiflexion; if foot is flat on floor, a steppage gait is produced. Tibialis posterior: excessive pronation of the foot.
Heel-off to toe-off	HIP: iliopsoas, adductor magnus, adductor longus for stability of limb position.	Undetermined	Undetermined
	KNEE: quadriceps required to control amount of knee flexion (eccentric contraction).	Quadriceps: excessive heel rise (knee flexion) at initial swing.	Typically not compensated for.
	ANKLE & FOOT: gastrocnemius, soleus, peroneus longus/brevis, flexor hallucis longus contract to plantar flex the foot.	Decreased or no push-off. Decreased contralateral step.	Slight lag in forward movement of swing leg; foot is lifted off of floor without push-off.
Acceleration to midswing	HIP: hip flexor activity to initiate swing (iliopsoas, rectus femoris, gracilis, sartorius, tensor fascia lata).	Diminished hip flexion causes inability to initiate forward movement of extremity.	Posterior lurch of trunk, circumduction, and/or hip hiking to bring limb forward and clear foot.
	KNEE: little or no activity in quadriceps; biceps femoris (short head) gracilis and sartorius act concentrically.	Biceps femoris: inadequate knee flexion	Increased hip flexion, circumduction, or hip hiking to clear foot.
	ANKLE & FOOT: dorsiflexors contract to bring the ankle into neutral and to prevent toe drag.	Foot drop and/or toe dragging	Increased hip and knee flexion to prevent toe drag, hip hiking, circumduction, or vaulting on opposite limb.
Midswing to deceleration	HIP: hip extensors and hamstrings.	Control forward movement of limb, stabilization of hip for stance.	
	KNEE: hamstrings eccentric contraction	Control extension movement of knee.	Knee snaps into extension.
	ANKLE & FOOT: dorsiflexors contract to maintain dorsiflexion.	Foot drop and/or toe dragging.	Early phase: increased hip and knee flexion to prevent toe drag, hip hiking, circumduction, or vaulting on opposite limb.

a. Muscle activation patterns: hip, knee and ankle flexors work concentrically to allow foot clearance. At the end of the phase the knee flexors begin to work eccentrically to control forward momentum of the tibia; ankle dorsiflexors work concentrically to clear the toe.

3. Deceleration (T): begins directly after swing phase when the limb is slowing down in preparation for heel strike. Terminal swing (RLA): begins when the tibia is perpendicular to the ground and ends when the foot touches the ground.
   a. Muscle activation patterns (see Table 12-2): hip flexors work concentrically early in the phase and hip extensors work eccentrically at the end to slow forward movement; knee flexors (hamstrings) work eccentrically to decelerate the limb; ankle dorsiflexors work concentrically/isometrically to prepare for heel strike.

Other Motions Occurring During Gait

1. Pelvic motion.
   a. The pelvis moves forward and backward (transverse pelvic rotation).
      (1) Forward rotation occurs during swing phase; approximately 4 degrees.
      (2) During weight-bearing or stance, the pelvis rotates 4 degrees for a total of 8 degrees.
   b. The pelvis moves up and down on the unsupported or swing side (lateral pelvic tilt) approximately 5 degrees.
      (1) Controlled by hip abductor muscles on stance limb.
      (2) The high point is at midstance.
      (3) The low point is during the period of double support.

2. Cadence is the number of steps taken over a period of time.
   a. The average is 110–120 steps per minute.
   b. Running causes the period of double support to disappear. Common cadence for running is 180 steps per minute.
   c. Increased cadence: results in a shorter step length and decreased duration of double support.

3. Step.
   a. Step length is the measured distance between the points of foot contact (preferably heel strike), of one extremity to the point of foot contact of the opposite extremity; measure in centimeters or inches.
   b. Step time is the number of seconds that elapse during one step.
   c. Step width is the distance between the feet (measured in centimeters or meters from one heel to the same point on the opposite heel); normal range is between 2.54 and 12.7 cm (2–4 inches).
      (1) This makes up the base of support.
      (2) Increases as stability demands rise; e.g., wide-based gait in older adults or very young children.

4. Stride.
   a. Stride length is the distance between two consecutive contact points of the same extremity.
   b. Stride time is the number of seconds that elapse during one stride (one complete gait cycle).

5. Velocity (walking speed) is the rate of motion in any direction or the distance per unit of time.
   a. The average walking speed is approximately 3 mph.
      (1) Affected by a person's height, weight, gender and physical ability.
   b. Velocity decreases with age, physical disability, balance deficit, etc.

6. Acceleration is the rate of change of the velocity with respect to time.

7. Energy cost of walking.
   a. Average oxygen consumption rate for comfortable walking is 12mL/kg x minutes.
   b. Metabolic cost of walking averages 5.5 Kcal/min on level surfaces.
   c. Energy costs dependent on.
      (1) Speed.
      (2) Stride length.
      (3) Body weight.
      (4) The type of surface, gradient.
   d. Increased energy costs occur with age, abnormal gait and or the use of an assistive device.

Common Gait Deviations: Stance Phase

1. Trunk and hip.
   a. Lateral bending of the trunk may be caused by a weak gluteus medius. This happens during the loading response of midstance.
      (1) Bending to the same side of the weakness is known as a Trendelenburg gait.
      (2) Patients may experience hip pain.
   b. Backward lean of the trunk is usually caused by a weak gluteus maximus. This happens during the loading response.
      (1) The patient will have difficulty going up stairs or ramps.
   c. Forward lean of the trunk may be caused by a weak quadriceps muscle, hip or knee flexion contracture or proprioceptive deficit. This happens during loading response and the first part of midstance.
   d. Excessive hip flexion usually caused by weak hip extensors or tight hip or knee flexors.
   e. Limited hip extension can be caused by tight or spastic hip flexors.

f. Limited hip flexion can be caused by weak hip flexors or tight hip extensors.

g. Abnormal synergistic activity generally occurs after a neurological insult (e.g., stroke): the patient may demonstrate excessive hip adduction combined with hip and knee extension, plantar flexion, scissoring or adducted gait pattern.

h. Antalgic gait (painful gait): this is a protective gait pattern. Stance time is usually limited on the painful limb resulting in uneven timing and/or uneven step lengths; the uninvolved limb will demonstrate a shortened step length since it must bear weight sooner than normal.

2. Knee.

a. Excessive knee flexion: the result of weak quadriceps (may see wobbling or buckling of knee) or knee flexion contracture.
   (1) The patient will have difficulty going down stairs or ramps.
   (2) The trunk may compensate by increasing forward bending.
   (3) May have difficulty with sit-to-stand.

b. Hyperextension of the knee: the result of a weak quadriceps muscle, plantar flexion contracture or extensor spasticity.

3. Ankle and foot.

a. Toe first: toes contact floor at heel strike, the result of weak dorsiflexors, spastic or tight plantar flexors, shortened leg length, a painful heel or a positive support reflex.

b. Foot slap: the foot makes floor contact with an audible slap, the result of weak dorsiflexors or hypotonia.
   (1) Patient may compensate for this deficit by using a steppage gait (excessive hip and knee flexion.

c. Foot flat: the entire foot contacts the ground at initial contact, the result of weak dorsiflexors, limited range of motion or immature gait pattern (neonatal).

d. Excessive dorsiflexion with uncontrolled forward motion of the tibia. This is the result of weak plantar flexors; known as a calcaneus gait.

e. Excessive plantar flexion (equinus gait). The heel does not touch the ground. May be caused by spasticity or contracture of the plantar flexors; the patient will have poor eccentric contraction and difficulty advancing the tibia.

f. Supination: excessive lateral contact of foot during stance with varus position of calcaneus. May occur in initial contact and correct at foot flat with weight acceptance or remain throughout stance.
   (1) Possible causes: weak spastic invertors, weak evertors, pes varus, genu varum.

g. Pronation: excessive medial contact of foot during stance with valgus position of calcaneus.
   (1) Possible causes: weak invertors, spasticity, pes planus, genu valgum.

h. Toes claw: the result of spastic toe flexors, possibly a hyperactive plantar grasp reflex.

i. Inadequate push-off: the result of weak plantar flexors, decreased range of motion or pain in the forefoot/toe.

Common Gait Deviations: Swing Phase

1. Trunk and hip.

a. Insufficient forward pelvic rotation (pelvic retraction): the result of weak abdominal muscles or weak flexor muscles (e.g., stroke).

b. Insufficient hip and knee flexion: the result of weak hip and knee flexors; inability to lift the leg and bring it forward.

c. Circumduction: the leg swings out to the side in abduction and external rotation, the result of weak hip or knee flexors.

d. Hip hiking: excessive action of the quadratus lumborum; a compensatory response for weak hip and knee flexors or extensor spasticity.

e. Steppage gait (excessive hip and knee flexion); a compensatory response to shorten the leg, the result of weak dorsiflexors (e.g., diabetic neuropathy of the peroneal nerve).

f. Abnormal synergistic activity resulting from a neurological insult.
   (1) Characterized by excessive hip and knee flexion with abduction.

g. Vaulting: swing leg is able to advance through the combination of elevation of the pelvis and plantar flexion of the stance limb.

2. Knee.

a. Insufficient knee flexion: the result of extensor spasticity, pain, decreased range of motion or weak hamstrings.

b. Excessive knee flexion: the result of flexor spasticity or a flexor withdrawal reflex.

3. Ankle and foot.

a. Foot drop (equinus): the result of weak or delayed contraction of the dorsiflexors or spastic plantar flexors.

b. Varus or inverted foot: the result of spastic invertors (anterior tibialis), weak peroneals or abnormal synergistic patterns (e.g., stroke).

c. Equinovarus: the result of spasticity of the posterior tibialis and/or the gastrocnemius/soleus; developmental abnormality.

Ambulatory Aids

Canes

1. Widen the base of support to improve balance; provide limited stability and unweighting (can unload forces on involved extremity by about 30%; can be used to relieve pain, antalgic gait.

2. Cane measurement: 20–30 degrees of elbow flexion is desirable; measure from the greater trochanter to a point 6 inches lateral to the toes.

3. Types: wood or aluminum (adjustable with push-pin lock).
   a. Standard, single point cane: handle and shaft may be standard (J-shaped) or offset.
   b. Quad cane: four contact points with the ground (a broader-based support) for increased stability. Slows gait.
      (1) Small-based quad cane (SBQC): useful for stairs, more support than standard cane and less support than LBQC.
      (2) Large-based quad cane (LBQC): provides more support than SBQC; can be difficult to use on the stairs.
   c. Walk cane (hemiwalker).
      (1) Very broad base with four-point contact. The legs furthest from the patient's body are angled to maintain floor contact to improve stability.
      (2) More stable than a quad cane.
      (3) Difficult to use on stairs.

4. Gait sequencing. The cane is held in the hand opposite the involved extremity.
   a. Advanced gait pattern: the involved extremity and the cane are advanced simultaneously, followed by the uninvolved extremity.
   b. Beginning gait pattern: the cane is advanced first, followed by the involved extremity (stepping to or through [past] the cane), then the uninvolved extremity; this results in a slower, more stable gait pattern.

Crutches

1. Used to increase the base of support, provide moderate degree of stability and/or relieve weight-bearing on the lower extremities.

2. Crutch measurement: 20–30 degrees of elbow flexion is desirable, 2–3 finger width clearance between the axillary pad and the axilla, tips located approximately 6 inches in front of and 2 inches lateral to the toes.
   a. In standing position, one can subtract 16 inches from the patient's height or measure from a point 2 inches below the axilla to a point 6 inches in front and 2 inches lateral to the foot.
   b. In supine, measure from the axilla to a point 6–8 inches lateral to the heel.
   c. In sitting, abduct the upper extremities to 90 degrees, flex one elbow and extend the other. Measure from the olecranon process of the flexed elbow to the tip of the middle finger of the opposite arm; this approximates overall crutch height.
   d. Forearm crutches: the cuff should cover the proximal third of the forearm, about 1.0–1.5 inches below the olecranon process of the elbow. Adjust height of crutch to allow for 20–25 degrees of elbow flexion.

3. Types of crutches.
   a. Axillary: made of aluminum or wood and generally have adjustable handgrip and crutch height. Adjust by wing nuts or push-button locks with telescoping legs. Axillary pads and handgrips are cushioned.
      (1) Provide increased trunk support over forearm crutches.
      (2) Can be awkward in small areas.
      (3) Create potential for damage to the radial nerve and axillary artery in the axilla if patient leans on axillary bar.
   b. Forearm (Lofstrand) crutches: have a forearm cuff and a handgrip; provide slightly less stability but increased ease of movement; frees hands for use without dropping the crutch (secured by forearm cuff).
      (1) Canadian crutches: have a triceps versus forearm cuff.

4. Crutch tips: rubber, about 1.5-inch diameter, provides suction to minimize slippage.

5. Platform attachment: can be added to and used on walkers or crutches. They provide for transfer of body weight through the forearm versus the hand/wrist.
   a. They are used when weight-bearing through the wrist and hand is contraindicated or difficult, or in patients with arthritis or patients who have suffered a fracture of the upper extremity, or in patients who lack grasp or wrist strength following neurological injury such as stroke.

Walkers

1. widen base of support, provide increased lateral and anterior stability and can reduce weight bearing on one or

both lower extremities; easy to use; frequently prescribed for patients with debilitating conditions, poor balance or lower extremity injury when use of crutches is precluded: e.g., elderly patients, poor balance or coordination. Negative features: no reciprocal arm swing, increased flexor posture.

2. Types of walkers.
   a. Rigid.
      (1) Standard walker.
   b. Folding (collapsible): facilitate mobility in community, cars.
   c. Rolling (wheeled): available with two or four wheels (four requires hand brake to aid stability and stopping); facilitates walking as a continuous movement with reciprocal lower extremity gait pattern; allows for increased speed.
      (1) May allow functional ambulation for patients who are unable to lift and move a conventional walker.
   d. Reciprocal walker: hinged, allows advancement of one side of walker at a time; used with reciprocal gait patterns, reciprocating orthoses. Less stable than standard or folding walker.
      (1) Useful for patients incapable of lifting the walker with both hands and moving it forward.

   e. Stair climbing walker: has two posterior extensions and additional handgrips off of the rear legs for use on stairs.
   f. Hemiwalker, Hemicane or walk cane: modified for use with one hand only. Used on unaffected side; provides large base of support; flared legs placed away from patient.

3. Attachments: fold-down seats, carrying baskets.

4. Measuring: same as for cane.

Bariatric Equipment

1. Assistive device: selection based on specific patient needs (safety, gait pattern, fatigue) and weight capacity of device. Heavy-duty walkers can be obtained and are used to assist with ambulation.
   a. Heavy duty mechanical lifts are used to help transfer patient (e.g., sit-to-stand).
   b. A stand pole may be used; patient grasps and pulls on it to assist with standing.

2. Typical gait changes include greater hip abduction and hip rotation, less knee flexion, pronated feet, difficulty weight shifting side-to-side with increased girth.

Gait Patterns and Guarding

Weight-bearing Status

1. Non weight-bearing (NWB): no weight-bearing is permitted; three-point gait pattern (see below) is required.

2. "Toe-touch" or "touch-down" weight-bearing (TTWB): the foot of the affected extremity is allowed to touch the ground for balance only; no weight-bearing is allowed.
   a. Encourage heel-strike; patient may use foot flat.

3. Partial weight-bearing (PWB): plantar surface of involved lower extremity contacts the floor; allowed percentage of patient's weight (e.g., 25%, 50%) is borne on involved extremity, while remaining weight is absorbed through the upper extremities as the uninvolved extremity takes a step.
   a. Typically used with three-point or modified three-point gait pattern (see below).

4. Weight-bearing as tolerated (WBAT): patient bears as much weight as can be tolerated without discomfort; used with multiple gait patterns.

5. Full weight-bearing (FWB): full weight is permitted on involved extremity.

Gait Sequencing

1. Two-point gait: one crutch and opposite extremity move together, followed by opposite crutch and extremity.
   a. Requires use of two assistive devices (canes or crutches).
   b. Allows for natural arm and leg motion during gait.
   c. Provides good support and stability from two opposing points of contact.

2. Three-point gait (non weight-bearing): both crutches and involved leg advance together—no weight is taken through involved limb and then uninvolved leg is advanced forward.
   a. Requires use of two assistive devices (crutches, canes) or a walker.
   b. Indicated for use with involvement of one extremity or lower extremity fracture.

3. Modified three-point gait (weight-bearing): both crutches and involved leg are advanced together and weight is taken through involved leg; uninvolved leg advances either to (in the instance of poorer balance) or through/past the assistive devices (better balance).
   a. Requires use of two assistive devices (crutches, canes) or a walker.
   b. Indicated for use with involvement of one extremity or lower extremity fracture.

4. Four-point gait: a slow, stable gait in which one crutch is advanced forward and placed on the floor, followed by advancement of the opposite leg; then the remaining crutch is advanced forward followed by the opposite remaining leg.
   a. Sequence: left crutch–right leg–right crutch– left leg.
   b. Requires use of two assistive devices (crutches, canes).
   c. Provides maximum stability with three points of support while one limb is moving; used for patients with poor balance.

5. Swing-to and swing-through are utilized when both lower extremities are involved, such as with paraplegia or spina bifida and when there is trunk instability.
   a. Swing-to: both crutches are advanced forward together, and weight is then shifted onto hands for support and both legs are swung (or dragged) forward to meet the crutches.
      (1) Requires the use of two crutches (typically Lofstrand) or a walker.
   b. Swing-through: both crutches are advanced forward together; weight is shifted onto the hands for support and both legs are swung forward beyond the point of the crutch placement; requires the use of two crutches.
      (1) Not as safe as swing-to pattern.
      (2) Requires better balance and strength than swing-to gait pattern.

6. Stairs.
   a. Ascent: the stronger (uninvolved) leg steps up first, followed by the assistive device and/then the involved leg.
   b. Descent: the assistive device and/then the weaker (involved) leg steps down first, followed by the uninvolved leg.
   c. Mnemonic to teach the patient: "The good go up to heaven, the bad go down to hell," "Up with the good, down with the bad."

Gait Patterns with Rigid Walkers

1. Patient instruction: all four legs of the walker should be picked up and placed down simultaneously (provides maximum stability) or rolled forward (wheeled walker); advance walker about an arm's length forward (back legs should be in line with patient's toes).

   a. Avoid: forward trunk flexion; stepping too close to or beyond forward edge of walker; rocking from back to front legs during gait.

2. Full weight-bearing: advance walker, then advance lower extremity (weaker first if applicable); follow with remaining lower extremity.

3. Partial weight-bearing: advance walker, then advance involved leg; transfer body weight through upper extremities and bear partial weight (as prescribed) on involved leg; advance uninvolved leg to (step-to) or past (step-through) involved leg.

4. Non weight-bearing: advance walker, then advance involved leg forward—do not place on ground; transfer full weight through upper extremities and move uninvolved leg forward with a small hop.

Guarding

1. Protects the patient from falling; requires the use of gait belt for initial training for most patients.

2. Use key points of control: shoulder, bilateral or unilateral pelvis, gait belt; do not grasp clothing or the patient's extremities.

3. Level surfaces: clinician stands slightly behind and lateral to the weaker or more involved side of the patient.
   a. Move feet out of sequence with the patient's feet so that when the patient's feet are moving, the clinician's feet are planted.

4. Stairs: clinician is positioned below the patient and takes steps out of sequence with patient as identified above.
   a. Ascent: stand behind and slightly toward involved side; hands on key points of control (identified above).
   b. Descent: stand in front and slightly toward involved side; hands on key points of control (identified above).

5. Loss of balance.
   a. Forward on stairs: clinician pulls the patient toward self, using the gait belt and a hand on patient's shoulder or trunk.
   b. Backward on stairs: clinician positions body behind patient and allows patient to lean against clinician's body.
   c. On level ground: clinician pulls patient toward self and steadies patient.

Use of Body-Weight Support (BWS) and a Motorized Treadmill

1. BWS: an overhead harness is used to support body weight.

a. Initially support is high (e.g., 40% of body weight), progresses to less weight support (30%, 20%, 10%) and eventually progresses to no BWS as patient is able.

b. BWS >55% is contraindicated as it interferes with gait cycle (unable to achieve flat foot during stepping).

2. Motorized treadmill training.

a. Progresses from treadmill walking with slow speeds (e.g., 0.6–0.8 mph) to faster, near-normal walking speeds (e.g., 2.6–2.8 mph).

b. Progresses from level treadmill to walking to slight incline walking.

c. Progresses from treadmill walking to overground walking.

3. Manual assistance: level of assistance decreases as training progresses (maxA, to modA, to minA, to no assistance). Assistance can include hands on pelvis (assisted pelvic motions and weight shift) and hands on lower extremity (LE) (assisted stepping).

4. BWS with motorized treadmill and robotic ambulation assistance can also be used to improve gait pattern and ambulatory status (e.g., Lokomat).

a. Currently being applied primarily for those with paraparesis or developmental disorders.

Wheelchairs

Components

1. Postural support system.

a. Seating.

(1) Sling seat; standard on wheelchairs. Hips tend to slide forward; tends to cause thighs to adduct and internally rotate; reinforces poor pelvic position (posterior pelvic tilt).

(2) Insert or contour seats: create a firm (stable) seating surface (wood or plastic padded with foam).

(a) Advantages: reduces the tendency for the patient to slide forward or sit with a posterior pelvic tilt (sacral sitting); improves neutral pelvic position, decreases hip internal rotation and adduction (especially important in instance of a hip replacement).

(3) Seat cushions: distribute weight-bearing pressures; assist in preventing decubitus ulcers in patients with decreased sensation, prolongs wheelchair sitting times. Patient required to perform pressure relief push-ups, typically every 15–20 minutes.

(a) Pressure-relieving contoured foam cushion: uses dense, layered foam. Accommodates moderate to severe postural deformity. Easy for caregivers to reposition patients, low maintenance. May interfere with slide transfers.

(b) Pressure-relieving fluid/gel or combination (fluid/gel plus foam). Can be custom molded. Accommodates moderate to severe postural deformity. Easy for caregivers to reposition patients. Requires some maintenance; heavier, more expensive.

(c) Pressure-relieving air cushion. Accommodates moderate to severe postural deformity. Lightweight, improved pressure distribution. Expensive; base may be unstable for some patients. Requires continuous maintenance.

(4) Adds to measurements to determine back height for wheelchair.

b. Back: support to the mid-scapular region is provided by most standard sling-back wheelchairs.

(1) Lower back height may increase functional mobility (i.e., sports chairs); may also increase back strain.

(2) High back height may be necessary for patients with poor trunk stability or with extensor tone/spasms.

(3) Insert or contour backs improve back extension and overall upright alignment.

(4) Lateral trunk supports: improve trunk alignment for patients with scoliosis, poor trunk stability, developmental disability.

(5) Power wheelchairs will require upper back support for the movement of initial acceleration.

c. Armrests.

(1) Full length: usually run the full length of the seat.

(2) Desk length: facilitates closer proximity to desk or table; typically one-half or one-fourth the length of the full-length armrests.

(3) Fixed height or adjustable height; can be raised to facilitate sit-to-stand transfers.

(4) Removable armrests facilitate side transfers.

(5) Wraparound (space saver) armrests reduce the overall width of the chair by 1.5 inches.

(6) Upper extremity support surfaces (tray or troughs) can be secured to the armrests; provide additional postural assistance for patients with decreased use of upper extremities.

d. Legrests comprised of calf pad and front rigging.
   (1) Fixed.
   (2) Swing-away and removable: facilitates ease in transfers, front approach to wheelchair when ambulating.
   (3) Elevating: indicated for LE edema control, postural support.
      (a) Contraindicated for patients with knee flexor (hamstring) hypertonicity or tightness.
e. Footrests/footplate.
   (1) Footplates: provide a resting base for feet; ankles are positioned in neutral with knees flexed to 90 degrees; footplates can be raised or removed to facilitate transfers.
   (2) Heel loops: help maintain foot position on footplate to prevent posterior sliding.
   (3) Straps (ankle, calf): can be added to stabilize the feet on the footplates.

2. **Wheeled mobility base.**
   a. Frame.
      (1) Rigid or folding.
         (a) Rigid frame facilitates stroke efficiency, increases distance per stroke.
         (b) Folding facilitates mobility in the community, ease of storage.
      (2) Available in heavy-duty, standard, light-weight, active-duty lightweight, ultra-lightweight construction.
         (a) Heavy-duty/wide width will accommodate bariatric patients.
         (b) Standard: seat width 18 inches, seat depth 16 inches and seat height 20 inches.
         (c) Hemiheight: decrease seat height to 17.5 inches. This allows for easier wheelchair propulsion with the lower extremities.
      (3) In general, the lighter the weight of the frame, the greater the ease of use.
      (4) The level of expected activity and environment should be taken into account when deciding on frame construction.
      (5) Functional mobility, cognition and physical need should be taken into consideration when deciding on a type of wheelchair.
   b. Wheels, handrims.
      (1) Casters are the small front wheels that swivel and are typically 8 inches in diameter; caster locks can be added to facilitate wheelchair stability during transfers.
      (2) Drive wheels: the large rear wheels used for propulsion; outer rim allows for handgrip and propulsion.
         (a) Projections may be attached to the rims (vertical, oblique or horizontal) to facilitate propulsion in patients with poor hand strength (e.g., quadriplegia); projections widen the chair and may limit maneuvering in the home.

      (b) Friction rims/leather gloves: increase handgrip function, ease of propulsion in patients with poor handgrip.
      (c) Construction of drive wheels are made with standard spokes or spokeless wheels.
   c. Tires.
      (1) Standard hard rubber tires are durable and low maintenance.
      (2) Pneumatic (air-filled) tires provide a smoother ride, increase shock absorption and require more maintenance. Recommended for community use and uneven terrain.
   d. Brakes.
      (1) Most brakes consist of a lever system with a cam.
      (2) Brakes must be engaged for all transfers in and out of the chair.
      (3) Extensions may be added to increase ease of reaching to lock and unlock; e.g., for upper extremity weakness, arthritis, neurological deficits.
   e. Additional attachments.
      (1) Seat belts (pelvic positioner): belt should grasp over the pelvis at a 45-degree angle to the seat.
      (2) Seat positioners.
         (a) Lateral or medial (adductor pommel) positioners can be added at hip and knee to maintain alignment of the lower extremities.
         (b) A seat wedge or tilt-in-space seat can be used for extensor spasm or thrusting.
      (3) Chest belt assists with sitting balance.
      (4) Seat back positioners provide added lateral alignment, control for scoliosis.
      (5) Antitipping device: a posterior extension attached to the lower horizontal supports prevents tipping backward in the chair.
         (a) Limits going up curbs or over threshold.
      (6) Hill-holder device: a mechanical brake that allows the chair to go forward, but automatically brakes when the chair goes in reverse.
         (a) Useful for patients who are not able to ascend a long ramp or hill without a rest.
      (7) Crutch/cane holder: a small cup at the base of the wheelchair with a strap at the top to allow transportation of ambulatory aids.

3. **Specialized wheelchairs.**
   a. Reclining back: indicated for patients who are unable to independently maintain an upright sitting position; includes extended back and typically elevating legrests; head and trunk supports may also be added.
      (1) Electric reclining back controls: sip/puff, hand, chin or head control power mechanism. Indicated for patients with high cervical cord lesions and other neurological deficits.
      (2) Used to redistribute weight-bearing on the buttocks if the patient is unable to perform active

wheelchair push-ups or pressure-relief maneuvers.

b. Tilt-in-space: entire seat and back may be tipped backwards (normal seat to back angle is maintained).
   (1) Indicated for patients with extensor spasms that may throw the patient out of the chair or for pressure relief.

c. One-arm drive: the drive mechanisms are located on one wheel, usually with two outer rims (or by push lever); the patient propels the wheelchair by pushing on both rims (or lever) with one hand.
   (1) Difficult for some patients to use, e.g., patients with left hemiplegia, cognitive/perceptual impairments.

d. Hemiplegic chair (Hemichair): a chair that is designed to be low to the ground, allowing propulsion with the uninvolved upper and lower extremities.

e. Amputee chair: wheelchair is modified by placing drive wheels posterior to the vertical back supports (~2 inches backward); increases the length of the base of support and posterior stability.
   (1) Prescribed for patients with bilateral lower extremity amputations whose center of gravity is now located more posterior when seated in a wheelchair.

f. Powered wheelchairs: utilize a power source (battery) to propel the wheelchair; prescribed for patients who are not capable of self-propulsion or who have very low endurance.
   (1) Microprocessors allow the control of the wheelchair to be adapted to various controls, i.e., joystick, head or chin controls.
   (2) Propulsion drives: changes in pressure on the control result in directly corresponding changes in speed.
   (3) Microswitching systems: speed is preset; controls turn system on and off, i.e., sip-n-puff tubes for individuals with quadriplegia.

g. Sports wheelchairs: lightweight reinforced frames for ease of maneuvering and increased ease in transporting (front and back seats in cars); lower seats and backs; tucked seating position; canted (slanted) drive wheels for increased speed, efficiency; small push rims.

h. Bariatric wheelchair: heavy duty, extrawide wheelchair designed to assist mobility for individuals who are obese.
   (1) Selection based on patient characteristics, safety and function.
   (2) The bariatric client has a center of body mass that is positioned several inches forward in comparison with the normal-sized person.
      (a) In order to ensure wheelchair stability, the rear axle is displaced forward in comparison with the standard wheelchair; forward position allows for more efficient arm push (full arm stroke with less wrist extension).
   (3) Bariatric wheelchair can be ordered with special adaptations:
      (a) Hard tires versus pneumatic tires for increased durability.
      (b) Adjustable backrest to accommodate excessive posterior bulk.
      (c) Reclining wheelchair to accommodate excessive anterior bulk, cardiorespiratory compromise (e.g., orthostatic hypotension).
      (d) Power application attached to a heavy-duty wheelchair to accommodate excessive fatigue.

Wheelchair Measurements

1. **General considerations.**
   a. Overall size of the wheelchair must be proportional to the size of the patient. Take into account demands of expected use and the environment in which the chair will be used.
   b. Measurements should be taken with the patient situated on a firm surface, either sitting or supine. Hips, knees and ankles positioned at 90 degrees of flexion.

2. **Six key measurements to properly fit someone for a wheelchair.**
   a. Seat width.
      (1) Measurement on the patient: measure the patient at the widest part of the hips.
      (2) Chair measurement: add 2 inches to the patient's measurement.
      (3) Potential problems.
         (a) Extrawide wheelchairs will result in added difficulties in reaching the drive wheels and propelling the chair.
         (b) The width of the wheelchair should accommodate the width of doorways; can use a narrowing device; requires coordination to turn the cranking device.
         (c) Wheelchairs that are too narrow will result in pressure and/or discomfort on the lateral pelvis and thighs; lateral space should allow for changes in bulk of clothing.
      (4) The bariatric client with a pear-shape body will have increased gluteal femoral weight distribution. Measurement should consider the widest portion of the seated position. Also consider room for weight shifting for pressure relief and possible use of lift devices.
   b. Seat depth.
      (1) Measurement on the patient: posterior buttock to the posterior aspect of the lower leg at the popliteal fossa.
      (2) Chair measurement: subtract 2–3 inches from the patient measurement (decreases pressure and swelling of feet).

(3) Potential problems.
    (a) Seat depth that is too short fails to support thigh adequately, results in increased pressure on the posterior thigh.
    (b) Seat depth that is too long may compromise tissues in the popliteal fossa causing edema and nerve pressure, results in kyphotic posture and/or posterior pelvis tilting and sacral sitting.

c. Leg length/seat to footplate length.
    (1) Measurement on the patient: from the bottom of the shoe (customary footwear) to just under the thigh in the popliteal fossa; when a seat cushion is used, the height must be subtracted from the patient's measurement.
    (2) Potential problems.
        (a) Excessive leg length will encourage sacral sitting and sliding forward in the chair; potential difficulty with clearing threshold at doorways.
        (b) If the leg length is too short, uneven weight distribution on the thighs and excessive weight on the ischium will occur, predisposing the patient to pressure sores.

d. Seat height.
    (1) No patient measurement is necessary.
    (2) Chair measurement: minimum clearance between the floor and the footplate is 2 inches, measuring from the lowest point on the bottom of the footplate.
    (3) Add 2 inches to the patient's leg length measurement.
    (4) If the patient will be propelling the chair with the lower extremities, this needs to be taken into consideration and the chair may need to be lowered.

e. Armrest height (hanging elbow height).
    (1) Measurement on the patient: from the seat platform to just below the elbow held at 90 degrees with the shoulder in neutral position.
    (2) Chair measurement: add 1 inch to the patient's hanging elbow measurement.
    (3) Potential problems.
        (a) Armrests that are too high will cause shoulder elevation.
        (b) Armrests that are too low will encourage leaning forward.

f. Back height: will vary depending upon the amount of support the patient needs.
    (1) Measurement on the patient: from the seat platform to the lower angle of the scapula, midscapula or top of shoulder, depending on the amount of support needed.
    (2) If the patient is going to use a seat cushion, the height of the cushion must be added to the patient measurement.

Table 12-3 ➤ STANDARD WHEELCHAIR DIMENSIONS (IN INCHES)

CHAIR STYLE	SEAT WIDTH	SEAT DEPTH	SEAT HEIGHT
Adult	18	16	20
Narrow adult	16	16	20
Slim adult	14	16	20
Hemi/low seat			17.5
Junior	16	16	18.5
Child	14	11.5	18.75
Tiny tot	12	11.5	19.5

(3) Potential problems.
    (a) Additional back height may increase difficulties in getting the chair into an automobile; may also prevent patient from hooking onto the push handle for stabilization or weight relief, e.g., the patient with quadriplegia.

3. Standard dimensions (Table 12-3).
a. Custom-made wheelchairs add significantly to the cost of a wheelchair; take into consideration prior to ordering.

Wheelchair Training

1. **Persons unfamiliar with wheelchair use will require instruction in use, safety and maintenance.**

2. **Instruction in good sitting posture and pressure relief is necessary to the patient and the caregiver.**
  a. Instruct in use of wheelchair cushions: care and maintenance, schedule of use, limitations of the cushion, correct placement in chair (which side is up, front, back, etc).
  b. Instruct in pressure-relief activities: arm push-ups, weight shifts—leaning to one side, then the other, amount of time required to off weight load ischial tuberosities.

3. **Wheelchair propulsion.**
  a. Instruct in manual wheelchair propulsion.
    (1) Both arms on drive (push) wheels, one arm on drive wheel/one foot pulls diagonally across floor under chair (e.g., the patient with hemiplegia).
        (a) In the case of a one-arm drive-equipped chair, place hand on both outer rims located on one side.
    (2) Propulsion: forward/backward, flat surfaces, uneven surfaces, ramp.
    (3) Turning: push harder with one hand than the other; for sharp turning pull one wheel backward and push the other forward at the same time.
    (4) Negotiation of obstacles, curbs, thresholds, etc.

b. Power chair training: focus on driving skills and safety; instruct in use of switches (on/off, turns), joystick and other controls to ensure maneuverability, safe stopping, speed control.

4. **Wheelchair management.**
   a. Instruct in use of wheel locks (brakes), foot supports (footplate, legrest) and elevation of legrests (if applicable).
   b. Instruct in routine maintenance of wheelchair; normal cleaning, power chair maintenance (battery).

5. **Community mobility.**
   a. Ramps.
      (1) Ascending: forward lean of head and trunk, use short quick hand strokes.
      (2) Descending: grip hand rims loosely, control chair's descent; or descend in wheelie position (steep ramp). Gloves recommended.
   b. Practice "wheelie".
      (1) Teach patient to "pop a wheelie." A lightweight wheelchair will make training easier.
         (a) The clinician assists the patient into a wheelie position as the patient learns how to come up onto and balance on the rear wheels with the front casters off the ground.
         (b) Moving into wheelie position: patient places hands well back on the hand-rims and moves head and trunk forward, then pulls rims forward abruptly and forcefully and then pulls back forcefully.
         (c) The patient practices holding/balancing in wheelie position while clinician guards by holding the handgrips.

(2) Balancing in wheelie position: consistent movement of the wheels forward and back helps maintain balance on wheels in wheelie position.
   (a) Chair tips further back when wheels are pushed forward; chair tips into upright position when wheels are pulled back.
c. Curb management.
   (1) Practice curb ascent: pop a wheelie and place the front casters up on the curb; the patient then leans forward and pushes forward forcefully on the handrims to get rear wheels up onto the curb.
      (a) Momentum and forward thrust of the head and trunk are used to assist.
   (2) Practice curb descent: descending backwards with forward head and trunk lean; descending forward in wheelie position.
d. Practice ascending/descending stairs. In wheelchair this requires assist of at least two, preferably three, people if attempting to ascend more than one step.
   (1) The wheelchair is facing the stairs backwards: one person stands behind the chair and tilts it back using the handgrips while the patient leans forward; two people are in front of the chair lifting with their hands on the frame of the chair. Remove legrests if possible—reduces weight of chair.
   (2) Practice in chair and on buttocks.
e. Instruct in how to fall safely and return to wheelchair.
f. Instruct in how to transfer into a car: place wheelchair inside car by pulling wheelchair behind the car seat, or use wheelchair lift (van equipped).

Transfer Training

Levels of Assistance

1. **Independent:** patient is consistently able to perform skill safely without any verbal or tactile cues.

2. **Standby or supervision:** patient requires supervision, verbal cues to complete the activity; clinician is within arm's reach for patient safety.

3. **Close guarding:** clinician positioned close but not touching the patient; minimal likelihood the patient will need assistance during activity. Can give verbal cues.

4. **Contact guarding:** clinician positioned in close guarding with hands on the patient (one hand should be positioned on the gait belt); high likelihood the patient will need verbal and tactile assistance during activity.

5. **Minimal assistance:** patient performs the majority (75%) of the effort to complete the activity; clinician provides 25% assistance.

6. **Moderate assistance:** patient performs approximately 50% of the effort required to complete the activity; clinician provides the other 50%.

7. **Maximal assistance:** patient performs less than 25% of the effort required to complete the activity; clinician provides the rest.

8. **Dependent:** total assist is required of one or more clinicians to complete the activity.

Transfer Activities

1. **Preparation.**
   a. Review the chart and identify any restrictions (limitations in upright posture, weight-bearing, etc.); identify if another person is required to assist; identify if orthostatic hypotension is likely.
   b. Gather equipment and assistance if needed.
   c. Place a gait belt on the patient; be sure to avoid placing over tubes, drains, etc.
   d. Ensure the patient has nonslip footwear on and provide the patient with glasses or corrective eyewear if necessary.
   e. Position equipment close and secure or lock brakes; plan the transfer toward the patient's strong side if applicable.
   f. Clear the area: remove or position excess equipment out of the way (over-bed tables, oxygen tanks, etc.).
   g. Ensure IV lines, catheter bags, drains, feeding tubes, etc., have sufficient length to complete the activity; avoid excess tugging and kinks in lines.

2. **Instruction.**
   a. Introduce yourself (and others if needed).
   b. Explain the activity, identify expectations of the patient and demonstrate when appropriate.
   c. Use explanations the patient can follow (e.g. single-step, two-step commands); avoid excess words and demonstrations.
   d. Synchronize actions using commands and counts.

3. **Dependent transfers.**
   a. Dependent lift transfer (football transfer).
      (1) Wheelchair is positioned parallel to surface.
      (2) Patient is flexed forward at hips in tucked position with hips and knees flexed.
      (3) Clinician locks patient's tucked knees between legs; places one hand under buttocks and one hand on transfer belt.
      (4) Patient is rocked forward and lifted using a backward weight shift with therapist in a semisquat position.
      (5) Clinician then pivots using small steps and gently lowers patient to support surface.
   b. Dependent stand-pivot transfer. Similar to above but the patient is standing with lower extremities extended and in contact with floor.
   c. Hydraulic lift transfer. Positioning and widening of base of device is critical to stability; correct positioning of patient harness paramount to safe transfer.

4. **Assisted Transfers.**
   a. Assisted stand-pivot transfer.
      (1) Used for patients who are unable to stand independently and can bear some weight on lower extremities (e.g., the patient with cerebrovascular accident [CVA], incomplete spinal cord injury [SCI] and hip fracture/replacement).
      (2) Wheelchair is placed parallel to surface (on the patient's sound or stronger side).
      (3) Clinician can block out one or both of the patient's knees to provide stability; support can be added by placing both hands on the patient (on gait belt and buttock, on both buttocks, both on upper back or one on buttock/one on upper back).
      (4) Patient rocks forward and pushes up into standing.
      (5) Clinician assists patient with forward weight shift and standing, pivoting toward chair and controlled lowering toward the support surface.
      (6) Variation: assisted squat-pivot transfer for patients who are unable to stand fully or with marked weakness of both lower extremities.
   b. Assisted transfer using a transfer (sliding) board.
      (1) Used for the patient with good sitting balance who can lift most but not all of weight of buttocks or the patient with complete level C5 SCI or CVA.
      (2) Wheelchair is placed parallel to surface.
      (3) Patient moves forward in chair and board is placed well under buttocks.
      (4) Patient performs transfer by doing a series of push-ups and lifts along board.
      (5) Clinician assists in lift (hands on buttocks, on transfer belt or one on buttock/one on belt).
      (6) Care must be taken not to pinch fingers under board or drag/traumatize skin.
      (7) Feet can remain on foot pedals (for patient with SCI) or be positioned on the floor.
      (8) The patient with complete level C6 SCI can be independent with transfer board on level surfaces.
   c. Push-up transfer (pop-over transfer).
      (1) Used for patient with good sitting balance who can lift buttocks clear of sitting surface; can be a progression in transfer training from using a transfer board.
      (2) The patient with complete C7 level SCI can be independent in transfers without a sliding board.
      (3) The patient utilizes head-hips relationship to successfully complete the transfer (movement of head in one direction results in movement of the hips in the opposite direction/toward the support surface).

Environmental Considerations for Wheelchair and Ambulatory Aid Users

Environmental Assessment

1. **Purpose.**
   a. To assess the degree of safety, function and comfort of the patient in the home, community and work environments.
   b. Provide recommendations to the patient and caregivers to ensure a barrier-free environment and the greatest level of functional independence and safety.

2. **Standard adult wheelchair dimensions for environmental access.**
   a. Width: 24–26 inches from rim to rim.
   b. Length: 42–43 inches.
   c. Height (push handles to floor): 36 inches.
   d. Height (armrest to floor): 29–30 inches.
   e. Footrests may extend for taller people.
   f. 360-degree turning radius requires space of 60 inches by 60 inches.
   g. 90-degree turning space needs a minimum of 36 inches.
   h. Minimum clearance for doorways and halls is 32 inches; ideal is 36 inches.
   i. Forward reach is 48 inches maximum height.

3. **Home.**
   a. Entrance: accessible; stairs with handrails, ramp and platform to allow for ease of door opening.
   b. Floors: nonskid surface, carpeting securely fastened to the floor, no throw rugs and low-pile carpeting preferable.
   c. Furniture arrangement: should allow sufficient room to maneuver easily with wheelchair or ambulating with an assistive device.
   d. Doors: thresholds should be flush or level (no doorsills); standard door width is 32 inches; outside door, swing area requires a minimum of 18 inches for walkers and 26 inches for wheelchairs.
   e. Stairs: uniform riser heights (7 inches high) with tread depth (a minimum of 11 inches); handrails, recommended height is 32 inches, 0.5–2.0 inches in diameter, securely fastened into a concrete wall or stud; nonskid surface; well lighted; color code with reds, oranges and yellows if visual impairments exist.
   f. Bedroom: furniture arrangement for easy maneuverability; a minimum of 3 feet on side of bed for wheelchair transfers; firm mattress; stable bed (no wheels); sufficient height to facilitate sit-to-stand transfers; phone accessibility; appropriate height for wall switches is 36–48 inches; outlets a minimum of 18 inches above the floorboard.
   g. Bathroom: toilet height seat should be 17–19 inches; tub seat or bench; nonskid surface or mat; grab bars securely fastened; optimal height of horizontal grab bars from 33–36 inches.
   h. Kitchen: appropriate height of counter tops for wheelchair users is no higher than 31 inches; counter depth of at least 24 inches; accessible equipment and storage areas.

4. **Community/workplace.**
   a. Steps: recommended 7–9 inches width with 7- to 9-inch riser height.
   b. Ramps: recommended ratio of slope to rise is 1:12 (for every inch of vertical rise, 12 inches of ramp is required); minimum of 36 inches wide with nonslip surface; handrail waist high for ambulatory patients (34–38 inches) and should extend 12–18 inches beyond the top and bottom of runs; ramp should have level landing at top and bottom.
   c. Parking (handicapped): parking space with adjacent 4-foot aisle for wheelchair maneuverability; accessible within a short distance of building; curb cutouts. Requires special permit or tag issued from the registry or department of motor vehicles.
   d. Building entrance: accessible; accessible elevator.
   e. Access to public telephones, drinking fountains and bathrooms.
   f. Ergonomic assessment of immediate work area: lighting, temperature, seating surface, height and size of work counter.
   g. Public transportation: accessible.

Orthotics

General Concepts

1. **Orthosis is a device used to.**
   a. Correct malalignment and prevent deformity.
   b. Restrict or assist motion.
   c. Transfer load to improve function.
   d. Reduce pain.

2. **Splint: a temporary device that may serve the same functions; materials generally not as durable, able to withstand prolonged use.**

3. **Three-point pressure principle: forms the mechanical basis for orthotic correction; a single force is placed at the area of deformity or angulation; two additional counterforces act in the opposing direction.**

4. **Alignment: correct alignment permits effective function.**
   a. Minimizes movement between limb and orthoses (pistoning).
   b. Minimizes compression on pressure-sensitive tissues.

Lower-Limb Orthoses: Components/Terminology

1. **Shoes: the foundation for an orthosis; shoes can reduce areas of concentrated pressure on pressure-sensitive feet.**
   a. Traditional leather orthopedic shoes or athletic sneakers can be worn with orthoses; attachments can be external (to the outer part of a leather shoe's sole) or internal (a molded shoe insert).
   b. Parts of a shoe.
      (1) Upper: portion of the shoe that covers the dorsum of foot; includes the stay (the part of the shoe through which the laces are woven).
         (a) A flap-type lace stay is preferable for use with ankle-foot orthoses (AFOs) as it provides for more adjustability.
      (2) Quarter: heel area of the shoe.
         (a) A reinforced counter is preferable for use with AFOs and orthoses.
         (b) A broad heel provides more stability.
         (c) A 1-inch heel will move the center of gravity forward and aid in transition through stance phase without interfering with knee alignment.
      (3) Sole: bottom portion of the shoe; contains the shank (longitudinal plate to reinforce the sole.
         (a) If using with an AFO, the sole should have two leather layers for its attachment.

         (b) A slight rise in the sole at the toe is termed "toe spring," which assists with the rocker effect during toe-off.
      (4) Toe box: reinforcement at toe of the shoe to protect toes.
         (a) Should be high enough for toes in the presence of toe deformity or hammer toe.

2. **Foot orthoses (FOs): may be attached to the interior of the shoe (e.g., an inserted pad) or exterior to the shoe (e.g., a Thomas heel).**
   a. Soft inserts (i.e., viscoelastic plastic or rubber pads or relief cutouts) reduce areas of high loading, restrict forces and protect painful or sensitive areas of the feet.
      (1) Metatarsal pad: located posterior to metatarsal heads; transfers pressure off the metatarsal heads and onto the metatarsal shafts; allows more push-off in weak or inflexible feet.
      (2) Cushion heel: cushions and absorbs forces at heel contact; used to relieve strain on plantar fascia in plantar fasciitis.
      (3) Heel-spur insert: may be viscoelastic plastic or rubber; sloped anteriorly to decrease load on heel; has concave relief to decrease pressure on heel spur.
   b. Longitudinal arch supports: prevent depression of the subtalar joint and correct for pes planus (flat foot); flat foot can be flexible or rigid.
      (1) UCBL (University of California Bio-mechanics Laboratory) insert: a semirigid plastic molded insert to correct for flexible pes planus.
      (2) Scaphoid pad: used to support the longitudinal arch at medial border of foot, apex at sustenaculum tali and navicular tuberosity; provides minimal support.
      (3) Thomas' heel: a heel wedge with an extended anterior medial border used to support the longitudinal arch and correct for flexible pes valgus (pronated foot).
   c. Posting.
      (1) Rearfoot posting: alters the position of the subtalar joint (STJ) or rearfoot from heel strike to foot flat. Must be dynamic, control but not eliminate STJ motion.
         (a) Varus post (medial wedge): limits or controls eversion of the calcaneus and internal rotation of the tibia after heel strike. Reduces calcaneal eversion during running.
         (b) Valgus post (lateral wedge): controls the calcaneus and subtalar joint that are excessively inverted and supinated at heel strike.

(2) Forefoot posting: supports the forefoot.
   (a) Medial wedge prescribed for forefoot varus.
   (b) Lateral wedge prescribed for forefoot valgus.
(3) Contraindicated in the insensitive foot.
  d. Heel lifts (or heel platform).
    (1) Accommodates for leg-length discrepancy; can be placed inside the shoe (up to 0.375 inch) or attached to the outer sole.
    (2) Accommodates for limitation in ankle joint dorsiflexion.

e. Rocker bar: located proximal to metatarsal heads; improves weight shift onto metatarsals.
f. Rocker bottom: builds up the sole over the metatarsal heads and improves push-off in weak or inflexible feet. May also be used with insensitive feet.

3. AFOs: consist of a shoe attachment, ankle control, uprights and a proximal leg band (Table 12-4).
  a. Shoe attachments.

Table 12-4 ➤ ANKLE FOOT ORTHOSES: INDICATIONS, ADVANTAGES AND DISADVANTAGES

NAME	INDICATION	DESCRIPTION	ADVANTAGES	DISADVANTAGES
ANKLE FOOT ORTHOSES (AFOs)				
Posterior Leaf Spring	Dorsiflexion assist	Plastic insert; "off the shelf" or custom fit. Posterior component attached to foot plate, secured in shoe and with calf band.	Relatively light compared to metal components. Can easily switch to different shoes.	May not provide enough assist in the instance of high plantar flexor tone.
ToeOFF® or Ypsilon™	Dorsiflexion assist	Brand name dorsiflexion assist AFOs. Consist of a foot plate secured in shoe, a lateral and lateral-to-medial upright secured with a calf band proximally. Made of carbon material. For use with mild to moderate foot drop.	ToeOFF® good for mild to severe foot drop accompanied with mild to moderate ankle instability. Ypsilon™ good for mild to moderate isolated foot drop; provides free ankle movements.	Not indicated for use with moderate to severe spasticity. Ypsilon™ not suitable in instance of ankle instability.
Plastic hinged ankle AFO; posterior stop metal upright	Dorsiflexion assist - through plantar flexion resistance.	Plastic hinged AFO: hinged ankle joint with a dorsiflexion assist (flexible rubber at ankle joint) and plantar flexion stop (posting at posterior upright). Metal upright joint shape prevents plantar flexion at heel strike. Metal uprights can be made of steel, aluminum, carbon graphite or titanium.	Helps prevent knee from hyperextending at heel strike.	May alter gait pattern by forcing knee flexion earlier than normally occurring following heel strike. Plastic AFO contraindicated in instance of fluctuating edema. Newer, lighter metals make for a more expensive AFO.
Solid ankle-foot orthosis	Full ankle control for dorsiflexion and plantar flexion, as well as medial/lateral motion.	Plastic AFO that encompasses posterior, medial and lateral calf areas as well as malleoli; may or may not be hinged. Hinged version may have plastic overlap at ankle, plastic rod ankle or metal ankle.	Hinged version increases cadence, step length and velocity. Metal ankle can be adjusted to alter excursion of ankle motion.	Heavier and bulkier than posterior leaf spring or hinged AFO. Contraindicated in instance of fluctuating edema.
Spiral AFO	Control of ankle motion in all planes; does not eliminate motion.	A single upright spirals up from foot plate medially around leg and stops at calf band. Typically made of polypropylene, nylon or carbon fiber.	Minimally conspicuous compared to larger AFOs.	Contraindicated in instance of fluctuating edema.
Floor Reaction Orthosis	Knee extension assist	Anterior upright portion attached to foot plate, provides knee extension force during stance phase.	Controls knee during stance phase to maintain extension.	Pressure on anterior tibia may be difficult to tolerate or cause tissue irritation.
Klenzak Joint AFO	Dorsiflexion assist	Solid stirrup and metal uprights attached to sole (heel area) of shoe with spring at ankle.	Spring can be adjusted for amount of assistance required.	Fixed to pair of shoes, not interchangeable. Heavy and bulky.
BiCAAL (bichannel adjustable ankle locks)	Full range of ankle dorsiflexion and plantar flexion control.	Metal uprights attached to sole of shoe with hinges. Hinges have ability for motion assist and resistance through use of pins and springs.	Full range of control for ankle motions, resistance and assistance.	Bulky and heavier than plastic AFOs. Attached directly to shoe, not interchangeable between shoes. Sole should have a rocker bottom bar to assist with roll over at late stance.
Valgus correction strap	Limits valgus movement of ankle.	Typically used with metal upright AFOs. A "T" strap attached to lateral border of shoe and secured around medial upright.	Uses three-point pressure system to control valgus movement at ankle.	

(1) Footplate: a molded plastic shoe insert; allows application of the brace before insertion into the shoe, ease of changing shoes of same heel height.

(2) Stirrup: a metal attachment riveted to the sole of the shoe; split stirrups allow for shoe interchange; solid stirrups are fixed permanently to the shoe and provide for maximum stability.

b. Ankle controls.

(1) Free motion: provides mediolateral stability while allowing free motion in dorsiflexion and plantar flexion.

(2) Solid ankle: allows no movement; indicated with severe pain or instability.

(3) Limited motion: allows motion to be restricted in one or both directions.

(a) Bichannel adjustable ankle lock (BiCAAL): an ankle joint with the anterior and posterior channels that can be fit with pins to reduce motion or springs to assist motion.

(b) Anterior stop (dorsiflexion stop): determines the limits of ankle dorsiflexion. In an AFO, if the stop is set to allow slight dorsiflexion (~5 degrees), knee flexion results; can be used to control for knee hyperextension; if the stop is set to allow too much dorsiflexion, knee buckling could result.

(c) Posterior stop (plantar flexion stop): determines the limits of ankle plantar flexion. In an AFO, if the stop is set to allow slight plantar flexion (~5 degrees), knee extension results; can be used to control for an unstable knee that buckles; if the stop is set to allow too much plantar flexion, recurvatum or knee hyperextension could result.

(d) Solid AFO: limits all foot and ankle motion.

(4) Dorsiflexion assistance.

(a) Spring assist (Klenzak's housing): double upright metal AFO with a single anterior channel for a spring assist to aid dorsiflexion.

(b) Posterior leaf spring (PLS): a plastic AFO that inserts into the shoe; at heel strike, the AFO posterior upright bends backward slightly and with toe-off assists in maintaining ankle in dorsiflexed/neutral position during swing phase. Widely used to compensate for drop foot; is lighter and less bulky than the Klenzak-type AFO; can be custom fitted or "off the shelf."

(5) Varus or valgus correction straps (T straps): control for varus or valgus forces at the ankle. Medial strap buckles around the lateral upright and corrects for valgus; lateral strap buckles around the medial upright and corrects for varus.

c. Uprights and attachments (bands or shells).

(1) Conventional AFOs have metal uprights (aluminum, carbon graphite or steel) and a hinged ankle joint allowing plantar flexion and dorsiflexion. Provides maximum support; if the patient's condition is changing (e.g., peripheral edema), conventional metal AFOs may be easier to alter to accommodate changes than molded AFOs.

(a) Double metal uprights extend upward from the ankle on both sides of the leg and attach to a calf band.

(b) Conventional AFO, calf band (metal with leather lining or plastic); provides for proximal stabilization on leg; anterior opening and buckle or Velcro closure.

(2) Molded AFOs are made of molded plastic and are lighter in weight and cosmetically more appealing; contraindicated for individuals with changing leg volume.

(a) Posterior leaf spring (PLS): has a flexible, narrow posterior shell; functions as dorsiflexion assist; holds foot at 90-degree angle during swing; displaced during stance; provides no medial-lateral stability.

(b) Modified AFO: has a wider posterior shell with trimlines just posterior to malleoli; footplate includes more of medial and lateral borders of foot; provides more medial-lateral stability (control of calcaneal and forefoot inversion and eversion).

(c) Solid ankle AFO: has widest posterior shell with trimlines extending forward to malleoli; controls (prevents) dorsiflexion, plantar flexion, inversion and eversion.

(d) Spiral AFO: a molded plastic AFO that winds (spirals) around the calf; provides limited control of motion in all planes.

(e) Hinged plastic AFOs are available.

(3) Specialized AFOs.

(a) Patellar tendon–bearing brim: allows for weight distribution on the patellar shelf similar to patellar tendon–bearing prosthetic socket; reduces weight-bearing forces through the foot.

(b) Tone-reducing orthosis: molded plastic AFO that applies constant pressure to spastic or hypertonic muscles (plantar flexors and invertors); snug fit is essential to achieve the benefits of reciprocal inhibition.

4. Knee-ankle-foot orthoses (KAFO): consists of a shoe attachment, ankle control, uprights, knee control and bands or shells for the calf and thigh.

a. Knee controls.

(1) Hinge joint: provides mediolateral and hyperextension control while allowing for flexion and extension.

(a) Offset: the hinge is placed posterior to the weight-bearing line (trochanter-knee-ankle,

TKA line); assists extension, stabilizes knee during early stance; patients may have difficulty on ramps where knee may flex inadvertently.

  (2) Locks.

    (a) Drop ring lock: ring drops over joint when knee is in full extension to provide maximum stability; a retention button may be added to hold the ring lock up, permit gait training with the knee unlocked.

    (b) Pawl lock with bail release: the pawl is a spring-loaded posterior projection (lever or ring) that allows the patient to unlock the knee by pulling up or hooking the pawl on the back of a chair and pushing it up; adds bulk and may unlock inadvertently with posterior knee pressure.

  (3) Knee stability.

    (a) Sagittal plane stability achieved by bands or straps used to provide a posteriorly directed force.

     • Anterior band or strap (knee cap): attaches by four buckles to metal uprights; may restrict sitting, increases difficulty in putting on KAFO.

     • Anterior bands: pretibial, suprapatellar or both.

    (b) Frontal plane controls: for control of genu varum or genu valgum; may be achieved by the addition of:

     • Posterior plastic shell;

     • Older braces utilize valgum (medial) or varum (lateral) correction straps which buckle around the opposite metal upright; less effective as controls than plastic shell.

b. Thigh bands.

  (1) Proximal thigh band.

  (2) Quadrilateral or ischial weight-bearing brim: reduces weight-bearing through the limb.

    (a) Patten bottom: a distal attachment added to keep the foot off the floor; provides 100% unweighting of the limb; a lift is required on the opposite leg or, used with Legg-Calvé-Perthes disease.

c. Specialized KAFOs.

  (1) Craig-Scott KAFO: commonly used appliance for individuals with paraplegia; consists of shoe attachments with reinforced foot plates, Bi-CAAL ankle joints set in slight dorsiflexion, pretibial band, pawl knee locks with bail release and single thigh bands.

  (2) Oregon orthotic system: a combination of plastic and metal components allows for triplanar control in sagittal, frontal and transverse planes.

  (3) Fracture braces: a KAFO device with a calf or thigh shell that encompasses the fracture site and provides support.

  (4) Functional electrical stimulation (FES) orthosis: orthotic use and functional ambulation is facilitated by the addition of electrical stimulation to specific muscles.

    (a) The pattern and sequence of muscle activation by portable stimulators is controlled by an externally worn miniaturized computer pack.

    (b) Requires full passive range of motion and good functional endurance.

    (c) Is in limited use with individuals with paraplegia, drop foot; also scoliosis.

d. Standing frames.

  (1) Standing frames: allow for standing without crutch support; may be stationary or attached to a wheeled mobility base.

  (2) Parapodium: allows for standing without crutch support; also allows for ease in sitting with the addition of hip and knee joints that can be unlocked; used with children with myelodysplasia.

5. Specialized knee orthoses (KOs).

a. Articulated knee orthoses: control knee motion and provide added stability.

  (1) Postsurgery KO protects repaired ligaments from overload.

  (2) Functional KO is worn long-term in lieu of surgery or during selected activities (sports competitions).

  (3) Examples include Lenox Hill, Pro-AM, Can-Am and Don Joy.

b. Swedish knee cage: provides mild control for excessive hyperextension of the knee.

c. Patella-stabilizing braces.

  (1) Improve patellar tracking; maintain alignment.

  (2) Lateral buttress (often made of felt) or strap positions patella medially.

  (3) A central patellar cutout may help positioning and minimizes compression.

d. Neoprene sleeves.

  (1) Nylon-coated rubber material.

  (2) Provide compression, protection and proprioceptive feedback.

  (3) Provide little stabilization unless metal or plastic hinges are added.

  (4) Retains body heat, which may increase local circulation.

  (5) A central cutout minimizes patellar compression.

  (6) Can be used in other areas of the body such as elbow, thigh and so on.

6. Hip-knee-ankle orthoses (HKAFOs): contain a hip joint and pelvic band added to a KAFO.

a. Hip joint: typically a metal hinge joint.

  (1) Controls for abduction, adduction and rotation.

  (2) Controls for hip flexion when locked, typically with a drop ring lock; a locked hip restricts gait pattern to either a swing-to or swing-through.

b. Pelvic attachments: a leather-covered, metal pelvic band; attaches the HKAFO to the pelvis between the greater trochanter and iliac crest.
  (1) Adds to difficulty in donning and doffing.
  (2) Adds weight and increases overall energy expenditure during ambulation.

7. **Specialized THKAFOs: contains a trunk band added to a HKAFO.**
  a. Reciprocating gait orthosis (RGO): utilizes plastic molded solid ankle orthoses with locked knees, plastic thigh shells, a hip joint with pelvic and trunk bands.
  b. The hips are connected by steel cables which allow for a reciprocal gait pattern (either four point or two point); when the patient leans on the supporting hip, it forces it into extension while the opposite leg is pushed into flexion allowing limb advancement.

8. **Specialized lower limb devices.**
  a. Denis Browne splint: a bar that connects two shoes which can swivel; used for correction of clubfoot or pes equinovarus in young children.
  b. Frejka pillow: keeps hips abducted; used for hip dysplasia or other conditions with tight adductors in young children.
  c. Toronto hip abduction orthosis: abducts the hip; used in treatment of Legg-Calvé-Perthes disease.

Spinal (Trunk) Orthoses: Components/ Terminology

1. **Corset: provides abdominal compression, increases intra-abdominal pressures.**
  a. Assists respiration in individuals with spinal cord injury; relieves pain in low-back disorders; provides sacroiliac support e.g. pregnancy.

2. **Lumbosacral orthoses (LSOs): control or limit lumbosacral motions.**
  a. Lumbosacral flexion extension lateral control orthoses, LS FEL (a Knight spinal orthosis): includes pelvic and thoracic bands to anchor the orthosis with two posterior uprights, two lateral uprights and an anterior corset.
  b. Plastic lumbosacral jacket: provides maximum support by spreading the forces over a larger area; more cosmetic but hotter.

3. **Thoracolumbosacral orthoses (TLSOs): control or limit thoracic and lumbosacral motions.**
  a. Thoracolumbosacral flexion extension control orthosis, TLS FE (a Taylor brace): includes components of a LS FEL with the addition of axillary shoulder straps to limit upper trunk flexion.
  b. Plastic thoracolumbosacral jacket: provides maximum support and control of all motions; used in

individuals recovering from spinal cord injury; allows for early mobilization out-of-bed and functional training.
  c. Jewett orthosis (TLSO): limits flexion, but encourages hyperextension (lordosis); used for compression fractures of the spine.

4. **Cervical orthoses (CO): control or limit cervical motion.**
  a. Soft collar: provides minimal levels of control of cervical motions or cervical pain, whiplash.
  b. Four-poster orthosis: has two plates (occipital and thoracic) with two anterior and two posterior posts to stabilize the head; used for moderate levels of control in individuals with cervical fracture/spinal cord injury.
  c. Halo orthosis: attaches to the skull by screws, four uprights connect from the halo to a thoracic band or plastic jacket; provides maximal control for individuals with cervical fracture/spinal cord injury; allows for early mobilization out-of-bed and functional training.
  d. Minerva orthosis: a rigid plastic appliance that provides maximum control of cervical motions; uses a forehead band without screws.

5. **Specialized trunk orthoses.**
  a. Milwaukee orthosis: a cervical, thoracic, lumbosacral orthosis (CTLSO) used to control scoliosis; it has a molded plastic pelvic jacket and one anterior and two posterior uprights extended to a superior neck or chest ring; pads and straps are used to apply pressure to areas of convexity of spinal curves; bulky, less cosmetic; may be used for all kyphotic and scoliotic curves of 40 degrees or less.
  b. Boston orthosis (TLSO): a low-profile, molded plastic orthosis for scoliosis; more cosmetic, can be worn under clothing; used for mid-thoracic or lower scoliosis curves of 40 degrees or less; also used to treat spondylolisthesis and conditions of severe trunk weakness or muscular dystrophy.

Upper-Limb (UE) Orthoses: Components/ Terminology

1. **Functional considerations: most UL orthoses are directed toward creating usable prehension, functional hand position.**

2. **Passive (static) positioning devices: generally made out of a variety of low-temperature plastics; i.e. orthoplast, Hexalite.**
  a. Resting splint (cock-up splint): an anterior or palmar splint that positions the wrist and hand in a functional position.
    (1) Wrist can be held in neutral or in 12–20 degrees of wrist extension.

(2) Fingers supported, all phalanges slightly flexed, with thumb in partial opposition and abduction.

(3) Used for patients with rheumatoid arthritis, fractures of carpal bones, Colles' fracture, carpal tunnel syndrome, stroke with paralysis, etc.

b. Dorsal wrist splint: frees the palm for feeling and grasping by the use of grips that curve around over the second and fifth metacarpal heads; allows for the attachment of dorsal devices (i.e., rubber bands) to make it a dynamic device.

c. Airplane splint: positions the patient's arm out to the side at about 90 degrees of abduction; the elbow is flexed to 90 degrees. The weight of the outstretched arm is borne on a padded lateral trunk bar and iliac crest band; a strap holds the device across the trunk; used to immobilize the shoulder following fracture or injury when strapping to the chest is not desirable or with burns.

3. Dynamic devices.

a. Wrist-driven prehension orthosis (flexor hinge orthosis): assists the patient in using wrist extensors to approximate the thumb and forefingers (grip) in the absence of active finger flexion; facilitates tenodesis grasp in the patient with quadriplegia.

b. Motor-driven flexor hinge orthosis: complex control systems that allow for grasp; not generally in widespread use.

Physical Therapy Intervention

1. Physical therapist assistant functions as a member of the team and provides patient education and instruction in the care and use of the orthotic device, breaking-in phase, donning/doffing, skin inspection, gait training, etc.

a. The PTA becomes an active member after the clinic team (physician orthotist and physical therapist) have evaluated and determined the appropriate orthosis for the patient.

b. The PTA has to have a good working knowledge of how the device was determined to be appropriate for the patient as well as what deviations the device is accommodating for.

2. Information for the assessment.

a. Preorthotic assessment and prescription evaluation include the following: joint mobility; sensation; strength and motor function; function level; cognitive status; compliance with wearing.

b. Information included in the orthotic prescription.

(1) The patient's needs and abilities are considered: level of impairments, functional limitations, disabilities and patient's current condition.

(2) Is it permanent or changing?

(3) Patient's acceptance of the disability.

(4) The patient's level of function and current lifestyle are considered.

(a) Community ambulator versus a household ambulator.

(b) Patient's recreational and work-related needs.

(5) The overall weight of the orthotic device in regard to the patient's energy capabilities.

(a) If energy consumption is too taxing for the patient, he or she will abandon the orthotic device in favor of using a wheelchair, e.g., patients with high level of paraplegia.

(6) Consideration of the patient's manual dexterity and mental capacity being able to don/doff and use the device. Is the device too difficult or complicated for the patient?

(7) Consider skin integrity: Can they tolerate a plastic device? Will they need a double-metal upright? e.g., in the case of fluctuating edema.

(8) Consider use of a temporary orthosis to assess likelihood of functional independence and reduce costs, e.g., patients with high level of paraplegia.

c. Orthotic assessment (check-out procedures). The PTA actively participates in the check-out process to ensure proper fit, function and construction of the orthosis.

(1) Static assessment: check alignment of lower limb orthosis.

(a) In midstance, the foot should be flat on the floor.

(b) Orthotic hip joint: 0.8 cm anterior and superior to greater trochanter.

(c) Medial knee joint: about 2 cm above joint space and adductor tubercle.

(d) Ankle joint: at tip of malleolus.

(e) Plastic shell or metal uprights, thigh and calf bands: conform to contours of limb.

(f) No undue tissue pressure or restriction of function.

(g) Check for redness of the skin after the orthosis is removed.

(2) Dynamic assessment:

(a) Fit and function during ADL, functional mobility skills (e.g., sit-to-stand).

(b) Fit and function during gait.

3. Orthotic training.

a. Instruct the patient in procedures for orthotic maintenance: routine skin inspection and care.

b. Ensure orthotic acceptance.

(1) Patient should clearly understand functions, limitations of an orthosis.

(2) Can use support groups to assist.

c. Teach proper application (donning-doffing) of the orthosis.

d. Teach proper use of the orthosis.

(1) Balance, gait and functional activities training.

e. Reassess fit, function and construction of the orthosis at periodic intervals; assess habitual use of the orthosis.

4. **Selected orthotic gait deviations.**
   a. Lateral trunk bending: patient leans toward the orthotic side during stance.
      (1) Possible causes: KAFO medial upright too high; insufficient shoe lift; hip pain, weak or tight abductors on the orthotic side; short leg; poor balance.
   b. Circumduction: during swing, leg swings out to the side in an arc.
      (1) Possible causes: locked knee, excessive plantar flexion (inadequate stop, plantar flexion contractures), weak hip flexors or dorsiflexors. All of these could also cause vaulting (rising up on the sound limb to advance the orthotic limb forward).
   c. Anterior trunk bending: patient leans forward during stance.
      (1) Possible causes: inadequate knee lock, weak quadriceps, hip or knee flexion contracture.
   d. Posterior trunk bending: patient leans backward during stance.
      (1) Possible causes: inadequate hip lock, weak gluteus maximus, knee ankylosis.
   e. Hyperextended knee: excessive extension during stance.
      (1) Possible causes: inadequate plantar flexion stop, inadequate knee lock, poor fit of calf band (too deep), weak quadriceps, loose knee ligaments or extensor spasticity, pes equinus.

   f. Knee instability: excessive knee flexion during stance.
      (1) Possible causes: inadequate dorsiflexion stop, inadequate knee lock, knee and/or hip flexion contracture, weak quadriceps or insufficient knee lock, knee pain.
   g. Foot slap: foot hits the ground during early stance.
      (1) Possible causes: inadequate dorsiflexor assist, inadequate plantarflexor stop, weak dorsiflexors.
   h. Toes first: on toes posture during stance.
      (1) Possible causes: inadequate dorsiflexor assist, inadequate plantarflexor stop, inadequate heel lift, heel pain, extensor spasticity, pes equinus, short leg.
   i. Flat foot: contact of entire foot at midstance.
      (1) Possible causes: inadequate longitudinal arch support, pes planus.
   j. Pronation: excessive medial foot contact during stance, valgus position of calcaneus.
      (1) Possible causes: transverse plane malalignment, weak invertors, pes valgus, spasticity, genu valgum.
   k. Supination: excessive lateral foot contact during stance, varus position of the calcaneus.
      (1) Possible causes: transverse plane malalignment, weak evertors, pes varus, genu varum.
   l. Excessive stance width: patient stands or walks with a wide base of support.
      (1) Possible causes: KAFO height of medial upright too high; HKAFO hip joint aligned in excessive abduction; knee is locked; abduction contracture; poor balance; sound limb is too short.

Prosthetics

General Concepts

1. **Prosthesis: a replacement of a body part with an artificial device; an artificial limb.**

2. **Lower extremity levels of amputation.**
   a. Transmetatarsal amputation: partial foot amputation.
   b. Ankle disarticulation (Syme's): amputation through the ankle joint; heel pad is preserved and attached to distal end of tibia for weight bearing.
   c. Transtibial amputation: below-knee (BK) amputation; ideally 20%–50% of the tibial length is spared; short transtibial is less than 20% of tibial length.
   d. Knee disarticulation: amputation through the knee joint, femur is intact.

   e. Transfemoral amputation: above-knee (AK) amputation; ideally 35%–60% of the femoral length is spared; short transfemoral is less than 35% of femoral length.
   f. Hip disarticulation: amputation of entire lower limb, pelvis is preserved.
   g. Hemipelvectomy: amputation of entire lower limb, lower half of the pelvis is resected.
   h. Hemicorporectomy: amputation of both lower limbs and pelvis below L4, L5 level.

3. **Upper extremity levels of amputation.**
   a. Transradial amputation: below-elbow (BE) amputation.
   b. Elbow disarticulation: amputation through the elbow joint.

c. Transhumeral amputation: above-elbow (AE) amputation.

d. Shoulder disarticulation: amputation through the shoulder joint.

4. **Components: all prosthetic devices contain a socket and terminal device with varying components in between.**

a. Sockets are custom-molded to the residual limb; total contact is desired with the load distributed to all the tissues; this assists with circulation and provides maximal sensory feedback.

   (1) Functions to.

     (a) Contain the residual tissues.

     (b) Provide a means to suspend the prosthetic limb.

     (c) Transfer forces from the prosthesis to the residual limb.

   (2) Selective loading: pressure-tolerant areas are built up to increase loading (i.e., build-ups for tendon-bearing areas), while pressure-sensitive areas are relieved to decrease loading (i.e., reliefs for bony prominences, nerves).

   (3) Types

     (a) A socket made of hard plastic with a soft polyethylene foam liner is the most common type; removable liners aid in ease of prosthetic donning and adjustment.

     (b) Flexible sockets: are made of soft, pliable thermoplastic material within a rigid frame; used for most AK sockets because of better suspension.

   (4) Socks.

     (a) Used in every suspension system except suction.

     (b) Provide a soft interface between the residual limb and the socket; minimize shear forces between socket and skin.

     (c) Changing sock thickness or adding more socks can assist in accommodating to changes in volume of residual limb, prevent pistoning.

     (d) Excessive thickness of socks (>15 ply) can alter fit and weight-bearing of the socket.

b. Terminal device (TD).

   (1) Functions to provide an interface between the amputee's prosthesis with the external environment.

   (2) Lower limb prosthesis: TD is a foot.

   (3) Upper limb prosthesis: TD is a hook or hand.

Lower-Limb Prosthetic Devices (LLPs)

1. **Partial-foot prosthesis.**

a. Plastic foot replacement: restores foot length, protects residual limb.

b. Function may be assisted by the addition of a rocker bottom or plastic calf shell.

2. **Transtibial (below-knee) prosthesis.**

a. Foot-ankle assembly.

   (1) Functions to.

     (a) Absorb shock at heel strike.

     (b) Plantarflex in early stance; permits metatarsophalangeal hyperextension in late stance.

     (c) Cosmetic replacement of foot.

   (2) SACH foot: (solid ankle cushion heel).

     (a) The most commonly prescribed foot; nonarticulated; contains an energy-absorbing cushion heel and internal wooden keel that limits sagittal plane motion; primarily allows plantar flexion.

     (b) Permits a very small amount of mediolateral (frontal plane) and transverse plane motion.

     (c) Assists in hyperextension of knee (knee stability) during stance.

   (3) SAFE foot (solid-ankle flexible): a flexible nonarticulated foot (similar to SACH); permits more nonsagittal plane motions; prescribed for more active individuals.

   (4) Single-axis foot: an articulated foot with the lower shank; motion is controlled by anterior and posterior rubber bumpers that limit dorsiflexion and plantar flexion; more stable (permits only sagittal plane motion); may be prescribed for individuals with bilateral transfemoral amputations.

   (5) Flex-foot: a leaf-spring shank (not a foot) used with an endoskeletal prosthesis; the long band of carbon fiber originates directly from the shank; stores energy in early stance for later use during push-off; prescribed for more active individuals.

   (6) Athletic foot: multiple companies design feet for active individuals; designs provide multiangle functionality that include progressive response to axial loading, hydraulic plantar flexion and dorsiflexion, independent toe/heel motions, adaptability to multiple surfaces (rocky, up hill, down hill, etc.).

b. Shank.

   (1) Functions to:

     (a) Provide leg length and shape.

     (b) Connect and transmit weight from socket to foot.

   (2) Exoskeletal: conventional components, usually made of wood with a plastic laminated finish; colored for cosmesis; durable.

   (3) Endoskeletal: contains a central metal shank (aluminum, titanium and other high-strength alloys) covered by soft foam and external stocking; offers improved cosmesis; modular components allows for increased ease of prosthetic adjustment.

c. Socket.
   (1) PTB socket (patellar tendon-bearing): a total contact socket that allows for moderate loading over the area of the patellar tendon.
   (2) Pressure-sensitive areas of the transtibial residual limb include.
       (a) Anterior tibia.
       (b) Anterior tibial crest.
       (c) Fibular head and neck.
       (d) Peroneal nerve.
   (3) Pressure-tolerant areas of the typical transtibial residual limb include.
       (a) Patellar tendon.
       (b) Medial tibial plateau.
       (c) Tibial and fibular shafts.
       (d) Distal end (rarely, may be sensitive).
d. Suspension.
   (1) Silicone sheath with a distal metal pin (also called a *shuttle lock*). The sheath clings to the skin; the sheathed residual limb is then guided into the socket where the distal pin attachment secures to the prosthesis.
   (2) Supracondylar suspension.
       (a) Cuff suspension: leather strap that buckles over the femoral condyles; commonly used, easily adjusted.
       (b) Transtibial suspension sleeve: sleeve that fits over the proximal end of the prosthetic socket and is pulled over the distal thigh. Disadvantage: requires strong hands to pull into place; is best used on limb that does not have excessive subcutaneous tissue.
   (3) Supracondylar socket suspension (SC). medial and lateral walls of the socket extend up and over the femoral condyles; a removable medial wedge assists in donning and removal; more cosmetic (no buckles or straps); provides increased mediolateral stability.
   (4) Supracondylar/suprapatellar (SC/SP): similar to SC but with a high anterior wall; assists in suspension of short residual limbs.
   (5) Thigh corset suspension: a hinged joint with metal uprights attached to a thigh corset; provides larger surface for weight-bearing; prescribed for individuals with sensitive skin on the residual limb; the knee joint allows for knee control (locks); pistoning may be a problem.

3. **Transfemoral (above-knee) prosthesis.**
   a. Knee unit.
      (1) Axis.
          (a) Single axis: permits knee motions to occur around a fixed axis; knee flexion is needed during late stance and swing and during sitting and kneeling.
          (b) Polycentric systems (multiple axis): changing axis of motion allows for adjustments

to the center of knee rotation; more stable than single-axis joints; complex, not widely used.
      (2) Friction devices: control knee motions; provide resistance to pendular motion at the knee.
          (a) Constant friction: continuous resistance is provided by a clamp acting on the knee mechanism; friction device can be easily adjusted by screws; usually prescribed for older individuals who do not vary their gait speeds greatly.
          (b) Variable friction: resistance can be regulated to the demands of the gait cycle; at early swing, high resistance is needed to prevent excessive heel rise; during midswing when the leg swings forward, friction demands are minimal; at late swing, friction is increased to prevent terminal swing impact.
          (c) Hydraulic knee units (fluid controlled) or pneumatic knee units (air controlled): adjusts resistance dynamically to the individual's walking speed; prescribed for younger, more active individuals; heavier, more complicated; increased maintenance, cost.
      (3) Knee stabilization in extension achieved by.
          (a) Prosthetic alignment: the knee center is aligned posterior to the trochanter-knee-ankle (TKA) line; a knee aligned further posterior will be very stable (will not flex easily); may be prescribed for short residual limbs; an unstable knee may occur if the knee falls anterior to the TKA line.
          (b) Manual lock: prescribed for individuals who require a constantly locked knee or experience weakness of hip extensors; difficulty with clearance of the leg during swing can be controlled by shortening the total prosthetic limb length about 1 cm.
          (c) Friction brake: a device that increases friction at midstance to prevent knee flexion, but permits smooth knee motion through the rest of the gait cycle.
          (d) Extension aid: an external elastic strap or internal coiled spring that assists in terminal knee extension during late swing.
   b. Socket.
      (1) Quadrilateral socket: most commonly prescribed AK socket; quadrilateral in shape.
          (a) Contains a broad horizontal posterior shelf for seating of the ischial tuberosity and gluteals.
          (b) The medial wall is the same height as the posterior wall while the anterior and lateral walls are 2.5–3.0 inches higher.
          (c) A posterior-directed force is provided by the anterior and lateral walls to ensure proper seating.

(d) Scarpa's bulge: an area built up on the anterior wall to distribute forces across the femoral triangle.

(e) Reliefs are provided for the adductor longus tendon, hamstring tendons and sciatic nerve, gluteus maximus and rectus femoris.

(2) Pressure-sensitive areas of the typical transfemoral residual limb:

(a) Distolateral end of the femur.

(b) Pubic symphysis.

(c) Perineal area.

(3) Pressure-tolerant areas of the typical transfemoral residual limb.

(a) Ischial tuberosity.

(b) Gluteals.

(c) Lateral sides of residual limb.

(d) Distal end (rarely, may be sensitive).

c. Suspension.

(1) Suction suspension: suction is employed to maximize contact and suspension; air is pumped out through a one-way air release valve located at the socket's bottom; suction suspension can be total or partial (individual wears a sock).

(2) Strap suspension: adjustable, readily accommodates to volume changes. Disadvantage: pistoning when it is the sole type of suspension.

(a) Silesian bandage: a strap that anchors the TKA prosthesis by reaching around the pelvis (below iliac crest); controls rotatory motions.

(3) Hinge suspension: hinged hip joint attached to a metal/leather pelvic band anchored around the pelvis.

(a) Adds controls for medial/lateral stability of hip (rotation, abduction/adduction).

(b) Reduces Trendelenburg gait deviation.

(c) Disadvantages: adds extra weight and bulk.

4. Knee disarticulation prosthesis.

a. Functional, allows weight-bearing on the distal end of the femur.

b. Problems with cosmesis, added thigh length with the knee joint attached, especially noticeable in sitting.

c. Lower shank is shortened to balance leg length in standing.

5. Hip disarticulation prosthesis.

a. Socket is molded to accommodate the pelvis; weight-bearing occurs on ischial seat, iliac crests.

b. Endoskeletal components frequently used, decreases weight of prosthesis.

c. Stability achieved with hip extension aid; posterior placement of knee joint with anterior placement of the hip joint to the weight-bearing line.

6. Immediate postoperative prosthesis (rigid dressing).

a. Plaster of Paris socket is fabricated in the operating room with the capability to attach a foot and pylon.

b. Advantages.

(1) Allows early, limited weight-bearing ambulation within days of surgery.

(2) Limits postoperative sequelae: edema, postoperative pain.

(3) Enhances wound healing.

(4) Allows for earlier fit of permanent prosthesis.

c. Limitations.

(1) Requires skilled application and close monitoring.

(2) Does not allow for daily wound inspection; contraindicated for older patients with cardiovascular compromise or diabetes and increased risk for wounds.

Upper-Limb Prosthetic Devices (ULPs)

1. Below-elbow (BE) prosthesis: contains a terminal device (TD), wrist and forearm socket, harness system.

2. Above-elbow (AE) prosthesis: in addition, contains an elbow and arm socket.

3. Conventional system: power for voluntary opening of the TD (hook or hand) is transmitted by a cable from a figure-of-eight shoulder harness to the TD, rubber bands are used for closure and prehensile strength; forearm rotation is done by manual prepositioning of the TD.

a. BE prosthesis: bilateral scapular abduction or ipsilateral flexion of the humerus is used to pull on the cable and force opening of the hook.

b. AE prosthesis (dual-control system): the same motions can be used to flex the elbow in the AE prosthesis; when the elbow locks (by scapular depression and humeral extension); the forces are then transmitted to operate the TD.

4. Externally powered system: microswitches (EMG myoelectric devices) are activated by the same motions as conventional power systems; small electric motors (battery-powered) are activated to operate the TD.

a. Improves ease of function, prehensile strength.

b. Adds weight; increased maintenance, cost.

Physical Therapy Assessment and Intervention

1. The PTA should be involved with the clinic team in order to have a good working knowledge of the patient's prosthetic and medical needs.

a. The clinic team is usually comprised of a physician, prosthetist and therapist/assistant.

2. Preprosthetic management.

a. Patient and prosthetic evaluation performed by the physical therapist to establish a plan of care for the patient.

b. Will be ongoing during the rehabilitation of the patient by both the PT and the PTA.

3. **Ongoing assessments performed by the PT and/or PTA.**
   a. Skin: inspect incision for healing, scar tissue, open wounds or erythema.
   b. Residual limb.
      (1) Circumference measurements: check for edema.
      (2) Shape should be cylindrical or conical; check for abnormalities; i.e., bulbous end, dog ears, adductor roll.
      (3) Sensation: monitor for phantom limb pain and need for desensitization treatment.
   c. AROM and PROM: examine for contractures that might interfere with prosthetic prescription; e.g., hip and knee flexion contractures.
   d. Strength: strength of residual limb as tolerated; also include strength assessment of sound limb, trunk and upper extremities needed for ADL.
   e. Functional status: assess the patient's functional ability (bed mobility, transfers, wheelchair use) and ability to perform activities of daily living.
   f. Assess cardiopulmonary status and tolerance for increased energy needed to ambulate with prosthesis.
      (1) Limitations of functional capacity: cardiovascular diseases; diabetes; the individual's fitness level and pain; obesity.

4. **Preprosthetic training.**
   a. Dressings.
      (1) Postoperative dressings applied to the residual limb: help to limit edema, increase healing, reduce postoperative pain, help to shape the residual limb.
      (2) Elastic wraps: flexible; soft bandaging; inexpensive; require frequent reapplication; always apply the greatest pressure distally; use figure-of-eight wrapping technique.
      (3) Stump shrinkers: flexible; soft; inexpensive; available in different sizes; pressure applied is consistent through wearing.
      (4) Semirigid dressings: Unna's paste dressing (zinc oxide, gelatin, glycerin and calamine); applied in operating room.
      (5) Rigid dressings: plaster of Paris dressings; applied in the operating room; a component of immediate postoperative fitting.
         (a) Allows for early ambulation with a temporary prosthesis (pylon and foot).
         (b) Good for patients who are young and who are good candidates for a permanent prosthesis.
   b. Desensitizing activities: pressure; rubbing; tapping; stroking; bandaging of the residual limb.
   c. Hygiene: inspection and care of the residual limb; keep limb dry and clean.
   d. Positioning for the prevention of contractures (positions to avoid).

   (1) Transfemoral: avoid hip flexion, abduction, external rotation; encourage prone-lying to decrease possibilities of contractures.
   (2) Transtibial: avoid hip flexion, abduction and external rotation; avoid knee flexion: encourage prone lying on a regular basis; use posterior board in the wheelchair to assist with maintaining knee extension.
   e. Flexibility exercises: full AROM and PROM; active stretching, especially in hip and knee extension; flexibility of sound limb and hip.
   f. Strengthening: utilize a general strengthening exercise program.
      (1) Hip extensors: especially for patient with transfemoral amputation.
      (2) Knee extensors: especially for a patient with transtibial amputation.
      (3) Hip abductors: for stance phase and pelvic stability.
      (4) Dynamic exercises: utilize gravity and body weight to provide resistance during functional mat activities.
   g. Functional mobility training.
      (1) Sit-to-stand transitions, transfers, standing.
      (2) Wheelchair independence.
      (3) Hopping on the sound limb; contraindicated for patients with arthritis or cardiac conditions.
      (4) Mobility in seated position. Scooting for patients with bilateral transfemoral amputation.
      (5) Early walking with crutches or walker. Consider early ambulation with a temporary prosthesis.
   h. Bilateral lower extremity amputation.
      (1) Wheelchair training will likely be patient's primary means of locomotion.
      (2) Prolonged wheelchair time will increase the possibilities of hip and knee flexion contractures; have patient perform prone-lying and extension stretching on a regular basis.
      (3) Energy expenditure during prosthetic ambulation is increased dramatically. The use of a temporary prosthesis would be helpful in determining the patient's ambulatory ability.
      (4) Bilateral transfemoral amputation: ambulation requires a walker secondary to the loss of proprioception and increased balance difficulty.
         (a) Loss of knee extensor function will result in difficulties with stair climbing, curbs and stepping.
         (b) Patients can be fitted with a shortened prosthesis consisting of a socket and foot component with no knee joints; increases ease of use and function; generally poor acceptance secondary to cosmesis.

4. **Prosthetic management.**
   a. Prosthetic checkout.
      (1) Prosthesis.

(a) Usually performed by the PT prior to or in conjunction with the PTA's first treatment with the patient.

(b) Ongoing assessments, recommendations for adjustment and ongoing treatment can be and are performed by the physical therapist assistant as well as the physical therapists.

(c) Initial inspection assures prosthesis is delivered as ordered and properly functioning (inspect both on and off the patient).

(2) Static assessment.

(a) Ongoing throughout rehabilitation.

(b) Alignment and comfort in standing, sitting.

(c) Leg length discrepancy: check pelvic level.

(d) Fit and suspension: pistoning when the pelvis is elevated.

(3) Dynamic assessment.

(a) Ongoing throughout rehabilitation.

(b) Sit-to-stand transitions.

(c) Gait: smooth; safe gait; absence of gait deviations; gait speeds decreased secondary to higher energy expenditure.

(d) Stairs and inclines: assess training progression.

(4) Inspection of the residual limb with the prosthesis off: proper loading; transient redness is to be expected in pressure tolerant areas after prosthetic use; no redness should be seen in pressure-sensitive areas.

b. Prosthetic training.

(1) Goals and interventions.

(a) Donning and doffing of the prosthesis: training specific to type of socket and type of suspension.

(b) Strengthening, flexibility exercises: emphasize hip and knee extension with the prosthesis on.

(2) Balance and coordination.

(a) Symmetrical stance and weight-bearing on prosthetic limb.

(b) Weight shifting to limits of the patient's stability.

(c) Dynamic balance control: stepping and weight-shifting (reaching, kicking) activities.

(3) Gait training.

(a) Conventional training: focus on smooth weight transfer from sound limb to prosthetic limb; reciprocal movement sequence.

(b) Biofeedback training: limb-loading devices to facilitate weight-bearing through the prosthesis.

(c) Training with the use of the least assistive device: parallel bars may be used initially; however, prolonged use may interfere with learning and independent ambulation with some patients.

(4) Functional activities training to include: transfers, stairs, curbs, ramps, down and up from the floor, proper falling techniques, recreational activities, regular inspection and maintenance of the prosthesis.

(5) Hygiene: care of stump socks, interior of the socket.

(6) Facilitate prosthetic acceptance.

5. Selected prosthetic gait deviations (Table 12-5).

a. Transfemoral amputation.

(1) Circumduction: the prosthesis swings out to the side in an arc. Possible causes: a long prosthesis, locked knee, small or loose socket, inadequate suspension, foot plantar flexed, abduction contracture, poor knee control.

(2) Abducted gait: prosthesis is laterally displaced to the side. Possible causes: crotch or medial wall discomfort, long prosthesis, low lateral wall or malalignment; tight hip abductors.

(3) Vaulting: the patient rises up on the sound limb to swing the prosthesis through. Possible causes: prosthesis too long; inadequate suspension; socket too small; prosthetic foot set in too much plantar flexion; too little knee flexion.

(4) Lateral trunk bending during stance: the trunk bends toward the prosthetic side. Possible causes: low lateral wall, short prosthesis, high medial wall, weak abductors, abductor contracture, hip pain, short amputation limb.

(5) Forward flexion during stance: the trunk bends forward. Possible causes: unstable knee unit, short ambulatory aids, hip flexion contracture.

(6) Lumbar lordosis during stance: exaggeration of the lumbar curve. Possible causes: insufficient support from anterior or posterior walls; painful ischial weight-bearing, hip flexion contracture; weak hip extensors or abdominals.

(7) High heel rise: during early swing the heel rises excessively. Possible causes: inadequate knee friction; too little tension in the extension aid.

(8) Terminal swing impact: the prosthesis comes to a sudden stop as the knee extends during late swing. Possible causes: insufficient knee friction or too much tension in the extension aid; patient fears that the knee will buckle; forceful hip flexion.

(9) Swing phase whips: at toe-off, the heel moves either medially or laterally. Possible causes: socket is rotated; knee bolt is rotated and foot is malaligned.

(10) Foot rotation at heel strike: as the heel contacts the ground, the foot rotates laterally, sometimes with vibratory motion. Possible causes: foot is malaligned; stiff heel cushion or plantar flexion bumper.

Table 12-5 ➤ PROSTHETIC GAIT ANALYSIS AND DEVIATIONS

BELOW-KNEE AMPUTATIONS

PORTION OF PHASE	DEVIATION	PROSTHETIC CAUSES	ANATOMIC CAUSES
Initial contact (early stance)	Excessive knee flexion	High shoe heel; insufficient plantar flexion; stiff heel cushion; socket too far anterior; socket excessively flexed; cuff tabs too posterior	Flexion contracture; weak quadriceps
	Insufficient knee flexion	Low shoe heel; excessive plantar flexion; soft heel cushion; socket too far posterior; socket insufficiently flexed	Extensor hyperreflexia; weak quadriceps; anterodistal pain; arthritis
Mid stance	Excessive lateral thrust	Excessive foot inset	
	Excessive medial thrust	Excessive foot outset	
Late stance	Early knee flexion: drop off	High shoe heel; insufficient plantar flexion; keel too short; dorsiflexion stop too soft; socket too anterior; socket excessively flexed; cuff tabs too posterior	Flexion contracture
	Delayed knee flexion: walking up hill	Low shoe heel; excessive plantar flexion; keel too long; dorsiflexion stop too stiff; socket too posterior; socket not flexed enough	Extensor hyperreflexia

ABOVE-KNEE AMPUTATIONS

PHASE	DEVIATION	PROSTHETIC CAUSES	ANATOMIC CAUSES
Stance	Abduction	Long prosthesis; abducted hip joint; inadequate lateral wall adduction; sharp or high medial wall	Abduction contracture; weak abductors; laterodistal pain; instability
Swing	Circumduction	Long prosthesis; locked knee unit; loose friction; inadequate suspension; small socket; loose socket; foot plantar flexed	Abduction contracture; poor knee control
Stance	Lateral bend	Short prosthesis; inadequate lateral wall adduction; sharp or high medial wall	Abduction contracture; weak abductors; hip pain; instability; short amputation limb
Stance	Forward flexion	Unstable knee unit; short walker or crutches	
Stance	Lordosis	Inadequate socket flexion	Hip flexion contracture; weak extensors
Heel off	Medial (lateral) whip	Faulty socket contour; knee bolt externally (internally) rotated; foot malrotated; prosthesis donned in malrotation	With sliding friction unit; fast pace
Heel contact	Foot rotation	Stiff heel cushion; malrotated foot	
Early swing	High heel rise	Inadequate friction; slack extension aid	
Late swing	Terminal impact	Inadequate friction; taut extension aid	Forceful hip flexion
Swing	Vaulting	See above: circumduction	With sliding friction unit; fast pace
Swing	Hip hike	See above: circumduction	
	Uneven step length	Uncomfortable socket; insufficient socket flexion	Hip flexion contracture instability

(11) Foot slap: excessive plantar flexion at heel strike. Possible cause: heel cushion or plantar flexion bumper is too soft.

(12) Uneven step length: patient favors sound limb and limits weight-bearing time on the prosthetic limb. Possible causes: socket discomfort or poor alignment; hip flexion contracture or hip instability.

b. Transtibial amputation.

(1) Excessive knee flexion during stance. Possible causes: socket may be aligned too far forward or tilted anteriorly; plantar flexion bumper is too hard, limiting plantar flexion; high-heel shoe, knee flexion contracture or weak quadriceps.

(2) Inadequate knee flexion during stance. Possible causes: socket may be aligned too far back or tilted posteriorly; plantar flexion bumper or heel cushion too soft low-heel shoe, anterodistal discomfort, weak quadriceps.

(3) Lateral thrust at midstance. Possible causes: foot is inset too much.

(4) Medial thrust at midstance. Possible causes: foot is outset too much.

(5) Drop-off or premature knee flexion in late stance. Possible causes: socket is set too far forward or excessively flexed; dorsiflexion bumper is too soft, resulting in excess dorsiflexion of the foot; prosthetic foot keel too short; knee flexion contracture.

(6) Delayed knee flexion during late stance: patient feels as if they were walking "up hill." Possible causes: socket is set too far back or lacks suffi-

cient flexion; dorsiflexion bumper is too stiff, causing excess plantar flexion; prosthetic foot keel too long.

Bariatric Equipment

Definition

1. Field of medicine dealing with the treatment of conditions and diseases of patients who are overweight, including education, exercise instruction and behavior modification. The word "bariatrics" is derived from the Greek "baros" meaning "weight" and "iatreia" meaning "medical treatment."

Patient Mobility

1. Transfers: utilize assistive devices that are available for patient and clinician safety.
   a. When safe and practical, as with any other functional activity, instruct the patient to assist as able. Use principles of transfer techniques to best position the patient for transfer activities.
   b. Utilize the mobility features available on newer bariatric beds (listed below).
      (1) Position the bed so the patient is in a sitting position prior to attempting a stand-pivot type transfer.
   c. Always use enough help to assist with transfers.
      (1) Follow general rules for multiperson assist transfers by assigning the "lead" person to direct the transfer activities and instruct the patient.

Equipment

1. Beds.
   a. Often mechanized for ease of use. Includes ability to raise/lower entire bed, convert to a chair, Trendelenburg's and reverse Trendelenburg's position.
      (1) Often include a built-in scale to weigh patient.
   b. Mattress may be a low-air-loss or air suspension. Contains several segmented bladders or compartments that are individually controlled for air pressure per patient needs (skin condition, mobility level, weight, etc.).
      (1) If cardiopulmonary resuscitation becomes necessary, a rigid board must be inserted between the patient and the mattress to ensure a firm surface.

c. Designed to accommodate weights of 300 to 1000 pounds.

2. Wheelchairs: consist of reinforced frame, larger width, adjustable legrests with calf supports. Can be found in sizes to accommodate patients up to 850 pounds.
   a. Specially made seat cushions can be found to accommodate patients up to 650 pounds.

3. Transfer Assist Devices: utilized to assist healthcare personnel safely transfer a bariatric patient.
   a. Supine sliding board: used to bridge the gap between surfaces that are relatively similar in height, for the supine sliding transfer of patients. These devices decrease the tissue pressures on the patient.
      (1) Note that sitting sliding board transfers are not recommended for this population due to the potential for tissue damage and difficulty maintaining the position of the board.
      (2) Transfer sheets may be used to accomplish this same transfer; however, they do not bridge the gap between surfaces and pose some risk for tissue damage.
   b. Air mattress transfer system: specially designed air mattress is placed under the patient for a supine, lateral sliding transfer.
      (1) The mattress has many small perforations on the underside that continuously release air when inflated and hooked to an airflow system, reducing friction between the surface of the air mattress and bedding, thus decreasing the effort needed to complete the transfer.
      (2) Some may be manufactured to be radiolucent to allow for magnetic resonance imaging (MRI) or x-ray.
   c. Bedside sling mechanical lift–floor-based lift: mechanical sling lift used to transfer the patient from bed to/from chair.
      (1) The sling lift used to transfer the bariatric patient should meet these requirements.
         (a) Lift capacity sufficient for the patient weight.
         (b) Base expandable to meet the width of a bariatric chair.
         (c) Sufficient clearance under the bariatric bed (typically 6 inches or less).

(d) Single spreader bar of 30 inches; quadrapoint spreader bar of 25 inches point-to-point.

(e) Lift boom to allow sufficient clearance and rotation of the patient.

(2) Two persons should be utilized to rotate the patient for the transfer and an additional person to maneuver the lift.

Standing lift device

1. Device secures the feet and legs of the patient while positioning the upper body weight over the blocked lower extremities.

2. Note the device does not allow for the lower extremity abduction deformity found in some bariatric patients. It is contraindicated if the weight-bearing status of the patient is limited.

Ceiling mounted lift

1. Installed directly into the ceiling and/or building support. Allow for greater lift capacities and do not pose the risk for tipping over as the bedside mechanical lift does.

2. Disadvantage: they are not portable between patients and can only be used at the location where they are installed.

Overhead A-frame lift device

1. A portable lift device that fits over the bed with its support on the floor; requires sufficient clearance around bed; lift capacities are virtually unlimited; maintenance is minimal; has the ability to lower the patient below floor height (lower into a walking pool).

2. Advantage: they are portable from department to department; some models can accommodate patients up to 1000 pounds.

Standing pole

1. A pole that is affixed to the floor and ceiling. The patient can use it to hang onto to help pull self into a standing position.

2. Other devices: reinforced equipment designed to support weights between 400 and 700 pounds.
   a. Walkers with increased width measurement; reinforced step stools.
   b. Stretcher chair: mechanized chair utilized to position the patient into a sitting position. A supine transfer technique may be used to transfer a patient to the stretcher chair. The chair is typically mechanized, can hold up to 1000 pounds, is up to 40 inches in width and typically has adjustable footrest.
   c. Treatment tables: specialized treatment tables provide additional features to assist in the safe handling and management of patients during therapy sessions. Features include: built-in transfer bars, adjustable/ motorized back support (including head supports) and seat belts.
   d. Facility considerations: the building in which units specifically designed to care for the bariatric patient must have floor load capacities sufficient to support the devices utilized.

3. Beds specifically designed for the bariatric patient are heavier than the typical hospital bed.

4. Elevators must be of sufficient load-bearing capacities and must be of sufficient width to accommodate beds and equipment necessary to transport and care for the patient.

5. Toilets: toilet should be floor-mounted model versus wall-hung toilet that is typically designed to support no more than approximately 300 pounds.

6. Other equipment: MRI scanners that are of appropriate size, computed tomographic (CT) scanners or tables, etc., must all be of sufficient load-bearing capacities and width to accommodate the bariatric patient.

Adhesive Taping

Purposes

1. Limit ROM of specific joint.

2. Support injured body segment or sprain, strain.

3. Secure protective devices such as felt, foam, gel or plastic padding, orthoplast or plastazote.

4. Keep dressings and bandages in place and secure.

5. Provide preventative support for a joint that is at risk.

6. Realign position and reduce pain; e.g., McConnell's treatment for patellofemoral pain.

7. May enhance proprioception.

Preparation

1. Part to be taped should be properly positioned and supported.

2. Select appropriate type and width of tape.

3. Body hair should be shaved; skin should be clean. Foam underwrap or stockinet may be used.

4. Lubricated pads should be placed over areas of potential blister formation from friction or heel and lace-area pads on the foot.

5. Occlusive dressings should be applied over wounds or skin conditions to be covered by tape.

6. Skin adherent such as benzoin should be applied to increase adhesion of the tape and aid in toughening the skin to decrease irritation.

Application

1. If the part has not been previously injured, it should be taped in a neutral position.

2. Injured ligaments should be held in a shortened position.

   a. Lateral or inversion ankle sprains should be taped in an everted position.
   b. Tape should follow body contours and be applied primarily from medial to lateral in the case of an inversion sprain.

3. Tape should be applied with even pressure with overlap of previous tape strip by one-half.

4. Circular strapping should be applied very cautiously because of potential circulatory compromise.

5. Avoid creases and folds.

6. If tape is too tight, adjust by removing or modifying strips or reapply.

Complications

1. Allergic reactions to the tape.

2. Skin irritation.

3. Reduced circulation.

4. If the tape is too tight, it might compromise the ability of the athlete, performing artist, patient, client, etc., to perform the skill intended.

5. Tape may lose its effectiveness in an hour or so and may need to be reapplied.

chapter 13

Teaching & Learning

KAREN E. RYAN

Focus Areas for Content Review:
- Principles and theories of teaching and learning.
- Strategies for patient/client education as a component of the plan of care.
- Communication strategies.
- Communication disorders, the implications on physical therapy and strategies to manages these issues.

Educational Theories

Learning Styles

1. **Description.**
   a. A preferred method (or style) by which an individual attains knowledge and processes it into new meaningful information.

2. **Kinesthetic learner.**
   a. Learns by doing.
   b. Prefers to have "hands-on" experiences.
   c. "Touch" helps enhance the learning experience.

3. **Visual learner.**
   a. Prefers the use of.
      (1) Diagrams.
      (2) Maps.
      (3) Pictures to enhance the learning experience.
   b. Written or spoken words will have less significance without visual aids.

4. **Auditory learner.**
   a. Prefers to take in information that is heard, versus read.
   b. May read text out loud to self to enhance understanding.

5. **Intuitive versus concrete learner.**
   a. Intuitive.
      (1) Abstract in thinking and speaking.
      (2) Deals well with theory.
      (3) Sees the big picture. May miss, or doesn't deal with, the details.
      (4) Often comes up with imaginative solutions.
   b. Concrete.
      (1) Prefers details, specifics and set patterns.
      (2) Does not deal well with theoretical information.
      (3) Sees things as black or white, not gray.
      (4) Solutions will be less imaginative.

6. **Active/independent versus passive/dependent learner.**
   a. Active/independent learner.
      (1) Actively seeks knowledge.
         (a) Participates in discussions.
         (b) Asks questions.
         (c) Draws conclusions.
         (d) Exhibits initiative.
         (e) Likes to work independently.
         (f) Thinks for self.
         (g) Has confidence in ability to learn.
   b. Passive/dependent learner.
      (1) Lets the learning experience "happen" to self.
      (2) Demonstrates little initiative.
         (a) Looks to the instructor for direction.
      (3) Lacks confidence in the ability to learn.

Learning Theories

1. **Behaviorism.**
   a. Theorists:
      (1) Skinner.
      (2) Watson.
      (3) Magner.
   b. Based on the stimulus-response model of behavior.
      (1) Behaviors can be shaped by "operant conditioning."
         (a) The learner is rewarded for good behaviors.
      (2) Correct behaviors are identified and rewarded.
         (a) Theory being that the correct behaviors will then be repeated with more and more frequency.
            • Good behaviors are immediately rewarded; no delay.
            • Rewards given must be meaningful to the individual.
            • Behaviors that are associated with punishment are less likely to continue occurring.
            • Eventually, incorrect behaviors will lessen and not reappear.
      (3) Incorrect behaviors are not rewarded.
   c. Learning takes place in a series of reinforced steps.
   d. Learning is arranged from simple to complex for the learner.
   e. The learner must actively participate.
      (1) Practice is important.
   f. The learning environment is managed to lead the student to correct behaviors.

2. **Cognitive.**
   a. Theorists:
      (1) Piaget.
      (2) Bruner.
   b. Theory is that the development of cognitive abilities occurs in stages of biological development.
      (1) Learning moves from specific concepts to complex thought processes.
   c. Piaget's four stages:
      (1) Sensorimotor stage (birth to 2 years).
         (a) Grasp objects.
         (b) Bring objects to mouth.
      (2) Preparational stage (2–7 years).
         (a) Manipulation of objects for simple tasks.
      (3) Concrete stage (7–11 years).
         (a) Beginning to understand/develop concepts.
      (4) Formal operations (11–14 years).
         (a) Full conceptualization.
         (b) Problem-solving begins.
   d. Cognitive educator.
      (1) Looks at learners as individuals within the classroom with differing needs and skills.

   (2) Focuses instruction to learner needs based on readiness to learn.
   (3) Organizes learning experiences so that the student gradually assumes greater responsibility to transfer information and problem solve.

3. **Humanism.**
   a. Emphasis placed on the "human potential" to learn.
   b. Is student-centered and based on the student's need.
      (1) Differences in student abilities are expected and respected.
   c. The instructor provides the learner with the correct tools for learning.
   d. The instructor creates the conditions in which learning takes place.
   e. Student shares in the responsibility for learning.
      (1) The student is self-directed.
         (a) Student's ability to self-assess is important.
   f. Critique of performance is to be constructive and meaningful.

4. **Adult learning (andragogy): the field of educating the adult learner.**
   a. Theorists.
      (1) Knowles.
      (2) Kidd.
   b. Characteristics of the adult learner.
      (1) Highly motivated and self-directed learner.
      (2) Motivated by activities that learner perceives as being directly related to the learner's need for learning (don't like to waste time).
      (3) Brings an accumulation of life experiences.
         (a) Can serve as a resource for fellow students.
         (b) Can also serve as obstacle to overcome.
            • May tend to be less flexible than the younger learner.
            • Wants to participate in the decision-making process as it relates to assessment of needs, setting goals, choosing activities.
         (c) May enjoy less structured opportunities to experiment with knowledge.
         (d) May choose ungraded learning opportunities as opposed to graded assignments.
         (e) Tends to be more interested in mastering or attaining knowledge versus simply achieving a grade.
   c. Teaching the adult student.
      (1) The instructor.
         (a) Selects activities in which the student can actively participate and in which the learning outcome is clear and meaningful.
         (b) Involves the student in decision-making and goal-setting.
         (c) Incorporates the learner's life experiences into classroom discussions.

Instruction

Description

1. **Instruction is the act of explaining or supplying information for the learner.**
   a. It involves supplying information as well as constructing the learning environment to help make it conducive for learning.

Instructional Activities

1. **Patient/client instruction.**
   a. Teaching a patient/client the necessary information or exercise for them to improve/maintain their condition.
   b. Takes on many forms.
      (1) Discussion.
      (2) Demonstration.
      (3) Return demonstration.
      (4) Illustration of written and video information.
   c. Should be designed to provide information to enhance the patient/client understanding of the diagnosis and specific rationale for interventions.
   d. Is enhanced through use of applicable.
      (1) Models.
      (2) Diagrams.
      (3) Illustrations.
      (4) Hands-on guidance of correct movement patterns.
   e. Outcome is often for patient/client to continue independently from treatment session to treatment session and after discharge.
   f. The patient/client is empowered to use this information to manage:
      (1) His or her condition.
      (2) Adaptation to home or work environment.

2. **Care provider instruction.**
   a. Specific goal is to instruct care provider in specific techniques.
      (1) Enhance.
      (2) Promote.
      (3) Produce identified outcomes with the patient/client.
         (a) Focused on safety for the provider and patient/client.
   b. Instruction can take on many forms, including:
      (1) Discussion.
      (2) Demonstration.
      (3) Return demonstration.
      (4) Illustration of written and video information.

3. **In-service.**
   a. Therapist and/or assistant prepare short educational programs designed to impart specific aspects of knowledge to peers.

4. **Clinical education.**
   a. Therapist and/or assistant participate in guiding the learning experiences of a student in the clinical environment.
   b. Typically occurs prior to the student's graduation from their formal educational program in the academic setting.
      (1) Takes the form of modeling clinical techniques.
      (2) Involves observing learner performance.
      (3) Requires structured critique and feedback of the learner's performance.
      (4) Experiences and expectations progress from basic to complex, building on previous learning.

Instructional Process

1. **Identify needs or goals of learner, or receiver, of the instruction to be given.**
   a. Instructional method chosen should meet those needs.
      (1) Needs may be emotional as well as physical.

2. **Assess barriers to learning.**
   a. Design a method that will take these needs into consideration:
      (1) Cognitive abilities of the learner.
      (2) Psychosocial readiness.
      (3) Support systems.
   b. Take into consideration the learner's preferred:
      (1) Learning style.
      (2) Motivation.
      (3) Energy level.

3. **Develop the teaching tool.**
   a. Create the teaching tool to meet the learner's needs.
      (1) Demonstration.
      (2) Handout.
      (3) Video.
   b. Create something that will actively involve the learner.
   c. Include humor when appropriate.

4. **Assess the outcome.**
   a. Did the program achieve the goal identified?
   b. Ask for clarification from the learner.
   c. Are they able to verbalize or demonstrate understanding of the information or technique back to you?

Instruction Modes

1. **Presentation/demonstration.**
   a. Present most important information first.
   b. Keep content brief and to the point.
   c. Emphasize the most important points.
   d. Organize the presentation into subsets of information.
   e. Be specific with instructions.
   f. Use a variety of methods/ways to present information.
   g. Present at a level the learner can comprehend.
   h. Provide hands-on demonstration of techniques or ideas when possible.
      (1) Use terminology easily understood by the audience.
         (a) Avoid technical terms for an audience of laypersons.
         (b) Limit unnecessary extraneous information that will distract the learner from the intended outcome.

2. **Lecture.**
   a. Keep it short.
   b. Involve the participants in discussions of key points.
   c. Build on information the learner already has processed.
   d. Add visual aids to enhance important points or concepts.
      (1) Diagrams.
      (2) Illustrations.
      (3) Models.
         (a) Provide handouts with important points outlined.
         (b) Identify these in the presentation.

3. **Written handout for exercise.**
   a. Should be specific about.
      (1) Repetitions.
      (2) Amount of resistance.
      (3) Positions for performing.
      (4) Number of sets or bouts per day.
   b. Include diagrams and identify affected and unaffected limbs as necessary.
   c. Include signs/symptoms of intolerance and when to decrease or stop activity.
   d. Include contact information for the therapist, PTA or clinic.

4. **Video.**
   a. Videos can be made to specifically meet the learner's needs.
   b. The video should include a review at the start of what the presentation includes.
      (1) Identify any equipment the participant will need.
      (2) Explein any technical terms used.
      (3) Speak clearly.
      (4) Focus the camera on critical aspects of the performance.
      (5) Limit unnecessary background distractions.

5. **Return demonstration.**
   a. Allows the presenter to assess how well the learner grasped the concepts presented.
   b. Performance activity.
      (1) Observe the learner's performance of the task.
         (a) Critique.
         (b) Praise.
         (c) Help refine the learner's performance until consistency is established.
   c. Cognitive information.
      (1) Ask the learner to explain the information as they understand it.
         (a) Critique.
         (b) Praise.
         (c) Help refine the learner's understanding until understanding is demonstrated.

Implementation of Instruction

1. **Patients/clients.**
   a. Assess the patients'/clients' abilities and learning styles; identify obstacles to learning.
      (1) The instructional method will need to adapt to a patients/client who has cognitive deficits or learning disabilities.
      (2) If language is a problem, identify resources available or adapt presentation.
      (3) Use a variety of teaching methods to involve several learning styles at the same time.
   b. Assess the patients'/clients' readiness to learn.
      (1) If they are uninterested in learning, your efforts will be unsuccessful.
         (a) Identify how the learning is relevant to the patients'/clients' needs.
         (b) Example.
            • Learning to roll in the bed will help lead to independence in bed mobility.
   c. Develop teaching methods to meet the patients'/clients' learning needs.
      (1) If they are visual learners, use handouts and diagrams.
      (2) If they are kinesthetic learners, develop a teaching method that allows them hands-on experiences.
      (3) Keep instructions simple and to the point.
         (a) Avoid extra or unnecessary information.
   d. Create an environment that the patients/client feel comfortable in.
      (1) Anxiety, pain and distractions will interfere with learning.
   e. Implement the instructional method.
      (1) Assess its success.

(2) Adapt it as necessary to meet the patients'/clients' needs.

f. Actively involve patients/clients.
   (1) Have them do a return demonstration of a task.
   (2) Or have them explain a procedure to you.

g. Review what has been learned and answer any questions.

2. **Families.**
   a. Assess the family members' abilities and learning styles.
      (1) Identify obstacles to learning.
      (2) The instructional method will need to adapt to the specific needs.
      (3) If language is a problem, identify resources available or adapt presentation.
      (4) Use a variety of teaching methods to involve several learning styles at the same time.
   b. Assess the family members' readiness to learn.
      (1) If they are uninterested in learning, your efforts will be unsuccessful.
         (a) Identify how the learning is relevant to their needs and the patient's/client's needs.
            • By learning to transfer the patient/client, they may be able to take their family member home, as opposed to moving them to a long-term care facility.
   c. Develop teaching methods to meet the family members' learning needs.
   d. Create an environment that the family and patient/client feel comfortable in.
      (1) Limit distractions, which will interfere with learning.
   e. Implement the instructional method.
      (1) Assess its success.
      (2) Adapt it as necessary to meet the patient's/client's needs.
   f. Actively involve the family member.
      (1) Have the family do a return demonstration of a task.
      (2) Or have them explain a procedure to you.

g. Review what has been learned and answer any questions.

3. **Healthcare providers.**
   a. Assess the needs of the healthcare provider and identify obstacles to learning.
      (1) The instructional method will need to meet their specific needs.
      (2) If language is a problem, identify resources available or adapt presentation.
      (3) Use a variety of teaching methods to involve several learning styles at the same time.
   b. Assess the healthcare provider's readiness to learn.
      (1) If they are uninterested in learning, your efforts will be unsuccessful.
         (a) Identify how the learning is relevant to their needs and the patient's/client's needs.
         (b) By learning to transfer the patient/client more therapeutically, they will cause less pain to the patient and will reinforce therapy goals.
         (c) By learning and using good body mechanics, they can limit their potential for pain or injury.
   c. Develop teaching methods to meet their learning needs and capture their interest.
   d. Create an environment that the healthcare provider feels comfortable in; create a fun, relaxed environment.
      (1) Limit distractions, which will interfere with learning.
   e. Implement the instructional method.
      (1) Assess its success.
      (2) Adapt it as necessary to meet the healthcare provider's needs.
   f. Actively involve the healthcare provider in the learning process.
      (1) Have the participants do a return demonstration of a task.
      (2) Or have them explain a procedure to you.
   g. Review what has been learned and answer any questions.

Motor Learning

Description

1. **Motor control is the ability of a participant to regulate or direct motor actions to accomplish a task.**
   a. Motor learning looks at the process the participant uses to practice and eventually "learn" the skills necessary to accomplish a task.

Phases of Motor Learning (Table 13-1)

1. **Cognitive phase.**
   a. The learner understands the goal of the tasks.
      (1) Develops strategies to perform the task.
      (2) Learners need to specifically think about how to perform the task.

Table 13-1 ➤ STAGES OF MOTOR LEARNING AND TRAINING STRATEGIES

CHARACTERISTICS	TRAINING STRATEGIES
Cognitive Stage The learner: • develops an understanding of task: cognitive mapping • assesses abilities, task demands • identifies stimuli, contacts memory • selects response, performs initial approximations of task • structures motor program • modifies initial responses	Highlight purpose of task in functionally relevant terms Demonstrate ideal performance of task to establish a **reference of correctness** Have patient verbalize task components and requirements Point out similarities to other learned tasks Direct attention to critical task elements **Select appropriate feedback** • Emphasize intact sensory systems, intrinsic feedback systems • Carefully pair extrinsic feedback with intrinsic feedback • High dependence on vision: have patient watch movement • **Knowledge of Performance (KP)**: focus on errors as they become consistent; do not cue on large number of random errors
"What to do" decision	• **Knowledge of Results (KR)**: focus on success of movement outcome Ask learner to evaluate performance, outcomes; identify problems, solutions Use reinforcements (praise) for correct performance, continuing motivation **Organize feedback schedule** • Feedback after every trial improves performance during early learning • Variable feedback (summed, fading, bandwidth designs) increases depth of cognitive processing, improves retention; may decrease performance initially; can begin to use by end of stage **Organize initial practice** • Stress controlled movement to minimize errors • Provide adequate rest periods (distributed practice) if task is complex, long or energy costly or if learner fatigues easily, has short attention, poor concentration • Use manual guidance to assist as appropriate • Break complex tasks down into component parts; teach both parts and integrated whole • Utilize bilateral transfer as appropriate • Use blocked (repeated) practice of same task to improve performance • Use variable practice (serial or random practice order) of related skills to increase depth of cognitive processing and retention; may decrease performance initially • Use mental practice to improve performance and learning, reduce anxiety **Assess, modify arousal levels as appropriate** • High or low arousal impairs performance and learning (inverted U theory) • Avoid stressors, mental fatigue **Structure environment** • Reduce extraneous environmental stimuli, distractors to ensure attention, concentration • Emphasize closed skills initially, gradually progressing to open
Associated Stage The learner: • practices movements • refines motor program: spatial and temporal organization • decreases errors, extraneous movements • Dependence on visual feedback decreases, increases for use of proprioceptive • Cognitive monitoring decreases	**Select appropriate feedback** • Continue to provide KP; intervene when errors become consistent • Emphasize proprioceptive feedback, "feel of movement" to assist in establishing an internal reference of correctness • Continue to provide KR; stress relevance of functional outcomes • Assist learner on improving self-evaluation, decision-making skills • Facilitation techniques; guided movements may be counterproductive during this stage of learning
"How to do" decision	**Organize feedback schedule** • Continue to provide feedback for continuing motivation; encourage patient to self-assess achievements • Avoid excessive augmented feedback • Focus on use of variable feedback (summed, fading, bandwidth) designs to improve retention **Organize practice** • Encourage consistency of performance • Focus on variable practice order (serial or random) of related skills to improve retention **Structure environment** • Progress toward open, changing environment • Prepare the learner for home, community, work environments Assess need for conscious attention, automaticity of movements
Autonomous Stage The learner: • practices movements • continues to refine motor responses; spatial and temporal highly organized • movements are largely error-free • minimal level of cognitive monitoring	**Select appropriate feedback** • Learner demonstrates appropriate self-evaluation, decision-making skills • Provide occasional feedback (KP, KR) when errors evident **Organize practice** • Stress consistency of performance in variable environments, variations of tasks (open skills) • High levels of practice (massed practice) are appropriate

(Continued on following page)

Table 13-1 ➤ continued

CHARACTERISTICS	TRAINING STRATEGIES
"How to succeed" decision	**Structure environment** • Vary environments to challenge learner • Ready the learner for home, community, work environments Focus on competitive aspects of skills as appropriate, e.g., wheelchair sports

From O'Sullivan S, Schmitz T. *Physical Rehabilitation—Assessment and Treatment.* 4th ed. FA Davis., Philadelphia, 2001:368, with permission.

2. Associative phase.
   a. Actions are perfected during this phase to produce the most efficient action.
      (1) The learner thinks about performing the steps to accomplish the task with greater refinement and precision.
         (a) Establishes an "internal reference of correctness" of the performance.

3. Automatic (autonomous) phase.
   a. The learner is able to accomplish the task with very little thinking; it is automatic.
      (1) The learner is able to perform the task with a high level of skill in a multitude of environments with a multitude of distracters.
         (a) Able to perform multiple tasks at the same time.

Implications for Intervention or Instruction

1. Learner readiness.
   a. Assess.
      (1) Motivation.
      (2) Fatigue.
      (3) Attention to task.
      (4) Cognitive abilities of the participant.
   b. Take into account that these variables may change from day-to-day, treatment to treatment.
      (1) Adjust interventions accordingly.

2. Identify the task and importance.
   a. Identify the task the learner is to accomplish.
   b. Break it into component parts.
   c. Identify the importance the task has for the learner's overall function.

3. Demonstration.
   a. Demonstrate the task for the participant to gain an appreciation for ideal performance.
   b. Break the task into component parts for practice.
   c. Provide hands-on facilitation of movements required to accomplish the task.

4. Progress from simple to complex in treatment approach.
   a. Identify components of a task and begin practice with those components.

      (1) Introduce multiple components when the learner is ready.
      (2) Progress to accomplishing the whole task without breaking it into component parts.
   b. Control the environment to assure success.
      (1) Decrease distractions.
      (2) Ensure level surfaces for transfer or ambulation if appropriate.

5. Feedback should vary with learner's ability to accomplish.
   a. Begin with greater verbal and tactile cues for successful accomplishment of task.
   b. Identify potential problem areas for the participant to be aware of and plan for.
   c. Eventually decrease the amount of verbal or tactile cues provided to assist the learner to accomplish the task.
   d. Allow the learner to make mistakes and correct self while maintaining a safe environment.
   e. Progress to environments in which the participant needs to plan the performance around obstacles and problem solve independently.

Assessment of Performance/Learning

1. As learning occurs.
   a. The level of accuracy in movements to accomplish the tasks will improve.
   b. The performance will become more automatic and require less cognitive awareness to accomplish.
   c. The speed of accurately performing the task will increase.

2. As skill retention occurs.
   a. The learner will be able to perform the skill after a period of not practicing the specific skill.

3. As skill variability occurs.
   a. The learner will be able to perform the skill in varied environments, from varied or modified positions.

4. Measuring outcomes.
   a. Identify level of independence in performing task.

CHAPTER 13

b. Identify level of function in performing task.

c. Identify the amount of effort required to accomplish task.

5. Performance fatigue.

a. Identify causes of performance decline or avoidance.

b. Provide reinforcements relevant to the learner.

c. Identify motivation for performance and consequences for nonperformance.

Communication

Verbal

1. Messages that are conveyed via voice from the sender to the receiver.

2. Level of understanding is dependent on:

a. The perception of the person receiving the message.

b. The clarity of the message sent.

c. The complexity of the message.

3. One-way versus two-way communication.

a. One-way.

  (1) Typically less effective.

    (a) Does not allow receiver to clarify the message.

    (b) Does not allow sender to question how message was interpreted.

b. Two-way.

  (1) Typically more effective.

    (a) Allows for both sender and receiver to clarify message.

    (b) Helps assure understanding of message intent.

Nonverbal

1. Description.

a. Includes those messages that are conveyed through mediums other than the spoken word.

2. Body language.

a. Postures and gestures that convey messages from the sender to the receiver and vice versa.

b. Open postures convey a willingness to receive a message.

  (1) Open postures.

    (a) Arms at sides.

    (b) Legs uncrossed.

    (c) Erect posture.

    (d) Face the sender.

    (e) Position yourself at eye level with the receiver.

c. Closed postures convey an unwillingness to receive a message.

  (1) Closed postures.

    (a) Arms and/or legs crossed.

    (b) Slumped posture.

    (c) Turned away from the sender.

d. There are many cultural influences and variations that have a bearing on body language.

  (1) Eye contact may or may not be appropriate.

    (a) A nod of the head does not mean the same thing in all cultures.

3. Facial expression/gestures and eye contact.

a. Can convey acceptance or rejection of thoughts and ideas presented.

  (1) Acceptance.

    (a) Smile.

    (b) Direct eye contact.

    (c) Head nodding.

  (2) Rejection.

    (a) Frown or flat expression.

    (b) Rolling the eyes.

    (c) Looking up, down or away from the sender.

    (d) Head shaking.

Effective Communication Strategies

1. Use active listening skills, "I statements," to clarify what you think you heard the patient/client tell you.

a. Restate the patient's problem as you heard them stated.

  (1) "You mean you don't feel as good today as you did yesterday?"

b. Reflect on what you heard the patient/client tell you, and on the feelings they implied in the message.

  (1) "You don't feel as good today as you did yesterday and that really concerns you."

c. Clarify or summarize the message you thought you heard the patient/client send you.

  (1) You would summarize the spoken words you heard your patient/client convey to you to clarify the message, thoughts and frustrations you heard.

(a) "When you started therapy you improved rapidly and thought you would continue to feel better each day. Now that you have had some days that you feel the same and the progress has slowed, you are concerned about how long this process will take."

2. **Ensure understanding of the patient/client goals right from the start of care.**
   a. What problem do they want help with?
   b. Accomplish this by asking questions to clarify what you think you hear the patient/client telling you.
   c. Focus on the patient/client, not your next appointment or the phone call you need to return.
   d. Develop trust with your patient/client.
      (1) Followup with questions, activities or ideas.

3. **Develop your ability to empathize or sympathize with your patient/client.**
   a. Definition.
      (1) Ability to identify with how the patient/client may be feeling.
         (a) Be empathetic with the patient's condition/situation, yet maintain a professional relationship.
   b. Resist pitying patient/clients.
      (1) This conveys an inequality between you and your patient.
         (a) Conveys that they are somehow less than you with this situation or condition.
   c. Do not offer reassurances. "It can't be all that bad," or "It's only for a short time."
      (1) This discounts the patient's feeling or thoughts and conveys an unwillingness to really listen.

4. **Develop rapport with your patient/client.**
   a. Use open body language when interacting with your patient/client.
   b. Be sure facial expressions convey a genuine interest in the patient and his or her needs.
   c. Listen actively to determine what the patient's/client's needs are.
      (1) Ask open-ended questions to gain a greater perspective.
   d. Speak in even, moderate tones using language the patient/client can understand.
      (1) Choose words and language sensitive to the patient's/client's level of understanding and cultural background.
   e. Respect their concerns, questions and ideas.
   f. Be honest about what you can do and cannot do for them.
      (1) Identify what the patient's responsibilities are to help him- or herself.
      (2) It is critical that patients/clients understand that part of the healing process lies in their hands as well as yours.

Speech/Language Disorders

1. **Description.**
   a. A language disorder related to brain damage.
      (1) The specific type of aphasia is related to the area of the brain that is damaged.

2. **Dysarthria.**
   a. Incoordination of the facial muscles, lips, tongue and jaw that results in apraxic speech production.
      (1) Results from damage to the central or peripheral nervous system.
      (2) Often the result of a cerebral vascular attack (CVA).
   b. Presentation.
      (1) The patient/client has difficulty pronouncing words.
      (2) Usually retains the ability to comprehend speech.
   c. Patient/client instruction.
      (1) Will not be able to verbally repeat instructions but can give a return demonstration of techniques learned.

3. **Expressive aphasia.**
   a. Word-finding difficulty or the inability to speak despite intact oral musculature.
   b. Presentation.
      (1) May be very frustrated secondary to not being understood.
   c. Guard against assuming that there is a problem with the thought process.
      (1) May be able to understand, but are unable to vocalize this.
   d. Test for accurate yes/no responses.
   e. Usually capable of problem-solving and learning from demonstration.

4. **Receptive aphasia.**
   a. Difficulty understanding spoken or written language despite intact auditory ability.
      (1) Most patients/clients are able to verbalize ideas accurately.
   b. Multilingual patients/clients may lose both their birth (primary) language and/or secondary language skills.
      (1) May only lose the secondary language.
         (a) If the secondary language is lost, instructions should be provided in the primary language.
   c. Guard against assuming they understand because they nod in response to questions or are able to speak well.
   d. Patient/client instruction.
      (1) Will respond better to.
         (a) Pictures.
         (b) Diagrams.
         (c) Physical demonstration.
         (d) Gestures.

5. Global aphasia.
   a. Characterized by loss of both expressive language and receptive language.
      (1) Cannot form clear spoken words or understand spoken or written words.
   b. Patient interaction.
      (1) Guard against the impression that the patient/client understands.
         (a) Gestures.
         (b) Voice tone changes.
         (c) Facial expression.
      (2) May seem to comprehend when they do not understand what is being asked.

Treatment Considerations with Aphasia

1. Seek assistance from the speech and language pathologist involved with the patient/client for effective communication strategies.

2. Help reinforce goals set by the pathologist by using these communication strategies during treatment sessions.

3. Patient posture, reflex movements and respiration can influence the ability to form words clearly.
   a. Treatment techniques should be directed at limiting influences that negatively affect the ability to communicate.

4. Eye contact with the patient/client can help improve communication efforts.

5. The assistant should.
   a. Be clear.
   b. Use concise instructions.
   c. Speak slowly.
   d. Consider timing.
      (1) Avoid wordiness with instructions.
         (a) If yes/no responses are accurate, use closed-ended questions to facilitate communication.

6. Present material to include multiple learning styles:
   a. Verbal.
   b. Kinesthetic.
   c. Visual.

7. Limit distracters during treatments.

8. Avoid talking "down" to the patients/clients as if they were children.

9. Avoid increasing voice volume as if the patients/clients were hard of hearing.

10. Use realistic testing and training situations.
    a. Carryover from hypothetical or simulated situations may be poor.
       (1) Therapists will often overestimate the patients'/clients' ability to comprehend.

11. Family education and involvement is essential.

12. Aphasia can improve over time.
    a. Could involve months or years.
       (1) Greatest gains will be seen in the initial rehabilitation phase.

Management, Safety and Professional Roles

JANE BALDWIN

Focus Areas for Content Review:

- Critical issues involved in patient/client safety; the responsibilities of healthcare providers to ensure that patient/client management safe environment and factors that influence patient/client safety.
- Emergency preparedness (e.g., CPR, first aid, disaster response)
- Proper body mechanics.
- Infection control procedures

- Legal issues (state practice acts; obligations for reporting abuse and neglect patient/client rights)
- Human resource legal issues (e.g., OSHA, sexual harassment)
- Standards of documentation
- Roles and responsibilities of PT, PTA other healthcare professionals and support staff.

Facility Department Management

Medical Records Management

1. **Documentation format/Problem Oriented Medical Record (POMR).**
   a. Record system for documentation.
      (1) Subjective.
         (a) Information from the patient or family member.
      (2) Objective.
         (a) Measurable outcomes that a PT or PTA gathers.
         (b) Measurements can be gathered during the evaluation, treatment sessions or reevaluations.
         (c) Document in objective, measurable, functional terms.
      (3) Assessment.
         (a) Analysis of problems, impairments and functional limitations including short- and long-term goals/outcomes as determined by the PT at evaluation.
         (b) Ongoing assessment is conducted by the PTA treating the patient on a weekly or daily basis.
         (c) Document patient's tolerance to treatment session.
         (d) Frequency of reporting is determined by the insurance or facility requirements.
      (4) Plan.
         (a) Specific treatment plan for the identified problems of the patient.
         (b) Determined by the PT on the initial evaluation.

2. **International Classification of Functioning, Disability and Health Resources (ICF) Model.**
   a. Developed by the World Health Organization (WHO) and endorsed by the American Physical Therapy Association (APTA) and other international organizations.
   b. The ICF model identifies dimensions of functioning (body functions and body structures, activities, participation) and dimensions of disability (impairments, activity limitations, participation restrictions). See Box 14-1 for complete definitions.
   c. ICF terms serve as a platform for choosing terminology to identify limitations the individual experiences at the level of the body, the environment or in society.

Box 14-1 ➤ TERMINOLOGY: FUNCTIONING, DISABILITY AND HEALTH

Health condition is an umbrella term for disease, disorder, injury or trauma and may also include other circumstances, such as aging, stress, congenital anomaly, or genetic predisposition. It may also include information about pathogenesis and/or etiology.

Body Functions are physiological functions of body systems (including psychological functions).

Body Structures are anatomical parts of the body such as organs, limbs and their components.

Impairments are the problems in body function or structure such as a significant deviation or loss.

Activity is the execution of a task or action by an individual.

Participation is involvement in a life situation.

Activity Limitations are difficulties an individual may have in executing activities.

Participation Restrictions are problems an individual may experience in involvement in life situations.

Contextual Factors represent the entire background of an individual's life and living situation.

- **Environmental Factors** make up the physical, social and attitudinal environment in which people live and conduct their lives, including social attitudes, architectural characteristics, legal and social structures.

- **Personal Factors** are the particular background of an individual's life, including gender, age, coping styles, social background, education, profession, past and current experience, overall behavior pattern, character and other factors that influence how disability is experienced by an individual.

Performance describes what an individual does in his/her current environment.

Capacity describes an individual's ability to execute a task or an action (highest probable level of functioning in a given domain at a given moment).

From *The World Health Organization. International Classification of Functioning, Disability, and Health Resources (ICF)*. World Health Organization, Geneva, 2002. http://www.who.int/classifications/en/

    d. ICF terminology represents a shift from terminology used in the medical model, which focuses on the condition or the disease affecting the individual.

3. **Various methods used for documentation depending on setting, state and federal regulations and third-party reimbursement requirements.**

4. **Reasons for documenting.**
   a. Record accurate and current status of the patient.
   b. Provide history or "story" of the patient's condition and treatments provided by the entire medical team.
   c. In physical therapy, is utilized as a system to track and document patient goals, expected outcomes and determine interventions for achievement of identified goals.
   d. Record patient response to interventions and assists in clinical decisions to determine whether interventions are appropriate and effective.
   e. Provide legal documentation.
      (1) This information can be subpoenaed if necessary.
   f. Utilized as a communication tool between PT and PTA, as well as other health care professionals.

5. **Guidelines for documentation (Appendix I).**
   a. All documentation must comply with jurisdictional and regulatory requirements.
   b. Compliance with all insurance and Medicare guidelines is required to ensure reimbursement.
   c. The patient's right to privacy must always be respected and protected.
   d. Release of any medical information must be authorized by the patient in writing.
      (1) The PTA always refers the person who is asking for medical information to the supervising PT.
   e. Records must be kept in a safe and secure place for a certain number of years, usually 7 years.

6. **Basic principles of documentation (Appendix I).**
   a. Documentation must be consistent with the APTA's Standards of Practice (Appendix II).
   b. All documents must be legible.
   c. Medically approved abbreviations or symbols can be used.
   d. All documentation should be written in blue or black ink.
   e. Mistakes should be crossed out with a single line through the error.
      (1) Should be initialed and dated by the assistant.
      (2) The mistake must be legible to anyone reviewing the chart.
   f. Obtaining informed consent for treatment prior to treatment is the responsibility of the physical therapist.
      (1) Must be signed by a competent adult.
      (2) Minor child or adult deemed incompetent: parent or appointed guardian must sign.
   g. Every treatment has to be documented.
      (1) Specifics of documentation vary greatly depending on setting, insurance guidelines and state and federal regulations.
   h. The patient's name, medical ID number and date of birth should be on each page.
   I. Date each entry and document the length of each visit.
   j. Sign each of your entries with first and last name as it reads on your PTA license and your professional designation (PTA).
   k. Record all communications with any of the team members.
      (1) Team members could include: physical therapists, nurses, physicians and/or social workers, etc.

7. **Progress notes.**
   a. Document specific treatment, equipment provided. Include signature of therapist or assistant providing care.
   b. Document patient response to treatment, functional progress, goals achieved, revision of goals and suggestions for treatment plan modification.

c. Interim progress notes can be written by:
  (1) Physical therapist (PT).
  (2) Physical therapist assistant (PTA).
  (3) Student (PT, PTA) notes must be cosigned by supervising therapist.

8. Reevaluation/Reassessment.

a. Completed as indicated by the supervising PT (minimally every 30 days for Medicare patients). Includes.
  (1) Restatement of initial problems.
  (2) Length of time patient has been treated.
  (3) Progress or regression since last assessment or initial evaluation (whichever occurred last).
  (4) Rationale for continued care.
  (5) Revision of goals and outcomes.
    (a) Discussed with PTA.
    (b) Patient is in agreement.
  (6) Revision of plan of care.
    (a) Discussed with PTA.
    (b) Patient is in agreement.
b. Must be written by the supervising PT.
c. Frequency of reevaluations/reassessments varies according to setting, insurance guidelines and state and federal regulations.

9. Discharge summary.

a. Must be written by the supervising PT.
b. The PTA can and should provide objective tests and measures to the PT.
c. Includes: progress toward goals and outcome achievements.

10. Discharge plan.

a. Must be written by supervising PT.
b. The PTA can and should provide input into discharge plan and participate in setting up follow-up and home services.

11. Common reasons for payment denials.

a. Insufficient/incomplete documentation. Missing data and insufficient detail and descriptions may cause a denial of payment.
b. Incorrect documentation. Wrong date of service, incorrect billing units, mismatched billing date with date in documentation. May result in denial of payment.
c. Medically unnecessary. Poor documentation that does not fully explain medical reason for interventions may result in denial of payment. If documentation reflects maintenance level of care and no continued progress, this may result in denial of payment.
d. Incorrect coding. Failure to document the proper CPT, ICD-9 or other codes may result in denial of payment.
e. Pay for performance. As pay for performance programs grow, poor documentation that does not reflect best practice may result in reduced payments for services.

12. Successful documentation practices.

a. Demonstrate progress toward goals in specific and functional terms.
b. Document medical necessity and reasons for skilled care.
c. If progress not being made, state confounding factors such as medical setbacks, exacerbations of condition, etc.
d. Documentation should stand up in court. Avoid jargon, obscure abbreviations.
  (1) Document in full words and avoid abbreviations if in doubt.
  (2) Write legibly.
  (3) Be factual and objective.
  (4) Sign and date all entries.

Risk Management

1. Physical therapist assistant role.

a. PTAs will be responsible to understand and follow specific risk management practices utilized at the facility where they work.
b. PTAs may be placed in roles of responsibility to monitor, enforce and review risk management practices.

2. A program that identifies, evaluates and takes corrective action against risk to staff or patients.

a. Identifies sites or causes of potential patient, employee or visitor injuries.
b. Identifies potential property loss or damage:
  (1) Financial loss.
  (2) Legal liability.

3. Identification of unusual occurrences or safety concerns is reported by all personnel via incident/occurrence reports.

a. Staff needs to report unusual occurrences.
  (1) Report in objective manner what happened and the result of the occurrence/incident.
  (2) Do not include opinions or judgments.
  (3) Report is submitted to supervisor and risk management team.
b. Reports are not used for punitive or corrective action.
c. Reports are used in the quality improvement process to change policy, procedures and attitudes.

4. Risk management in physical therapy practice.

a. Equipment maintenance.
  (1) Yearly check and documentation of electrical equipment.
  (2) Procedure for identifying, marking and reporting malfunctioning equipment.
b. Ongoing staff education.
  (1) Safety training for all staff in the use of equipment.
  (2) Basic life support certification.
  (3) Infection control.
c. Daily check of emergency cart.

CHAPTER 14

5. **Occurrence/incident and sentinel event reporting.**
  a. Occurrence/incident report is used to document events that involve patients and/or staff which result in harm and/or potential for harm to patient and/or staff.
    (1) Are not part of the medical record, nor should they be mentioned in the medical record.
    (2) Used to document additional information, circumstances, contributing factors that would not be appropriate to include in the medical record.
    (3) Only facts are documented in an occurrence/incident report. No subjective data is given. Statements of what people said should be in quotes. Document factors leading up to the event, what occurred during the event and actions taken after the event.
    (4) Used as part of an internal quality improvement program. May be used to evaluate systems and processes that may have contributed to the event in order to evaluate and improve underlying causes or contributing factors.
    (5) May be used as part of an individual employee performance appraisal.
  b. A sentinel event is a specific patient-related occurrence in which an unexpected finding or outcome can be analyzed to improve processes, systems or therapist/assistant performance to reduce the likelihood of reoccurrence.
    (1) Sentinel events signal the need for immediate investigation and response.
    (2) A sentinel event is an unexpected occurrence involving death or serious physical or psychological injury or the risk thereof.
    (3) Includes any process variation for which a recurrence would carry a significant chance of a serious adverse outcome.
    (4) Is part of a comprehensive quality assurance and improvement program to analyze and improve processes, systems or therapist performance to reduce the likelihood of reoccurrence.
    (5) Many regulatory and accrediting agencies require sentinel event reporting and analysis be done, particularly on specific types of events.

6. **Assuring patient safety and reducing risk in the healthcare environment.**
  a. Efforts taken to decrease risk in physical therapy.
    (1) Equipment maintenance, e.g., biannual check of electrical equipment.
    (2) Staff education, e.g., safety training for new equipment.
    (3) Proper procedure for identifying and notification of malfunctioning equipment.
    (4) Regular check of essential safety equipment.
    (5) Policies to clean equipment and reduce potential for spreading infections.
  b. Patient and staff safety: review all occurrence/incident reports.
  c. Identify risk factors in patient care or therapist safety; e.g., if there are greater than three staff back injuries, implement an in-service on proper body mechanics.
  d. Proper and timely reporting of adverse patient reactions or occurrences (sentinel event) as required by federal and/or state statute. May include:
    (1) Adverse drug reaction.
    (2) Abuse or neglect of patient.
    (3) Outbreak of disease which may affect public safety, e.g., influenza.
    (4) Violence against patient and/or staff.
  e. Annual certification/recertification of staff in cardiopulmonary resuscitation (CPR).

Policy and Procedures

1. **Policy and procedure manual.**
  a. Provides extensive information on what is to be accomplished and how it is to be accomplished in an organization, physical therapy department and/or specific units or clinics.
  b. Policy and procedure manuals are required by:
    (1) The Joint Commission of Accreditation of Healthcare Organizations (JCAHO).
    (2) Commission on Accreditation of Rehabilitation Facilities (CARF).

2. **Policies are broad statements that are used as a guide in decision-making such as.**
  a. Operational policies.
    (1) Billing policies.
    (2) Medical record management.
    (3) Quality assurance and improvement activities.
  b. Human resources policies.
    (1) Vacation/time off.
    (2) Probationary period as a new employee.
    (3) Leave of absence/maternity leave.
    (4) Dress code.
  c. Policies vary greatly depending on facility and its organizational structure.

3. **Procedures.**
  a. Procedures are specific guides to job behaviors for all personnel such as:
    (1) Safety and emergency procedures.
    (2) Equipment management.
    (3) Hand washing.
    (4) Hazardous waste management.
    (5) Disciplinary action.
    (6) Reporting of abuse.
  b. Policies outline specific procedures that all employees need to follow.
  c. Disregard for policies and procedures can lead to disciplinary action and possible termination.

Quality Assurance/Continuous Quality Improvement

1. **Quality assurance (QA).**
   a. Monitor quality.
   b. Monitor appropriateness of care.
   c. Resolve identified problems/inconsistencies.

2. **Continuous quality improvement (CQI).**
   a. Can also be known as continuous performance improvement (CPI).
   b. Systematic process that involves ongoing, deliberate and continuous monitoring of systems and processes affecting patient care to attain the best quality outcomes possible.

3. **Utilization review (UR).**
   a. Monitors quality of services delivered and appropriateness of care.
   b. Resolves identified problems with the quality of service and care delivered.
   c. Can be done in a variety of ways.
      (1) Peer review.
         (a) A system in which quality, appropriateness and effectiveness of work/treatments are reviewed by peers.
         (b) Results are educational, not punitive.
         (c) The goal is to improve the quality of care.
         (d) Focuses on how well services are performed in the delivery of care under review.
         (e) Determines if the patient's needs have been met.
      (2) Concurrent review.
         (a) Review of documentation of ongoing treatment.
         (b) Determine if services rendered are necessary, appropriate and comprehensive in relation to the patient's needs.
      (3) Retrospective reviews.
         (a) Conducted after services have been rendered.
         (b) Method to ensure appropriate care was given.
         (c) Time-consuming and expensive method for third-party payers.
      (4) Professional review organization (PRO).
         (a) A group of reviewers who evaluate the appropriateness of services and quality of care under reimbursement and/or state licensure requirements.
         (b) Reviews services provided to Medicare and Medicaid beneficiaries and some managed care plans.
         (c) Determines the appropriateness of services delivered to patients.
   4. Prospective review.
      a. Evaluation of proposed treatment plan including specifics of how care will be provided.

   b. Used by third-party payers to approve physical therapy services.
5. Program evaluation.
   a. Assessment of the management of patients with a specific diagnosis.
   b. Objectives are established for patients and program, e.g., total hip replacement (THR) rehab.
   c. Outcomes are evaluated in terms of range of motion (ROM), strength, gait, function, etc.
   d. Comparisons made between therapists, facilities, units, etc.
   e. Programs modified and improved according to findings.

6. **CQI projects.**
   a. Once an area of concern or deficit is identified, a plan or process to correct the situation is developed.
   b. Projects are not only identified for direct patient care but can be related to operational procedures.
   c. The process of developing this plan.
      (1) Prioritize the outcomes that need to change or be achieved.
      (2) Conduct a more thorough review of the care/procedures.
      (3) Identify problems or areas of concern.
      (4) Develop a plan to change patient care or procedures.
      (5) Implement the plan.
      (6) Monitor plan and changes in behavior.
      (7) Assess if changes result in desired outcome.

Human Resource Responsibilities

1. **Interview.**
   a. Performed by director, supervisor and possible representative from human resources.
   b. Purpose is to meet prospective employees/employers.
      (1) Exchange questions and answers for both the employer and candidate to make an informed decision.
      (2) Questions asked are informational for both the employee and candidate requiring details and not just "yes" or "no": e.g., "Give me an example of how you handled the last stressful situation you experienced with a coworker."
      (3) No questions can be asked about age, race, religion, sexual orientation, marital status, number of children, political views, etc.
      (4) May ask about academic record, educational program, past performance but must obtain permission from candidate.
   c. Many employers require criminal background checks, which require candidate's permission.
   d. Employers look for the following.
      (1) Decision-making skills.
      (2) Communication skills.

CHAPTER 14

(3) Interpersonal skills (body language, tact, ability to work with others).

(4) Leadership.

(5) Employment record.

(6) Personal goals/direction.

e. Interviewer should provide.

(1) Organizational structure.

(2) Benefits (e.g., health insurance, vacation time, sick time, tuition reimbursement).

(3) Career ladder.

(4) Salary.

(5) Job description.

f. Documents reviewed for employment.

(1) Application.

(2) Previous experience.

(3) Transcript from educational program.

(4) Resume.

(5) References.

2. **Job descriptions.**

a. General summary of responsibilities.

(1) Includes overview of position, supervisory structure, both administrative and clinical.

b. Specific job responsibilities.

(1) Task-specific responsibilities.

(2) Performance standards established.

(3) Outlines skilled and non skilled duties.

(4) Outlines supervisory relationships.

(a) Position title.

(b) Department division.

(c) Supervisor's title (administrative).

(d) Supervisor's title (clinical).

c. Job specifications.

(1) Educational requirements.

(2) Licensure requirements.

(3) Essential job functions (physical and cognitive).

(a) Lifting requirements.

(b) Transferring requirements.

(c) Positioning/ambulatory requirements.

(d) Reading/writing/comprehension. requirements.

(e) Communication requirements.

d. Expectations regarding ability to organize and plan time; overall work habits.

e. Required problem-solving skills.

3. **Performance review/appraisal.**

a. Assesses an employee's performance in relation to objective performance criteria.

b. Written report, discussed with employee in person.

(1) Usually have probationary period of 90 days at start of employment.

(2) Reviews are often performed annually.

c. Reviews correlate to job description as well as organizational goals.

d. Feedback should be objective and specific.

e. Outcome of performance review may be used for promotion and raises.

f. Performance reviews may identify areas needing improvement.

4. **Continuing education.**

a. Ongoing educational activities to foster life-long learning.

(1) Enhances clinical knowledge.

(2) Exposes, instructs and teaches therapists/assistants new techniques and technologies.

b. Educational programs can be delivered a variety of ways.

(1) On-site programs.

(a) In-services.

(b) Journal clubs.

(c) Case presentations.

(2) Off-site programs.

(a) Continuing education programs.

(b) National and state physical therapy meetings.

(c) Special interest group–sponsored courses.

c. Frequency can vary according to time and resources.

d. Employers should support and may subsidize staff member's attendance. Should promote professionalism, educational development and continued competence.

5. **OSHA (Occupational Safety and Health Administration).**

a. Federal agency whose role is to assure safe and healthful working conditions for working men and women.

b. Provides funds for research, information, education and training in the field of occupational safety and health.

c. Any workplace needs to comply with OSHA standards pertaining to such things as blood-borne pathogens, needle sticks and construction safety.

d. Respond to worker's complaints of unsafe work conditions.

e. Performs inspections of workplaces.

(1) Inspects physical aspect of work environment.

(2) Meets with and interviews workers.

(3) Reviews policies and procedures addressing worker safety.

(4) Philosophy of continuous quality improvement. Policies are constantly reviewed to assure optimal safety for workers in the workplace.

(5) Areas specific to physical therapy that OSHA addresses.

(a) Bloodborne pathogens.

(b) Ergonomics.

(c) Slips/falls.

(d) Hazardous chemicals.

(e) Equipment hazards.

6. **Sexual harassment.**

a. All employees are protected through both state and federal laws through the EEOC (Equal Employment Opportunity Commission).

b. Sexual advances, requests for sexual favors and verbal or physical conduct of a sexual nature.
  (1) Submission to or rejection of such advances is made (explicitly or implicitly) a term or condition of employment and/or may affect promotions or other things such as vacations, etc.
  (2) Such advances have the purpose or effect of unreasonably interfering with an individual's work performance by creating an intimidating, hostile, humiliating or sexually offensive work environment.
c. Either sex may be the harasser.
d. Sexual harassment may occur regardless of the intentions of the harasser.
e. Harasser can be the victim's supervisor, a supervisor in another area, a coworker or a nonemployee.
f. Harasser's conduct must be unwelcome.
g. Examples of sexual harassment.
  (1) Sexual jokes.
  (2) Leering, whistling and brushing against the body.
  (3) Display of sexually graphic art, cartoons, objects.
  (4) Request for sexual favors in exchange for job benefits.
h. Employee education and prevention is the best tool against sexual harassment.
I. Individual can file a complaint through the human resources department.
j. Unlawful to retaliate against an individual for filing a complaint.

Emergency Preparedness

1. All work places must have emergency plans that address emergencies within the facility as well as how to respond to emergencies outside the facility.

2. Work places must have written emergency plans.
  a. Available for employees to review at any time.
  b. Procedures for reporting fire or other emergency.
  c. Procedures for emergency evacuation, including type of evacuation and exit route assignments.
  d. Procedures to account for all patients and employees after evacuation.
  e. Procedures to be followed by employees performing rescue or medical duties.

3. Work places must also have an alarm system that has a distinctive signal for each purpose (e.g., fire, evacuation, tornado).

4. Employee training must occur. An employer must designate and train employees to assist in a safe and orderly evacuation of patients and other employees.

5. Employers must review the emergency action plan with employees on a yearly basis or when the following occurs.
  a. Changes are made to the plan.
  b. When the plan is developed or the employee is assigned initially to a job.
  c. When the employee's responsibilities under the plan change.

6. Facilities also have emergency plans to respond to external emergencies.
  a. Local disasters (train wreck, multiple car wreck on major highway, chemical spill).
  b. Natural disasters (floods, earthquakes, forest fires).
  c. Terrorist attacks.

7. Drills to cover both internal and external disasters occur on a regular basis.

8. Employees are to follow facility specific procedures when drills occur and in case of a true disaster.

Patient Safety and Protection

Fall Risk and Prevention

1. Reducing falls and identifying those who are at risk for falls are initiatives of many organizations/facilities.

2. Programs identify best practices in fall prevention to people who are risk for falling.

3. Physical therapy plays an integral role in those programs.
  a. Identifying risk factors of a facility's environment.
    (1) Call light, TV control, phone, etc., are within reach of patient.
    (2) Spills are cleaned up quickly.
    (3) Room is well lit.
    (4) IVs, catheters, etc., are secure and out of way.
    (5) Patient is frequently checked.
  b. Identifying risk factors in the home environment.
    (1) Scatter rugs removed.
    (2) All stairs have sturdy handrails.
    (3) Rooms are well lit and night lights are used.
    (4) Bathroom has needed adaptations, e.g., raised toilet seat, grab bars.
    (5) Area rugs are secured down with tape and/or nonskid treads.
    (6) Phone is within easy reach.

(7) All clutter is removed from hallways and stairs.

(8) Phone and electrical cords are tucked away.

(9) Chairs are sturdy, have arms and are easy to get in and out.

(10) Frequently used items in kitchens and closets are stored at waist level.

c. Screening of individuals for characteristics that make them a risk to fall.

(1) Visual deficit.

(2) Lower extremity weakness.

(3) Balance deficit.

(4) History of falls.

(5) Over 80 years of age.

(6) Use of assistive device.

(7) Depression and/or cognitive impairment.

(8) Decreased sensation in lower extremities.

(9) Multiple prescription medications.

4. Performing standardized balance tests to identify the level or risk for falls. Such tests can include:

a. Berg Balance Scale.

b. Timed Up and Go (TUG).

c. Functional Reach.

d. Dynamic Gait Index.

e. Tinetti Assessment Tool.

5. Development and implementation of physical therapy programs to address and resolve individual's deficits.

6. Assessment of environment and modifying environment key to preventing falls.

Use of Equipment

1. Equipment is used to prevent injury to both patient and caregiver.

2. Many states/jurisdictions now have minimal lift guidelines in place; various jurisdictions have different laws and guidelines. Facility-specific guidelines may also be in place.

a. If patient is more than a minimal-assist transfer, a mechanical lift is used.

b. Intent is to minimize back injuries of the worker.

c. Want to promote an environment where the usage of assistive equipment is encouraged and expected.

3. Various types of equipment can assist with lifting/transfers.

a. Slide boards.

b. Total mechanical lift.

c. Hoyer lift.

d. Sit-Stand Mechanical Lift (SARA lift).

e. Transfer/gait belt.

4. Equipment can help caregivers be more efficient and increase the confidence of the patient.

5. Injury prevention should be facility's philosophy.

6. Proper training regarding lifting, proper body mechanics and use of equipment is needed for all caregivers.

Use of Restraints

1. JCAHO and other regulators determined facilities should be as "restraint-free" as possible.

2. Guiding principle is to create a physical, social and cultural safe environment that preserves patient rights yet protects patients from injury.

3. Environment limits restraint usage by preventive and alternative strategies (bed alarms, sitters).

4. The decision to use a restraint is based on a comprehensive review of the patient/resident with concern for safety.

a. A restraint will be used when it is deemed that there is greater risk to the patient/resident if no restraint is used.

5. If restraints are needed, less restrictive method is used.

6. Use of restraints is evaluated regularly and restraint is discontinued at earliest possible time.

Patient/Client Rights

1. Health Insurance Portability and Accountability Act (HIPAA).

a. Federal law established in 1996 applies to health information created or maintained by healthcare providers.

b. Assures privacy of all healthcare information, especially information that is electronic.

(1) Gives individuals rights over their health information.

(2) Sets rules and limits of who can look at and receive health information.

c. All the following must abide by law.

(1) All healthcare providers: physicians, nurses, physical therapists/assistants, pharmacists, etc.

(2) Health insurance companies, Health Maintenance Organizations (HMOs), employer group health plans.

(3) Medicare and Medicaid.

d. Information that is protected.

(1) Information entered in the medical record.

(2) Conversations among caregivers and between patient and caregivers.

(3) Billing information.

e. Information can be shared in order to.

(1) Provide appropriate care and coordination of care.

(2) Pay physicians, facilities and other individuals who provided care.

(3) Protect public (i.e., report cases of flu or whooping cough).

(4) Complete required reports to authorities (i.e., gunshot wounds to police).

f. Information cannot be shared in order to.

(1) Give information to the employer.

(2) Develop marketing or advertising campaigns.

(3) Share notes about mental health or psychiatric counseling.

g. Providers who must comply with this law.

(1) Take reasonable steps to keep health information secure.

(2) Instruct and train staff as to how information may and may not be used and shared.

2. Americans with Disabilities Act (ADA).

a. Signed into law in July 1990, the ADA is wide-ranging legislation intended to make society more accessible to people with disabilities.

b. The ADA's protection applies primarily to "disabled" individuals.

c. An individual is considered disabled if he/she meets at least one of the criteria:

(1) Has a physical or mental impairment that substantially limits one or more of his/her major life activities.

(2) Has a record of such an impairment.

(3) Is regarded as having such impairment.

d. Other individuals protected by the ADA.

(1) Parents of an individual with a disability.

(2) Those that are coerced or subjected to retaliation for assisting people with disabilities in asserting their rights under the ADA.

e. The ADA is divided into five titles.

(1) Employment: business must provide reasonable accommodations such restructuring jobs, altering the layout of work-stations or modifying equipment.

(2) Public services: state and local government, commuter authorities cannot deny to people with disabilities services, programs or activities that are available to people without disabilities. Public transportation must be accessible to individuals with disabilities.

(3) Public accommodations: all new construction and modifications must be accessible to individuals with disabilities. Public accommodations include facilities such as restaurants, hotels, grocery stores, retail stores, etc.

(4) Telecommunications: companies offering telephone service to the general public must have telephone relay service to individuals who use telecommunication devices for the deaf Text Telephone (TTYs) or similar devices.

f. Employment rules apply to those who employ 15 or more employees.

g. Public accommodations rules apply to all, no matter the size, including all governmental offices.

3. Individuals with Disabilities Education Act (IDEA).

a. Originally enacted in 1975, allowing children with disabilities from birth through age 21 to receive a free, appropriate education in the least restrictive environment.

b. Federal funding is given to individual school systems to help cover the cost of educating students with special needs.

c. IDEA mandates that students receive related services (e.g., PT, occupational therapist [OT], speech therapist) to meet their educational needs.

d. Related services must be provided by qualified personnel.

e. Students who qualify for services must be evaluated every three years and an Individual Educational Plan (IEP) must be devised.

(1) Parent/guardian must approve and sign off on the IEP.

(2) Team meeting including the parent and student (when appropriate) must take place to discuss plan and outcomes.

f. Related services such as PT are provided to the student to meet their educational needs and to allow the student to access their school environment.

4. Abuse and neglect.

a. PTs and PTAs are mandated reporters of neglect and/or abuse of children, elders and the disabled in all 50 states.

b. Each state may have specific reporting systems and requirements.

c. All 50 states have a hotline to report abuse/neglect.

d. Facilities will have specific protocols to report such findings.

e. States have varying levels of knowledge that trigger a report.

(1) Some states may require only a "reasonable suspicion."

(2) Other states may require a higher threshold of "know or suspect."

f. All states have legislation that provides for immunity from prosecution arising out of the reporting abuse/neglect.

g. In most states a person who reports suspected child abuse in "good faith" is immune from criminal and civil liability.

h. Victims are not likely to report abuse, as they are often dependent on the abuser.

i. Elder abuse/neglect.

(1) Individuals 50 years of age or older.

(2) Any action that constitutes the willful infliction of injury, unreasonable confinement, intimidation

or cruel punishment with resulting physical harm, pain or mental anguish.

    (3) Denial of goods or services (e.g., food, medical care) to an elder with the intent to cause physical harm, mental anguish or mental illness.

    (4) Abuse/neglect can be physical, emotional, medical, financial and/or sexual.

    (5) Signs of abuse/neglect.

      (a) Unexplained physical injuries.

      (b) Withdrawal.

      (c) Increased agitation.

      (d) Increased depression.

      (e) Malnutrition.

      (f) Substandard care or poor physical hygiene.

5. Sexual harassment/advances.

  a. It is unlawful and unethical for a PT or PTA to have a sexual relationship with a patient/client.

  b. Sexual harassment can be in the form of.

    (1) Sexual jokes.

    (2) Leering, whistling, rude and unwanted sexual comments.

    (3) Display of sexually graphic art, cartoons, objects.

    (4) Request for sexual favors in exchange for treatment.

    (5) Inappropriate touching or physical exam given diagnosis.

  c. Even if contact is consensual, it is still unethical.

  d. If patient/client makes advances to the PT/PTA the practitioner has to be clear that those actions are inappropriate.

    (1) Caution should be taken; work with those patients in an open area with others in the area.

      (a) If situation continues, care should be transferred to another therapist.

  e. PTs and PTAs are obligated to report any caregivers who engage in sexual activity with their patients/clients.

First Aid

1. External bleeding.

  a. Minor bleeding.

    (1) Usually clots within 10 minutes.

    (2) If patient/client taking aspirin or non-steroidal anti-inflammatory drugs (NSAIDs), clotting time may be longer.

  b. Severe bleeding characteristics.

    (1) Blood spurting from a wound.

    (2) Blood fails to clot even after measures to control bleeding have been taken.

    (3) Arterial bleed: high pressure, spurting, red blood.

    (4) Venous bleed: low pressure, steady flow, dark red or maroon blood.

    (5) Capillary bleed: low pressure, oozing, dark red blood.

  c. Controlling external bleeding.

    (1) Use standard precautions such as wearing gloves.

    (2) Apply gauze pads using firm pressure. If no gauze available, use a clean cloth, towel, a gloved hand or patient's own hand. If blood soaks through, do not remove any gauze; add additional layers.

    (3) Elevate the part if possible unless it is deformed or it causes significant pain when elevated.

    (4) Apply a pressure bandage, such as roller gauze, over the gauze pads.

    (5) If necessary, apply pressure with the heel of your hand over pressure points. The femoral artery in the groin and the brachial artery in the medial aspect of the upper arm are two such points.

    (6) Monitor A, B, Cs and overall status of the patient. Administer supplemental oxygen if nearby. Seek more advanced care as necessary.

2. Internal bleeding.

  a. Could be the result of a fall, blunt force, trauma or a fracture rupturing a blood vessel or organ.

  b. Severe internal bleeding may be life threatening.

  c. Characteristics.

    (1) Ecchymosis (black and blue) in the injured area.

    (2) Body part, especially the abdomen, may be swollen, tender and firm.

    (3) Skin may appear blue, gray or pale and may be cool or moist.

    (4) Respiratory rate is increased.

    (5) Pulse rate is increased and weak.

    (6) Blood pressure is decreased.

    (7) Patient may be nauseated or vomit.

    (8) Patient may exhibit restlessness or anxiety.

    (9) Level of consciousness may decline.

  d. Management of internal bleeding.

    (1) If minor, follow RICE procedure: rest, ice, compression, elevation.

    (2) Major internal bleeding.

      (a) Summon advanced medical personnel.

      (b) Monitor A, B, Cs and vital signs.

      (c) Keep the patient comfortable and quiet. Prevent either overheating or getting chilled.

      (d) Reassure patient or victim.

      (e) Administer supplemental oxygen if available and nearby.

3. Shock (hypoperfusion).

  a. Failure of the circulatory system to perfuse vital organs.

  b. At first, blood is shunted from the periphery to compensate.

    (1) Victim may lose consciousness as the brain is affected.

    (2) Heart rate increases resulting in increased oxygen demand.

    (3) Organs ultimately fail when deprived of oxygen.

(4) Heart rhythm is affected, ultimately leading to cardiac arrest and death.

c. Types and causes of shock.

(1) Hemorrhagic: severe internal or external bleeding.

(2) Psychogenic: emotional stress causes blood to pool in body away from the brain.

(3) Metabolic: loss of body fluids from heat or severe vomiting or diarrhea.

(4) Anaphylactic: allergic reaction from drugs, food or insect stings.

(5) Cardiogenic: MI or cardiac arrest results in pump failure.

(6) Respiratory: respiratory illness or arrest results in insufficient oxygenation of the blood.

(7) Septic: severe infections cause blood vessels to dilate.

(8) Neurogenic: traumatic brain injury (TBI), spinal cord injury (SCI) or other neural trauma causes disruption of autonomic nervous system resulting in disruption of blood vessel dilation/constriction.

d. Signs and symptoms.

(1) Pale gray or blue, cool skin.

(2) Increased weak pulse.

(3) Increased respiratory rate.

(4) Decreased blood pressure.

(5) Irritability or restlessness.

(6) Diminishing level of consciousness.

(7) Nausea or vomiting.

e. Care for shock.

(1) Obtain a history if possible.

(2) Examine the victim for airway, breathing, circulation and bleeding.

(3) Assess level of consciousness.

(4) Determine skin characteristics and perform capillary refill test of finger tips.

(a) Capillary refill: squeeze fingernail for 2 seconds. In healthy individuals, the nail will blanch and turn pink when pressure is released. If nail bed does not refill and turn pink within 2 seconds, the cause could be that blood is being shunted away from the periphery to vital organs or to maintain core temperature.

(5) Treat any specific condition if possible: control bleeding, splint a fracture, Epi-Pen for anaphylaxis and so on.

(6) Keep the victim from getting chilled or overheated.

(7) Elevate the legs 12 inches unless there is suspected spinal injury or painful deformities of the lower extremities.

(8) Reassure the victim and continue to monitor A, B, Cs.

(9) Administer supplemental oxygen if nearby.

(10) Do not give any food or drink.

(11) Summon more advanced medical care.

Basic Life Support and CPR (Box 14-2)

Box 14-2 ➤ BASIC LIFE SUPPORT (BLS) AND CARDIOPULMONARY RESUSCITATION (CPR)

Most victims of sudden cardiac arrest (SCA) experience ventricular fibrillation (VF), requiring resuscitation and defibrillation performed within the first 5 minutes after collapse. CPR is critical both before and after defibrillation. Current CPR guidelines for healthcare (HC) providers include the following:

1. For sudden collapse in victims of all ages, HC providers should call for help (911 or if in hospital a "code" and get an automated external defibrillator [AED] [when readily available]), return to the victim and begin CPR and use the AED.
2. For unresponsive victims of all ages (e.g., asphyxial arrest), the HC provider should deliver about five cycles of CPR (about 2 minutes) before calling for help and getting the AED. Upon return, begin CPR and use the AED.
3. Initial Breathing: the HC provider should open the airway (use head-tilt/chin-lift maneuver) and deliver two rescue breaths. If trauma is suspected, use jaw thrust to open airway; do not tilt head.
   - Pinch nose shut and seal lips around the victim's mouth or mouth and nose if an infant.
   - Mouth-to-Mouth Rescue Breathing: deliver two rescue breaths at 1-second/breath that make the chest rise.
   - Mouth-to-Barrier Device Breathing: place pocket face mask over victim's mouth and nose. Continue to tilt head and lift chin, give two slow rescue breaths into opening of pocket mask.
   - For individuals with respiratory arrest and a perfusing rhythm (pulses), provide rescue breaths without chest compressions at 10–12 breaths per minute for the adult and 12–20 breaths per minute for the infant (less than 1 year) and child (1–8 years). Recheck pulse every 2 minutes.
4. After two rescue breaths, the HC provider should feel for a pulse (carotid pulse). If no pulse within 10 seconds, the provider should begin cycles of chest compressions and ventilations.
   - Overall compression rate is about 100/minute for adults, infants and child.
   - Compression-ventilation ratio is 30:2 for all adults (one or two rescuers); 30:2 for single rescuer (child); 15:2 for infant (two rescuers).
   - Victim must be supported on a hard surface.
   - Compression landmarks: place heel of one hand on the lower half of the sternum between the nipples; the other hand is placed on top of first hand. For the infant, use two fingers to compress the chest just below the nipple line.
   - Push hard and fast and release completely; compression depth should be 1.5–2.0 inches for adults; approximately one third to one half the depth of the chest for an infant and child. Minimize interruptions in compressions.
   - Reevaluate patient's pulse after 1 minute and every 1–3 minutes thereafter. If pulse returns but not breathing, continue with rescue breathing only.

(Continued on following page)

Box 14-2 ➤ CONTINUED

- Continue with CPR until advanced life support (ALS) providers take over, or victim starts to move.

     Lay rescuers should immediately begin cycles of chest compressions and ventilations after delivering two rescue breaths for an unresponsive victim. Lay rescuers are not taught to assess for pulse or signs of circulation for an unresponsive victim. Lay rescuers are not taught to provide rescue breathing without chest compressions.

5. Defibrillation AED.
   - All basic life support providers should be trained to use AED/defibrillator.

     Whenever defibrillation is attempted, rescuers must coordinate good CPR with defibrillation to minimize interruptions in chest compressions and to ensure immediate resumption of chest compressions after shock delivery.
   - When any rescuer witnesses an out-of-hospital arrest and an AED is immediately available on-site, the rescuer should use the AED as soon as possible. HC providers who treat cardiac arrest in hospitals and other facilities with AEDs on-site should provide immediate CPR and should use the AED/defibrillator as soon as it is available.
   - When an out-of-hospital cardiac arrest is not witnessed by EMS personnel, they may give about five cycles of CPR before checking the ECG rhythm and attempting defibrillation.
   - If not shockable, resume CPR immediately for five cycles. Check rhythm every five cycles.
   - For children (1–8 years old) use pediatric AED system if available. Defibrillation not recommended for infants < 1 year of age.
   - Continue until ALS providers take over or victim starts to move.

6. Foreign-Body Airway Obstruction (choking).
   - Examine for signs of airway obstruction by a foreign body. "Are you choking?" "Can you speak?"
   - Universal distress signal: victim clutches his or her neck with the thumb and index finger.
   - Difficulty speaking, high-pitched sounds while inhaling.
   - Poor, ineffective coughs.
   - Bluish skin color (cyanosis).
   - Procedure for obstructed airway.
   - If victim is conscious and standing, use Heimlich's maneuver. Make a fist with one hand, place thumb side of fist on victim's abdomen, below breast bone and above navel. Grasp around victim with other hand and provide quick upward thrusts into the victim's abdomen. Repeat until object is expelled.
   - For child, use back slaps and chest thrusts.

From: *2005 American Heart Association Guidelines for Cardiopulmonary Resuscitation and Emergency Cardiovascular Care.* Circulation 112:IV–12–IV-17, 2005.

Illegal Practice and Malpractice

Statutory Laws

1. **Passed by the legislature and impacting physical therapy.**
   a. Licensure laws.
   b. Workers' Compensation Acts.
   c. Medicare/Medicaid.
   d. Americans with Disabilities Acts (ADA).

Goals of Statutory Laws Impacting Physical Therapy

1. **Professional licensing laws are enacted by all states.**
   a. Protect the consumer against practitioners who are incompetent.
   b. Determine the minimal standards of educational preparation and the scope of practice.
      (1) Graduation from an accredited program or its equivalent in physical therapy.
      (2) Successful completion of a national licensing examination.
      (3) Ethical and legal standards relating to continuing practice of physical therapy.
      (4) Each state determines criteria to practice and issues a license.

Nondiscrimination Laws

1. **Prevent a facility from discrimination against employees regarding race, color, religion, gender or national origin.**

2. **Title VII of the Civil Rights Act of 1964 prohibits employment discrimination based on:**
   a. Race.
   b. Color.
   c. Sex.
   d. Religion.
   e. National origin.

3. The Age Discrimination and Employment Act of 1967.
a. Prohibits employers from discriminating against persons from 40–70 years of age in any area of employment.

4. 1973 Rehabilitation Act.
a. Prohibits employment discrimination based on disability in:
(1) Federal executive agencies.
(2) All institutions receiving Medicare, Medicaid and other federal support.

5. The Americans with Disability Act (ADA), 1990.
a. Prevents discrimination against people with disabilities.
b. Ensures their integration into mainstream life.
c. The definition "disabilities" encompasses a wide range of physical and mental conditions.
d. Requires businesses of 15 or more employees to reasonably accommodate the needs of persons with disabilities to facilitate their economic independence in both the public and private sector.
e. Equal Employment Opportunity Commission (EEOC) oversees issues and interprets regulations.
f. Reasonable accommodations in the workplace by removing barriers must be made unless it would cause "undue hardship."
(1) Installing an elevator so the individual could access the upper floors may be considered an undue hardship.

Common Law

1. Has evolved from legal decisions and impacts in physical therapy in several areas.

Injury Prevention

Overview

1. Back injuries are one of the leading causes of lost work days among healthcare workers.

2. Patient lifts and transfers were found to be the most common causes of reported back injury among healthcare workers.

3. Common back musculoskeletal injuries.
a. Strained ligaments.
b. Strained muscles.
c. Injury to muscle or ligaments from repetitive motions.

2. Malpractice.
a. Physical therapists and physical therapist assistants are personally responsible for negligence and other acts that may result in harm to a patient through professional/patient relationships.
b. Negligence.
(1) Failure to do what a reasonably competent practitioner would have done under similar circumstances.
(2) To find a practitioner negligent, harm must have occurred to the patient.
(3) Every individual is liable for his/her own negligence.
c. Supervisors or superiors may also be found "vicariously" negligent because of the actions of their workers if they provided faulty supervision or inappropriate delegation of responsibilities.
d. Patients may contribute to their own negligence if they do not follow directions from the assistant or therapist.
e. The institution usually is found "vicariously" negligent if a patient was harmed as a result of an environmental problem.
(1) Slippery floor.
(2) Fall in a poorly lit hall.
f. The institution is also liable if an employee was incompetent or not properly licensed.
g. Statute of limitations is a legal time limit in which an injured party can make a claim of medical malpractice.
(1) Time limitation is from 1–4 years after the injury occurred.
h. A physical therapist assistant may be asked to be an expert witness or testify in a malpractice case for.
(1) The plaintiff (victim).
(2) The defendant (accused).

4. Common causes of injury.
a. Single high-load incident.
b. Awkward postures for lifting or for sustained periods of time.
c. Fatigue; not taking breaks when tired.
d. Repetitive and sustained activities in one direction.
e. Stressful situations with increased workload demand.

5. Prevention is the key by use of proper body mechanics, appropriate equipment and other safety principles.

6. Assessment of the situation prior to lift or transfer is key in preventing injuries.

a. Determine level of assistance patient requires.
b. Assess the environment.
   (1) Transfer/patient area should be free of clutter.
   (2) Transfer/patient area should allow easy access to patients and visitors.
   (3) Adjustments in technique may be needed in small areas such as bathrooms.
   (4) Bed or wheelchair should be moved to allow access from both sides.
   (5) Proper footwear is needed for both patient and healthcare worker.
   (6) If floor too slippery due to high polish or wet (e.g., floor of tub/shower) cover with nonslip material.

7. Reducing the chances of injury requires a combination of equipment, training and policy.

Body Mechanics: General Concepts

1. Back should be held in a neutral position to maintain the spine's natural curves.
   a. This position protects the back and tolerates larger compressive forces.

2. Avoid twisting.
   a. Discs are weaker and more vulnerable when flexing is combined with twisting.
   b. Move feet to maintain alignment of the hips and shoulders.

3. Keep weight close to the body (center of gravity, lower abdominal area).
   a. Supporting weight at increased distances from the center of gravity increases stresses placed on the spine.

4. Utilize slow planned movements.
   a. Jerking movements limit the ability of the body to recruit all the muscles necessary for a safe lift.

5. Bend at the hips and lift with the legs.
   a. The large muscles of the legs have greater strength and power than the back muscles to do the lifting.
   b. Tighten the lower abdominal muscles to provide more support to the lower back.

6. Maintain a wide base of support for improved balance.

7. Push rather than pull heavy loads; when possible, push a heavy load instead of lifting and carrying the load.

Body Mechanics: Inpatient Care

1. Consider use of a mechanical lift given the patient's size and the amount of assistance he or she is able to offer.

2. Ask for help from another healthcare worker when necessary.

3. Keep in mind all of the body mechanic principles when lifting/transferring a patient.

4. Assess and set up the environment prior to the transfer.

5. Explain procedure to patient/client and assure comprehension.

6. Instruct the patient to do as much as they can themselves.

7. If needed, lift in stages; use slide board to assist and give a surface to rest on.

8. If a patient or object slips, lower gently to the floor.

9. If in doubt, ask for "stand by" assistance.

Body Mechanics: Instructions for Patient/Client

1. Patients and caregiver instructions for safe handling should cover the following.
   a. Correct and safe use of transfer equipment, e.g., wheelchairs, sliding boards, gait belt.
   b. Correct positioning of equipment, patient/client, helper.
   c. Body mechanics guidelines for the helper.
   d. Mechanical principles to assist in transfer and bed mobility activities, e.g., "nose over the toes" to assist in standing, weight shift away from direction of scoot on sliding board.

Other Injury Prevention Information

1. Purchase furniture and equipment with patient handling and patient use in mind.

2. Furniture and equipment should have removal arm rests and leg rest to assist with ease of transfers.

3. Beds should always be lowered or raised in order to make transfers easy.

4. Bathrooms, toilets and showers should be designed and set up so pushing and pulling of shower chairs is as easy as possible.

5. Ensure that staff is properly trained.

6. Consider use of mechanical aid with transfers.

7. Exercise such as strength training, stretching and conditioning helps prevent muscle sprains, low back pain and improves flexibility, all in order to help prevent injuries.

Roles and Responsibilities

PT/PTA Relationship

1. The physical therapist and physical therapist assistant work as a team.

2. The PT is the only individual who can clinically direct and supervise a PTA; the PTA always needs to practice under the direction of a PT.

3. Each jurisdiction has specific guidelines/rules as to what type of supervision a PTA requires and how often that supervision needs to occur.

4. Various practice environments and facilities will have different policies as to the required supervision of the PTA.

5. The PTA must follow the plan of care established by the PT.

6. In working as a team member, the PTA works closely with other healthcare professionals (see below).

7. In working with and discussing patient care with other professionals, the PTA must convey the prognosis, plan of care, goals and outcomes established by the PT.

Principles of Collaboration

1. Definition: a team is a group of equally important individuals with a common interest, collaborating to develop shared goals, building trusting relationships to achieve these shared goals.

2. Members of the healthcare team.
   a. The patient/client/consumer.
   b. Patient family members.
   c. Significant others.
   d. Caregivers.
   e. Healthcare professionals.
   f. Insurance company or assigned liaison.

3. Professional members on the team will vary with practice setting.

4. The consumer, family member, significant other and/or caregiver role on the team have become increasingly important as the focus on healthcare has changed.
   a. Collaboration with these individuals is mandated by law.

5. Factors that influence and increase the effectiveness of a functioning team:
   a. Identifying member's skills and knowledge level.
   b. Team members' commitment to the patient's goals.
   c. Team members must be effective communicators to all other team members.
   d. Membership composition must address all of the patient's medical needs.
   e. Members must share a common language.
   f. Members have to be effective leaders.

Caregiver Definition and Roles

1. Physical therapy director.
   a. Oversees the function of the department.
   b. Ensures policies and procedures are carried out effectively.
   c. Acts as a liaison with the facility administration.
   d. Sets goals and strategic plans for the department.

2. Physical therapy supervisor.
   a. Qualified experienced clinician with a variety of skills.
      (1) Good clinical knowledge of tasks performed.
      (2) Ability to motivate subordinates and communicate effectively with supervisors.
      (3) Ability to evaluate staff and give oral and written feedback effectively.
      (4) Ability to delegate tasks to appropriate staff.

3. Physical therapist (PT).
   a. A skilled healthcare professional who is licensed by the state jurisdiction.
   b. Every PT is licensed by each state or jurisdiction following successful performance on the national physical therapy examination.
   c. Role of the PT:
      (1) Examines patients.
      (2) Evaluates data.
      (3) Establishes diagnosis.
      (4) Establishes prognosis.
      (5) Establishes plan of care.
      (6) Executes interventions.
      (7) Supervises treatment.
   d. PTs can delegate portions of treatments to PTAs.
   e. PTs have the authority to supervise and direct supportive personnel (PTA and PT aides or techs) in designated tasks.
   f. Reevaluates and adjusts the patient's plan of care as indicated.

g. Performs and documents initial/reevaluation/final evaluation, establishes discharge and follow-up plans.

4. Physical therapist assistant (PTA).
   a. A PTA is a technically educated healthcare provider who assists the PT in the provision of physical therapy.
   b. The PTA is a graduate of a PTA associate degree program accredited by the Commission on Accreditation in Physical Therapy Education (CAPTE).
   c. Required to pass a national examination in most jurisdictions.
   d. Utilization of the physical therapist assistant:
      (1) The PT is directly responsible for the actions of the PTA related to patient/client management (Appendices II and III).
      (2) The PTA may perform selected physical therapy interventions under the direction and at least general (the PT is not required to be on-site during patient care) supervision of the PT.
         (a) Some state bylaws require direct or on-site supervision (refer to individual state bylaws for clarification).
         (b) The ability of the PTA to perform the selected interventions as directed shall be assessed on an ongoing basis by the supervising PT.
         (c) The PTA may modify an intervention in accordance with changes in patient/client status within the scope of the established plan of care.
   e. In all practice settings, the performance of selected interventions by the PTA must be consistent with safe and legal PT practice and shall be predicated on the following factors:
      (1) The complexity and acuity of the patient's/client's needs.
      (2) The proximity and accessibility to the PT.
      (3) The supervision available in the event of an emergency or during critical events.
      (4) The type of setting in which the service is provided.
   f. The PTA is also expected to work within outlined ethical guidelines. These are outlined in APTA documents and may also be found in individual state documents (Appendix III).
   g. Supervision of the PTA in off site settings: The following requirements must be observed (Appendix III).
      (1) A PT must be accessible by telecommunications to the PTA at all times while the PTA is treating patients/clients.
      (2) There must be regularly scheduled and documented conferences with the PTA regarding the patient/client.
         (a) The frequency is determined by the needs of the patient/client and the needs of the PTA.

   (3) When the PTA is involved in the care of a patient/client, supervisory visits by the PT will be made:
      (a) Upon the PTA's request for a reexamination.
      (b) When a change in the treatment plan of care is needed.
      (c) Before any planned discharge.
      (d) In response to a change to the patient's/client's medical status.
   (4) Supervisory visits should occur at least once a month.
      (a) Or at a higher frequency when established by the PT, in accordance with the needs of the patient.
   (5) Supervisory visits should include.
      (a) An on-site reexamination of the patient/client by the physical therapist.
      (b) On-site review of the plan of care with appropriate revision or termination.

5. Physical therapy aide.
   a. Is a nonlicensed worker.
      (1) Specifically trained under the direction of a PT or PTA.
         (a) When permissible by the individual state practice act, PTAs can supervise physical therapy aides.
   b. Functions only with continuous on-site supervision of a PT or PTA.
   c. Performs designated routine tasks related to the operation of the physical therapy service.
   d. Job responsibilities.
      (1) Patient transportation.
      (2) Equipment maintenance.
      (3) Secretarial or housekeeping duties.
         (a) May set up patients for treatments where permissible by state law (e.g., assist in application of heat, cold or participate in basic whirlpool treatments).
   e. Medicare and some insurance companies do not reimburse for the services provided by the physical therapy aide.

6. PT and PTA students.
   a. Performs duties commensurate with level of education.
   b. PT or PTA clinical instructor (CI) is responsible for all actions and duties of the affiliating student and must provide on-site supervision at all times.
   c. All student documentation must be cosigned by clinical instructor.
   d. Patients must be informed that they will be treated by a student and have the right to refuse treatment.

7. Home health aide (HHA).
   a. A nonlicensed worker.
      (1) Provide personal care and home management services.
         (a) Assist patients to remain in the home setting.

b. Responsibilities.
 (1) Bathing.
 (2) Grooming.
 (3) Light housework.
 (4) Shopping.
 (5) Cooking.
 (6) Provide supervision/assistance to the patient to perform a home exercise program (HEP) after receiving instruction/supervision from the PT and/or PTA.
c. Home health aides are supervised directly by nursing or the physical therapist.

8. **Occupational therapist (OTR/L).**
 a. A skilled healthcare professional who is licensed by the state jurisdiction.
 b. Required to pass a national examination.
 c. Responsibilities.
  (1) Provides education and training in activities of daily living.
  (2) Development and fabrication of orthoses (splints).
  (3) Provides training, recommendations and selecting of adaptive equipment.
  (4) Provides therapeutic activities.
   (a) Functional performance.
   (b) Cognitive/perceptual function.

9. **Occupational therapist assistant (COTA).**
 a. A skilled technician holding an associate's degree who is licensed by the state jurisdiction.
 b. Required to pass a national examination.
 c. Works under the supervision of the occupational therapist in carrying out established treatment plans. COTA relationship follows similar guidelines to the PT/PTA.

10. **Speech-language pathologist (speech therapist).**
 a. A skilled healthcare professional licensed in the state jurisdiction.
  (1) Has completed 1 year of supervised field experience.
 b. Required to pass a national examination.
 c. Develops and conducts treatments to.
  (1) Restore or improve communication of patients with language and speech impairments:
   (a) Physiological deficits.
   (b) Neurological disturbances.
   (c) Defective articulation.
 d. Works closely with occupational therapy to correct swallowing problems and cognitive processing deficits.

11. **Certified orthotist.**
 a. Designs, fabricates and fits orthoses prescribed by physicians.
  (1) Braces.
  (2) Splints.
  (3) Cervical collars.
  (4) Corsets.
  (5) Orthotics/shoe inserts.
 b. Successfully completed the examination by the American Orthotist and Prosthetist Association.

12. **Certified prosthetist.**
 a. Designs, fabricates and fits prostheses for patients with partial or total absence of a limb.
 b. Successful passage on the examination by the American Orthotist and Prosthetist Association.

13. **Certified respiratory therapy technician (CRRT) (respiratory therapist).**
 a. Technically trained with an associate's degree from an accredited program.
 b. Administers treatment as prescribed and supervised by a physician.
  (1) Pulmonary function tests.
  (2) Treatments: nebulizers, aerosols, oxygen therapy.
  (3) Maintains all respiratory equipment and assists patient with its use (e.g., ventilators, continuous positive airway pressure [CPAP]).

14. **Registered nurse (RN).**
 a. Skilled healthcare professional who is a graduate of an accredited program and who has successfully passed a licensure exam.
 b. Primary liaison between patient and physician.
 c. Supervises other levels of nursing care (e.g., licensed practical nurse (LPN), certified nursing assistants, home health aides).
 d. Makes referrals under the direction of the physician.
 e. Dispenses medication but cannot change drug dosages.

15. **Social worker.**
 a. Skilled healthcare professional who is a graduate of an accredited program and after 1 year of practical field work are licensed or registered by the state.
 b. Can serve as a family and patient counselor.
 c. Can serve as a case manager coordinating patient's care and transition from one setting to another.
  (1) Assist family/patient with applications for financial assistance.
  (2) Assist family/patient with search of nursing home or other facilities for transfer of care.
  (3) Assures all discharge plans and referrals are in place.
  (4) Advocate for patient in family and dealing with outside agencies and procuring continued services (e.g., insurance companies, home health agencies).
  (5) Mediates between family/patient and team surrounding discharge plans and ongoing care.

16. **Rehabilitation counselor (vocational counselor).**
 a. Technically educated healthcare worker.
 b. Counsels individuals with physical and/or cognitive disabilities.

c. Administers vocational testing which can assist in determining optimal occupational choices for an individual.

d. Will assist individuals with job placement and may arrange job-specific training.

17. **Audiologist.**
   a. Skilled healthcare professional who is a graduate of an accredited program and has successfully passed a licensure exam.
   b. Specialist in hearing disorders:
      (1) Uses audiometric tests to assess sensitivity of sense of hearing and of hearing loss.
      (2) Uses speech audiometric tests to assess the ability to understand the spoken word.

18. **Physiatrist.**
   a. A physician specializing in physical medicine and rehabilitation.
   b. Completes board certification as a specialist.
   c. Primary focus is maximal restoration of physical, psychological, social, vocational function and to alleviate pain.
   d. Often serves as the attending physician on inpatient rehab units.

19. **Primary care physician (PCP).**
   a. Serves to manage routine healthcare needs.
   b. Can be an internist, family medicine physician or general practitioner.
   c. Can serve as "gate keepers" of medical care.
      (1) Many times, individuals need a referral from their PCP prior to seeing any specialist, including physical therapist.

20. **Physician assistant (PA, PA-C) or nurse practitioner (NP).**
   a. Skilled healthcare professional who is a graduate of an accredited program and who has successfully passed a licensure exam.
   b. Considered a "physician extender."
   c. Under supervision of the physician, can perform routine diagnostic, preventive, therapeutic interventions.
   d. Can practice in a variety of settings.
   e. Able to provide physical therapy referral and prescribe certain medications.
   f. Nurse practitioner must complete RN training and pass licensure board prior to training as a nurse practitioner.

21. **Athletic trainer.**
   a. Skilled healthcare professional who is a graduate of an accredited program and who has successfully passed a national certification exam.
   b. Integral provider of care to athletes.
      (1) Works with athletes to prevent injuries.
      (2) Works with athletes after an injury for rehabilitation and return to sport.
   c. Setting for delivery of care: public schools, colleges and universities, professional athletic teams and private or hospital-based clinics.
      (1) If working in private or hospital-based clinics, various jurisdictions have various rules and regulations of how an athletic trainer can be used in the clinic.

APPENDIX I

American Physical Therapy Association

DOCUMENTATION AUTHORITY FOR PHYSICAL THERAPY SERVICES—*May 2007*

Physical therapy examination, evaluation, diagnosis, prognosis and plan of care (including interventions) shall be documented, dated and authenticated by the physical therapist who performs the service. Interventions provided by the physical therapist or selected interventions provided by the physical therapist assistant under the direction and supervision of the physical therapist are documented, dated and authenticated by the physical therapist or, when permissible by law, the physical therapist assistant.

Other notations or flow charts are considered a component of the documented record but do not meet the requirements of documentation in or of themselves.

Students in physical therapist or physical therapist assistant programs may document when the record is additionally authenticated by the physical therapist or, when permissible by law, documentation by physical therapist assistant students may be authenticated by a physical therapist assistant.

Excerpts from the American Physical Therapy Association's Board of Directors Guidelines for Documentation. Last updated December 2008.

GUIDELINES: PHYSICAL THERAPY DOCUMENTATION OF PATIENT/CLIENT MANAGEMENT

General Guidelines

- Documentation is required for every visit/encounter.
- All documentation must comply with the applicable jurisdictional/regulatory requirements.
- All handwritten entries shall be made in ink and will include original signatures. Electronic entries are made with appropriate security and confidentiality provisions.
- Charting errors should be corrected by drawing a single line through the error and initialing and dating the chart or through the appropriate mechanism for electronic documentation that clearly indicates that a change was made without deletion of the original record.
- All documentation must include adequate identification of the patient/client and the physical therapist or physical therapist assistant.
- The patient's/client's full name and identification number, if applicable, must be included on all official documents.
- All entries must be dated and authenticated with the provider's full name and appropriate designation:
- Documentation of examination, evaluation, diagnosis, prognosis, plan of care and discharge summary must be authenticated by the physical therapist who provided the service.
- Documentation of intervention in visit/encounter notes must be authenticated by the physical therapist or physical therapist assistant who provided the service.
- Documentation by physical therapist or physical therapist assistant graduates or other physical therapists and physical therapist assistants pending receipt of an unrestricted license shall be authenticated by a licensed physical therapist, or, when permissible by law, documentation by physical therapist assistant graduates may be authenticated by a physical therapist assistant.
- Documentation by students (SPT/SPTA) in physical therapist or physical therapist assistant programs must be additionally authenticated by the physical therapist or, when permissible by law, documentation by physical therapist assistant students may be authenticated by a physical therapist assistant.
- Documentation should include the referral mechanism by which physical therapy services are initiated:
  - Self-referral/direct access.
  - Request for consultation from another practitioner.
- Documentation should include indication of no-shows and cancellations.

Visit/Encounter

- Documentation of each visit/encounter shall include the following elements:
  - Patient/client self-report (as appropriate).
  - Identification of specific interventions provided, including frequency, intensity and duration as appropriate. Examples include:
    - Knee extension, three sets, 10 repetitions, 10# weight.
    - Transfer training bed to chair with sliding board.
    - Equipment provided.
  - Changes in patient/client impairment, functional limitation and disability status as they relate to the plan of care.
  - Response to interventions, including adverse reactions, if any.
  - Factors that modify frequency or intensity of intervention and progression goals, including patient/client adherence to patient/client-related instructions.
  - Communication/consultation with providers/patient/client/family/ significant other.
  - Documentation to plan for ongoing provision of services for the next visit(s), which is suggested to include, but not be limited to:
    - The interventions with objectives.
    - Progression parameters.
    - Precautions, if indicated.

CHAPTER 14

APPENDIX II

American Physical Therapy Association House of Delegates

STANDARDS OF PRACTICE FOR PHYSICAL THERAPY June 2003 PREAMBLE

The physical therapy profession's commitment to society is to promote optimal health and function in individuals by pursuing excellence in practice. The American Physical Therapy Association attests to this commitment by adopting and promoting the following *Standards of Practice*

for Physical Therapy. These Standards are the profession's statement of conditions and performances that are essential for provision of high quality professional service to society and provide a foundation for assessment of physical therapist practice.

Ethical/Legal Considerations

Ethical Considerations

The physical therapist practices according to the *Code of Ethics* of the American Physical Therapy Association.

The physical therapist assistant complies with the *Standards of Ethical Conduct for the Physical Therapist Assistant* of the American Physical Therapy Association.

Legal Considerations

The physical therapist complies with all the legal requirements of jurisdictions regulating the practice of physical therapy.

The physical therapist assistant complies with all the legal requirements of jurisdictions regulating the work of the assistant.

Administration of the Physical Therapy Service

Statement of Mission, Purposes and Goals

The physical therapy service has a statement of mission, purposes and goals that reflects the needs and interests of the patients/clients served, the physical therapy personnel affiliated with the service and the community.

Organizational Plan

The physical therapy service has a written organizational plan.

Policies and Procedures

The physical therapy service has written policies and procedures that reflect the operation, mission,

purposes and goals of the service and are consistent with the Association's standards, policies, positions, guidelines and *Code of Ethics*.

Administration

A physical therapist is responsible for the direction of the physical therapy service.

Fiscal Management

The director of the physical therapy service, in consultation with physical therapy staff and appropriate administrative personnel, participates in the planning for and allocation of resources. Fiscal planning and management of the service is based on sound accounting principles.

Improvement of Quality of Care and Performance

The physical therapy service has a written plan for continuous improvement of quality of care and performance of services.

Staffing

The physical therapy personnel affiliated with the physical therapy service have demonstrated competence and are sufficient to achieve the mission, purposes and goals of the service.

Staff Development

The physical therapy service has a written plan that provides for appropriate and ongoing staff development.

Physical Setting

The physical setting is designed to provide a safe and accessible environment that facilitates fulfillment of the mission, purposes and goals of the physical therapy service. The equipment is safe and sufficient to achieve the purposes and goals of physical therapy.

Collaboration

The physical therapy service collaborates with all disciplines as appropriate.

Patient Client Management

Patient/Client Collaboration

Within the patient/client management process, the physical therapist and the patient/client establish and maintain an ongoing collaborative process of decision-making that exists throughout the provision of services.

Initial Examination/Evaluation/Diagnosis/Prognosis

The physical therapist performs an initial examination and evaluation to establish a diagnosis and prognosis prior to intervention.

Plan of Care

The physical therapist establishes a plan of care and manages the needs of the patient/client based on the examination, evaluation, diagnosis, prognosis, goals and outcomes of the planned interventions for identified impairments, functional limitations and disabilities.

The physical therapist involves the patient/client and appropriate others in the planning, implementation and assessment of the plan of care.

The physical therapist, in consultation with appropriate disciplines, plans for discharge of the patient/client taking into consideration achievement of anticipated goals and expected outcomes and provides for appropriate follow-up or referral.

Intervention

The physical therapist provides or directs and supervises the physical therapy intervention consistent with the results of the examination, evaluation, diagnosis, prognosis and plan of care.

Reexamination

The physical therapist reexamines the patient/client as necessary during an episode of care to evaluate progress or change in patient/client status and modifies the plan of care accordingly or discontinues physical therapy services.

Discharge/Discontinuation of Intervention

The physical therapist discharges the patient/client from physical therapy services when the anticipated goals or expected outcomes for the patient/client have been achieved. The physical therapist discontinues intervention when the patient/client is unable to continue to progress toward goals or when the physical therapist determines that the patient/client will no longer benefit from physical therapy.

including the results of the initial examination and evaluation, diagnosis, prognosis, plan of care, interventions, response to interventions, changes in patient/client status relative to the interventions, reexamination and discharge/discontinuation of intervention and other patient/client management activities.

Communication/Coordination/Documentation

The physical therapist communicates, coordinates and documents all aspects of patient/client management

Education

The physical therapist is responsible for individual professional development. The physical therapist assistant is responsible for individual career development.

The physical therapist and the physical therapist assistant, under the direction and supervision of he physical therapist, participate in the education of students.

The physical therapist educates and provides consultation to consumers and the general public regarding the purposes and benefits of physical therapy.

The physical therapist educates and provides consultation to consumers and the general public regarding the roles of the physical therapist and the physical therapist assistant.

Research

The physical therapist applies research findings to practice and encourages, participates in and promotes

activities that establish the outcomes of patient/client management provided by the physical therapist.

Community Responsibility

The physical therapist demonstrates community responsibility by participating in community and community agency activities, educating the public, formulating public policy or providing pro bono physical therapy services.

APPENDIX III

American Physical Therapy Association House of Delegates

DIRECTION AND SUPERVISION OF THE PHYSICAL THERAPIST ASSISTANT—
June 2005

Physical therapists have a responsibility to deliver services in ways that protect the public safety and maximize the availability of their services. They do this through direct delivery of services in conjunction with responsible utilization of physical therapist assistants who assist with selected components of intervention. The physical therapist assistant is the only individual permitted to assist a physical therapist in selected interventions under the direction and supervision of a physical therapist.

Direction and supervision are essential in the provision of quality physical therapy services. The degree of direction and supervision necessary for assuring quality physical therapy services is dependent upon many factors, including the education, experiences and responsibilities of the parties involved, as well as the organizational structure in which the physical therapy services are provided.

Regardless of the setting in which the physical therapy service is provided, the following responsibilities must be borne solely by the physical therapist:

1. **Interpretation of referrals when available.**

2. **Initial examination, evaluation, diagnosis and prognosis.**

3. **Development or modification of a plan of care which is based on the initial examination or reexamination and which includes the physical therapy goals and outcomes.**

4. **Determination of when the expertise and decision-making capability of the physical therapist requires the physical therapist to personally render physical therapy interventions and when it may be appropriate to utilize the physical therapist assistant. A physical therapist shall determine the most appropriate utilization of the physical therapist assistant that provides for the delivery of service that is safe, effective and efficient.**

5. **Reexamination of the patient/client in light of their goals and revision of the plan of care when indicated.**

6. **Establishment of the discharge plan and documentation of discharge summary/status.**

7. **Oversight of all documentation for services rendered to each patient/client.**

The physical therapist remains responsible for the physical therapy services provided when the physical therapist's plan of care involves the physical therapist assistant to assist with selected interventions. Regardless of the setting in which the service is provided, the determination to utilize physical therapist assistants for selected interventions requires the education, expertise and professional judgment of a physical therapist as described by the *Standards of Practice, Guide to Professional Conduct and Code of Ethics.*

In determining the appropriate extent of assistance from the physical therapist assistant (PTA), the physical therapist considers:

• The PTA's education, training, experience and skill level.
• Patient client criticality, acuity, stability and complexity.
• The predictability of the consequences.
• The setting in which the care is being delivered.
• Federal and state statutes.
• Liability and risk management concerns.
• The mission of physical therapy services for the setting.
• The needed frequency of reexamination.

Physical Therapist Assistant

Definition The physical therapist assistant is a technically educated healthcare provider who assists the physical therapist in the provision of physical therapy. The physical therapist assistant is a graduate of a physical therapist assistant associate degree program accredited by the Commission on Accreditation in Physical Therapy Education (CAPTE).

Utilization The physical therapist is directly responsible for the actions of the physical therapist assistant related to patient/client management. The physical therapist assistant may perform selected physical therapy interventions under the direction and at least general supervision of the physical therapist. In general supervision, the physical therapist is not required to be on-site for direction and supervision, but must be available at least by telecommunications. The ability of the physical therapist assistant to perform the selected interventions as directed shall be assessed on an ongoing basis by the supervising physical therapist. The physical therapist assistant makes modifications to selected interventions either to progress the patient/client as directed by the physical therapist or to ensure patient/client safety and comfort.

The physical therapist assistant must work under the direction and at least general supervision of the physical therapist. In all practice settings, the performance of selected interventions by the physical therapist assistant must be consistent with safe and legal physical therapist practice and shall be predicated on the following factors: complexity and acuity of the patient's/client's needs; proximity and accessibility to the physical therapist; supervision available in the event of emergencies or critical events; and type of setting in which the service is provided.

When supervising the physical therapist assistant in any off-site setting, the following requirements must be observed:

1. A physical therapist must be accessible by telecommunications to the physical therapist assistant at all times while the physical therapist assistant is treating patients/clients.

2. There must be regularly scheduled and documented conferences with the physical therapist assistant regarding patients/clients, the frequency of which is determined by the needs of the patient/client and the needs of the physical therapist assistant.

3. In those situations in which a physical therapist assistant is involved in the care of a patient/client, a supervisory visit by the physical therapist will be made:

a. Upon the physical therapist assistant's request for reexamination, when a change in the plan of care is needed, prior to any planned discharge and in response to a change in the patient's/client's medical status.

b. At least once a month, or at a higher frequency when established by the physical therapist, in accordance with the needs of the patient/client.

c. A supervisory visit should include:
   i. An on-site reexamination of the patient/client.
   ii. On-site review of the plan of care with appropriate revision or termination.
   iii. Evaluation of need and recommendation for utilization of outside resources.

APPENDIX IV

American Physical Therapy Association House of Delegates

STANDARDS OF ETHICAL CONDUCT FOR THE PHYSICAL THERAPIST ASSISTANT AND GUIDE FOR CONDUCT OF THE PHYSICAL THERAPIST ASSISTANT—June 2000

Note: These are the current documents valid through June 30, 2010. Effective July 1, 2010 revised Standards and Guidelines will be in effect. Please see APPENDIX V.

Preamble

This document of the American Physical Therapy Association sets forth standards for the ethical conduct of the physical therapist assistant. All physical therapist assistants are responsible for maintaining high standards of conduct while assisting physical therapists. The physical therapist assistant shall act in the best interest of the patient/client. These standards of conduct shall be binding on all physical therapist assistants.

STANDARD 1

A physical therapist assistant shall respect the rights and dignity of all individuals and shall provide compassionate care.

STANDARD 2

A physical therapist assistant shall act in a trustworthy manner towards patients/clients.

STANDARD 3

A physical therapist assistant shall provide selected physical therapy interventions only under the supervision and direction of a physical therapist.

STANDARD 4

A physical therapist assistant shall comply with laws and regulations governing physical therapy.

STANDARD 5

A physical therapist assistant shall achieve and maintain competence in the provision of selected physical therapy interventions.

STANDARD 6

A physical therapist assistant shall make judgments that are commensurate with their educational and legal qualifications as a physical therapist assistant.

STANDARD 7

A physical therapist assistant shall protect the public and the profession from unethical, incompetent and illegal acts.

Guide for Conduct of the Physical Therapist Assistant
This *Guide for Conduct of the Physical Therapist Assistant* (Guide) is intended to serve physical therapist assistants

in interpreting the *Standards of Ethical Conduct for the Physical Therapist Assistant* (Standards) of the American Physical Therapy Association (APTA). The Guide provides guidelines by which physical therapist assistants may determine the propriety of their conduct. It is also intended to guide the development of physical therapist assistant students. The Standards and Guide apply to all physical therapist assistants. These guidelines are subject to change as the dynamics of the profession change and as new patterns of healthcare delivery are developed and accepted by the professional community and the public. This Guide is subject to monitoring and timely revision by the Ethics and Judicial Committee of the Association.

Interpreting Standards The interpretations expressed in this Guide reflect the opinions, decisions and advice of the Ethics and Judicial Committee. These interpretations are intended to guide a physical therapist assistant in applying general ethical principles to specific situations. They should not be considered inclusive of all situations that a physical therapist assistant may encounter.

STANDARD 1

A physical therapist assistant shall respect the rights and dignity of all individuals and shall provide compassionate care.

1.1 Attitude of a physical therapist assistant

    A. A physical therapist assistant shall recognize, respect and respond to individual and cultural difference with compassion and sensitivity.

    B. A physical therapist assistant shall be guided at all times by concern for the physical and psychological welfare of patients/clients.

    C. A physical therapist assistant shall not harass, abuse or discriminate against others.

STANDARD 2

A physical therapist assistant shall act in a trustworthy manner towards patients/clients.

2.1 Trustworthiness

    A. The physical therapist assistant shall always place the patient's/client's interest(s) above those of the physical therapist assistant. Working in the patient's/client's best interest requires sensitivity to the patient's/client's vulnerability and an effective working relationship between the physical therapist and the physical therapist assistant.

    B. A physical therapist assistant shall not exploit any aspect of the physical therapist assistant–patient/client relationship.

    C. A physical therapist assistant shall clearly identify him/herself as a physical therapist assistant to patients/clients.

    D. A physical therapist assistant shall conduct him/herself in a manner that supports the physical therapist–patient/client relationship.

    E. A physical therapist assistant shall not engage in any sexual relationship or activity, whether consensual or nonconsensual, with any patient/client entrusted to his/her care.

    F. A physical therapist assistant shall not invite, accept or offer gifts or other considerations that affect or give an appearance of affecting his/her provision of physical therapy interventions. See section 6.3.

2.2 Exploitation of Patients

A physical therapist assistant shall not participate in any arrangements in which patients/clients are exploited. Such arrangements include situations where referring sources enhance their personal incomes by referring to or recommending physical therapy services.

2.3 Truthfulness

    A. A physical therapist assistant shall not make statements that he/she knows or should know are false, deceptive, fraudulent or misleading.

    B. Although it cannot be considered unethical for a physical therapist assistant to own or have a financial interest in the production, sale or distribution of products/services, he/she must act in accordance with law and make full disclosure of his/her interest to patients/clients.

2.4 Confidential Information

    A. Information relating to the patient/client is confidential and shall not be communicated to a third party not involved in that patient's/client's care without the prior consent of the patient/client, subject to applicable law.

    B. A physical therapist assistant shall refer all requests for release of confidential information to the supervising physical therapist.

STANDARD 3

A physical therapist assistant shall provide selected physical therapy interventions only under the supervision and direction of a physical therapist.

3.1 Supervisory Relationship

    A. A physical therapist assistant shall provide interventions only under the supervision and direction of a physical therapist.

    B. A physical therapist assistant shall provide only those interventions that have been selected by the physical therapist.

    C. A physical therapist assistant shall not provide any interventions that are outside his/her education, training, experience or skill, and shall notify the responsible physical therapist of his/her inability to carry out the intervention. See sections 5.1 and 6.1.B.

    D. A physical therapist assistant may modify specific interventions within the plan of care established by the physical therapist in response to changes in the patient's/client's status.

E. A physical therapist assistant shall not perform examinations and evaluations, determine diagnoses and prognoses or establish or change a plan of care.

F. Consistent with the physical therapist assistant's education, training, knowledge and experience, he/she may respond to the patient's/client's inquiries regarding interventions that are within the established plan of care.

G. A physical therapist assistant shall have regular and ongoing communication with the physical therapist regarding the patient's/client's status.

STANDARD 4

A physical therapist assistant shall comply with laws and regulations governing physical therapy.

4.1 Supervision

A physical therapist assistant shall know and comply with applicable law. Regardless of the content of any law, a physical therapist assistant shall provide services only under the supervision and direction of a physical therapist.

4.2 Representation

A physical therapist assistant shall not hold him/herself out as a physical therapist.

STANDARD 5

A physical therapist assistant shall achieve and maintain competence in the provision of selected physical therapy interventions.

5.1 Competence

A physical therapist assistant shall provide interventions consistent with his/her level of education, training, experience and skill. See sections 3.1.C and 6.1.B.

5.2 Self-assessment

A physical therapist assistant shall engage in self-assessment in order to maintain competence.

5.3 Development

A physical therapist assistant shall participate in educational activities that enhance his/her basic knowledge and skills.

STANDARD 6

A physical therapist assistant shall make judgments that are commensurate with his/her educational and legal qualifications as a physical therapist assistant.

6.1 Patient Safety

A. A physical therapist assistant shall discontinue immediately any interventions(s) that, in his/her judgment, may be harmful to the patient/client and shall discuss his/her concerns with the physical therapist.

B. A physical therapist assistant shall not provide any interventions that are outside his/her education, training, experience or skill and shall notify the responsible physical therapist of his/her inability to carry out the intervention. See sections 3.1.C and 5.1.

C. A physical therapist assistant shall not perform interventions while his/her ability to do so safely is impaired.

6.2 Judgments of Patient/Client Status

If in the judgment of the physical therapist assistant, there is a change in the patient/client status he/she shall report this to the responsible physical therapist. See section 3.1.

6.3 Gifts and Other Considerations

A physical therapist assistant shall not invite, accept or offer gifts, monetary incentives or other consideration that affect or give an appearance of affecting his/her provision of physical therapy interventions. See section 2.1.F.

STANDARD 7

A physical therapist assistant shall protect the public and the profession from unethical, incompetent and illegal acts.

7.1 Consumer Protection

A physical therapist assistant shall report any conduct that appears to be unethical or illegal.

7.2 Organizational Employment

A. A physical therapist assistant shall inform his/her employer(s) and/or appropriate physical therapist of any employer practice that causes him or her to be in conflict with the Standards of Ethical Conduct for the Physical Therapist Assistant.

B. A physical therapist assistant shall not engage in any activity that puts him or her in conflict with the Standards of Ethical Conduct for the Physical Therapist Assistant, regardless of directives from a physical therapist or employer.

APPENDIX V

Standards of Ethical Conduct for the Physical Therapist Assistant —valid July 1, 2010.
American Physical Therapy Association's House of Delegates document:

STANDARDS OF ETHICAL CONDUCT FOR THE PHYSICAL THERAPIST ASSISTANT AND GUIDE FOR CONDUCT OF THE PHYSICAL THERAPIST ASSISTANT

Preamble

The Standards of Ethical Conduct for the Physical Therapist Assistant (Standards of Ethical Conduct) delineate the ethical obligations of all physical therapist assistants as determined by the House of Delegates of the American Physical Therapy Association (APTA). The Standards of Ethical Conduct provide a foundation for conduct to which all physical therapist assistants shall adhere. Fundamental to the Standards of Ethical Conduct is the special obligation of physical therapist assistants to enable patients/clients to achieve greater independence, health and wellness and enhanced quality of life.

No document that delineates ethical standards can address every situation. Physical therapist assistants are encouraged to seek additional advice or consultation in instances where the guidance of the Standards of Ethical Conduct may not be definitive.

STANDARDS:

Standard #1: Physical therapist assistants shall respect the inherent dignity and rights of all individuals.

1A. Physical therapist assistants shall act in a respectful manner toward each person regardless of age, gender, race, nationality, religion, ethnicity, social or economic status, sexual orientation, health condition or disability.

1B. Physical therapist assistants shall recognize their personal biases and shall not discriminate against others in the provision of physical therapy services.

Standard #2: Physical therapist assistants shall be trustworthy and compassionate in addressing the rights and needs of patients/clients.

2A. Physical therapist assistants shall act in the best interests of patients/clients over the interests of the physical therapist assistant.

2B. Physical therapist assistants shall provide physical therapy interventions with compassionate and caring behaviors that incorporate the individual and cultural differences of patients/clients.

2C. Physical therapist assistants shall provide patients/clients with information regarding the interventions they provide.

2D. Physical therapist assistants shall protect confidential patient/client information and, in collaboration with the physical therapist, may disclose confidential information to appropriate authorities only when allowed or as required by law.

Standard #3: Physical therapist assistants shall make sound decisions in collaboration with the physical therapist and within the boundaries established by laws and regulations.

3A. Physical therapist assistants shall make objective decisions in the patient's/client's best interest in all practice settings.

3B. Physical therapist assistants shall be guided by information about best practice regarding physical therapy interventions.

3C. Physical therapist assistants shall make decisions based upon their level of competence and consistent with patient/client values.

3D. Physical therapist assistants shall not engage in conflicts of interest that interfere with making sound decisions.

3E. Physical therapist assistants shall provide physical therapy services under the direction and supervision of a physical therapist and shall communicate with the physical therapist when patient/client status requires modifications to the established plan of care.

Standard #4: Physical therapist assistants shall demonstrate integrity in their relationships with patients/clients, families, colleagues, students, other healthcare providers, employers, payers and the public.

4A. Physical therapist assistants shall provide truthful, accurate and relevant information and shall not make misleading representations.

4B. Physical therapist assistants shall not exploit persons over whom they have supervisory, evaluative or other authority (e.g., patients/clients, students, supervisees, research participants or employees).

4C. Physical therapist assistants shall discourage misconduct by healthcare professionals and report illegal or unethical acts to the relevant authority, when appropriate.

4D. Physical therapist assistants shall report suspected cases of abuse involving children or vulnerable adults to the supervising physical therapist and the appropriate authority, subject to law.

4E. Physical therapist assistants shall not engage in any sexual relationship with any of their patients/clients, supervisees or students.

CHAPTER 14

4F. Physical therapist assistants shall not harass anyone verbally, physically, emotionally or sexually.

Standard #5: Physical therapist assistants shall fulfill their legal and ethical obligations.

5A. Physical therapist assistants shall comply with applicable local, state and federal laws and regulations.

5B. Physical therapist assistants shall support the supervisory role of the physical therapist to ensure quality care and promote patient/client safety.

5C. Physical therapist assistants involved in research shall abide by accepted standards governing protection of research participants.

5D. Physical therapist assistants shall encourage colleagues with physical, psychological or substance-related impairments that may adversely impact their professional responsibilities to seek assistance or counsel.

5E. Physical therapist assistants who have knowledge that a colleague is unable to perform his or her professional responsibilities with reasonable skill and safety shall report this information to the appropriate authority.

Standard #6: Physical therapist assistants shall enhance their competence through the lifelong acquisition and refinement of knowledge, skills and abilities.

6A. Physical therapist assistants shall achieve and maintain clinical competence.

6B. Physical therapist assistants shall engage in life-long learning consistent with changes in their roles and responsibilities and advances in the practice of physical therapy.

6C. Physical therapist assistants shall support practice environments that support career development and lifelong learning.

Standard #7: Physical therapist assistants shall support organizational behaviors and business practices that benefit patients/clients and society.

7A. Physical therapist assistants shall promote work environments that support ethical and accountable decision-making.

7B. Physical therapist assistants shall not accept gifts or other considerations that influence or give an appearance of influencing their decisions.

7C. Physical therapist assistants shall fully disclose any financial interest they have in products or services that they recommend to patients/clients.

7D. Physical therapist assistants shall ensure that documentation for their interventions accurately reflects the nature and extent of the services provided.

7E. Physical therapist assistants shall refrain from employment arrangements, or other arrangements, that prevent physical therapist assistants from fulfilling ethical obligations to patients/clients.

Standard #8: Physical therapist assistants shall participate in efforts to meet the health needs of people locally, nationally or globally.

8A. Physical therapist assistants shall support organizations that meet the health needs of people who are economically disadvantaged, uninsured and underinsured.

8B. Physical therapist assistants shall advocate for people with impairments, activity limitations, participation restrictions and disabilities in order to promote their participation in community and society.

8C. Physical therapist assistants shall be responsible stewards of healthcare resources by collaborating with physical therapists in order to avoid overutilization or under-utilization of physical therapy services.

8D. Physical therapist assistants shall educate members of the public about the benefits of physical therapy.

Proviso: The Standards of Ethical Conduct for the Physical Therapist Assistant as substituted will take effect July 1, 2010, to allow for education of APTA members and nonmembers.

Guide for Conduct of the Physical Therapist Assistant
This *Guide for Conduct of the Physical Therapist Assistant* (Guide) is intended to serve physical therapist assistants in interpreting the *Standards of Ethical Conduct for the Physical Therapist Assistant* (Standards) of the American Physical Therapy Association (APTA). The Guide provides guidelines by which physical therapist assistants may determine the propriety of their conduct. It is also intended to guide the development of physical therapist assistant students. The Standards and Guide apply to all physical therapist assistants. These guidelines are subject to change as the dynamics of the profession change and as new patterns of healthcare delivery are developed and accepted by the professional community and the public. This Guide is subject to monitoring and timely revision by the Ethics and Judicial Committee of the Association.

Interpreting Standards The interpretations expressed in this Guide reflect the opinions, decisions and advice of the Ethics and Judicial Committee. These interpretations are intended to guide a physical therapist assistant in applying general ethical principles to specific situations. They should not be considered inclusive of all situations that a physical therapist assistant may encounter.

Reference to Standards of Ethical Conduct for the Physical Therapist Assistant In light of the recent amendments to the *Standards of Ethical Conduct for the Physical Therapist Assistant* and in lieu of setting forth in the Guide interpretations of the *Standards of Ethical Conduct for the Physical Therapist Assistant*, the Ethics and Judicial Committee does hereby refer Physical Therapist Assistants to the *Standards of Ethical Conduct for the Physical Therapist Assistant*.

chapter *15*

Research and Evidence-Based Practice

PATTY PENNELL

Evidence-Based Practice

Definition of Evidence-Based Practice

1. Evidence-based medicine is the conscientious, explicit and judicious use of current best evidence in making decisions about the care of individual patients.

2. The practice of evidence-based medicine means integrating individual clinical expertise, and the wishes, desires and goals of the patient or client with the best available external clinical evidence from systematic research.

Incorporating Clinical Decisions Into Practice

1. Clinicians who are considered evidence-based practitioners.
   a. Consistently read clinically relevant research.
   b. Identify relevancy of research to tests, measures, interventions and approaches used in patient management.
   c. Utilize research results to select interventions based on the evidence to support their use.

Research Resources

PubMed

1. MEDLINE database of citations, abstracts and some full-text articles on life sciences and biomedical topics.

2. The US National Library of Medicine at the National Institutes of Health maintains this database.

Cochrane Library

1. A collection of databases in medicine and other healthcare specialties.

2. Provided by the Cochrane Collaboration and other organizations.

The Cumulative Index to Nursing and Allied Health Literature (CINAHL)

1. The professional source for full-text articles from more than 580 journals in nursing and allied health.

EBCSOhost

1. A fee-based search engine providing access to reference databases.

2. Including: Academic Search Premier, America: History & Life, ATLA Religion Database, Business Source Premier, Catholic Periodical and Literature Index.

Google Scholar

1. A freely accessible Web search engine that indexes full-text articles.

2. Includes scholarly literature across an array of publishing formats and disciplines.

Stages of Scientific Method

Scientific Method

1. Definition: principles and procedures for the systematic pursuit of knowledge involving:
   a. The recognition and formulation of a problem.
   b. The collection of data through observation and experiment.
   c. The formulation and testing of a hypothesis.

Literature Review

1. Involves the surveying of scholarly articles, books and other sources (e.g., dissertations, conference proceedings) relevant to a particular issue, area of research or theory, providing a description, summary and critical evaluation of each work.

2. Purpose is to offer an overview of significant literature published on a topic.

Hypothesis Development

1. A tentative assumption made to draw out and test its logical or empirical consequence.

2. Specifies the purpose of a study.

Method

1. Criteria for and methods of subject selection.

2. Description and number of subjects.

3. Measurement methods.

4. Data analysis procedure.

Data Collection

1. Data are collected and recorded.

2. Information is placed in a usable form for analysis.

Table 15-1 ➤ ELECTRONIC MEDICAL DATABASES

PubMed—US National Library of Medicine's search service to Medline and Pre-Medline (database of medical and biomedical research)	http://www.ncbi.nlm.nih.gov/pubmed/
APTA Open Door - Hooked on Evidence (database of evidence-based physical therapy practice)	http://www.apta.org/AM/Template.cfm?Section=Research&Template=/MembersOnly
Cochrane Database of Systemic Reviews (Cochrane Reviews) (database of systematic reviews of RCTs; primary source for clinical effectiveness information)	http://www.www.cochrane.org/reviews
CINAHL (database of nursing and allied health research)	http://www.cinahl.com
Physiotherapy Evidence Database (PEDro) (database of physical therapy RCTs, systematic reviews, and evidence-based clinical practice guidelines)	http://www.pedro.fhs.usyd.edu.au/index.html
The Sheffield Evidence for Effectiveness and Knowledge	http://www.shef.ac.uk/seek/infosearch.htm#guide
The Centre for Health Evidence	http://www.cche.net/usersguides/start.asp#Tracking
ERIC (database of education research)	http://www.eric.ed.gov/
Ovid (database of health and lifescience research)	http://www.ovid.com
DARE (database of abstracts of reviews of evidence from medical journals)	http://www.york.ac.uk/inst/crd/crddatabases.htm
RehabDATA (database of disability and rehabilitation research)	http://www.naric.com/research
Center for International Rehabilitation Research Information and Exchange (database of rehabilitation research)	http://www.cirrie.buffalo.edu?

Results

1. Narrative description of statistical outcomes.

2. Tables and figures to summarize findings.

3. Support or reject hypothesis.

Discussion

1. Interpretation of statistical outcomes.

2. Discussion of clinical significance.

3. Comparison of results with work of others.

4. Critique of the study limitations and strengths.

5. Suggestions for further study.

Methods

Types of Research

1. Descriptive research.
   a. Involves questionnaires, interviews or direct observations.
   b. Designed to document conditions, attitudes or characteristics of individuals or groups of individuals.
   c. Forms of descriptive research.
      (1) Case study: a form of descriptive research that typically involves in-depth description of an individual's conditions or response to treatment.
      (2) Developmental research: the description of developmental change and the sequencing of behaviors in people over time.
      (3) Longitudinal study: a researcher follows a cohort of subjects over time, performing repeated measurements.

2. Normative research: describes typical or standard values for characteristics of a given population.

3. Qualitative research: seeks to describe the complex nature of humans and how individuals perceive their own experiences with a specific social event.

4. Exploratory research.
   a. Systematic investigation of relationships among two or more variables.
   b. Usually guided by a set of hypotheses that help with measurements and interpretation of findings.

5. Correlation research.
   a. Correlation: a measure of the degree of association among variables.
   b. Correlation research describes the nature of existing relationships among variables.

6. Experimental research.
   a. Attempts to define cause-and-effect relationship through group comparison.
   b. True experimental design: random assignment into experimental group (receives treatment) and control group (no treatment).
   c. Subject design (repeated measures): subjects serve as their own control.
      (1) Randomly assigned to treatment or no treatment groups.

7. Causal comparative research.
   a. Attempts to define cause-and-effect relationship through group comparisons.

Data Collection Techniques

1. Surveys: a series of questions that are posed to a group of respondents.
   a. Interview: researcher asks the respondent specific questions.
   b. Questionnaires: structured surveys that are self-administered.
   c. Self report: survey data that are collected via either an oral interview or a written questionnaire.

2. Direct observation.

Variables

1. Independent variable: the activity or factor that brought about change in the independent variable; the cause or treatment.

2. Dependent variable: the change or the difference in behavior that results from the intervention (independent variable); the outcome that is being measured.

Important Terminology

1. **Validity:** the degree to which an instrument measures what it is intended to measure.

2. **Reliability:** the degree of consistency with which an instrument or rater measures a variable.

3. **Interrater reliability:** the degree to which two or more raters can obtain the same ratings for a given variable.

4. **Intrarater reliability:** the degree to which one rater can obtain the same rating on multiple occasions of measuring.

Definitions and Grading of Evidence

Definitions

1. **Systematic review including meta-analysis.**
   a. A review in which the primary studies are summarized, critically appraised and statistically combined.
   b. Usually quantitative in nature with specific inclusion and exclusion criteria.
   c. Pros.
   d. Cons.

2. **Randomized Control Trial/Study.**
   a. An experimental study in which participants are randomly assigned to either an experimental or control group to receive different interventions or a placebo.

3. **Case report (study).**
   a. A type of descriptive research in which only one individual is studied in depth.
   b. Often done retrospectively (after intervention has been performed or completed).

Levels of Evidence

1. **Graded on a scale from level 1 to level 5.**
   a. Each level is also associated with a letter grade: A, B, C, D.
   b. Rank ordered with level 1A being the highest grade, and level 5D the lowest.

2. **Level 1, grade A and B criteria.**
   a. Include randomized, large, multicenter systematic review.
   b. Substantial agreement of size and direction of treatment effects; treatment effects are precisely defined.

3. **Level 2, grade A and B criteria.**
   a. Systematic review with homogeneity of the comparison groups.
   b. Is prospective (patients are identified before outcomes are achieved).
   c. A quality study would include more than 80% follow-up of patients enrolled in study.

4. **Level 3, grade A and B criteria.**
   a. Systematic review with homogeneity of case–control studies (case comparisons).
   b. Retrospective: patients identified for study after outcomes have been achieved.

5. **Level 4 and 5.**
   a. Considered poor quality; information gleaned from these should not necessarily be used to direct patient intervention or physical therapy practice.
   b. Examples include.
      (1) Case-series and poor-quality cohort and case–control studies.
      (2) Largely dispersive studies.
      (3) Expert opinion.
      (4) Observations not made on patients.

Outcome Measurement Tools

Tools Used to Assess Musculoskeletal Pain

1. **DASH (Disabilities of the Arm, Shoulder and Hand).**
   a. A 30-item, self-report questionnaire.
   b. Designed to measure physical function and symptoms in people with any of several musculoskeletal disorders of the upper limb.

2. **Oswestry Disability Index.**
   a. A 10-item questionnaire used to measure the function of people with low back pain.

3. **NDI (Neck Disability Index).**
   a. Used to measure function of patients with neck pain.
   b. Modified from the Oswestry Disability Index.
   c. A self-report questionnaire that measures physical function and symptoms; has been proven to be valid and reliable.

Balance Measurement Tools

1. **Berg Balance Scale.**
   a. A test of 14 balance tasks that are made up of activities from everyday living.
   b. Provides baseline data predictive of falls in the elderly.
   c. High validity scores; high inter- and intrarater reliability scores.

2. **Performance Oriented Mobility Assessment (POMA; Tinetti).**
   a. A test assessing dynamic and static balance as well as gait.
   b. Provides baseline data predictive of falls in the elderly.
   c. High validity scores; high interrater reliability scores, lower intrarater reliability scores.

3. **Timed Up and Go Test (TUG).**
   a. A test consisting of timing the performance of standing up, walking 10 feet (3 m), turning around, returning to and sitting in a chair.
   b. Provides baseline data predictive of falls in the elderly.
   c. Expert consensus on validity, lower validity scores when compared with other balance tests; high inter- and intrarater reliability scores.

Computer Simulated Examinations

Examinations are on the enclosed compact disk. Follow the procedure to complete the simulated examinations on the disk. After you complete the examinations, your performance will be analyzed in six domains and five categories. Then you may refer to the following questions with correct answers and rationales.

Questions with Answers and Rationales

DOMAINS

- **I.** Cardiovascular, Pulmonary
- **II.** Musculoskeletal
- **III.** Neuromuscular
- **IV.** Integumentary
- **V.** Other Systems, Metabolic-Endocrine, GI, Multisystem
- **VI.** Devices, Modalities, Evidence-based Practice, Administration, Ethics, Teaching

CATEGORIES

- **A.** Clinical Applications
- **B.** Data Collection
- **C.** Interventions
- **D.** Equipment, Devices, Modalities
- **E.** Safety, Professional Roles, Teaching, Evidence-based Practice

CRITICAL REASONING STRATEGIES

 Inductive Reasoning

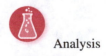 Inference

Analysis

Deductive Reasoning

Evaluation

Examination A

A patient sustained a fracture to the left proximal humerus, which is now healed. Treatment is proceeding well except that the left scapula protracts, elevates early and moves excessively with shoulder flexion. Physical therapy intervention should emphasize:

CHOICES:

1. stretching of scapular stabilizers and strengthening of the pectoralis major and minor muscles to regain muscle balance.
2. scapulothoracic mobilization and strengthening of the pectoralis major and minor muscles to regain normal scapulo-humeral rhythm.
3. glenohumeral mobilization and strengthening of scapular stabilizers to regain normal scapulohumeral movement.
4. glenohumeral mobilization, and strengthening of the rotator cuff muscles to regain muscle balance.

CORRECT ANSWER: 3

RATIONALE:

Compensation for glenohumeral restrictions is often exhibited as excessive scapular movement. Therefore, mobilization of the glenohumeral joint and strengthening of scapular stabilizers is needed to regain normal scapulohumeral motion.

TYPE OF REASONING: INDUCTIVE

One must determine the best therapeutic approach for a patient with excessive scapular movement. This requires knowledge of the diagnosis and therapeutic approaches for it, which is an inductive reasoning skill. For this case, the assistant should emphasize glenohumeral mobilization and strengthening the scapular stabilizers. If answered incorrectly, review intervention approaches for excessive scapular movement.

A2 | Cardiovascular/Pulmonary | Clinical Applications

A physical therapist assistant is supervising the exercise of cardiac rehabilitation outpatient class on a very hot day, with temperatures expected to be above 90°F. The class is scheduled for 2 p.m. and the facility is not air conditioned. The **BEST** strategy is to:

CHOICES:

1. decrease the exercise intensity by slowing the pace of exercise.
2. increase the warm-up period to equal the total aerobic interval in time.
3. keep the same time of the exercise class because of scheduling requirements.
4. shift to intermittent exercise but decrease the rest time.

CORRECT ANSWER: 1

RATIONALE:

Clinical decisions should focus on reducing the environmental costs of exercising (change the time of day of the exercise class to reduce the heat stress) or reducing the overall metabolic costs of the activity (decrease the pace of exercise, add more rest periods). Altering the warm-up period does not lower the overall cost of the aerobic exercise period.

TYPE OF REASONING: EVALUATIVE

One must determine a best course of action for a group of clients exercising in hot temperatures. The test taker must weigh the potential courses of action and outcomes to arrive at a correct conclusion, which is an evaluative reasoning skill. For this case, the best strategy is to decrease the exercise intensity by slowing the pace of exercise. If answered incorrectly, review cardiac rehabilitation guidelines, including exercise in warmer temperatures.

A3 | Devices, Admin, etc. | Equipment, Modalities

A patient has a transtibial amputation and has recently been fitted with a patellar tendon–bearing (PTB) socket. During gait training, the physical therapist assistant instructs the patient to walk several times in the parallel bars and then sit down and take the prosthesis off. Upon inspection of the skin the assistant should NOT expect to find redness in the pressure-sensitive area of the:

CHOICES:

1. anterior tibia and tibial crest.
2. patellar tendon and tibial tuberosity.
3. medial tibial and fibular plateaus.
4. medial and lateral distal ends of the residual limb.

CORRECT ANSWER: 1

RATIONALE:

In a PTB socket, reliefs are provided for pressure-sensitive areas: the anterior tibia and tibial crest, fibular head and peroneal nerve. All the other choices are considered pressure-tolerant areas.

TYPE OF REASONING: INFERENTIAL

One must infer or draw a reasonable conclusion about gait training with a PTB socket and areas that are not likely to show redness after walking. This requires one to determine what may not occur with the patient, necessitating an inferential reasoning skill. For this situation, one should not expect to find redness on the anterior tibia and tibial crest. If answered incorrectly, review properties of a PTB socket and pressure relief.

A4 | Devices, Admin, etc. | Equipment, Modalities

The plan of care indicates ultrasound treatment for a muscle spasm of the piriformis. The piriformis is compressing the sciatic nerve and producing pain in the posterior hip region. The pain has been worsening over the past 3 months. What is the **MOST** beneficial ultrasound setting for this case?

CHOICES:

1. 1 MHz pulsed at 1.0 w/cm.²
2. 3 MHz continuous at 1.0 w/cm.²
3. 3 MHz pulsed at 1.0 w/cm.²
4. 1 MHz continuous at 1.0 w/cm.²

CORRECT ANSWER: 4

RATIONALE:

One MHz of continuous ultrasound provides deep heating to a depth of 3 cm to 5 cm. At this frequency, attenuation (absorption) is less in superficial tissues. This allows more energy to be absorbed; thus, more heat is produced in deeper tissue layers. Continuous ultrasound is applied to achieve thermal effects (e.g., for chronic pain) and pulsed ultrasound is used when nonthermal effects are desired (e.g., for acute soft-tissue injuries).

TYPE OF REASONING: INDUCTIVE

This question requires one to determine the most beneficial ultrasound setting for a patient with a muscle spasm of the piriformis. This requires clinical judgment to arrive at a correct conclusion, necessitating inductive reasoning skill. For this scenario, it is most beneficial to administer ultrasound at 1 MHz continuously at 1.0 w/cm² to achieve desired deep-heating thermal effects. If answered incorrectly, review ultrasound guidelines for patients with chronic pain.

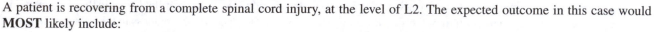

A5 | Neuromuscular | Clinical Applications

A patient is recovering from a complete spinal cord injury, at the level of L2. The expected outcome in this case would **MOST** likely include:

CHOICES:

1. a spastic or reflex bladder.
2. some recovery of function because damage is to peripheral nerve roots.
3. loss of motor function and pain and temperature sensation below the level of the lesion with light touch, proprioception and position sense preserved.
4. greater loss of upper-extremity function than of lower-extremity function with early loss of pain and temperature sensation.

CORRECT ANSWER: 2

RATIONALE:

A spinal cord lesion below L1 is a cauda equina lesion (injury to peripheral roots and nerves). Because some regeneration is possible, some recovery in function can be expected. A spastic or reflex bladder is associated with upper motor neuron injury. Other choices describe the deficits associated with anterior cord syndrome or central cord syndrome.

TYPE OF REASONING: INFERENTIAL

One must determine the most likely outcome for a patient with a complete spinal cord injury to arrive at a correct conclusion. Questions that require the test taker to project what may occur in the future often require inferential reasoning skill. For this case, the patient would most likely demonstrate some recovery of function because damage is to peripheral nerve roots. If answered incorrectly, review outcomes for cauda equina spinal cord injuries.

A6 | Devices, Admin, etc. | Safety, Roles, Teaching, EBP

A physical therapist assistant is gait training a patient with left hemiplegia who has recently been fitted with a new ankle–foot orthosis. The assistant is overwhelmed with too many patients and asks the physical therapist assistant student to take over. This is the student's first affiliation (second day) and the student has never performed tissue inspection for a patient with an ankle–foot orthosis. The assistant will be in the same vicinity treating other patients. This task should be:

CHOICES:

1. given to the student who could call out to the supervisor if problems arose.
2. given to the physical therapist in charge of the case.
3. given to another physical therapist assistant who is working in a nearby treatment room.
4. not be completed now and the patient should be sent back to his room.

CORRECT ANSWER: 2

RATIONALE:

Physical therapy students should not perform advanced tasks for the first time without any instruction or direct supervision. This might be unsafe for the patient. The task of tissue inspection is most appropriately performed by an experienced physical therapist assistant or physical therapist. In this case, the physical therapist is the most appropriate practitioner to perform the examination.

TYPE OF REASONING: EVALUATIVE

This question requires one to determine a best course of action when staffing issues are present in a busy clinic and a student is present. This requires one to weigh the courses of action and determine an appropriate response, which requires evaluative reasoning skill. For this case, because the student has not performed the task before, the task of tissue inspection should be given to the physical therapist in charge of the case. If answered incorrectly, review student supervisory guidelines.

A7 | Musculoskeletal | Interventions

A patient has been diagnosed with acute synovitis of the temporomandibular joint. Which intervention would be MOST BENEFICIAL to help resolve early stage acute inflammation?

CHOICES:

1. application of an intraoral appliance and phonophoresis.
2. joint mobilization and postural awareness.
3. instruction to eat a soft-food diet and phonophoresis.
4. temporalis stretching and joint mobilization.

CORRECT ANSWER: 3

RATIONALE:

Phonophoresis and education regarding consumption of only soft food could help resolve the acute inflammatory process in the temporomandibular joint. Application of an intraoral appliance occurs only when the acute inflammation is not resolved or bruxism continues. Joint mobilization should not be attempted with an acute inflammation.

TYPE OF REASONING: INDUCTIVE

One must utilize knowledge of intervention approaches for the temporomandibular joint to arrive at a correct conclusion. This necessitates clinical judgment, which is an inductive reasoning skill. For this situation, the most beneficial intervention approach is instruction to eat a soft-food diet and phonophoresis. If answered incorrectly, review intervention approaches for patients with acute synovitis of the temporomandibular joint.

A8 | Neuromuscular | Data Collection

An appropriate fine motor behavior that should be established by 9 months of age would be the ability to:

CHOICES:

1. pick up a raisin with a fine pincer grasp.
2. build a tower of 4 blocks.
3. hold a cup by the handle while drinking.
4. transfer objects from one hand to another.

CORRECT ANSWER: 4

RATIONALE:

Transferring objects from one hand to another is a task developmentally appropriate for an 8- or 9-month-old. Using a fine pincer grasp and building a tower of 4 blocks are skills that develop later. Holding a cup by the handle while drinking usually occurs by 12 months of age.

TYPE OF REASONING: DEDUCTIVE

For this question, the test taker must recall developmental guidelines of infants in fine motor skills to arrive at a correct conclusion. This requires recall of factual information, which is a deductive reasoning skill. For this case, a 9-month-old infant should demonstrate transfer of objects from one hand to another. Review developmental milestones of infants, especially fine motor skills, if answered incorrectly.

A9 | Devices, Admin, etc. | Safety, Roles, Teaching, EBP

A patient who is to undergo surgery for a chronic shoulder dislocation asks the physical therapist assistant to explain the rehabilitation following a scheduled surgical reconstructive procedure. The assistant's **BEST** response is to:

CHOICES:

1. explain in detail about the surgical procedure.
2. tell the patient to ask the surgeon for information about the procedure and appropriate rehabilitation.
3. explain how patients typically respond to the surgery and outline the progression of exercises.
4. refer the patient to a physical therapy clinical specialist who is an expert on shoulder reconstructive rehabilitation.

CORRECT ANSWER: 3

RATIONALE:

The physical therapist assistant should assess the needs of the patient and provide appropriate information based on the expected rehabilitation process. Physical therapist assistants should be knowledgeable about rehabilitation following orthopedic surgeries. Do not "pass the buck" unless the information is outside the assistant's scope of work. Information about the surgical procedure is in the realm of the surgeon. Rehabilitation is the physical therapy domain.

TYPE OF REASONING: EVALUATIVE

One must determine the best course of action when explaining the rehabilitation process to a patient about to undergo surgery. One must evaluate the courses of action provided and determine the one that effectively addresses the patient's needs. This is an evaluative reasoning skill. For this scenario, the assistant should explain how patients typically respond to the surgery and outline the progression of exercises. If answered incorrectly, review scope of practice guidelines for the physical therapist assistant.

A10 | Cardiovascular/Pulmonary | Data Collection

To correctly measure the circumference of a patient's calf following a knee arthroplasty a physical therapist assistant should measure beginning at the:

CHOICES:

1. area of the greatest edema, then 2 inches proximal and 2 inches distal.
2. inferior angle of the greater trochanter of that extremity and continuing distally until the inferior angle of the lateral malleolus.
3. inferior angle of the lateral malleolus, and in 2- to 4-inch increments proximally, stopping proximal to the edematous area.
4. bend of the knee and proceeding distally every 2 cm, stopping distal to the edematous area.

CORRECT ANSWER: 3

RATIONALE:

Circumferential measurement must be based from a bony landmark that is reproducible for future measurements; the option above including the greater trochanter does begin with a bony landmark; however, it includes the entire thigh and would not be necessary for edema in the gastric area. Soft tissues change with changes in edema and are not a reproducible landmark from which to base measurements. The measurements should include areas immediately proximal and distal to the edematous area. Circumferential measurements are best taken with an anthropometric measuring tape that has a pressure gauge on one end to ensure consistent pressure on the tape during measurement.

TYPE OF REASONING: DEDUCTIVE

This question requires the test taker to recall the procedures for circumferential measurement of a patient's calf following a total knee arthroplasty. This necessitates the recall of guidelines and procedures, which is a deductive reasoning skill. For this case, the assistant should measure beginning at the inferior angle of the lateral malleolus, and in 4-inch increments proximally, stopping proximal to the edematous area. If answered incorrectly, review the circumferential measurement procedures for the lower extremity.

A11 | Neuromuscular | Interventions

A patient with a complete T10 paraplegia is receiving initial ambulation training. The patient has received bilateral knee–ankle–foot orthoses and is being trained with axillary crutches. Because a reciprocal gait pattern is problematic for the patient, the **BEST INITIAL** gait pattern to teach is:

CHOICES:

1. 4-point.
2. swing-to.
3. 2-point.
4. swing-through.

CORRECT ANSWER: 2

RATIONALE:

A swing-to gait pattern is indicated for individuals with limited use of both lower extremities and trunk instability. It is slower and more stable than a swing-through gait pattern (a gait pattern this patient can be progressed to after initial training). This patient is unable to perform a reciprocal gait.

TYPE OF REASONING: INDUCTIVE

This question requires the test taker to determine the best initial gait pattern for a patient with T10 paraplegia. This requires knowledge of the diagnosis and typical gait patterns to arrive at a correct conclusion. This necessitates inductive reasoning skill. For this case, the assistant should teach a swing-to gait pattern. Review gait patterns and gait training for patients with T10 paraplegia if answered incorrectly.

A12 | Devices, Admin, etc. | Safety, Roles, Teaching, EBP

After mastectomy, a patient receiving home care cannot accept the loss of her breast. She reports being weepy all the time with loss of sleep. She is constantly tired and has no energy to do anything. The **BEST** action the assistant can take is to:

CHOICES:

1. contact the supervising physical therapist and suggest a psychological consult.
2. tell the nurse case manager to monitor the patient closely.
3. tell her depression is common at first, but will resolve with time.
4. have her spouse observe her closely for possible suicidal tendencies.

CORRECT ANSWER: 1

RATIONALE:

The patient is experiencing grief over her loss. Significant persistent symptoms are an indication for referral to a qualified professional (psychologist) to help her deal with her loss. She is no longer an inpatient; thus, a nurse case manager would not be able to regularly monitor her behavior. Depression does not necessarily resolve with time and is not an expected consequence of mastectomy. The patient has not expressed any suicidal tendencies. If so, after being informed by the assistant, the therapist would need to contact the physician immediately.

TYPE OF REASONING: EVALUATIVE

For this question, the test taker must determine a best course of action for a patient experiencing grief over the loss of her breast. This requires evaluative reasoning skill, as the test taker must weigh the courses of action to determine the best approach for the patient. For this case, the assistant should contact the supervising physical therapist and suggest a psychological consult. If answered incorrectly, review approaches for assisting patients dealing with grief and loss.

A13 | Other Systems | Clinical Applications

An individual with a body mass index (BMI) of 33 kg/m^2 is referred to an outpatient exercise program. The physical therapist assistant recognizes that this patient is at increased risk for:

CHOICES:

1. hyperthermia during exercise.
2. hypothermia during exercise.
3. rapid weight loss during the initial weeks.
4. increased anxiety and depression.

CORRECT ANSWER: 1

RATIONALE:

A patient with a BMI of 33 kg/m^2 is obese (BMI > 30 kg/m^2) and is at increased risk for hyperthermia during exercise (as well as orthopedic injury). Weight loss is the result of complex interplay between diet and exercise and not the result of exercise alone. A balanced program of exercise and diet will produce effects over time, not just in the initial weeks. An appropriately prescribed exercise program should decrease anxiety and depression.

TYPE OF REASONING: DEDUCTIVE

One must recall the risk factors for patients with obesity and engagement in exercise to arrive at a correct conclusion. This is factual information, necessitating deductive reasoning skill. For this scenario, patients with obesity are at an increased risk for hyperthermia during exercise. Review exercise guidelines for patients with obesity and risk factors if answered incorrectly.

A14 | Devices, Admin, etc. | Safety, Roles, Teaching, EBP

In a research study in which there is a skewed distribution with extreme scores on a balance measure that deviate from the performance of the total group, the **MOST** accurate representation of central tendency is:

CHOICES:
1. mean.
2. mode.
3. median.
4. standard deviation.

CORRECT ANSWER: 3

RATIONALE:
The mean is a measure of central tendency that is calculated by adding up all the scores and dividing the total by the number of scores. The median is the middle score and the mode is the most frequently occurring score. The most accurate measure of performance in skewed distribution with extreme scores is the median. Standard deviation is not a measure of central tendency.

TYPE OF REASONING: DEDUCTIVE
One must recall research guidelines including measures of central tendency to arrive at a correct conclusion. This is factual information and recall of a research definition, which is a deductive reasoning skill. For this case, the most accurate representation of central tendency is median. If answered incorrectly, review research terminology, especially median scores.

A15 | Devices, Admin, etc. | Equipment, Modalities

A patient is recovering from a right cerebrovascular accident (CVA) resulting in severe left hemiplegia and visuospatial deficits. Additionally, there is a large diabetic ulcer on the left foot with pitting edema. The **MOST** appropriate wheelchair prescription for this patient would be a:

CHOICES:
1. hemiplegic chair with elevating leg rest on the left.
2. powered wheelchair with joystick and elevating leg rests.
3. lightweight active duty wheelchair with elevating leg rests.
4. one-arm drive chair with elevating leg rest on the left.

CORRECT ANSWER: 1

RATIONALE:
A one-arm drive wheelchair has both drive mechanisms located on one wheel. The patient can propel the wheelchair by using one hand. It is contraindicated in patients with cognitive or perceptual deficits (as in this case). A hemiplegic chair has a low seat height ($17^1/_2$ inches compared with the standard seat height of $19^1/_2$ inches) and is the best choice for this patient. The patient propels it by using both the sound hand and the lower extremity. The electric wheelchair with joystick might also work but is significantly more expensive, less transportable and would require increased maintenance. An elevating leg rest is needed to complete the wheelchair prescription.

TYPE OF REASONING: INDUCTIVE
This question requires one to utilize clinical judgment to determine the most appropriate wheelchair prescription for a patient with a CVA and hemiplegia. This requires knowledge of wheelchair prescription guidelines and clinical judgment, which is an inductive reasoning skill. For this case, the most appropriate wheelchair is a hemiplegic chair with elevating leg rest on the left. If answered incorrectly, review wheelchair prescription guidelines for patients with CVA and hemiplegia.

A16 | Devices, Admin, etc. | Equipment, Modalities

A patient fractured the right mid-tibia in a skiing accident 3 months ago. After cast removal, a severe foot drop was noted. The plan of care includes electrical stimulation orthotic substitution. The physical therapist assistant should set up the functional electrical stimulation to contract the appropriate muscles during:

CHOICES:

1. heel-off (terminal stance).
2. swing phase.
3. foot flat (loading response).
4. toe-off (preswing).

CORRECT ANSWER: 2

RATIONALE:

Foot drop is a swing phase deficit. Stimulation of the dorsiflexor muscles during the swing phase places the foot in a more neutral position and prevents the toes from contacting the ground and interfering with the gait pattern.

TYPE OF REASONING: ANALYTICAL

One must analyze the deficits of the patient to determine the appropriate use of functional electrical stimulation during gait training. This requires analytical reasoning skill. For this situation, the functional electrical stimulation should be set up to contract the muscles during the swing phase. If answered incorrectly, review functional electrical stimulation guidelines for use with patients with foot drop.

A17 | Devices, Admin, etc. | Safety, Roles, Teaching, EBP

A physical therapist assistant has weeping dermatitis on the back of the hand. The assistant is scheduled to treat a patient with HIV for management of a wound. The assistant should:

CHOICES:

1. double glove and treat as scheduled.
2. use sterile precautions with mask and gloves.
3. continue with treatment as scheduled but wash hands thoroughly before and after.
4. refrain from patient care but arrange for treatment by another practitioner.

CORRECT ANSWER: 4

RATIONALE:

Blood and Body Fluid Precautionary Guidelines from the Centers for Disease Control and Prevention (CDC) state that a healthcare worker with exudative lesions or weeping dermatitis should refrain from all direct patient care and from handling patient-care equipment until the condition resolves.

TYPE OF REASONING: EVALUATIVE

One must utilize judgment to determine a best course of action when the assistant has weeping dermatitis and is scheduled to treat a patient with human immunodeficiency virus. This requires the test taker to weigh the courses of action to arrive at a correct conclusion. This necessitates evaluative reasoning skill. For this case, the assistant should refrain from treating the patient but arrange for treatment by another practitioner. If answered incorrectly, review CDC guidelines for treating patients with human immunodeficiency virus when one has weeping dermatitis.

A18 | Devices, Admin, etc. | Safety, Roles, Teaching, EBP

The initial evaluation for a patient with a right cerebrovascular accident (CVA) identifies that the patient has a profound deficit of homonymous hemianopsia. The **BEST INITIAL** strategy to assist the patient in compensating for this deficit is to:

CHOICES:

1. teach the patient to turn the head to the affected left side.
2. provide constant reminders, printed notes on the left side, telling the patient to look to the left.
3. place items, eating utensils on the patient's left side.
4. rearrange the room so while the patient is in bed the left side is facing the doorway.

CORRECT ANSWER: 1

RATIONALE:

A patient with homonymous hemianopsia needs to be made aware of his/her deficit and instructed to turn the head to the affected left side (a compensatory training strategy). The question asks for **Initial strategies**. Initial strategies include placing items on the right (unaffected side) or positioning the patient so that the doorway is on the right (unaffected side) so that the patient can successfully interact with the environment. Later, as there is ability to compensate, items can be moved to midline and finally to the affected left side. Placing items on the left (affected side) initially is too advanced for an initial strategy.

TYPE OF REASONING: INDUCTIVE

This question requires one to determine a best initial strategy for patient with a CVA and homonymous hemianopsia to arrive at a correct conclusion. This requires inductive reasoning skill. For this patient the assistant's best initial strategy is to teach the patient to turn the head to the affected left side. If answered incorrectly, review compensatory training strategies for patients with homonymous hemianopsia.

A19 | Neuromuscular | Clinical Applications

A patient with multiple sclerosis exhibits moderate fatigue during a 30-minute exercise session. When the patient returns for the next regularly scheduled session 2 days later, the patient reports going home after the last session and immediately going to bed. The patient was exhausted and unable to get out of bed until the late afternoon of the next day. The physical therapist assistant's **BEST** strategy is to:

CHOICES:

1. treat the patient in a warm, relaxing environment.
2. utilize a massed practice schedule.
3. utilize a distributed practice schedule.
4. switch the patient to a pool therapy program.

CORRECT ANSWER: 3

RATIONALE:

Common problems in multiple sclerosis include fatigue and heat intolerance. Exercise intensity should be reduced and a distributed practice schedule used in which rest times equal or exceed exercise times. A massed practice schedule in which the exercise time exceeds the rest time is contraindicated. A cool environment (e.g., cooling suit) can reduce heat intolerance and fatigue that commonly accompanies exercise. A warm environment or pool therapy in a warm pool are contraindicated as both can increase fatigue.

TYPE OF REASONING: INDUCTIVE

One must utilize clinical judgment to determine a best strategy for a patient with multiple sclerosis. This requires inductive reasoning skill. For this case, given the patient's experience with the previous treatment session, the best strategy is to utilize a distributed practice schedule. Review treatment scheduling for patients with multiple sclerosis to prevent fatigue if answered incorrectly.

A20 | Integumentary | Clinical Applications

A patient with a venous stasis ulcer near the left medial malleolus is referred for physical therapy. Skin changes consistent with stasis dermatitis are evident in the lower extremity. Palpation reveals patent femoral, popliteal and pedal pulses. An enlarged and dilated greater saphenous vein is evident in the standing position. The **MOST** important nonoperative physical therapy intervention for venous stasis ulcers is:

CHOICES:

1. daily walking for 30 to 60 minutes.
2. elastic wraps and daily exercises.
3. daily warm water baths and exercise.
4. compression therapy with exercise.

CORRECT ANSWER: 4

RATIONALE:

Compression therapy is the mainstay of nonoperative treatment of venous stasis ulcers and works with exercise to facilitate movement of excess fluid from the lower extremity. Dressings are applied before compression bandages. Pliable, non-stretchable dressing wraps (e.g., Unna boot) or custom-fitted graduated compression stockings can be used to assist in venous circulation. Elastic wraps are easy to apply but provide only light support and do little to assist circulation. Prolonged hydrotherapy is contraindicated for venous ulcers. Skin changes associated with venous disease include pigmentation, venous eczema and lipodermatosclerosis.

TYPE OF REASONING: INDUCTIVE

One must recall the treatment guidelines for patients with venous stasis ulcers to arrive at a correct conclusion. This necessitates clinical judgment, which is an inductive reasoning skill. For this situation, the most important nonoperative intervention is compression therapy with exercise. If answered incorrectly, review treatment guidelines for patients with venous stasis ulcers, including nonoperative approaches.

A21 | Neuromuscular | Clinical Applications

A patient recovering from stroke is having difficulty bearing weight on the left lower extremity. The patient is unable to advance the tibia forward and abbreviates the end of the stance phase on the left going directly into swing phase. Which factor following stroke is MOST LIKELY to result in failure to advance the lower extremity when walking?

CHOICES:

1. weakness or contracture of hip extensors.
2. spasticity or contracture of the plantar flexors.
3. spasticity of the anterior tibialis muscle.
4. weakness or contracture of the dorsiflexors.

CORRECT ANSWER: 2

RATIONALE:

Forward advancement of the tibia from midstance to heel-off is controlled by eccentric contraction of the plantar flexors; from heel-off to toe-off the plantar flexors contract concentrically. Either spasticity or contracture of the plantar flexors would limit this forward progression. Patients compensate by going right into swing, typically with a circumducted gait or with increased hip and knee flexion because there is no push-off. This is commonly seen in the patient with stroke.

TYPE OF REASONING: INFERENTIAL

One must infer or draw a reasonable conclusion about the most likely reason for failure to advance the lower extremity when walking after stroke. A test taker must determine what may be true of this situation, necessitating inferential reasoning skill. For this scenario, the likely reason for this failure is spasticity or contracture of the plantar flexors. If answered incorrectly, review gait patterns for patients with stroke, especially failure to advance the affected leg.

A22 | Other Systems | Data Collection

A physical therapist assistant observing functional activities of a child who is 4½ years old would **NOT** ordinarily expect the child to demonstrate the ability to perform:

CHOICES:
1. skilled tandem walking.
2. jumping down off a step.
3. toe-walking.
4. jumping from two feet.

CORRECT ANSWER: 1

RATIONALE:
The ability to perform tandem walking typically develops at 5+ years of age; one would not expect a 4½ year-old child to be able to perform this skill. The ability to perform jumping from two feet and jumping down off a step typically develop between the ages of 3 and 4 years of age. A physical therapist assistant performing an intervention with this child could expect the child to be able to perform the jumping tasks.

TYPE OF REASONING: INFERENTIAL
This question requires the test taker to infer or draw a reasonable conclusion about the functional activities of a child and abilities not likely to be seen for a child this age. This requires inferential reasoning skill. For this case, one should not expect to see skilled tandem walking at 4½ years of age. If answered incorrectly, review developmental milestones of young children, including motor skills of 4 year-olds.

A23 | Devices, Admin, etc. | Safety, Roles, Teaching, EBP

The **MOST** appropriate feedback strategy for a physical therapist assistant to utilize when providing gait training for a patient who has been receiving gait training for 3 weeks is:

CHOICES:
1. immediate feedback given after each practice trial.
2. intermittent feedback given at scheduled intervals, every other practice trial.
3. continuous feedback with ongoing verbal cuing during gait.
4. occasional feedback given when consistent errors appear.

CORRECT ANSWER: 4

RATIONALE:
In learning a psychomotor skill, the patient needs to be able to actively process information and self-correct responses. Occasional feedback provides the best means of allowing for introspection and is appropriate for later practice (associated and autonomous phases of motor learning).

TYPE OF REASONING: INDUCTIVE
This question requires the test taker to determine a best approach when one is providing feedback for a patient during gait training. This requires clinical judgment, which is an inductive reasoning skill. For this situation, after 3 weeks of gait training, the assistant should provide occasional feedback when consistent errors appear. Review gait training guidelines and the use of feedback to improve performance if answered incorrectly.

A24 | Cardiovascular/Pulmonary | Clinical Applications

A patient has class III heart disease and is continually in and out of congestive heart failure. Digitalis (digoxin) has been prescribed to improve the patient's heart function. The patient will demonstrate understanding of the adverse side effects of this medication by recognizing the importance of informing the physical therapist assistant of which of the following symptoms during exercise?

CHOICES:

1. confusion and memory loss.
2. slowed heart rate.
3. involuntary movements and shaking.
4. weakness and palpitations.

CORRECT ANSWER: 4

RATIONALE:

Class III heart disease is characterized by marked limitation of physical activity; the patient is comfortable at rest but less than ordinary physical activity causes fatigue, palpitations, dyspnea or anginal pain. Digitalis (digoxin) is frequently used to treat congestive heart failure (it slows heart rate and increases force of myocardial contraction). Adverse side effects of digitalis can include muscle weakness and supraventricular or ventricular arrhythmias, including ventricular fibrillation, without premonitory signs.

TYPE OF REASONING: INFERENTIAL

One must infer the response by the patient that indicates that the patient understands the adverse side effects of digitalis medication. This requires the test taker to determine what may be true of a situation, which is an inferential reasoning skill. For this case, the patient understands the adverse side effects of the medication if the patient knows to report symptoms of weakness and palpitations. If answered incorrectly, review side effects of digitalis medication.

A25 | Devices, Admin, etc. | Safety, Roles, Teaching, EBP

A physical therapist assistant is working with a patient with active hepatitis B infection. Transmission of the disease is **MOST** effectively minimized if the assistant:

CHOICES:

1. washes hands before and after treatment.
2. wears gloves during any direct contact with blood or body fluids.
3. has the patient wear a gown and mask during treatment.
4. has the patient wear gloves to prevent direct contact with the therapist.

CORRECT ANSWER: 2

RATIONALE:

Standard precautions specify that healthcare workers wear gloves when they come into direct contact with blood or body fluids. Healthcare workers should wear moisture-resistant gowns and masks for protection from the splashing of blood, other body fluids or respiratory droplets. Although hand washing is important, it is not as important as wearing gloves when direct contact is made with blood or body fluids.

TYPE OF REASONING: INFERENTIAL

One must determine the most effective means of minimizing exposure to the hepatitis B virus to arrive at a correct conclusion. This requires recall of guidelines regarding standard precautions first and then determining the most effective approach according to these guidelines, which is an inferential reasoning skill. For this situation, the most effective means of minimizing risk is to wear gloves during any direct contact with blood or body fluids. Review standard precautions for the hepatitis B virus if answered incorrectly.

A26 | Devices, Admin, etc. | Equipment, Modalities

A patient reports pain (7/10) and limited range of motion of the right shoulder as a result of chronic overuse. The therapist has identified procaine hydrochloride iontophoresis as part of physical therapy intervention for this patient's problems. To administer this substance, it would be appropriate to use:

CHOICES:
1. continuous biphasic current with the medication under the anode.
2. continuous monophasic current with the medication under the anode.
3. continuous monophasic current with the medication under the cathode.
4. interrupted biphasic current with the medication under the cathode.

CORRECT ANSWER: 2

RATIONALE:
Because like charges are repelled, the positively charged medication would be forced into the skin under the positive electrode (anode). A continuous, unidirectional current flow is very effective in repelling ions into the skin. A pulsed or bidirectional current generates less propulsive force owing to the discontinuous nature of the current. Procaine is a positive medicinal ion and will be repelled from the anode (positive pole).

TYPE OF REASONING: DEDUCTIVE
One must recall the guidelines for use of iontophoresis to arrive at a correct conclusion. This is factual information, which necessitates deductive reasoning skill. For this case, it is best to administer the substance with continuous monophasic current with the medication under the anode. If answered incorrectly, review iontophoresis guidelines and the use of medication for treatment of pain.

A27 | Cardiovascular/Pulmonary | Clinical Applications

A **CONTRAINDICATION** to initiating joint mobilization on a patient with chronic pulmonary disease is:

CHOICES:
1. reflex muscle guarding.
2. long-term corticosteroid therapy.
3. concurrent inhalation therapy.
4. functional chest wall immobility.

CORRECT ANSWER: 2

RATIONALE:
Very often patients with chronic pulmonary disease have been managed with corticosteroid therapy. Long-term steroid use affects ligamentous integrity, which often produces joint hypermobility.

TYPE OF REASONING: DEDUCTIVE
One must recall the contraindications for joint mobilization in patients with chronic pulmonary disease to arrive at a correct conclusion. This necessitates the recall of factual guidelines, which is a deductive reasoning skill. For this situation, a contraindication to joint mobilization for a patient with chronic pulmonary disease is long-term corticosteroid therapy. If answered incorrectly, review contraindications for joint mobilization treatment, especially for patients with chronic pulmonary disease.

A28 | Devices, Admin, etc. | Safety, Roles, Teaching, EBP

A physical therapist assistant has been delegated the responsibility of dealing with departmental equipment safety. Which task would be beyond the scope of the assistant's responsibilities?

CHOICES:
1. training all staff to do "simple" repairs on all electrical equipment if a breakdown should occur.
2. supervising new staff and students in the use of all newly purchased equipment.
3. documenting all preventive maintenance and keeping this information on file.
4. conducting educational sessions for staff regarding the indications and contraindications for all equipment.

CORRECT ANSWER: 1

RATIONALE:
Electrical equipment is repaired by the manufacturer or local vendor, or in some cases, the maintenance department—not by physical therapy staff.

TYPE OF REASONING: EVALUATIVE
This question requires the test taker to use knowledge of the physical therapy scope of practice to determine a best course of action when managing equipment safety. This requires evaluative reasoning skill. For this case, it is NOT within the scope of practice for the assistant to train all staff to do simple repairs on all electrical equipment if a breakdown should occur. If answered incorrectly, review scope of practice guidelines.

A29 | Integumentary | Data Collection

An elderly and frail resident of an extended-care facility presents with hot, red and edematous skin over the shins of both lower extremities. The patient also has a mild fever. The physical therapist assistant should report to the physical therapist suspicion of:

CHOICES:
1. dermatitis.
2. cellulitis.
3. herpes simplex infection.
4. scleroderma.

CORRECT ANSWER: 2

RATIONALE:
Cellulitis is an inflammation of the cellular or connective tissue in or close to the skin. It is characterized by skin that is hot, red and edematous. Fever is a common finding. Dermatitis produces red, weeping, crusted skin lesions, but is not commonly accompanied by fever. Location on shins makes herpes an unlikely choice and there are no skin eruptions or vesicles. Scleroderma is a collagen disease producing tight, drawn skin.

TYPE OF REASONING: ANALYTICAL
This question provides symptoms and the test taker must determine the most likely problem. Questions of this nature often require analysis of the symptoms, which is an analytical reasoning skill. For this scenario, the symptoms are indicative of cellulitis and should be reported to the physical therapist by the assistant. If answered incorrectly, review signs and symptoms of cellulitis.

A30 | Devices, Admin, etc. | Equipment, Modalities

A 12 year-old child presents with pain (4/10) and limited knee range of motion (5°–95°) following surgical repair of the medial collateral ligament and anterior cruciate ligaments. In this case, the modality that can be used with **PRECAUTION** is:

CHOICES:

1. premodulated interferential current.
2. continuous short-wave diathermy.
3. high-rate transcutaneous electrical stimulation.
4. low-dose ultrasound.

CORRECT ANSWER: 4

RATIONALE:

Because the epiphyseal plates do not close until the end of puberty, ultrasound energy should be applied with caution around the epiphyseal area because of the potential for causing bone growth disturbances. However, there is no documented evidence that ultrasound creates any direct untoward effects on the growth plates, especially if applied at low dosage. Electrical stimulation or deep thermotherapy would have no deleterious effects on the epiphyseal plates because no mechanical effects on hard tissue are associated with their use.

TYPE OF REASONING: INDUCTIVE

This question requires one to utilize clinical judgment to determine the treatment modality that can be used with precaution on a 12 year-old. This necessitates inductive reasoning skill. For this case, low-dose ultrasound can be used with caution around the epiphyseal area. If answered incorrectly, review use of ultrasound in children and precautions.

A31 | Musculoskeletal | Clinical Applications

A weight lifter exhibits marked hypertrophy after embarking on a strength training regime. Hypertrophy can be expected to occur following at least:

CHOICES:

1. 1 to 2 weeks of training.
2. 3 to 4 weeks of training.
3. 2 to 3 weeks of training.
4. 6 to 8 weeks of training.

CORRECT ANSWER: 4

RATIONALE:

Hypertrophy is the increase in muscle size as a result of resistance training and can be observed following at least 6 to 8 weeks of training. Individual muscle fibers are enlarged, contain more actin and myosin, and have more, larger myofibrils.

TYPE OF REASONING: INFERENTIAL

One must infer or draw a reasonable conclusion about the likely expectation of hypertrophy with strength training. This requires one to determine what may be true of a situation, necessitating inferential reasoning skill. For this situation, one can expect hypertrophy after 6 to 8 weeks of training. If answered incorrectly, review outcomes of strength training and hypertrophy.

A32 | Musculoskeletal | Clinical Applications

A diagnosis of bicipital tendonitis has been made following an evaluation of a patient with shoulder pain. The **BEST** shoulder position to expose the tendon of the long head of the biceps for application of phonophoresis would be:

CHOICES:

1. lateral (external) rotation and extension.
2. medial (internal) rotation and abduction.
3. horizontal adduction.
4. abduction.

CORRECT ANSWER: 1

RATIONALE:

The long head of the biceps is best exposed in shoulder lateral (external) rotation and extension owing to its attachment at the supraglenoid tubercle of the scapula, which is at the medial aspect of the shoulder joint. Medial (internal) rotation and abduction places the long head of the biceps deep to the anterior deltoid and pectoralis major muscles. The anterior surface of the shoulder, including the long head of the biceps, loses exposure with horizontal adduction.

TYPE OF REASONING: INDUCTIVE

This question requires the test taker to utilize clinical judgment to determine the best shoulder position for application of phonophoresis to the long head of the biceps. This is an inductive reasoning skill. For this scenario, the long head of the biceps is best exposed in shoulder lateral rotation and extension. Review treatment guidelines for bicipital tendonitis and use of phonophoresis if answered incorrectly.

A33 | Musculoskeletal | Data Collection

The initial evaluation indicates that a patient has a weak gluteus maximus. What gait deviation would the physical therapist assistant expect to see with this patient during stance phase?

CHOICES:

1. lateral bending of the trunk to the same side.
2. lateral bending of the trunk to the opposite side.
3. backward trunk lean.
4. forward trunk lean.

CORRECT ANSWER: 3

RATIONALE:

A backward trunk lean is the substitution pattern most commonly used by a person with a weak gluteus maximus. This position helps to maintain hip extension by relying on the tension of the hip joint capsule and ligaments. A lateral trunk lean to the same side is a common gait deviation demonstrated by a patient with a weak gluteus medius. A lateral trunk lean to the opposite side may be demonstrated by the presence of a weak hip flexor. A forward trunk lean may be a function of a weak quadriceps or a hip or knee flexion contracture.

TYPE OF REASONING: INFERENTIAL

This question requires the test taker to draw a reasonable conclusion about the likely gait deviation expected for a patient with a weak gluteus maximus. This necessitates inferential reasoning skill as the test taker is determining what may be true for a patient. In this case, one should expect a backward trunk lean during the stance phase. If answered incorrectly, review substitution patterns for patients with a weak gluteus maximus.

A34 | Integumentary | Clinical Applications

A patient is transferred to a burn clinic with deep partial-thickness burns over 30% of the body. Healing of this type of burn is characterized by:

CHOICES:
1. blisters and minimal edema with spontaneous healing.
2. depressed skin area that heals with grafting and scarring.
3. moderate edema with spontaneous healing and minimal grafting.
4. marked edema with slow healing and extensive hypertrophic scarring.

CORRECT ANSWER: 4

RATIONALE:

Deep partial thickness burns involve destruction of the epidermis with damage of the dermis down into the reticular area. Appearance is mixed red/white color with sluggish capillary refill. Superficial sensation is decreased while sense of deep pressure is retained. The burn will heal spontaneously in 3 to 5 weeks if no infection develops (infection can convert the burn to full-thickness). There is marked edema with excessive scarring (hypertrophic). Superficial burns heal with minimal edema whereas superficial partial-thickness burns heal spontaneously with moderate edema and minimal scarring; they do not require grafting. Full-thickness burns require skin grafting; appearance is depressed with significant scarring.

TYPE OF REASONING: INFERENTIAL

This question provides a diagnosis and the test taker must infer the likely presentation of symptoms. Questions of this nature often require inferential reasoning skill. For this situation, healing of this burn is characterized by marked edema with slow healing and extensive hypertrophic scarring. Review burn healing guidelines for patients with deep partial thickness burns if answered incorrectly.

A35 | Devices, Admin, etc. | Equipment, Modalities

A patient with a complete spinal cord injury at the T6 level is being discharged home after 2 months of rehabilitation. In preparation for discharge, the rehabilitation team visits the home and finds three standard-height steps going into the home. A ramp will have to be constructed for wheelchair access. The recommended length of the ramp should be:

CHOICES:
1. 60 inches (5 feet).
2. 192 inches (16 feet).
3. 252 inches (21 feet).
4. 120 inches (10 feet).

CORRECT ANSWER: 3

RATIONALE:

The architectural standard for rise of a step is 7 inches (steps may vary from 7 to 9 inches). The recommended ratio of slope to rise is 1:12 (an 8% grade). For every inch of vertical rise, 12 inches of ramp will be required. A straight ramp will have to be 252 inches or 21 feet long.

TYPE OF REASONING: DEDUCTIVE

This question requires one to recall guidelines for the construction of a wheelchair ramp to arrive at a correct conclusion. Questions of this nature, where factual information is used to make decisions, often require deductive reasoning skill. For this case, guidelines indicate that the ramp should be 252 inches or 21 feet long. If answered incorrectly, review of Americans with Disabilities Act guidelines for wheelchair ramp construction.

A36 | Cardiovascular/Pulmonary | Clinical Applications

A patient with diagnosis of left-sided heart failure, class II, is referred for physical therapy. During exercise, this patient can be expected to demonstrate:

CHOICES:

1. severe, uncomfortable chest pain with shortness of breath.
2. weight gain with dependent edema.
3. anorexia and nausea with abdominal pain and distention.
4. dyspnea with fatigue and muscular weakness.

CORRECT ANSWER: 4

RATIONALE:

Left-sided heart failure is the result of the left ventricle failing to pump enough blood through the arterial system to meet the body's demands. It produces pulmonary edema and disturbed respiratory control mechanisms. Patients can be expected to demonstrate progressive dyspnea (exertional at first, then paroxysmal nocturnal dyspnea), fatigue and muscular weakness, pulmonary edema, cerebral hypoxia and renal changes. Severe chest pain and shortness of breath are symptoms of impending myocardial infarction. The other choices describe symptoms associated with right-sided ventricular failure.

TYPE OF REASONING: INFERENTIAL

This question provides a diagnosis and the test taker must infer the likely symptoms. Questions of this nature often require inferential reasoning skill as one is determining what may be true for a patient. For this situation, the patient can be expected to demonstrate dyspnea with fatigue and muscular weakness. If answered incorrectly, review signs and symptoms of left-sided heart failure.

A37 | Musculoskeletal | Interventions

A physical therapist assistant is instructing a physical therapist assistant student in proper positioning to prevent the typical contractures in a patient with a transfemoral amputation. The assistant stresses positioning the patient in:

CHOICES:

1. prone-lying with the residual limb in neutral rotation.
2. a wheelchair with a gel cushion and adductor roll.
3. supine-lying with the residual limb resting on a small pillow.
4. side-lying on the residual limb.

CORRECT ANSWER: 1

RATIONALE:

The typical contractures with a transfemoral amputation are hip flexion (typically from too much sitting in a wheelchair). The residual limb also rolls out into abduction and lateral (external) rotation. When the patient is in bed, hip extension should be emphasized (e.g., prone-lying). When the patient is sitting in the wheelchair, neutral hip rotation should be emphasized (e.g., using an abductor roll). Time in extension (prone, supine or standing) should counterbalance time sitting in a wheelchair.

TYPE OF REASONING: INDUCTIVE

One must utilize clinical judgment to determine positioning guidelines for a patient with transfemoral amputation. This requires inductive reasoning skill. For this situation, it is important to position the patient in the prone-lying position with the residual limb in neutral rotation to prevent contractures. If answered incorrectly, review positioning guidelines for patients with transfemoral amputations and prevention of contractures.

A38 | Other Systems | Clinical Applications

A physical therapist assistant is following the plan of care to provide gait training for a patient who is insulin dependent. In a review of the patient's medical record, the assistant notices that the blood glucose level for that day is 310 mg/dL. The assistant's **BEST** course of action is to:

CHOICES:
1. refrain from ambulating the patient, reschedule for tomorrow before other therapies.
2. ambulate the patient as planned but monitor closely for signs of exertional intolerance.
3. postpone therapy and consult with the nurse as soon as possible.
4. talk to the nurse about walking the patient later on that day after lunch.

CORRECT ANSWER: 3

RATIONALE:
Normal fasting plasma glucose is less than 115 mg/dL whereas a fasting plasma glucose level greater than 126 mg/dL on more than one occasion is indicative of diabetes. This patient is hyperglycemic with high glucose levels (equal to or greater than 250 mg/dL). Clinical signs that may accompany this condition include ketoacidosis (acetone breath) with dehydration, weak and rapid pulse, nausea/vomiting, deep and rapid respirations (Kussmaul's respirations), weakness, diminished reflexes and paresthesias. The patient may be lethargic and confused and may progress to diabetic coma and death if not treated promptly with insulin. Physical therapy intervention is contraindicated; exercise can lead to further impaired glucose uptake. Coordination with the nurse is crucial so that the patient's blood glucose levels drop to a point that is safe for ambulation.

TYPE OF REASONING: EVALUATIVE
This question requires one to evaluate the courses of action presented to determine the best course of action to effectively address the patient's symptoms. This requires evaluative reasoning skill. For this scenario the assistant's best course of action is to postpone therapy and consult with the nurse as soon as possible. If answered incorrectly, review intervention approaches for patients with hyperglycemia.

A39 | Musculoskeletal | Interventions

An infant was referred to physical therapy for right torticollis. The **MOST** effective method to stretch the muscle is by positioning the head and neck into:

CHOICES:
1. flexion, left side-bending, and left rotation.
2. extension, right side-bending, and left rotation.
3. flexion, right side-bending, and left rotation.
4. extension, left side-bending, and right rotation.

CORRECT ANSWER: 4

RATIONALE:
The right sternocleidomastoid produces left lateral (external) rotation and flexion of the cervical spine. The right sternocleidomastoid is in lengthened position with the head turned to the right and the cervical spine extended.

TYPE OF REASONING: INDUCTIVE
One must use knowledge of intervention approaches for torticollis to arrive at a correct conclusion. This necessitates clinical judgment, which is an inductive reasoning skill. For this situation, the most effective method to stretch the muscle is by positioning the head and neck into extension, left side-bending and right rotation. If answered incorrectly, review intervention approaches for torticollis.

A40 | Neuromuscular | Interventions

A patient is recovering from a stroke and demonstrates good recovery in the lower extremity (out-of-synergy movement control). Timing deficits are apparent during gait. Isokinetic training can be used to improve:

CHOICES:

1. rate control at slow movement speeds.
2. rate control at varying movement speeds.
3. both reaction and movement times.
4. initiation of movement.

CORRECT ANSWER: 2

RATIONALE:

Patients during the later stages of recovery from stroke frequently exhibit problems with rate control. They are able to move at slow speeds but as speed of movement increases, control decreases. An isokinetic device can be an effective training modality to remediate this problem.

TYPE OF REASONING: INFERENTIAL

One must determine the intervention approach that will be most beneficial for a patient with a stroke and timing deficits during gait to arrive at a correct conclusion. This requires inferential reasoning skill. For this situation, isokinetic training can be used to improve rate control at varying movement speeds. If answered incorrectly, review gait training guidelines for patients with stroke, especially for those with rate control problems.

A41 | Musculoskeletal | Interventions

An older adult patient with a transfemoral amputation is having difficulty wrapping the residual limb. The physical therapist assistant should:

CHOICES:

1. suggest the use of a shrinker.
2. redouble efforts to teach proper Ace bandage wrapping.
3. apply a temporary prosthesis immediately.
4. consult with the vascular surgeon about the application of an Unna's paste dressing.

CORRECT ANSWER: 1

RATIONALE:

A shrinker is a suitable alternative to elastic wraps. It is important to select the right size shrinker to limit edema and accelerate healing. An Unna's paste dressing is applied at the time of initial surgery. Use of a temporary prosthesis should be a prosthetic team decision and is based on additional factors such as age, balance, strength, cognition and so forth.

TYPE OF REASONING: INDUCTIVE

This question necessitates clinical judgment to determine the best course of action for a patient who is having difficulty with residual limb wrapping. This is an inductive reasoning skill. For this case, the assistant should suggest the use of a shrinker rather than elastic wraps. If answered incorrectly, review care for the residual limb, especially the use of shrinkers.

A42 | Cardiovascular/Pulmonary | Interventions

A physical therapist assistant is assisting a patient who has a segment of a lobe of the lung removed. The assistant should facilitate chest expansion during exercise by instructing the patient to:

CHOICES:

1. breathe in through the nose and raise the shoulders with inhalation.
2. round the shoulders forward with inhalation.
3. lean forward and rest the forearms on the thighs or on a countertop with inhalation.
4. breathe in through the nose and push the ribs out against hands placed on the lower ribs.

CORRECT ANSWER: 4

RATIONALE:

Breathing patterns to encourage chest expansion include the patient performing lateral costal breathing, or expanding the ribs with inhalation. Although patients should be encouraged to breathe in through their nose, they should be discouraged from raising their shoulders with inhalation as this encourages use of accessory musculature. Forward bending and supporting the forearms on the thigh or on a countertop helps to facilitate relaxation for persons with obstructive or restrictive breathing conditions. This position is often used to decrease dyspnea. The forward rounded shoulder position should be discouraged.

TYPE OF REASONING: INDUCTIVE

One must utilize clinical judgment to determine the best approach for facilitating chest expansion during exercise. This requires knowledge of therapeutic procedures for chest expansion exercises, which is an inductive reasoning skill. For this case, the assistant should instruct the patient to breathe in through the nose and push the ribs out against hands placed on the lower ribs. Review chest expansion exercises if answered incorrectly.

A43 | Neuromuscular | Data Collection

The physical therapist evaluation identifies that a patient has scored low on the Berg Balance Scale. The physical therapist assistant understands that this assessment best identifies the patient's ability to:

CHOICES:

1. hold a single-limb standing position without losing balance.
2. perform multiple daily activities including turning, stepping up or down, and reaching.
3. reach forward without losing balance.
4. rise from a chair, walk and return to a chair and sit back down.

CORRECT ANSWER: 2

RATIONALE:

The Berg Balance Scale assessment identifies the patient's ability to maintain posture and control during a variety of daily activities, such as stepping onto and off a step, turning and looking over a shoulder, and stooping to pick something off the floor. The Timed Up and Go test assess the patient's ability to rise from a chair, walk 3 m, and return to and sit back down in a chair. Higher scores on both of these assessments represent better balance and postural control. Single limb stance and the Forward Reach test specific measures of balance control that assess the patient's ability to perform those specific tasks.

TYPE OF REASONING: DEDUCTIVE

One must recall the parameters of the Berg Balance Scale to arrive at a correct conclusion. This necessitates the recall of factual information, which is a deductive reasoning skill. For this situation, the Berg Balance Scale identifies the patient's ability to perform multiple daily activities including turning, stepping up or down, and reaching. If answered incorrectly, review the Berg Balance Scale and assessment parameters.

A44 | Cardiovascular/Pulmonary | Interventions

A patient had a myocardial infarction 4 weeks ago. Resistive training using weights to improve muscular strength and endurance is appropriate:

CHOICES:

1. if exercise intensities are kept below 85% maximal voluntary contraction.
2. if exercise capacity is greater than 5 METs with no anginal symptoms or ST segment depression.
3. during all phases of rehabilitation after 4 to 6 weeks if judicious monitoring of heart rate is used.
4. only during post–acute phase III cardiac rehabilitation.

CORRECT ANSWER: 2

RATIONALE:

Resistance training is typically initiated after patients have completed 4 to 6 weeks of supervised cardiorespiratory endurance exercise. Lower intensities are prescribed. Careful monitoring of blood pressure is necessary as blood pressure will be higher and heart rate lower than for aerobic exercise. Contraindications to resistance training include unstable angina, uncontrolled arrhythmias, recent history of congestive heart failure, left ventricular outflow obstruction, severe valvular disease and uncontrolled hypertension. Patients should demonstrate an exercise capacity greater than 5 METs without anginal symptoms or ST segment depression (Source: American College of Sports Medicine: *Guidelines for Exercise Testing and Prescription*, Ed 6).

TYPE OF REASONING: INDUCTIVE

One must have knowledge of cardiac rehabilitation guidelines for patients with myocardial infarction to arrive at a correct conclusion. This knowledge is coupled with clinical judgment, which necessitates inductive reasoning skill. For this situation, resistive training using weights to improve muscular strength and endurance is appropriate if the exercise capacity is greater than 5 METs with no anginal symptoms or ST segment depression. If answered incorrectly, review cardiac rehabilitation guidelines and use of resistive training.

A45 | Devices, Admin, etc. | Equipment, Modalities

A patient diagnosed with lumbar spinal root impingement caused by narrowing of the intervertebral foramen has been referred to physical therapy. The physical therapist has indicated use of mechanical traction in the plan of care. What is the lowest percentage of body weight that should be considered for the **INITIAL** traction force?

CHOICES:

1. 25%.
2. 15%.
3. 55%.
4. 85%.

CORRECT ANSWER: 1

RATIONALE:

To overcome the coefficient of friction of the body moving horizontally over the surface of a table, the traction force should be at least 25% of the body weight when one is using a split table or 50% when one is using a non-split table. The minimum 25% for initial treatment would provide sufficient joint distraction by stretching the ligamentous tissue and widening the intervertebral foramen.

TYPE OF REASONING: DEDUCTIVE

This question requires the test taker to recall the guidelines for the use of mechanical traction. This necessitates the recall of factual guidelines, which is a deductive reasoning skill. For this case, the lowest percentage of body weight that should be considered for the initial traction force is 25%. If answered incorrectly, review mechanical traction guidelines and configuration of traction force.

A46 | Neuromuscular | Interventions

The **MOST** appropriate physical therapy intervention to use at school during class for an older child with decreased sitting balance, but normal tone would be:

CHOICES:

1. sitting on a therapy ball while performing desktop activities.
2. sitting in an adaptive wheelchair with lateral supports and lap tray.
3. standing on a static prone-stander with lap tray.
4. sitting in an appropriate height chair with lateral postural supports.

CORRECT ANSWER: 2

RATIONALE:

The goal of school physical therapy is to directly facilitate the educational process—for example, interacting in class, viewing the blackboard, etc. The adaptive wheelchair is the best choice for this child because it allows the child to move around in the classroom while maintaining a stable position. Sitting on a therapy ball is too advanced. The prone-stander is restrictive and does not promote sitting.

TYPE OF REASONING: INDUCTIVE

One must utilize clinical judgment to determine the most beneficial intervention approach for a child with decreased sitting balance. This necessitates inductive reasoning skill. For this case, the most appropriate approach is sitting in an adaptive wheelchair with the lateral supports and lap tray. If answered incorrectly, review school-based intervention approaches for children with decreased sitting balance.

A47 | Neuromuscular | Clinical Applications

A patient with Parkinson's disease demonstrates a highly stereotyped gait pattern characterized by impoverished movement. Which activity could present a danger if used by the physical therapist assistant?

CHOICES:

1. standing, using body weight support from a harness.
2. sidestepping and cross stepping using light touch-down support of hands.
3. gait training using a rolling walker.
4. rhythmic stepping using a motorized treadmill.

CORRECT ANSWER: 3

RATIONALE:

The patient with Parkinson's disease typically presents with postural deficits of forward head and trunk with hip and knee flexion contractures. Gait is narrow-based and shuffling. A festinating gait typically results from persistent forward posturing of the body near the forward limits of stability. A rolling walker is contraindicated because it would increase forward postural deformities and festinating gait. All other choices are appropriate training activities to improve upright standing balance and gait.

TYPE OF REASONING: INFERENTIAL

This question requires one to determine what may present a danger to a patient with Parkinson's disease to arrive at a correct conclusion. This requires inferential reasoning skill. For this situation, gait training with the use of a rolling walker could present a danger as this can increase forward postural deformities and festinating gait. If answered incorrectly, review contraindications for assistive device use with patients with Parkinson's disease.

A48 | Neuromuscular | Clinical Applications
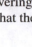

A physical therapist assistant working with a patient recovering from a stroke would need to implement additional safety precautions during treatment if the chart review revealed that the patient had:

CHOICES:
1. anosognosia.
2. ideational apraxia.
3. unilateral neglect.
4. ideomotor apraxia.

CORRECT ANSWER: 1

RATIONALE:

Anosognosia is a more severe form of neglect with lack of awareness and denial of the severity of one's paralysis. With ideomotor apraxia, a patient cannot perform a task upon command but can do the task when on his or her own. With ideational apraxia, a patient cannot perform a requested task at all. Unilateral neglect might lead the patient to ignore something positioned on the involved side.

TYPE OF REASONING: INFERENTIAL

One must infer or draw a reasonable conclusion about the level of safety precautions required for a patient with a stroke. This requires inferential reasoning skill. For this case, a patient with anosognosia would require additional safety measures during treatment to address the severity of the patient's neglect and denial of severity of paralysis. If answered incorrectly, review safety guidelines for patients with stroke, including patients with anosognosia.

A49 | Devices, Admin, etc. | Equipment, Modalities

A patient with a transfemoral amputation has been fitted with a prosthesis that utilizes a quadrilateral socket. The physical therapist assistant is performing gait training activities. Following gait training the assistant should examine pressure tolerance areas of the residual limb with the device off. These include:

CHOICES:
1. ischial tuberosity and lateral sides of residual limb.
2. adductor magnus and medial side of residual limb.
3. distolateral end of femur and ischial seat.
4. perineal area and medial side of the residual limb.

CORRECT ANSWER: 1

RATIONALE:

A quadrilateral socket in a transfemoral amputation is designed to selectively load tissues that are pressure tolerant. The ischial tuberosity, gluteals and lateral sides of the residual limb are pressure-tolerant areas.

TYPE OF REASONING: DEDUCTIVE

This question requires the test taker to recall the pressure-tolerant areas of the quadrilateral socket to arrive at a correct conclusion. This necessitates the recall of factual information, which is a deductive reasoning skill. For this scenario, the pressure-tolerant areas include the ischial tuberosity and lateral sides of the residual limb. If answered incorrectly, review pressure tolerance areas for a quadrilateral socket.

A50 | Musculoskeletal | Interventions

An older adult patient has been confined to bed for a period of 2 months and now demonstrates limited range of motion in both lower extremities. Range in hip flexion is 5° to 115° and knee flexion is 10° to 120°. The physical therapist has indicated that flexibility activities should be implemented to improve the range of motion in preparation of standing activities. The **MOST** appropriate intervention to improve flexibility and ready this patient for standing is:

CHOICES:

1. manual passive stretching, 10 repetitions each joint, 2 times a day.
2. tilt table standing, 20 minutes daily.
3. mechanical stretching using traction and 5-lb weights, 2 hours, twice daily.
4. hold–relax techniques followed by passive range of motion, 10 repetitions, 2 times a day.

CORRECT ANSWER: 3

RATIONALE:

Prolonged mechanical stretching involves a low-intensity force (generally 5 lb to 15 lb) applied over a prolonged period (30 minutes to several hours). It is generally the most effective way to manage long-standing flexion contractures. Manual passive stretching and tilt table standing are shorter duration stretches that are not likely to be effective in this case. Hold–relax techniques can be used to improve flexibility in the presence of shortening of muscular elements but are not likely to be effective in this case because of the short duration and long-standing contracture affecting connective tissue elements.

TYPE OF REASONING: INDUCTIVE

This question requires the test taker to have knowledge of muscle stretching guidelines for patients with prolonged periods of immobility to arrive at a correct conclusion. This necessitates clinical judgment, which is an inductive reasoning skill. For this situation, the most appropriate intervention is mechanical stretching using traction and 5-lb weights, twice per day. If answered incorrectly, review muscle stretching procedures for patients with prolonged immobility.

A51 | Devices, Admin, etc. | Safety, Roles, Teaching, EBP

A physical therapist assistant has recently attended a professional conference on myofascial release. The assistant has been asked to share this information with colleagues during an in-service session. The assistant's **BEST INITIAL** activity is to:

CHOICES:

1. ask colleagues to select a suitable time and place for the in-service.
2. provide a comprehensive packet of handouts in advance of the in-service.
3. organize a PowerPoint presentation and prepare a handout.
4. survey colleagues about their current level of knowledge by using a brief questionnaire.

CORRECT ANSWER: 4

RATIONALE:

To better share the information, the assistant needs to determine what information and skills colleagues currently have. A brief questionnaire is an effective means to achieve this goal. The other choices demonstrate planning of the learning experience **WITHOUT** benefit of a needs assessment.

TYPE OF REASONING: INDUCTIVE

One must utilize clinical judgment to determine the best initial approach to providing an in-service to colleagues to arrive at a correct conclusion. This necessitates inductive reasoning skill. For this situation, the assistant should survey colleagues about their current level of knowledge before providing the in-service. If answered incorrectly, review guidelines for planning in-services.

A52 | Musculoskeletal | Clinical Applications

To prepare a patient with an incomplete T12 paraplegia for ambulation with crutches, the upper-quadrant muscles that would be **MOST** important to strengthen include the:

CHOICES:

1. upper trapezius, rhomboids and levator scapulae.
2. deltoid, triceps and wrist flexors.
3. middle trapezius, latissimus dorsi and triceps.
4. lower trapezius, latissimus dorsi and triceps.

CORRECT ANSWER: 4

RATIONALE:

The upper-quadrant muscles that are most important to strengthen for crutch gaits include the lower trapezius, latissimus dorsi and triceps. Shoulder depression and elbow extension strength is crucial for successful crutch gait.

TYPE OF REASONING: INDUCTIVE

This question requires the test taker to determine the most important muscles to strengthen in the upper quadrant for a patient with T12 paraplegia. This requires clinical judgment, which is an inductive reasoning skill. For this case, the assistant should strengthen the lower trapezius, latissimus dorsi and triceps in preparation for crutch use. If answered incorrectly, review gait training approaches for patients with T12 injury, especially crutch use and musculature needed.

A53 | Cardiovascular/Pulmonary | Data Collection

A physical therapist assistant is discussing an aerobic exercise program with a pregnant woman. The assistant should inform the patient that she:

CHOICES:

1. should discontinue aerobic exercise until after she gives birth.
2. must limit her participation in aerobic exercise to the first and second trimesters and then discontinue it.
3. may notice that she reaches her maximum or preferred work level more quickly than she did prior to pregnancy.
4. should limit her aerobic exercise to bicycling or swimming.

CORRECT ANSWER: 3

RATIONALE:

A woman who has an established aerobic exercise program will likely continue to tolerate her exercise program during pregnancy; she may, however, notice that she reaches her desired workout level or maximum exercise capacity more quickly than she did prior to pregnancy. A woman does not have to discontinue her aerobic exercise program during pregnancy, nor does she have to limit participation to the first and second trimesters. Women who do not participate in a regular aerobic program prior to pregnancy may tolerate swimming, walking or biking more easily than running.

TYPE OF REASONING: DEDUCTIVE

This question requires one to recall the guidelines for exercise with pregnancy to arrive at a correct conclusion. This necessitates the recall of factual information, which is a deductive reasoning skill. For this situation, the assistant should inform the woman that she may notice that she reaches her maximum work level more quickly than she did prior to pregnancy. If answered incorrectly, review exercise guidelines during pregnancy.

A54 | Musculoskeletal | Clinical Applications

Following major surgery of the right hip, a patient walks with a Trendelenburg gait. The initial evaluation reveals right hip abductor weakness and range-of-motion limitations in flexion and lateral (external) rotation. The plan of care includes functional electrical stimulation to help improve the gait pattern. Stimulation should be initiated for the:

CHOICES:

1. right abductors during swing on the right.
2. right abductors during stance on the right.
3. left abductors during stance on the right.
4. left abductors during swing on the right.

CORRECT ANSWER: 2

RATIONALE:

During the stance phase of gait, the hip abductors of the support limb are activated to maintain the pelvis in a relative horizontal position. This allows the opposite foot to clear the floor during swing. Stimulation of the right abductors throughout swing or the left hip abductors during swing or stance would not compensate for the weakness of the right hip abductors during the support period.

TYPE OF REASONING: INDUCTIVE

This question requires one to determine the best placement for functional electrical stimulation to improve gait pattern. This requires knowledge of functional electrical stimulation protocols as well as clinical judgment, which is an inductive reasoning skill. For this case, the assistant should focus on the right abductors during stance on the right to improve the Trendelenburg gait. If answered incorrectly, review functional electrical stimulation guidelines to improve Trendelenburg gait.

A55 | Musculoskeletal | Clinical Applications

A physical therapist assistant is working with a patient who has a diagnosis of supraspinatus impingement with possible tear. The patient has been receiving physical therapy care for 4 weeks. Early **subacute** physical therapy intervention should be progressed to include:

CHOICES:

1. active assistive pulley exercises.
2. modalities to reduce pain and inflammation.
3. small-amplitude oscillations performed to the limit of tissue resistance to the glenohumeral joint.
4. resistance exercises for the affected muscles.

CORRECT ANSWER: 1

RATIONALE:

During the **early subacute phase**, active assistive pulley exercises are indicated to promote healing of the supraspinatus muscle and maintain active range of motion of the glenohumeral joint. Acute physical therapy intervention would focus on reduction of pain and inflammation. Oscillations to the limit of tissue resistance and resistance exercises are too vigorous at this stage.

TYPE OF REASONING: INDUCTIVE

One must determine the best approach for treating a supraspinatus impingement to arrive at a correct conclusion. This requires clinical judgment and knowledge of therapeutic approaches, which is an inductive reasoning skill. For this case, the assistant should progress to active assistive pulley exercises. If answered incorrectly, review treatment approaches for supraspinatus impingement, especially for the subacute phase.

A56 | Devices, Admin, etc. | Safety, Roles, Teaching, EBP

Two therapists are asked to perform a test on the same group of patients by using the Functional Independence Measure (FIM). The results of both sets of measurements reveal differences in therapists' scores but **NOT** in the repeat measurements. This is indicative of a problem in:

CHOICES:
1. concurrent validity.
2. intrarater reliability.
3. interrater reliability.
4. construct validity.

CORRECT ANSWER: 3

RATIONALE:

Interrater reliability is the degree to which two or more independent raters can obtain the same rating for a given variable. In this case, two therapists obtained different FIM scores for the same group of patients, indicating a problem in interrater reliability. Intrarater reliability is the consistency of an examiner on repeat tests. Issues of validity (Does the test measure what it says it measures?) are not relevant.

TYPE OF REASONING: DEDUCTIVE

This question requires the test taker to recall the parameters of interrater reliability to arrive at a correct conclusion. This is factual information, which requires deductive reasoning skill. For this case, the description of the differences in the therapists' scores indicates a problem with interrater reliability. If answered incorrectly, review research guidelines, including interrater reliability.

A57 | Neuromuscular | Interventions

A patient is recovering from a complete spinal cord injury with C5 tetraplegia. The physical therapist assistant is performing passive range of motion exercises on the mat when the patient complains of a sudden pounding headache and double vision. The assistant notices that the patient is sweating excessively, and assesses the patient's blood pressure, getting a reading of 240/95 mmHg. The assistant's **BEST** course of action is to:

CHOICES:
1. lie the patient down immediately, elevate the patient's lower extremities and then call for a nurse.
2. place the patient in a supported sitting position and continue to monitor blood presure before calling for help.
3. sit the patient up, check/empty catheter bag and then call for emergency medical assistance.
4. lie the patient down, open the patient's shirt and monitor the respiratory rate closely.

CORRECT ANSWER: 3

RATIONALE:

The patient is exhibiting autonomic dysreflexia (an emergency situation). The assistant should first sit the patient up and check for irritating or precipitating stimuli (e.g., a blocked catheter). The next step is to call for emergency medical assistance. Placing the patient supine can aggravate the situation.

TYPE OF REASONING: EVALUATIVE

This question requires one to determine a best course of action to effectively address the patient's symptoms from the choices provided. This requires one to have an understanding of the significance of the problem. This requires evaluative reasoning skill. For this scenario, the assistant should sit the patient up, check and empty the catheter bag, and then call for emergency medical assistance. If answered incorrectly, review signs and symptoms of autonomic dysreflexia and intervention approaches.

A58 | Devices, Admin, etc. | Equipment, Modalities

An external shoe modification that shifts weight bearing from the metatarsal joints to the metatarsal shafts is a:

CHOICES:

1. Thomas heel.
2. scaphoid pad.
3. metatarsal pad.
4. metatarsal bar.

CORRECT ANSWER: 4

RATIONALE:

A metatarsal bar is an external modification indicated to take pressure off the metatarsal heads and improve push off. The metatarsal pad is an internal shoe modification that does the same thing. Scaphoid pads and Thomas heels help to manage flexible flat foot.

TYPE OF REASONING: DEDUCTIVE

This question requires one to recall the device that shifts weight-bearing from the metatarsal joints to the metatarsal shafts to arrive at a correct conclusion. This is factual recall of information, which is a deductive reasoning skill. For this case, the device described is a metatarsal bar. If answered incorrectly, review shoe modifications, especially external and internal shoe modifications.

A59 | Integumentary | Interventions

A child with full-thickness burns to both upper extremities is developing hypertrophic scars. The BEST intervention to manage these scars is:

CHOICES:

1. primary excision followed by autografts.
2. application of custom-made pressure garments.
3. application of compression wraps.
4. application of occlusive dressings.

CORRECT ANSWER: 2

RATIONALE:

Following burns, edema and hypertrophic scarring can be effectively controlled with pressure garments. Surgery is an option of last resort. Custom garments are the best choice. Pressure should be maintained 23 hours per day, often for 6 to 12 months. Surgery is the option of last choice. Compression wraps (elastic bandages) and occlusive dressings have no impact on hypertrophic scarring.

TYPE OF REASONING: INDUCTIVE

One must use knowledge of hypertrophic scarring management guidelines to arrive at a correct conclusion. This requires clinical judgment, which is an inductive reasoning skill. For this situation, the best intervention to manage the scars is application of custom-made pressure garments. If answered incorrectly, review burn treatment guidelines, including management of hypertrophic scarring.

A60 | Cardiovascular/Pulmonary | Clinical Applications

A patient with chronic obstructive pulmonary disease has developed respiratory acidosis. The physical therapist instructs a physical therapist assistant who is participating in the care to monitor the patient closely for:

CHOICES:

1. disorientation.
2. tingling or numbness of the extremities.
3. dizziness or lightheadedness.
4. hyperreflexia.

CORRECT ANSWER: 1

RATIONALE:

A patient with respiratory acidosis may present with many symptoms of increased carbon dioxide levels in the arterial blood. Significant acidosis may lead to disorientation, stupor or coma. The other choices are signs and symptoms of respiratory alkalosis or a decrease of carbon dioxide in the arterial blood.

TYPE OF REASONING: DEDUCTIVE

One must recall the risk factors for patients with chronic obstructive pulmonary disease and respiratory acidosis to arrive at a correct conclusion. This is factual information, which necessitates deductive reasoning skill. For this situation, the patient is at risk for disorientation and the patient should be monitored closely for this symptom. If answered incorrectly, review risk factors for respiratory acidosis in patients with chronic obstructive pulmonary disease.

A61 | Other Systems | Clinical Applications

Which of the following is an appropriate exercise modification for a woman who is 15 weeks into her pregnancy?

CHOICES:

1. encouraging unilateral exercise of the lower extremities.
2. standing rather than supine lower-extremity resistive band exercises.
3. avoiding quadruped exercise activities.
4. placing a small wedge under right hip during supine exercise.

CORRECT ANSWER: 4

RATIONALE:

After the first trimester a pregnant women should avoid supine positioning for greater than 5 minutes at a time. When performing supine exercises, placement of a wedge under the right hip helps to decrease the effects of uterine compression on abdominal vessels and improves cardiac output. Asymmetrical stretching or strengthening activities of the lower extremities can contribute to joint instability, especially of the lower back and sacroiliac joint area. Quadruped positioning is an appropriate modification for prone activities; however, note that hip extension activities should be limited to midline and hip extension beyond midline should be avoided as this position can place asymmetrical forces through the sacroiliac joint and lower back area.

TYPE OF REASONING: INDUCTIVE

One must utilize clinical judgment to determine the best exercise modification for a patient who is 15 weeks pregnant. This requires knowledge of exercise guidelines during pregnancy, which is an inductive reasoning skill. For this case, the assistant should recommend placing a small wedge under the right hip during supine exercise. If answered incorrectly, review exercise modifications during pregnancy.

A62 | Devices, Admin, etc. | Equipment, Modalities

When working with a patient who is obese, what equipment would a physical therapist assistant use to assist in transferring the patient from sit to stand?

CHOICES:

1. sliding board.
2. gait belt.
3. standing pole.
4. bariatric wheelchair.

CORRECT ANSWER: 3

RATIONALE:

A standing pole provides the patient something to grip and pull on allowing them to assist the assistant in transferring from sit to stand. A sliding board assists in transferring from one surface to another. A gait belt is used for all transfers and may not be safe for use by the bariatric patient. A bariatric wheelchair will not assist in getting from a sitting to a standing position.

TYPE OF REASONING: INFERENTIAL

This question requires one to determine what may be true for a patient who is obese and needs assistance during a transfer. This requires knowledge of adaptive devices for patients who are obese to arrive at a correct conclusion. For this situation, the likely equipment to be used for the transfer is a standing pole. If answered incorrectly, review assistive devices for transfer skills with bariatric patients.

A63 | Neuromuscular | Clinical Applications

A patient with complete C6 tetraplegia should be instructed to initially transfer with a sliding board by using:

CHOICES:

1. shoulder depressors and triceps, keeping the hands flexed to protect tenodesis grasp.
2. pectoral muscles to stabilize elbows in extension and scapular depressors to lift the trunk.
3. shoulder extensors, lateral (external) rotators and anterior deltoid to position and lock the elbow.
4. serratus anterior to elevate the trunk with elbow extensors stabilizing.

CORRECT ANSWER: 3

RATIONALE:

The patient with complete C6 quadriplegia will lack triceps and should be taught to lock the elbow for push-up transfers by using shoulder lateral (external) rotators and extensors to position the upper extremity; the anterior deltoid locks the elbow by reverse actions (all of these muscles are functional).

TYPE OF REASONING: INDUCTIVE

One must utilize knowledge of sliding board transfer skills for patients with tetraplegia to arrive at a correct conclusion. This requires inductive reasoning skill. For this case, the patient should be instructed to use shoulder extensors, lateral (external) rotators and anterior deltoid to position and lock the elbow during the transfer. If answered incorrectly, review transfer techniques for patients with tetraplegia, especially C6 injuries.

A64 | Devices, Admin, etc. | Safety, Roles, Teaching, EBP

A physical therapist assistant volunteered to teach a stroke education class on positioning techniques for family members and caregivers. At the conclusion of the class, caregivers will be expected to utilize the skills taught. The **BEST** choice of teaching method is to utilize:

CHOICES:

1. assistant demonstration, caregiver practice and follow-up individual discussion.
2. assistant demonstration with caregiver role-playing patient.
3. multimedia (PowerPoint and handouts) that accompany an oral presentation.
4. question and answer addressing the specific individual concerns of the caregivers.

CORRECT ANSWER: 1

RATIONALE:

A variety of teaching methods including demonstration, practice and discussion has the best chance of reinforcing learning in a diverse group. Using only one type of teaching methodology is not likely to be as successful in meeting the needs of all the group members. Psychomotor skills are best learned by practice, not lecture or just question and answer. Feedback should include both knowledge of performance and knowledge of results.

TYPE OF REASONING: INDUCTIVE

One must determine the best approach for teaching caregivers positioning techniques to arrive at a correct conclusion. This requires clinical judgment, which is an inductive reasoning skill. For this case, the assistant should demonstrate the skills, facilitate caregiver practice and follow-up with individual discussion. If answered incorrectly, review training techniques and guidelines for caregivers.

A65 | Devices, Admin, etc. | Safety, Roles, Teaching, EBP

A patient with active tuberculosis is referred for physical therapy. Which of the following is an appropriate precaution?

CHOICES:

1. the patient must wear a tight-fitting mask while being treated in his or her room.
2. the assistant must wash hands only upon leaving the patient's room.
3. the assistant must wear a tight-fitting mask, gown and gloves while treating the patient.
4. the patient must be in a private, negative-pressurized room.

CORRECT ANSWER: 4

RATIONALE:

The assistant should wash hands upon entering and leaving every patient's room. When the patient is suspected of having tuberculosis, the patient should be in a private, negative-pressurized room. The room is considered a potentially infective environment and the assistant should don a tight-fitting mask prior to entering the room. Gown and gloves are not always necessary. The patient only needs to wear a mask if there is a need to leave the room (for a medical test, etc.). Refer to transmission-based precautions.

TYPE OF REASONING: DEDUCTIVE

One must recall the guidelines for standard precautions when working with patients who have active tuberculosis. This is factual information and recall of guidelines, which is a deductive reasoning skill. For this case, the assistant should realize that the patient should be in a private, negative-pressurized room. If answered incorrectly, review transmission-based guidelines for patients with tuberculosis in this text book.

A66 | Musculoskeletal | Clinical Applications

The plan of care for a patient following acute whiplash of the cervical spine calls for initiating cervical stabilization exercises. The patient is tolerating cervical nodding exercises and has a pain rating of 5 out of 10 (10 being the worst pain). The physical therapist assistant should begin by having the patient maintain a cervical nod while performing active shoulder flexion to:

CHOICES:
1. 90° while sitting on a ball.
2. 180° while supine.
3. 90° while supine.
4. 180° while standing.

CORRECT ANSWER: 3

RATIONALE:
Because the patient is only tolerating a cervical nod and has a pain rate of 5, the exercises should be progressed slowly. The correct progression from maintaining a cervical nod is to initiate partial shoulder range of motion with the head and trunk in a supported position. Further progressions will include full range motion of the shoulders in a supported position, with decreasing trunk support as the patient tolerates.

TYPE OF REASONING: INDUCTIVE
This question requires the test taker to utilize knowledge of intervention approaches for whiplash injury to arrive at a correct conclusion. This necessitates inductive reasoning skill, as clinical judgment is paramount to choosing a correct solution. For this case, the assistant should begin by performing active shoulder flexion to 90° while supine. If answered incorrectly, review intervention approaches for whiplash injuries.

A67 | Musculoskeletal | Interventions

A patient has undergone surgery and subsequent immobilization to stabilize the olecranon process. The patient now exhibits an elbow flexion contracture. In this case, an absolute **CONTRAINDICATION** for joint mobilization would be:

CHOICES:
1. soft end-feel.
2. springy end-feel.
3. empty end-feel.
4. firm end-feel.

CORRECT ANSWER: 3

RATIONALE:
An empty end-feel (no real end-feel) may be indicative of severe pain and muscle guarding associated with pathological conditions. Springy and firm end-feels may be expected after elbow surgery. Soft end-feel is an indication of range limited because of tissue compression (e.g., in knee flexion there is contact between the posterior lower extremity and the posterior thigh).

TYPE OF REASONING: DEDUCTIVE
This question requires the test taker to recall the contraindications for joint mobilization to arrive at a correct conclusion. This necessitates the recall of factual guidelines, which is a deductive reasoning skill. For this situation, the contraindication for joint mobilization is an empty end-feel. If answered incorrectly, review joint mobilization guidelines and contraindications.

A68 | Devices, Admin, etc. | Safety, Roles, Teaching, EBP

A physical therapist assistant is providing early stage gait training for a patient after a left total hip arthroplasty. The patient is using crutches and is practicing on a level surface. The assistant should guard the patient by standing slightly:

CHOICES:
1. behind and to the intact side, one hand on the gait belt.
2. in front of the patient, walking backward, with one hand on the gait belt and one hand on the shoulder.
3. behind and to the left side, one hand on the gait belt.
4. behind the patient with both hands on the gait belt.

CORRECT ANSWER: 3

RATIONALE:

The correct guarding technique to protect a patient from falling is to stand slightly behind and to one side (the involved or left side).

TYPE OF REASONING: INDUCTIVE

One must recall the guidelines for guarding techniques during gait training to arrive at a correct conclusion. This necessitates clinical judgment, which is an inductive reasoning skill. For this scenario, the assistant should stand behind and to the left side with one hand on the gait belt. If answered incorrectly, review gait training guidelines for patients with total hip arthroplasties, especially with the use of crutches.

A69 | Musculoskeletal | Interventions

A patient has lumbar spinal stenosis encroaching on the spinal cord. The physical therapist assistant should educate the patient to **AVOID**:

CHOICES:
1. bicycling on hills.
2. use of a rowing machine.
3. Tai Chi activities.
4. swimming using a crawl stroke.

CORRECT ANSWER: 4

RATIONALE:

Continuous positioning in spinal extension increases symptoms in patients with spinal stenosis. Activities such as swimming using a crawl stroke place the spine in this position. All other activities described do not require the patient to maintain a continuous extended spinal position.

TYPE OF REASONING: ANALYTICAL

One must analyze the activities presented to determine the activity that will increase symptoms for a patient with spinal stenosis because of continuous positioning in spinal extension. This requires analytical reasoning skill. For this case, swimming using a crawl stroke should be avoided to prevent an increase in symptoms. If answered incorrectly, review contraindications for functional activities in patients with spinal stenosis.

A70 | Devices, Admin, etc. | Equipment, Modalities

A patient with post-polio syndrome is being treated in outpatient physical therapy with symptoms of myalgia and increasing fatigue. The patient has been using a knee–ankle–foot orthosis for 10 years. During gait training the physical therapist assistant observes the patient rise up on the sound extremity to advance the extremity with the orthosis forward. The vaulting observed in this case is MOST LIKELY the result of weakness of the:

CHOICES:

1. quadriceps on the affected extremity.
2. iliopsoas on the affected extremity.
3. gluteus medius on sound extremity.
4. gastrocsoleus on the sound extremity.

CORRECT ANSWER: 2

RATIONALE:

This patient is vaulting (rising up on the sound extremity to advance the orthosis extremity forward). This is most likely because of weakness of the iliopsoas (hip flexors) on the affected extremity. This gait deficit increases the energy demands of gait and is most likely contributing to fatigue. The myalgia and fatigue are also direct impairments of post-polio syndrome. The quadriceps muscle may assist with hip flexion; however, weakness of it is more likely to result in a steppage-type gait deviation. Weakness of the gluteus medius on the sound extremity would likely result in lateral trunk bending to the sound side. The gastrocsoleus on the sound extremity is most likely overdeveloped secondary to the current gait deviation.

TYPE OF REASONING: INFERENTIAL

This question requires one to infer or draw a reasonable conclusion about the likely muscle that is weak and causing vaulting during ambulation. Therefore, one must determine what may be true for a patient, which is an inferential reasoning skill. For this case, the iliopsoas muscle on the affected extremity is most likely weakened. If answered incorrectly, review causes of vaulting during walking.

A71 | Devices, Admin, etc. | Equipment, Modalities

An athlete presents with pain (5/10) and muscle spasm of the left upper trapezius as the result of a strain that occurred 2 weeks previously. The plan of care indicates the use of a combination of ultrasound and electrical stimulation. The MOST appropriate treatment parameters would be:

CHOICES:

1. continuous ultrasound with intense motor-level electrical stimulation.
2. continuous ultrasound and comfortable sensory-level electrical stimulation.
3. pulsed ultrasound with motor-level electrical stimulation.
4. pulsed ultrasound at 50% duty cycle with comfortable motor-level electrical stimulation.

CORRECT ANSWER: 2

RATIONALE:

Continuous ultrasound is indicated to create increased temperatures in the tissues; sensory level stimulation will help contribute to decreasing muscle spasm. Pulsed ultrasound is not indicated as this in not an acute injury. Motor-level stimulation at this subacute phase may be irritating to the tissues that are still in the healing phase and is better indicated to reduce long-standing muscle spasm.

TYPE OF REASONING: DEDUCTIVE

One must recall the guidelines for the use of ultrasound and electrical stimulation for the treatment of pain and muscle spasm to arrive at a correct conclusion. This requires the recall of protocols and guidelines, which is a deductive reasoning skill. For this situation, the most appropriate treatment parameters are continuous ultrasound and comfortable sensory-level electrical stimulation. If answered incorrectly, review protocols for electrical stimulation and ultrasound for pain and muscle spasm.

A72 | Devices, Admin, etc. | Safety, Roles, Teaching, EBP

A researcher states that he expects that there will be a significant difference between 20- and 30 year-olds after a 12-week exercise training program using exercise heart rates and myocardial oxygen consumption as measures of performance. The kind of hypothesis that is being used in this study is a (an):

CHOICES:
1. quasi-experimental hypothesis.
2. research hypothesis.
3. null hypothesis.
4. nondirectional hypothesis.

CORRECT ANSWER: 2

RATIONALE:
The null hypothesis is a statistical hypothesis that states that there is no relationship (or difference) between variables. Any relationship found will be a chance relationship, not a true one. A research hypothesis predicts an expected relationship between variables (e.g., 20 year-olds will demonstrate improved measures of performance compared with 30 year-olds). Quasi-experimental means that the subjects cannot be randomly assigned to groups. Nondirectional means that a direction of change cannot be predicted.

TYPE OF REASONING: DEDUCTIVE
One must recall the definition of a research hypothesis to arrive at a correct conclusion. This necessitates the recall of factual information, which is a deductive reasoning skill. For this case, the prediction for this study presented is that of a research hypothesis. If answered incorrectly, review research terminology, especially research hypotheses.

A73 | Neuromuscular | Interventions

A patient has a 3 year history of multiple sclerosis. One of the disabling symptoms is persistent and severe diplopia, which leaves the patient frequently nauseated and immobile. An appropriate intervention strategy to assist the patient in successfully participating in rehabilitation would be to:

CHOICES:
1. provide the patient with special glasses that magnify images.
2. instruct the patient to close both eyes and practice movements without visual guidance.
3. provide the patient with a soft neck collar to limit head and neck movements.
4. patch one eye.

CORRECT ANSWER: 4

RATIONALE:
Double vision (diplopia) can be managed by patching of one eye. Patients are typically on an eye-patching schedule that alternates the eye that is patched. Loss of depth perception can be expected with eye-patching but is not as disabling as diplopia.

TYPE OF REASONING: INFERENTIAL
One must determine an intervention approach that will effectively address the patient's deficits. This requires one to determine what will be most beneficial for a patient, which is an inferential reasoning skill. For this scenario, the most effective intervention strategy for the patient's diplopia is to patch one eye. If answered incorrectly, review intervention approaches for diplopia for patients with multiple sclerosis.

A74 | Neuromuscular | Interventions

The **MOST** appropriate positioning strategy for a patient recovering from acute stroke who is in bed and who demonstrates a flaccid upper extremity is:

CHOICES:

1. supine with the affected upper extremity flexed with hand resting on stomach.
2. side-lying on the sound side with the affected shoulder protracted, and upper extremity extended resting on a pillow.
3. supine with the affected elbow extended and upper extremity positioned close to the side of the trunk.
4. side-lying on the sound side with the affected upper extremity flexed overhead.

CORRECT ANSWER: 2

RATIONALE:

Most patients with stroke recover from the flaccid stage and develop spasticity. Positioning for the patient with early stroke stresses (1) protection against ligamentous strain and the development of a painful subluxed shoulder and (2) positions counter to the typical spastic posture of flexion and adduction with pronation. Side-lying with the affected upper extremity supported on a pillow with the shoulder protracted and elbow extended accomplishes both of these goals. The other positions do not.

TYPE OF REASONING: INDUCTIVE

One must utilize clinical judgment to determine the most appropriate positioning strategy for a patient with acute stroke. This is an inductive reasoning skill. For this case, the most appropriate positioning strategy is side-lying on the sound side with the affected shoulder protracted, and upper extremity extended resting on a pillow. If answered incorrectly, review positioning strategies for a patient with stroke.

A75 | Other Systems | Clinical Applications

A physical therapist assistant is gait training an older adult in the home setting who has had a recent total hip arthroplasty. The patient is complaining of new tenderness in the groin, anterior hip and thigh area. The assistant should recognize that tenderness in these areas can also be an indication of:

CHOICES:

1. constipation.
2. diarrhea.
3. inflammatory bowel disease.
4. gastritis.

CORRECT ANSWER: 1

RATIONALE:

Constipation can cause abdominal pain and tenderness in the anterior hip, groin or thigh area. The assistant working with a patient who is homebound should recognize that a decreased activity level and the addition of pain medications can both lead to constipation. The identified tenderness is not a likely symptom of diarrhea, inflammatory bowel disease or gastritis.

TYPE OF REASONING: ANALYTICAL

This question provides a group of symptoms and the test taker must determine the most likely cause for these symptoms. This requires one to analyze the various symptoms to draw a correct conclusion, which is an analytical reasoning skill. For this case, the symptoms are indicative of constipation. If answered incorrectly, review signs and symptoms of constipation.

A76 | Integumentary | Data Collection

A patient presents with a large plantar ulcer that will be debrided. The foot is cold, pale and painless. The condition that would **MOST LIKELY** result in this clinical presentation is:

CHOICES:
1. chronic arterial insufficiency.
2. chronic venous insufficiency.
3. acute arterial insufficiency.
4. deep venous thrombosis.

CORRECT ANSWER: 2

RATIONALE:

Venous ulcers are often painless, or present with minimal pain compared with arterial ulcers, which are painful (claudication and rest pain). Chronic venous insufficiency is also characterized by thickening, coarsening and brownish pigmentation of the skin around the ankles. The skin is usually thin, shiny, and cyanotic. Deep venous thrombosis may be asymptomatic initially. When symptoms occur, patients typically report a dull ache, tightness or pain in the calf.

TYPE OF REASONING: ANALYTICAL

This question provides symptoms for a patient with a plantar ulcer and one must determine the most likely cause for such symptoms. This requires analytical reasoning skill, as symptoms are analyzed to reach a conclusion. For this situation, the symptoms indicate chronic venous insufficiency. If answered incorrectly, review signs and symptoms of chronic venous insufficiency.

A77 | Devices, Admin, etc. | Equipment, Modalities

A patient has been referred for physical therapy following a fracture of the femur 6 months ago. The cast was removed, but the patient was unable to volitionally contract the quadriceps. To address this problem the therapist indicates utilization of electrical stimulation to the quadriceps muscle in the plan of care. The **MOST** appropriate electrode size and placement for the physical therapist assistant to select is:

CHOICES:
1. large electrodes, closely spaced.
2. small electrodes, closely spaced.
3. large electrodes, widely spaced.
4. small electrodes, widely spaced.

CORRECT ANSWER: 3

RATIONALE:

Large electrodes are used on large muscles to disperse the current (minimize current density under the electrode) enabling a more comfortable delivery of current. Widely spaced electrodes permit the current to travel deeper into the muscle to stimulate a greater number of deeper muscle fibers.

TYPE OF REASONING: DEDUCTIVE

One must recall the guidelines for electrode size and placement for electrical stimulation to arrive at a correct conclusion. This necessitates the recall of factual protocols and guidelines, which is a deductive reasoning skill. For this case, the therapist should select large electrodes, widely spaced. If answered incorrectly, review electrical stimulation guidelines for stimulation of the quadriceps, especially electrode size and placement.

A78 | Neuromuscular | Data Collection

A patient suffered a severe traumatic brain injury and multiple fractures following a motor vehicle accident. The patient is recovering in the intensive care unit. The physical therapy referral requests passive range of motion and positioning. On day 1 the patient is semi-alert and drifts in and out during treatment. On day 2 the patient is less alert and the status is changing. Signs and symptoms of a possible life-threatening situation that would require emergency consultation with nursing and the physician include:

CHOICES:
1. developing irritability and disorientation.
2. decreasing function of eye movements.
3. rigidity in the neck muscles.
4. decreasing consciousness with slowing of pulse.

CORRECT ANSWER: 4

RATIONALE:
Signs of increased intracranial pressure secondary to cerebral edema and brain herniation include decreasing consciousness with slowing of pulse. The other choices are signs and symptoms associated with traumatic brain injury. All of the problems listed are serious. The correct choice is life-threatening.

TYPE OF REASONING: INFERENTIAL
One must infer or draw a reasonable conclusion about the symptoms that would indicate a life-threatening emergency and need for emergency consultation to arrive at a correct conclusion. This requires inferential reasoning skill. For this situation, symptoms of decreasing consciousness with slowing of pulse are indicative of an emergency and need for consultation, as they are signs of increased intracranial pressure. If answered incorrectly, review signs and symptoms of intracranial pressure and emergency procedures for patients with traumatic brain injuries.

A79 | Neuromuscular | Clinical Applications

A physical therapist assistant is working with a patient who has neurapraxia involving the ulnar nerve secondary to an elbow fracture. Based on knowledge of this condition, the assistant expects that:

CHOICES:
1. regeneration is likely in 6 to 8 months.
2. nerve dysfunction will be rapidly reversed, generally in 2 to 3 weeks.
3. regeneration is likely after 1 to 1½ years.
4. regeneration is unlikely because surgical approximation of the nerve ends was not performed.

CORRECT ANSWER: 2

RATIONALE:
Neurapraxia is a mild peripheral nerve injury (conduction block ischemia) that causes transient loss of function. Nerve dysfunction is rapidly reversed, generally within 2 to 3 weeks. An example is a compression injury to the radial nerve from falling asleep with the upper extremity over the back of a chair (Saturday night palsy).

TYPE OF REASONING: INFERENTIAL
This question provides a diagnosis and one must infer the likely progression of recovery to arrive at a correct conclusion. This requires one to determine what may be true for a patient, which is an inferential reasoning skill. For this case, one should expect that nerve dysfunction will be rapidly reversed, generally in 2 to 3 weeks. If answered incorrectly, review ulnar nerve neurapraxia and progression of recovery.

A80 | Other Systems | Clinical Applications

A home health physical therapist assistant is working with an older adult patient. On this day the patient is confused with shortness of breath and generalized weakness. Given the patient's history of hypertension and hyperlipidemia, the assistant should immediately contact the supervising physical therapist with information that:

CHOICES:

1. mental changes are indicative of early Alzheimer's disease.
2. the patient may be experiencing unstable angina.
3. the patient forgot to take his or her hypertension medication.
4. the patient may be presenting with early signs of myocardial infarction.

CORRECT ANSWER: 4

RATIONALE:

An elderly patient with a cardiac history may present with initial symptoms of mental confusion, the result of oxygen deprivation to the brain during developing myocardial infarction. The shortness of breath and generalized weakness may also be attributable to generalized circulatory insufficiencies coexisting with the developing myocardial infarction.

TYPE OF REASONING: ANALYTICAL

This question provides a group of symptoms and the test taker must determine the most likely cause for them. This requires analytical reasoning skill. For this case, the patient's symptoms are most indicative of early signs of myocardial infarction, given the history of hypertension and hyperlipidemia. If answered incorrectly, review early signs and symptoms of myocardial infarction.

A81 | Musculoskeletal | Clinical Applications

A baseball pitcher is being seen following surgical repair of a glenoid labrum lesion of the pitching upper extremity. In follow-up care, the assistant needs to pay attention to the pitching motion. The phase of the throwing motion that puts the **GREATEST** stress on the labrum and capsule is:

CHOICES:

1. wind-up.
2. cocking.
3. acceleration.
4. deceleration.

CORRECT ANSWER: 2

RATIONALE:

During the cocking phase, the upper extremity is taken into the end range of humeral lateral (external) rotation. At that point, the anterior aspects of the capsule and labrum are acting as constraints to prevent excessive anterior glide of the humerus.

TYPE OF REASONING: ANALYTICAL

One must analyze the conditions presented when pitching and utilize knowledge of stress factors for the labrum and capsule during pitching to arrive at a correct conclusion. This requires analytical reasoning skill. For this case, the greatest stress during pitching occurs during the cocking phase. If answered incorrectly, review effects of pitching on glenoid labrum and capsule stress.

A82 | Integumentary | Interventions

A frail older adult is confined to bed in a nursing facility and has developed a small superficial wound over the sacral area. Because only small amounts of necrotic tissue are present, the physical therapist has decided to use autolytic wound débridement. This is **BEST** achieved with:

CHOICES:

1. wound irrigation using a syringe.
2. transparent film dressing.
3. wet-to-dry gauze dressing with antimicrobial ointment.
4. sharp débridement.

CORRECT ANSWER: 2

RATIONALE:

Autolytic wound débridement allows the body's natural enzymes to promote healing by trapping them under a synthetic, occlusive dressing. Moisture-retentive dressings are applied for short durations (less than 2 weeks). Choices include transparent film dressings, hydrocolloid or hydrogel dressings. The other answers are wound management techniques; however, they are not autolytic.

TYPE OF REASONING: ANALYTICAL

One must recall the parameters for autolytic wound débridement and effective approaches to arrive at a correct conclusion. This requires one to analyze the approaches presented to determine the approach that will be most effective for wound healing. For this situation, transparent film dressing is best. If answered incorrectly, review wound healing guidelines for superficial wounds, especially autolytic wound débridement and dressings.

A83 | Musculoskeletal | Clinical Applications

The plan of care includes strengthening for a patient who reports subpatellar pain after participation in an aerobic exercise program for two weeks. The physical therapist's examination shows a large Q angle, pain with palpation at the inferior pole of the patella and mild swelling at both knees. The intervention should promote:

CHOICES:

1. vastus medialis muscle strengthening.
2. lateral patellar tracking.
3. vastus lateralis strengthening.
4. hamstring strengthening.

CORRECT ANSWER: 1

RATIONALE:

Q angles greater than 15° could be indicative of abnormal lateral patellar tracking. Vastus medialis muscle strengthening can reduce the tendency for the patella to track laterally. Vastus lateralis strengthening can promote greater lateral patellar tracking and further irritation of the patellofemoral joint. Vastus lateralis strengthening may promote an outward pull or dislocation of the patella. Hamstring strengthening does not directly affect tracking of the patella. In the closed chain, problems at the hip or foot can also contribute to patellofemoral pain syndrome.

TYPE OF REASONING: INDUCTIVE

One must utilize clinical judgment to determine a best course of action for a patient with subpatellar pain and a large Q angle. This requires inductive reasoning skill. For this case, the assistant should focus intervention efforts on vastus medialis strengthening. If answered incorrectly, review intervention approaches for subpatellar pain and large Q angle.

A84 | Neuromuscular | Clinical Applications

A physical therapist assistant is working with a patient in the patient's home. The patient is being seen for right hemiparesis. The physical therapy evaluation indicates that the patient demonstrates good recovery; both involved extremities are categorized as out-of-synergy. The patient is ambulatory with a small-based quad cane. The activity that would be **MOST** appropriate for a patient at this stage of recovery is:

CHOICES:
1. supine, bending the hip and knee up to the chest with some hip abduction.
2. sitting, marching in place (alternate hip flexion movements).
3. standing, picking the foot up behind and slowly lowering it.
4. standing, small-range knee extension movements to gain quadriceps control.

CORRECT ANSWER: 3

RATIONALE:

This stage of recovery is characterized by some movement combinations that do not follow paths of either flexion or extension obligatory synergies. Knee flexion in standing is an out-of-synergy movement. All other choices represent synergistic movements: the supine and sitting options are flexion synergy movements whereas the other standing option focuses on knee extensor movement within an extended position.

TYPE OF REASONING: INDUCTIVE

One must determine the most appropriate activity for a patient with hemiparesis and decline in spasticity. This requires knowledge of rehabilitation guidelines for patients with spasticity to arrive at a correct conclusion. This requires inductive reasoning skill. For this case, the most appropriate activity for a patient is standing, picking the foot up behind and slowly lowering it. If answered incorrectly, review rehabilitation guidelines for patients with spasticity.

A85 | Neuromuscular | Data Collection

A physical therapist assistant who has moved a patient's joint through its available range of motion, then stops to hold the joint in flexion, and asks the patient to identify the position of the joint is testing:

CHOICES:
1. tactile localization.
2. kinesthesia.
3. proprioception.
4. pressure perception.

CORRECT ANSWER: 3

RATIONALE:

Proprioception tests are performed by positioning a patient's affected joint into a position, following an instructional trial, and asking the patient to verbally (or visually using the uninvolved extremity) report which position the joint is in. Kinesthesia awareness is tested by moving the patient's affected joint through a portion of its range of motion and asking the patient to identify the range of movement performed. Tactile localization is assessing the patient's ability to identify the location of a touch stimulus provided by the clinician, e.g., radial condyle, web space of hand. Pressure perception is tested by applying pressure to a specific location using a finger tip or cotton swab and asking the patient to respond "yes" or "no" when they feel pressure.

TYPE OF REASONING: DEDUCTIVE

One must recall the testing procedures for proprioception to arrive at a correct conclusion. This necessitates the recall of factual procedures and guidelines, which is a deductive reasoning skill. For this situation, the test procedure described is that of proprioception. If answered incorrectly, review proprioception testing procedures.

A86 | Cardiovascular/Pulmonary | Clinical Applications

What is a preferred treatment position when one is providing strengthening exercises for a patient who is diagnosed with pulmonary edema?

CHOICES:

1. supine with the lower extremities elevated.
2. sitting with the lower extremities dangling.
3. side-lying.
4. prone with the head down.

CORRECT ANSWER: 2

RATIONALE:

The sitting position helps decrease the work of breathing and reduces venous return. Supine lying is a more difficult position for breathing. The side-lying or prone positions do not alleviate the difficulty with breathing.

TYPE OF REASONING: INDUCTIVE

This question requires one to determine the best position for strengthening exercises for a patient with pulmonary edema. This necessitates clinical judgment, which is an inductive reasoning skill. For this situation, the assistant should position the patient in sitting with the lower extremities dangling. If answered incorrectly, review positioning techniques for patients with pulmonary edema.

A87 | Devices, Admin, etc. | Equipment, Modalities

A patient with bilateral short transfemoral amputations will require a wheelchair for functional mobility in the home and community. An important feature for the wheelchair is:

CHOICES:

1. placement of the drive wheels 2 inches anterior to the vertical back supports.
2. lowering the seat height by 3 inches.
3. increasing the seat depth by 2 inches to accommodate the length of the residual extremities.
4. placement of the drive wheels 2 inches posterior to the vertical back supports.

CORRECT ANSWER: 4

RATIONALE:

Placement of the drive wheels 2 inches posterior to the vertical back supports is an appropriate modification for a patient with bilateral transfemoral amputations. This increases the length of the base of support and provides increased posterior stability. Lowering the seat height by 3 inches is an appropriate modification for a patient following a cardiovascular accident, who will use his or her sound extremities for wheelchair propulsion. Increasing the seat depth is not appropriate.

TYPE OF REASONING: INDUCTIVE

One must utilize knowledge of wheelchair prescription guidelines to arrive at a correct conclusion. This requires inductive reasoning skill. For this case, it is important for a patient with bilateral transfemoral amputations to have a wheelchair with placement of the drive wheels 2 inches posterior to the vertical back supports. If answered incorrectly, review wheelchair prescription guidelines for patients with bilateral transfemoral amputations.

A88 | Musculoskeletal | Clinical Applications

In treating a patient with a diagnosis of right shoulder impingement syndrome, the plan of care is focused on regaining normal scapular–humeral rhythm. The **FIRST** priority of the treatment should be to:

CHOICES:
1. implement a stretching program for the shoulder girdle musculature.
2. instruct the patient in proper postural alignment.
3. achieve complete active range of motion in all shoulder motions.
4. modulate all pain.

CORRECT ANSWER: 2

RATIONALE:
Without regaining normal postural alignment and scapular–humeral rhythm, the patient will continue to impinge the supraspinatus and/or biceps tendon at the acromion and never regain normal function of the shoulder. It is unlikely that all pain would be controlled. Appropriate active range of motion exercises and/or stretching could be the focus after posture has been corrected.

TYPE OF REASONING: INDUCTIVE
This question requires the test taker to determine a first priority in treatment of a patient with shoulder impingement syndrome. This requires knowledge of the diagnosis and appropriate intervention approaches, which is an inductive reasoning skill. For this situation, the priority should be to instruct the patient in proper postural alignment. If answered incorrectly, review intervention approaches for patients with shoulder impingement syndrome.

A89 | Musculoskeletal | Data Collection

Drooping of the shoulder, winging of the same scapula and inability to shrug the shoulder is **MOST LIKELY** caused by:

CHOICES:
1. muscle imbalance.
2. a lesion of the long thoracic nerve.
3. a lesion of the spinal accessory nerve.
4. strain of the serratus anterior.

CORRECT ANSWER: 3

RATIONALE:
Although this winging of the scapula could be found with all of the above answers, the shoulder drooping and inability to shrug the shoulder is secondary to a lesion of the spinal accessory nerve (cranial nerve XI), which innervates the trapezius muscle.

TYPE OF REASONING: ANALYTICAL
This question provides a group of symptoms and one must determine the most likely cause for them. This requires analysis of the symptoms to reach a correct conclusion, which is an analytical reasoning skill. For this case, the symptoms indicate a lesion of the spinal accessory nerve. If answered incorrectly, review signs and symptoms of spinal accessory nerve lesion.

A90 | Other Systems | Clinical Applications

An elderly and frail patient is being seen for balance instability and frequent falls. The patient arrives for a therapy session complaining of pain and tingling in the forehead, cheek and jaw on the left side of the face. An inspection of the face and trunk reveals the eruption of vesicles in the distribution of the T2 dermatome. The assistant's best course of action is to:

CHOICES:

1. discuss this with the physical therapist with potential referral to the primary physician.
2. utilize a hot pack to help relieve the pain and continue with balance training.
3. advise the patient to take a pain reliever and contact the physician if the pain worsens.
4. instruct the patient in cervical stretches to help relax the muscles on the left side of the neck.

CORRECT ANSWER: 1

RATIONALE:

This patient is exhibiting signs of a herpes zoster infection (varicella zoster virus [VZV]). This is also known as shingles; the same virus causes chickenpox in children. Varicella zoster virus affects the sensory ganglia of the spinal cord or cranial nerves (commonly the trigeminal nerve, cranial nerve V [CNV], and thoracic dermatomes). Early inflammation produces pain and tingling; late symptoms include postherpetic neuralgia (severe aching or burning pain) that can persist for months or years. The physical therapist assistant should recognize these early symptoms and immediately notify the physical therapist who will likely recommend an immediate physician visit. The physician will likely order antiviral medications (e.g., acyclovir) to control the virus; this may also help with pain. Oral medications can be used to control pain; however, recommending this is not within the scope of the assistant. Other interventions listed can be used to relieve pain but may be contraindicated without a full diagnostic workup and referral.

TYPE OF REASONING: EVALUATIVE

This question provides symptoms and the test taker must determine an appropriate course of action based on these symptoms. One must weigh the merits of the potential courses of action to arrive at a correct conclusion, which is an evaluative reasoning skill. For this situation, the assistant should discuss the symptoms with the physical therapist with potential referral to the primary physician, as the symptoms indicate VZV infection. Review signs and symptoms of VZV infection if answered incorrectly.

A91 | Devices, Admin, etc. | Equipment, Modalities

A patient with spastic hemiplegia is referred to physical therapy. The physical therapy evaluation indicates that the patient is having difficulty in rising to a standing position as a result of co-contraction of the hamstrings and quadriceps. The plan of care calls for the use of biofeedback as an adjunct to help break up this pattern. For knee extension, the biofeedback protocol should consist of:

CHOICES:

1. high-detection sensitivity with electrodes placed close together.
2. low-detection sensitivity with electrodes placed far apart.
3. high-detection sensitivity with electrodes placed far apart.
4. low-detection sensitivity with electrodes placed close together.

CORRECT ANSWER: 4

RATIONALE:

When the electrodes are close together, the likelihood of detecting undesired motor unit activity from adjacent muscles (crosstalk) decreases. By setting the sensitivity (gain) low, the amplitude of signals generated by the hypertonic muscles would decrease and keep the electromyograph output from exceeding a visual or auditory range.

TYPE OF REASONING: DEDUCTIVE

This question requires the test taker to recall the guidelines for use of biofeedback for patients with abnormal co-contraction to arrive at a correct conclusion. This is factual information, which is a deductive reasoning skill. For this case, the biofeedback protocol should consist of low-detection sensitivity with electrodes placed close together. If answered incorrectly, review biofeedback guidelines and electrode placement.

A92 | Musculoskeletal | Clinical Applications

A patient sustained a T10 spinal cord injury 4 years ago and is now referred for an episode of outpatient physical therapy. In the initial examination the physical therapist documented redness over the ischial seat that persisted for 10 minutes when the patient was not sitting. The plan of care includes strengthening and instruction in functional activities. Which of the following activities should the physical therapist assistant include in the therapy session to meet the plan of care?

CHOICES:
1. supine chest press with 20-pound barbell.
2. half-standing transfers between surfaces.
3. bilateral upper-extremity dips in the parallel bars.
4. seated, gravity-resisted triceps curls with 10 pounds.

CORRECT ANSWER: 3

RATIONALE:

Bilateral upper-extremity dips in the parallel bars will best strengthen the musculature needed to assist the patient to improve the ability to perform wheelchair push-ups to relieve pressure on the ischial tuberosities. Excessive ischial pressure and redness from prolonged sitting require an aggressive approach. Supine chest presses and gravity-resisted triceps curls only incorporate the triceps muscles and do not incorporate the latissimus; therefore, they are not as comprehensive in muscle recruitment as the parallel bar dips are. Performing the half-standing transfers for the patient is not functional training.

TYPE OF REASONING: INDUCTIVE

This question requires the test taker to determine a best therapeutic approach for a patient with ischial redness. This requires clinical judgment, which is an inductive reasoning skill. For this case, the assistant should include bilateral upper-extremity dips in the parallel bars to strengthen the muscles needed to perform wheelchair push-ups. If answered incorrectly, review pressure relief techniques and exercises for patients with ischial redness.

A93 | Devices, Admin, etc. | Safety, Roles, Teaching, EBP

A physical therapist assistant working in a long-term care facility witnesses a resident's family member collapse to the floor. Immediately after calling for help the assistant should:

CHOICES:
1. open the victim's airway and deliver two rescue breaths.
2. get an automated external defibrillator (AED) and begin cardiopulmonary resuscitation (CPR) and use of AED.
3. roll the victim over and deliver two quick abdominal thrusts.
4. deliver about 5 cycles (2 minutes) of CPR before calling for help.

CORRECT ANSWER: 2

RATIONALE:

When a sudden collapse is witnessed, for victims of all ages, healthcare providers should call for help (emergency response system outside of a care facility, or call for a code [or as directed in policy and procedure manual] in a care facility) and get an AED when readily available. In this instance the assistant is working in a long-term care facility; most likely an AED is immediately available. When an unresponsive victim is found, a healthcare provider should assess ABCs (airway, breathing and consciousness) and initiate CPR if appropriate after calling for help and getting an AED. Abdominal thrusts are only delivered if it is determined that the victim has choked on something.

TYPE OF REASONING: EVALUATIVE

This question requires one to weigh the courses of action presented and then make a determination of the action that will best address the person's immediate needs. This requires evaluative reasoning skill. For this situation, the assistant should get an AED and begin CPR and use of AED after calling for help. If answered incorrectly, review CPR and first responder guidelines.

A94 | Neuromuscular | Data Collection

During treatment in an outpatient rehabilitation center for an 18-month-old child with developmental delay and an atrioventricular shunt for hydrocephalus, the mother tells the assistant that the child vomited several times this morning, was irritable and is now lethargic. The assistant's **BEST** course of action is to:

CHOICES:

1. call for emergency transportation and notify the physical therapist immediately.
2. apply cold washcloths to try to rouse the child.
3. place the child in a side-lying position and monitor vital signs.
4. have the mother give the child clear liquids because the child vomited.

CORRECT ANSWER: 1

RATIONALE:

These signs could be the result of increased cerebral edema because of a clogged or infected shunt. Medical attention should be obtained immediately to avoid damage to the brain.

TYPE OF REASONING: EVALUATIVE

This question requires one to weigh the symptoms presented and then determine the best course of action that effectively addresses the issue at hand. This requires evaluative reasoning skill. For this case, the assistant should call for emergency transportation and notify the physical therapist immediately, as the symptoms indicate possible cerebral edema. Review signs and symptoms of cerebral edema, as well as first aid guidelines, if answered incorrectly.

A95 | Musculoskeletal | Interventions

A woman recently delivered twins. After delivery she developed a 4-cm diastasis recti abdominis. The **BEST INITIAL** intervention for this problem is to teach:

CHOICES:

1. pelvic tilts and bilateral straight leg raising.
2. pelvic floor exercises and sit-ups.
3. gentle stretching of hamstrings and hip flexors.
4. protection and splinting of the abdominal musculature.

CORRECT ANSWER: 4

RATIONALE:

Diastasis recti abdominis is a condition in which there is a lateral separation or split of the rectus abdominis. It is important to teach protection (splinting) of the abdominal musculature. Patients should be instructed to avoid full sit-ups or bilateral straight leg raising. Pelvic floor exercises are done but are not remediation for diastasis recti.

TYPE OF REASONING: INDUCTIVE

One must utilize clinical judgment to determine the best initial intervention for a patient with diastasis recti abdominis. Questions of this nature often require inductive reasoning skill. For this situation, the best initial intervention is teaching protection and splinting of the abdominal musculature. If answered incorrectly, review intervention guidelines for diastasis recti abdominis.

A96 | Neuromuscular | Clinical Applications

A patient has a 2 year history of amyotrophic lateral sclerosis and exhibits moderate functional deficits. The patient is still ambulatory with bilateral canes but is limited in endurance. When implementing the physical therapy plan of care, the physical therapist assistant should be careful to prevent:

CHOICES:

1. radicular pain and paresthesias.
2. overwork and damage in weakened, denervated muscle.
3. further ataxia.
4. further functional loss as a result of myalgia.

CORRECT ANSWER: 2

RATIONALE:

Amyotrophic lateral sclerosis is a progressive degenerative disease that affects both upper and lower motor neurons. An important early goal of physical therapy is to maintain the patient's level of conditioning while preventing overwork damage in denervated muscle (lower motor neuron injury). Myalgia is common in lower motor neuron lesions. It can be ameliorated but not prevented. Ataxia and radicular pain are not associated with amyotrophic lateral sclerosis.

TYPE OF REASONING: INDUCTIVE

One must utilize clinical judgment to determine therapeutic approaches that the assistant should prevent. This requires knowledge of the diagnosis to arrive at a correct conclusion, which is an inductive reasoning skill. For this situation, the assistant should prevent overworking and damaging the weakened, denervated muscle. If answered incorrectly, review therapeutic approaches for patients with amyotrophic lateral sclerosis and precautions for exercise.

A97 | Devices, Admin, etc. | Equipment, Modalities

A patient has extensive full-thickness burns to the dorsum of the right hand and forearm and is being fitted with a resting splint to support the wrists and hands in a functional position. An appropriately constructed splint positions the wrist and hand in:

CHOICES:

1. neutral wrist position with slight finger flexion and thumb flexion.
2. slight wrist extension with fingers supported and thumb in partial opposition and abduction.
3. slight wrist flexion with interphalangeal joint extension and thumb opposition.
4. neutral wrist position with interphalangeal joint extension and thumb flexion.

CORRECT ANSWER: 2

RATIONALE:

A resting splint that positions the wrist and hand in a functional position includes 10° to 20° of wrist extension, fingers supported and thumb in partial opposition and abduction.

TYPE OF REASONING: DEDUCTIVE

This question requires one to recall the guidelines for hand splinting after burns. This is factual information, requiring deductive reasoning skill. For this case, the functional hand splinting position includes slight wrist extension with fingers supported, and thumb in partial opposition and abduction. Review splinting guidelines for patients with hand burns if answered incorrectly.

A98 | Neuromuscular | Interventions

A young child with Down syndrome and moderate developmental delay is being treated at an early intervention program. Daily training activities that should be considered include:

CHOICES:

1. stimulation to postural extensors in sitting using rhythmic stabilization.
2. locomotor training using body weight support and a motorized treadmill.
3. holding and weight shifting in sitting and standing using tactile and verbal cueing.
4. rolling activities, initiating movement with stretch and tracking resistance.

CORRECT ANSWER: 3

RATIONALE:

Children with Down syndrome typically present with generalized hypotonicity. The low tone is best managed by weight-bearing activities in antigravity postures. Typical responses include widened base-of-support and co-contraction to gain stability. Proprioceptors are not in a high state of readiness and the child may be slow to respond to proprioceptive facilitation techniques (i.e., stretch, resistance, rhythmic stabilization). Verbal cueing for redirection is generally the best form of feedback to use along with visually guided postural control. With developmental delay this child is not ready for intensive locomotor training.

TYPE OF REASONING: INDUCTIVE

One must have knowledge of therapeutic activities for children with Down syndrome to arrive at a correct conclusion. This requires clinical judgment, which is an inductive reasoning skill. For this case, the assistant should focus on holding and weight shifting in sitting and standing using tactile and verbal cueing. Review treatment activities for children with Down syndrome if answered incorrectly.

A99 | Neuromuscular | Data Collection

A patient with multiple sclerosis demonstrates strong bilateral lower-extremity extensor spasticity in the typical distribution of antigravity muscles. This patient should be expected to demonstrate:

CHOICES:

1. sitting with the pelvis laterally tilted with increased weight-bearing on ischial tuberosities.
2. sacral sitting with increased extension and adduction of lower extremities.
3. sitting with both legs abducted and laterally (externally) rotated.
4. skin breakdown on the ischial tuberosities and lateral malleoli.

CORRECT ANSWER: 2

RATIONALE:

Spasticity is typically strong in antigravity muscles. In the lower extremities this is usually the hip and knee extensors, adductors and plantar flexors. Strong extensor tone results in sacral sitting with the pelvis tilted posteriorly.

TYPE OF REASONING: INFERENTIAL

One must determine what may be true for a patient with multiple sclerosis to arrive at a correct conclusion. This requires inferential reasoning skill. For this situation, the patient is likely to present with sacral sitting with increased extension and adduction of lower extremities. If answered incorrectly, review signs and symptoms of multiple sclerosis, especially effects of spasticity on functional positioning.

A100 | Neuromuscular | Clinical Applications

A patient with multiple sclerosis (MS) has been on prednisolone for the past 4 weeks. The medication is now being tapered off. This is the third time this year that the patient has received this treatment for an MS exacerbation. The physical therapist assistant recognizes that possible adverse effects of this medication are:

CHOICES:

1. weight gain and hyperkinetic behaviors.
2. hypoglycemia and nausea or vomiting.
3. muscle wasting, weakness and osteoporosis.
4. spontaneous fractures with prolonged healing or mal-union.

CORRECT ANSWER: 3

RATIONALE:

This patient is receiving systemic corticosteroids to suppress inflammation and the normal immune system response during an MS attack. Chronic treatment leads to adrenal suppression. There are numerous adverse reactions and side effects that can occur. Those affecting the patient's capacity to exercise include muscle wasting and pain, weakness and osteoporosis. Weight loss is common (anorexia) with nausea and vomiting. Adrenal suppression produces hyperglycemia, not hypoglycemia. Spontaneous fractures are not typical.

TYPE OF REASONING: DEDUCTIVE

One must recall the potential adverse effects of prednisolone to arrive at a correct conclusion. This requires recall of factual guidelines, which is a deductive reasoning skill. For this case, one should expect the potential adverse effects to include muscle wasting, weakness and osteoporosis. If answered incorrectly, review adverse effects of prednisolone.

A101 | Neuromuscular | Clinical Applications

A patient suffered carbon monoxide poisoning from a work-related factory accident and is left with permanent damage to the basal ganglia. Intervention for this patient will need to address expected impairments of:

CHOICES:

1. motor paralysis with the use of free weights to increase strength.
2. muscular spasms and hyperreflexia with the use of ice wraps.
3. impaired sensory organization of balance with the use of standing balance platform training.
4. motor planning with the use of guided and cued movement.

CORRECT ANSWER: 4

RATIONALE:

The basal ganglia functions to convert general motor activity into specific, goal-directed action plans. Dysfunction results in problems with motor planning and scaling of movements and postures (e.g., bradykinesia). Patients benefit from initial guided movement and task-specific training. Proprioceptive, tactile and verbal cues can also be used prior to and during a task to enhance movement. The other listed deficits (choices) are not typically seen with basal ganglia disorders.

TYPE OF REASONING: INFERENTIAL

This question requires the test taker to determine what symptoms are likely to be present and best intervention approaches for a patient with basal ganglia damage. This requires inferential reasoning skill. For this case, one should expect impairments in motor planning and should choose guided and cued movement. If answered incorrectly, review signs and symptoms of basal ganglia damage, as well as intervention approaches for this diagnosis.

A102 | Neuromuscular | Clinical Applications

While evaluating the gait of a patient with right hemiplegia, the physical therapist assistant notes foot drop during midswing on the right. The **MOST LIKELY** cause of this deviation is:

CHOICES:

1. inadequate contraction of the ankle dorsiflexors.
2. excessive extensor synergy.
3. decreased proprioception of foot and ankle muscles.
4. excessive flexor synergy.

CORRECT ANSWER: 1

RATIONALE:

Weakness or delayed contraction of the ankle dorsiflexors or spasticity in the ankle plantar flexors may cause foot drop during midswing. Excessive extensor synergy would cause plantar flexion during stance. Decreased proprioception of the foot and ankle muscles would cause difficulties with foot placement and balance during stance. A strong flexor synergy can cause dorsiflexion with hip and knee flexion during swing.

TYPE OF REASONING: ANALYTICAL

This question requires the test taker to analyze the symptoms for a patient with right hemiplegia and foot drop during midswing and determine a likely cause for the deviation. Questions of this nature often require analytical reasoning skill. For this situation, the most likely cause is inadequate contraction of the ankle dorsiflexors. Review causes of foot drop in patients with hemiplegia if answered incorrectly.

A103 | Devices, Admin, etc. | Equipment, Modalities

The use of ultrasound in the area of a joint arthroplasty is permissible even if the surrounding area contains:

CHOICES:

1. plastic implants.
2. infected tissue.
3. metal implants.
4. neoplastic lesions.

CORRECT ANSWER: 3

RATIONALE:

Several studies have shown the safe use of ultrasound over metal implants. The acoustical energy is dispersed throughout the metal and is absorbed into the surrounding tissue. There is no significant heating within the implant. The other choices are contraindications for the use of ultrasound.

TYPE OF REASONING: DEDUCTIVE

One must recall the guidelines for the use of ultrasound under certain conditions. This requires the recall of guidelines, which is a deductive reasoning skill. For this scenario, it is permissible to use ultrasound over metal implants. If answered incorrectly, review guidelines for safe use of ultrasound.

A104 | Neuromuscular | Data Collection

A physical therapist assistant observes genu recurvatum while gait training a patient with hemiplegia. The patient has been using a posterior leaf spring orthosis since discharge from subacute rehabilitation 4 weeks ago. The patient has strong synergies in the lower extremity and **NO** out-of-synergy movement. The **MOST LIKELY** cause of this deviation is:

CHOICES:

1. extensor spasticity.
2. hip flexor weakness.
3. dorsiflexor spasticity.
4. hamstring weakness.

CORRECT ANSWER: 1

RATIONALE:

A hyperextended knee can be caused by extensor spasticity, quadriceps weakness (a compensatory locking of the knee) or by plantar flexion contractures or deformity. The most likely cause in this case is extensor spasticity, which is consistent with strong obligatory synergies.

TYPE OF REASONING: ANALYTICAL

This question reveals deficits and the test taker must analyze the symptoms to determine a likely cause for them. Questions of this nature require analytical reasoning skill. For this situation, the most likely cause is extensor spasticity. Review causes of extensor spasticity in patients with hemiplegia if answered incorrectly.

A105 | Cardiovascular/Pulmonary | Data Collection

During a home visit a physical therapist assistant is providing postural drainage in the Trendelenburg position to a adolescent with cystic fibrosis. The patient suddenly experiences right-sided chest pain and shortness of breath. On auscultation, there are **NO** breath sounds on the right. The assistant should:

CHOICES:

1. continue treating as it is possibly a mucous plug.
2. reposition patient with the head of the bed flat as the Trendelenburg position is causing shortness of breath.
3. place the right lung in a gravity-dependent position to improve perfusion.
4. call emergency medical services as it may be a pneumothorax.

CORRECT ANSWER: 4

RATIONALE:

The combined signs and symptoms of absent breath sounds, sudden onset of chest pain and shortness of breath indicate a pneumothorax, especially in a adolescent (growth spurt) with pathological changes of lung tissue. This is an emergency situation.

TYPE OF REASONING: EVALUATIVE

This question requires one to weigh the courses of action presented to determine the action that will effectively address the patient's symptoms. This requires evaluative reasoning skill. For this situation, the assistant should call emergency medical services as it may be a pneumothorax. Review first aid approaches for patients with pneumothorax if answered incorrectly.

A106 | Neuromuscular | Interventions

A patient with an 8 year history of Parkinson's disease is referred for physical therapy. The initial evaluation identifies the patient as having significant rigidity, decreased passive range of motion in both upper extremities in the typical distribution and frequent episodes of akinesia. The exercise intervention that **BEST** deals with these problems is:

CHOICES:

1. quadruped position, upper-extremity proprioceptive neuromuscular facilitation (PNF) D2 flexion and extension.
2. resistance training, free weights for shoulder flexors at 80% of one repetition maximum.
3. modified plantigrade, isometric holding, stressing upper-extremity shoulder flexion.
4. PNF bilateral symmetrical upper extremity D2 flexion patterns, rhythmic initiation.

CORRECT ANSWER: 4

RATIONALE:

The patient with Parkinson's disease typically develops elbow flexion and shoulder adduction contractures of the upper extremities along with a flexed, stooped posture. Bilateral symmetrical upper-extremity PNF D2F patterns encourage shoulder flexion and abduction with elbow extension, and upper-trunk extension (all needed motions). Both quadruped and modified plantigrade positions encourage postural flexion.

TYPE OF REASONING: INDUCTIVE

One must utilize clinical judgment to determine the best intervention approach for a patient with Parkinson's disease. This is an inductive reasoning skill. For this case, the assistant should use PNF bilateral symmetrical upper-extremity D2 flexion patterns and rhythmic initiation to address the patient's deficits. If answered incorrectly, review intervention approaches for patients with Parkinson's disease, especially PNF approaches.

A107 | Neuromuscular | Clinical Applications

A patient is referred for rehabilitation following a middle cerebral artery stroke. Based on this diagnosis an assistant can expect that the patient will present with:

CHOICES:

1. contralateral hemiplegia with thalamic sensory syndrome and involuntary movements.
2. contralateral hemiparesis and sensory deficits, with the upper extremity more involved than the lower extremity.
3. decreased pain and temperature to the face and ipsilateral ataxia with contralateral pain and thermal loss of the body.
4. contralateral hemiparesis and sensory deficits, with the lower extremity more involved than the upper extremity.

CORRECT ANSWER: 2

RATIONALE:

A cerebrovascular accident (CVA) affecting the middle cerebral artery will result in symptoms of contralateral hemiparesis and hemisensory deficits with greater involvement of the upper extremity than the lower extremity. Contralateral hemiplegia with thalamic sensory syndrome and involuntary movements are characteristic of a CVA affecting the posterior cerebral artery syndrome (central territory). Decreased pain and temperature to the face and ipsilateral ataxia, with contralateral pain and thermal loss of the body are characteristic of a CVA affecting the vertebral artery, posterior inferior cerebellar artery (lateral medullary syndrome). Contraleteral hemiparesis and sensory deficits, with the lower extremity more involved than the upper extremity, are characteristic of a CVA affecting the anterior cerebral artery.

TYPE OF REASONING: DEDUCTIVE

This question requires the test taker to recall the symptoms of middle cerebral artery stroke to arrive at a correct conclusion. This necessitates recall of factual information, which is a deductive reasoning skill. For this diagnosis, the assistant should expect contralateral hemiparesis and sensory deficits, with the upper extremity more involved than the lower extremity. If answered incorrectly, review signs and symptoms of middle cerebral artery stroke.

A108 | Cardiovascular/Pulmonary | Data Collection

The cardiac rehabilitation team is conducting education classes for a group of patients. The focus is on risk factor reduction and successful lifestyle modification. A participant asks the physical therapist assistant to explain these cholesterol findings: Total cholesterol is 220 mg/dL, high-density liproprotein (HDL) cholesterol is 24 mg/dL, and low-density lipoprotein (LDL) cholesterol is 160 mg/dL. The assistant explains that these readings indicate:

CHOICES:

1. that the levels of HDL, LDL and total cholesterol are all abnormally high.
2. that LDL and HDL cholesterol levels are within normal limits and total cholesterol should be below 200 mg/dL.
3. that the levels of HDL, LDL and total cholesterol are all abnormally low.
4. the levels of LDL and total cholesterol are abnormally high and the level of HDL cholesterol is abnormally low.

CORRECT ANSWER: 4

RATIONALE:

Increased total blood cholesterol levels (>200 mg/dL) and levels of LDLs (>130 mg/dL) increase the risk of coronary artery disease (CAD); conversely, low concentrations of HDLs (<40 mg/dL for men and <50 mg/dL for women) are also harmful. The link between CAD and triglycerides is not as clear.

TYPE OF REASONING: ANALYTICAL

One must analyze the information presented to determine the significance of this information. This requires analytical reasoning skills, as pieces of information are assessed to draw a conclusion. For this situation, the findings indicate that the levels of LDL and total cholesterol are abnormally high and the HDL level is abnormally low. If answered incorrectly, review normal and abnormal blood cholesterol parameters.

A109 | Other Systems | Clinical Applications

When working with a patient in a pool who is submerged to chest level, the physical therapist assistant recognizes that:

CHOICES:

1. the patient will be able to better regulate body temperature in the water.
2. exercises will be more easily performed with the body part submerged more deeply in the water.
3. the patient's center of gravity (buoyancy in the water) moves higher, closer to the area of the sternum.
4. the more quickly the patient moves the easier the exercises will be.

CORRECT ANSWER: 3

RATIONALE:

When the patient is submerged in the pool, the patient's center of gravity moves to the area of the sternum. Buoyancy devices will alter this center of gravity, e.g., a buoyancy device placed posteriorly will cause the patient to lean forward. Temperature regulation is more challenging while submerged as less skin is exposed to allow heat dissipation through evaporation. Once the body part has overcome the surface tension and has been submerged in the water it will need to overcome the effects of buoyancy and viscosity; being submerged more deeply does not necessarily mean the exercise is harder to perform. Performing an exercise more quickly increases the water turbulence and drag thus making the exercise more difficult.

TYPE OF REASONING: INDUCTIVE

One must utilize clinical judgment to make a determination of the effects of submersion in water to chest level. This requires inductive reasoning skill. For this case, the effects include the center of gravity moving higher and closer to the area of the sternum. If answered incorrectly, review effects of submersion in water on buoyancy and center of gravity.

A110 | Cardiovascular/Pulmonary | Interventions

A patient is being treated for secondary lymphedema of the right upper extremity as a result of a radical mastectomy and radiation therapy. The BEST physical therapy method to help reverse pitting edema that is reversible is:

CHOICES:

1. isokinetics, extremity positioning in elevation and massage.
2. active range of motion and extremity positioning in a functional upper extremity/hand position.
3. isometric exercises, extremity positioning in elevation and compression bandaging.
4. intermittent pneumatic compression, extremity elevation and massage.

CORRECT ANSWER: 4

RATIONALE:

Lymphedema following surgery and radiation is classified as secondary lymphedema. Stage 1 means that there is pitting edema that is reversible with elevation. The arm may be normal size first thing in the morning with edema developing as the day goes on. It can be effectively managed by external compression and extremity elevation. Manual lymph drainage (massage and passive range of motion) are also appropriate interventions. Exercise and positioning alone would not provide the needed lymph drainage; isometric exercise is contraindicated.

TYPE OF REASONING: INDUCTIVE

One must utilize knowledge of lymphedema intervention approaches to arrive at a correct conclusion. This requires clinical judgment, which is an inductive reasoning skill. For this situation, the best method to reverse the pitting edema is intermittent pneumatic compression, extremity elevation and massage. If answered incorrectly, review intervention approaches for lymphedema, especially reversible pitting edema.

A111 | Cardiovascular/Pulmonary | Interventions

A postsurgical patient is receiving a regimen of postural drainage three times a day. The physical therapist assistant working with the patient should suggest reducing the frequency of treatment if the:

CHOICES:

1. consistency of the sputum changes.
2. patient becomes febrile.
3. patient experiences decreased postoperative pain.
4. amount of productive secretions decreases.

CORRECT ANSWER: 4

RATIONALE:

The purpose of postural drainage is to help remove secretions. If the amount diminishes, this might be an indicator that the treatment has been successful and that the frequency of treatment can be reduced. The other choices of fever, sputum consistency and pain do not provide a rationale to decrease treatment frequency.

TYPE OF REASONING: INDUCTIVE

This question requires the test taker to utilize knowledge of postural drainage guidelines and treatment approaches to arrive at a correct conclusion. This necessitates clinical judgment, which is an inductive reasoning skill. For this case, the assistant should suggest reducing the frequency of treatment if the amount of productive secretions decreases. Review postural drainage treatment approaches and frequency of treatment if answered incorrectly.

A112 | Cardiovascular/Pulmonary | Interventions

A patient with coronary artery disease received inpatient cardiac rehabilitation following a mild myocardial infarction. The patient is now enrolled in an outpatient exercise class that utilizes intermittent training. The **MOST** appropriate initial spacing of exercise and rest intervals to safely stress the aerobic system is:

CHOICES:
1. 1:1.
2. 5:1.
3. 2:1.
4. 10:1.

CORRECT ANSWER: 3

RATIONALE:

Presuming that the exercise goals for inpatient cardiac rehabilitation are met, an exercise-to-rest ratio of 2:1 can be used with this patient to begin exercise in an **outpatient setting** in a safe manner. An exercise-to-rest ratio of 1:1 is appropriate for an initial prescription for inpatient rehabilitation programs with a goal of achieving a 2:1 ratio. Ratios of 5:1 or 10:1 are too stressful to begin outpatient rehabilitation. A 5:1 ratio may be a goal for later exercise programming.

TYPE OF REASONING: INDUCTIVE

One must utilize clinical judgment and knowledge of cardiac rehabilitation guidelines to arrive at a correct conclusion. This requires inductive reasoning skill. For this case, the most appropriate initial spacing of exercise and rest intervals is 2:1. Review cardiac rehabilitation guidelines for patients with mild myocardial infarctions in outpatient settings if answered incorrectly.

A113 | Musculoskeletal | Clinical Applications

The **BEST INITIAL** intervention to improve functional mobility in an individual with a stable humeral neck fracture is:

CHOICES:
1. active resistive range of motion.
2. isometrics for all shoulder musculature.
3. pendulum exercises.
4. modalities to decrease pain.

CORRECT ANSWER: 3

RATIONALE:

This individual will typically be immobilized with a sling for a period of 6 weeks. After 1 week the sling should be removed to have the patient perform pendulum exercises to prevent shoulder stiffness. Resistive exercises are not indicated during this early period. Heat modalities may be effective in reducing pain but do not improve mobility.

TYPE OF REASONING: INDUCTIVE

This question requires the test taker to determine a best initial intervention approach for a patient with a stable humeral neck fracture. This requires clinical judgment, which is an inductive reasoning skill. For this scenario, the assistant should perform pendulum exercises for the initial intervention approach. Review intervention approaches for patients with stable humeral neck fractures if answered incorrectly.

A114 | Musculoskeletal | Clinical Applications

A dancer with unilateral spondylolysis at L4 is referred for physical therapy. The patient reports generalized low back pain when standing longer than 1 hour. Interventions for the subacute phase should include strengthening exercise for the:

CHOICES:

1. abdominals working from neutral to full flexion.
2. multifidi working from neutral to full extension.
3. abdominals working from full extension to full flexion.
4. multifidi working from full flexion back to neutral.

CORRECT ANSWER: 4

RATIONALE:

Performing strengthening exercises to the multifidi from flexion to neutral will not stress the pars defect. Abdominal strengthening will not provide the segmental stability needed with this condition. Lumbar extension beyond neutral and rotation will tend to aggravate the condition in the early stages of rehabilitation.

TYPE OF REASONING: INDUCTIVE

For this question, the test taker must utilize knowledge of spondylolysis and intervention approaches to arrive at a correct conclusion. This requires inductive reasoning skill. For this situation, the assistant should include strengthening exercises for the multifidi working from full flexion back to neutral. Review intervention approaches in the subacute phase of rehabilitation for patients with spondylolysis if answered incorrectly.

A115 | Musculoskeletal | Clinical Applications

A patient has fixed forefoot varus malalignment. Possible compensatory motion(s) or posture(s) might include:

CHOICES:

1. genu recurvatum.
2. excessive subtalar pronation.
3. ipsilateral pelvic lateral (external) rotation.
4. hallux varus.

CORRECT ANSWER: 2

RATIONALE:

Possible compensatory motions or postures for forefoot varus malalignment include plantar flexed first ray; hallux valgus; excessive midtarsal or subtalar pronation or prolonged pronation; excessive tibial, tibial and femoral, or femoral and pelvic medial (internal) rotation; and/or all with contralateral lumbar spine rotation.

TYPE OF REASONING: INFERENTIAL

This question requires the test taker to infer or draw a reasonable conclusion about the likely compensatory motions for a patient with fixed forefoot varus malalignment. This requires inferential reasoning skill. For this situation, the patient is likely to demonstrate excessive subtalar pronation. Review compensatory motions for fixed forefoot varus malalignment if answered incorrectly.

A116 | Integumentary | Clinical Applications

A patient comes into outpatient physical therapy following rotator cuff surgery. The physical therapist assistant initiates resistance band resistive exercise at the beginning of the session then proceeds with soft tissue mobilization and stretching to increase range of motion. Near the end of the therapy session the patient reports having watery eyes and an itchy feeling in the hands. Upon inspection the assistant notes a skin rash on the patient's palms and slight facial swelling. The **MOST LIKELY** cause is:

CHOICES:
1. atopic dermatitis.
2. rosacea.
3. latex allergy.
4. stasis dermatitis.

CORRECT ANSWER: 3

RATIONALE:
The patient is likely experiencing an immediate hypersensitivity to latex (type I hypersensitivity). Symptoms typically include contact dermatitis and, if severe, swelling and respiratory changes. The assistant should identify this as a latex sensitivity to the patient and have the patient follow up with the physician. The assistant should provide the patient with latex-free resistance band. Atopic dermatitis is a chronic inflammatory skin disease. Rosacea is a chronic form of acne with a vascular component (erythema, telangiectasis). In stasis dermatitis, skin is dry and thin with shallow ulcers that develop on the lower legs as a result of venous insufficiency.

TYPE OF REASONING: ANALYTICAL
This question provides a group of symptoms and the test taker must determine the most likely cause. Questions of this nature often require analytical reasoning skill. For this case, the symptoms the patient experienced after exercise are consistent with a latex allergy. If answered incorrectly, review signs and symptoms of latex allergies.

A117 | Cardiovascular/Pulmonary | Clinical Applications

A patient has an episode of syncope in the physical therapy clinic. The physical therapist asks the physical therapist assistant to check to see whether the patient is experiencing orthostatic hypotension. The assistant will do this by:

CHOICES:
1. checking heart rate (HR) and blood pressure (BP) in supine position after 5 minutes rest, then repeating in semi-Fowler position.
2. palpating the carotid arteries and taking HR; using the supine position for BP measurements.
3. checking HR and BP at rest, and after 3 and 5 minutes of cycle ergometry exercise.
4. checking resting BP and HR in sitting, then repeating measurements after standing for 1 minute.

CORRECT ANSWER: 4

RATIONALE:
Orthostatic hypotension is a fall in BP with elevation of position, i.e., from supine to sitting or sitting to standing. A small increase or no increase in heart rate upon standing may suggest baroreflex impairment. An exaggerated increase in HR upon standing may indicate volume depletion.

TYPE OF REASONING: DEDUCTIVE
This question requires one to recall the procedures for testing orthostatic hypotension. This is a factual procedure, which is a deductive reasoning skill. For this situation, the assistant should check resting BP and HR in sitting, then repeat measurements after standing for 1 minute. If answered incorrectly, review testing procedures for orthostatic hypotension.

A118 | Integumentary | Clinical Applications

An inpatient with a grade 3 diabetic foot ulcer is referred for physical therapy. Panafil is being applied to the necrotic tissue twice a day. The wound has **NO** foul smell; however, the physical therapist assistant notes a green tinge on the dressing. In this case, the assistant should:

CHOICES:

1. document the finding and contact the therapist immediately.
2. begin a trial of acetic acid to the wound.
3. document the finding and continue with treatment.
4. fit the patient with a total contact cast.

CORRECT ANSWER: 3

RATIONALE:

A greenish tinge to the dressing is expected with the use of Panafil. Panafil is a keratolytic enzyme used for selective débridement. A greenish or yellowish exudate can be expected. If the exudate were green and had a foul smell, *Pseudomonas aeruginosa* should be suspected and acetic acid would be the topical agent of choice. A total contact cast can be used only after the wound is free of necrotic tissue.

TYPE OF REASONING: EVALUATIVE

This question requires the test taker to determine a best course of action for and significance of a wound dressing with a green tinge on it. This requires one to weigh the merits of the courses of action, which is an evaluative reasoning skill. For this case, because a greenish tinge is expected with the use of Panafil, the assistant should document the finding and continue with treatment.

A119 | Devices, Admin, etc. | Safety, Roles, Teaching, EBP

A physical therapist assistant is performing a home assessment to examine the fall risk of an older adult patient who lives alone and has had two recent falls. The activity that represents the **MOST** common risk factor associated with falls in older adults is:

CHOICES:

1. climbing on a stepstool to reach overhead objects.
2. walking with a roller walker with hand brakes.
3. dressing while sitting on the edge of the bed.
4. turning around and sitting down in a chair.

CORRECT ANSWER: 4

RATIONALE:

Most falls occur during normal daily activity. Getting up or down from a bed or chair, turning, bending, walking and climbing or descending stairs all are high-risk activities. Only a small percentage of individuals fall during clearly hazardous activities (e.g., climbing the stepstool). Proper use of an assistive device reduces the risk of falls.

TYPE OF REASONING: INFERENTIAL

This question necessitates one to infer or draw a reasonable conclusion about the most likely risk factor for falls in the elderly. This requires inferential reasoning skill, as one must determine what is likely to be true for a population. For this scenario, the most common risk factor is turning around and sitting down in a chair. If answered incorrectly, review risk factors for falls in the elderly.

A120 | Other Systems | Clinical Applications

During surgery to remove an apical lung tumor, the long thoracic nerve was injured. Muscle weakness is 3+/5. The plan of care indicates strengthening exercises for the weak muscles. The **BEST INITIAL** exercises are:

CHOICES:

1. standing, upper-extremity overhead lifts using hand weights.
2. supine, upper-extremity overhead lifts using weights.
3. sitting, upper-extremity overhead lifts using a pulley.
4. standing, wall push-ups.

CORRECT ANSWER: 4

RATIONALE:

The long thoracic nerve supplies the serratus anterior muscle. With a muscle grade of fair plus (3+/5), the patient can begin functional strengthening by using standing wall push-ups, with resistance provided by the patient's own body. The other exercises would not be optimal for strengthening a fair plus serratus anterior.

TYPE OF REASONING: INDUCTIVE

This question requires clinical judgment to determine the best initial exercise approach for a patient with long thoracic nerve injury. This necessitates knowledge of muscles innervated by the long thoracic nerve and effective exercise approaches, which is an inductive reasoning skill. For this case, the therapist should instruct the patient in wall push-ups in standing. If answered incorrectly, review exercises for the serratus anterior and long thoracic nerve injury.

A121 | Musculoskeletal | Clinical Applications

A college soccer player sustained a hyperextension knee injury when kicking the ball with the opposite lower extremity. The physician in the emergency room discharged the patient with a diagnosis of "knee sprain." The patient was sent to physical therapy the **NEXT** day for rehabilitation. The therapist's initial evaluation identifies a positive Lachman's test for anterior cruciate ligament (ACL) integrity. The type of exercise that is indicated in the acute phase of treatment is:

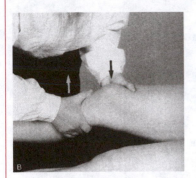

Magee D (2002) Orthopedic Physical Assessment, 4th ed. Philadelphia, W. B. Saunders, Figure 12-27B, page 700, with permission.

CHOICES:

1. agility exercises.
2. closed-chain terminal knee extension exercises.
3. open-chain terminal knee extension exercises.
4. plyometric functional exercises.

CORRECT ANSWER: 2

RATIONALE:

The test that was conducted was a Lachman's test to determine integrity of the ACL. A positive test suggests laxity of the anterior cruciate ligament. Quick cutting or lateral movements that occur in agility training and heavy joint loading that occurs with plyometric exercise should be avoided until the muscular restraints that reduce excessive anterior translation of the affected tibiofemoral joint are strengthened. Open-chain knee extension may place excessive load on the ACL. Closed-chain terminal knee extension exercises are safe and effective secondary to the dynamic stability inherent with this type of exercise.

TYPE OF REASONING: ANALYTICAL

One must analyze the symptoms presented to determine the appropriate approach for the acute phase of treatment. This requires analytical reasoning skill. For this case, the exercise approach that is indicated is closed-chain terminal knee extension exercises. If answered incorrectly, review treatment approaches for laxity of the ACL.

A122 | Musculoskeletal | Clinical Applications

A patient with a transtibial amputation is learning to walk with a patellar tendon–bearing prosthesis and is having difficulty maintaining prosthetic stability from heel-strike (initial contact) to foot-flat (loading response). The muscles that are **MOST LIKELY** weak during stance phase are the:

CHOICES:
1. knee extensors.
2. back extensors.
3. hip flexors.
4. knee flexors.

CORRECT ANSWER: 1

RATIONALE:

The quadriceps is maximally active at heel strike (initial contact) to stabilize the knee and counteract the flexion moment.

TYPE OF REASONING: INFERENTIAL

One must infer or draw a reasonable conclusion about the likely muscles that are weakened when a patient is demonstrating difficulty maintaining prosthetic stability from heel-strike to foot-flat. This requires inferential reasoning skill. For this situation, the most likely weak muscles are the knee extensors. Review gait deviations with the use of a patellar tendon–bearing prosthesis if answered incorrectly.

A123 | Devices, Admin, etc. | Equipment, Modalities

A physical therapist assistant is applying high-volt pulsed current to the vastus medialis to improve patellar tracking during knee extension. The patient reports that the current is uncomfortable. To make the current more tolerable to the patient, yet maintain a good therapeutic effect, the assistant should consider adjusting the:

CHOICES:
1. pulse rate.
2. current intensity.
3. pulse duration.
4. current polarity.

CORRECT ANSWER: 3

RATIONALE:

Decreasing the pulse duration reduces the electrical charge of each pulse, making the current more comfortable by decreasing the total current applied while maintaining the full therapeutic effect.

TYPE OF REASONING: DEDUCTIVE

This question requires one to recall the guidelines for use of high-volt pulsed current and adjustments made to provide comfort for the patient. This is factual information, which is a deductive reasoning skill. For this scenario, the assistant should adjust the pulse duration to make the current more comfortable for the patient. If answered incorrectly, review high-volt pulsed current treatment guidelines.

A124 | Other Systems | Clinical Applications

An older adult who is a wheelchair-dependent resident of a community nursing home has a diagnosis of organic brain syndrome, Alzheimer's disease type, stage 2. During an afternoon treatment session, the patient demonstrated limited interaction and mild agitation, and tried to wheel the chair down the hall. As it was late in the day, the assistant decided to resume the treatment the next morning. The patient was **MOST LIKELY** exhibiting:

CHOICES:

1. frustration because of an inability to communicate.
2. disorientation to time and date.
3. sundowning behavior.
4. inattention as a result of short-term memory loss.

CORRECT ANSWER: 3

RATIONALE:

A patient with stage 2 Alzheimer's disease can be expected to exhibit impaired cognition and abstract thinking, sundowning (defined as extreme restlessness, agitation and wandering that typically occur in the late afternoon), inability to carry out activities of daily living, impaired judgment, inappropriate social behavior, lack of insight, repetitive behavior and a voracious appetite. Inability to communicate is characteristic of stage 3. Short-term memory loss and disorientation to time and date are early signs of the disease (stage 1).

TYPE OF REASONING: ANALYTICAL

This question provides a group of symptoms and the test taker must determine the most likely cause for them. This requires analysis of the symptoms, which is an analytical reasoning skill. For this situation, the symptoms exhibited are most consistent with sundowning behavior. Review signs and symptoms of sundowning behavior in patients with Alzheimer's disease if answered incorrectly.

A125 | Other Systems | Clinical Applications

An older, frail adult is receiving physical therapy in the home environment to improve general strength and mobility. The patient has a 4 year history of taking NSAIDs (aspirin) for joint pain and recently began taking a calcium-channel blocker. The physical therapist assistant should be aware of adverse side effects, which could include:

CHOICES:

1. increased sweating, fatigue, chest pain.
2. stomach pain, hypertension, confusion.
3. weight increase, hyperglycemia, hypotension.
4. paresthesias, incoordination, bradycardia.

CORRECT ANSWER: 2

RATIONALE:

With advanced age, the capacity of the individual to break down and convert drugs diminishes secondary to decreased liver and kidney function, reduced hepatic and renal blood flow, etc. Some drugs additionally slow metabolism (e.g., calcium-channel blockers). NSAIDs are associated with potential gastrointestinal (GI) effects (stomach pain, peptic ulcers, GI hemorrhage), peripheral edema, and easy bruising and bleeding. NSAIDs can also lessen the effects of antihypertensive drugs. Central nervous system effects can include headache, dizziness, lightheadedness, insomnia, tinnitus, confusion and depression. The other choices are not expected adverse effects.

TYPE OF REASONING: DEDUCTIVE

This question requires one to recall the adverse side effects of taking both NSAIDs and calcium-channel blockers to arrive at a correct conclusion. This necessitates the recall of factual information, which is a deductive reasoning skill. For this case, the adverse side effects could include stomach pain, hypertension and confusion. Review adverse effects of NSAIDs and calcium-channel blockers if answered incorrectly.

A126 | Musculoskeletal | Data Collection

A patient presents with pain, joint swelling, subcutaneous olecranon nodules and increased erythrocyte sedimentation rate. These findings are characteristic of:

CHOICES:

1. rheumatoid arthritis.
2. fibromyalgia.
3. systemic lupus erythematosus.
4. osteoarthritis.

CORRECT ANSWER: 1

RATIONALE:

Rheumatoid arthritis (RA) is characterized by morning stiffness, pain and relatively symmetric joint involvement. Laboratory abnormalities in RA include positive serum rheumatoid factor and elevated erythrocyte sedimentation rate. Articular and extraarticular manifestations include weight loss, malaise, nodulosis and vasculitis. Synovial fluid analysis reveals elevated white blood cell count and protein count. Osteoarthritis, or degenerative joint pain, and fibromyalgia both produce pain but do not produce the laboratory findings reported above or nodulosis. Systemic lupus erythematosus (SLE) is an immunologic disorder characterized by inflammatory lesions in multiple organ systems. It is diagnosed by client history (multiple organ involvement, especially of skin, joints, serous membranes), systemic symptoms (e.g., fever, malaise, fatigability) and appearance of skin rash (erythema). Erythrocyte sedimentation rate is elevated in patients with SLE; however, nodulosis and joint malformations are not expected.

TYPE OF REASONING: ANALYTICAL

This question requires the test taker to analyze a group of symptoms to make a determination of the characteristics and likely problem. This requires analytical reasoning skill. For this situation, the symptoms are characteristic of rheumatoid arthritis. If answered incorrectly, review signs and symptoms of rheumatoid arthritis.

A127 | Cardiovascular/Pulmonary | Clinical Applications

A patient is exercising in a phase III outpatient cardiac rehabilitation program that utilizes circuit training. One of the stations utilizes weights. The patient lifts a 5-lb weight, holds it for 20 seconds and then lowers it slowly. The physical therapist assistant corrects the activity and tells the patient to reduce the length of the static hold. The static exercise can be expected to produce:

CHOICES:

1. abnormal oxygen uptake.
2. lower heart rate and arterial blood pressure.
3. higher heart rate and arterial blood pressure.
4. reduced normal venous return to the heart and elevated blood pressure.

CORRECT ANSWER: 3

RATIONALE:

Dynamic exercise facilitates circulation whereas isometric (static) exercise hinders blood flow, producing higher heart rates and arterial blood pressures. The Valsalva maneuver that accompanies breath-holding produces increased intrathoracic pressure, which, in turn, hinders normal venous return to the heart. Breath-holding is more likely with isometric exercise but is not always present. There was no mention of breath-holding in this scenario.

TYPE OF REASONING: INFERENTIAL

One must infer the likely effects of static exercise for a patient in a cardiac rehabilitation program to arrive at a correct conclusion. This requires inferential reasoning skill, as one must determine what is likely to be true for a patient. For this case, the static exercise can produce a higher heart rate and arterial blood pressure. If answered incorrectly, review effects of static exercise on patients in cardiac rehabilitation programs.

A128 | Other Systems | Clinical Applications

A teenaged child with a 4 year history of type 2 diabetes is insulin dependent and wants to participate in cross-country running. The physical therapist assistant who has previously worked with the athlete in the clinic advises the athlete to measure plasma glucose concentrations before and after running and to:

CHOICES:
1. consume a carbohydrate after practice to avoid hyperglycemia.
2. increase insulin dosage immediately before running.
3. consume a carbohydrate before or during practice to avoid hypoglycemia.
4. avoid carbohydrate-rich snacks within 12 hours of a race.

CORRECT ANSWER: 3

RATIONALE:

During exercise of increasing intensity and duration, plasma concentrations of insulin progressively decrease. Exercise-induced hypoglycemia is the likely result. Hypoglycemia can also occur up to 4 to 6 hours after exercise. To counteract these effects, the individual may need to reduce insulin dosage or increase carbohydrate intake before or after running. Consuming a carbohydrate product before or during the race will have a preventive modulating effect on hypoglycemia.

TYPE OF REASONING: EVALUATIVE

For this question, the test taker must weigh the information provided in the form of advice given to a patient and determine which advice is best aligned with the patient's diagnosis and current needs. This requires evaluative reasoning skill. For this case, the assistant should advise the patient to consume a carbohydrate before or during practice to avoid hypoglycemia. Review exercise guidelines for patients with type 2 diabetes and intervention approaches for exercise-induced hypoglycemia.

A129 | Devices, Admin, etc. | Equipment, Modalities

An athlete presents with pain and muscle spasm of the upper back (C7–T8) extending to the lateral border of the scapula. This encompasses a 10 cm by 10 cm area on both sides of the spine. If the ultrasound unit only has a 5 cm^2 sound head, the physical therapist assistant should treat:

CHOICES:
1. the entire area in 5 minutes.
2. the entire area in 10 minutes.
3. each side allotting 2.5 minutes for each section.
4. each side allotting 5 minutes for each section.

CORRECT ANSWER: 4

RATIONALE:

The total treatment area is too large for the 5 cm^2 sound head to produce adequate tissue heating. Moving the transducer too fast to cover both sides adequately in the allotted time does not allow sufficient time for the acoustic energy to produce heat because the head is not in a given area long enough. Increasing the treatment time will not affect the rate of heat production. Sonating the two areas independently will allow more time for the tissue temperature to rise during the treatment time in each area. Two and a half minutes is too brief to produce sufficient tissue heating.

TYPE OF REASONING: INDUCTIVE

This question requires one to utilize clinical judgment to determine a best course of action when one is providing ultrasound treatment over a large surface area. This requires knowledge of ultrasound guidelines and judgment about a best approach, which is an inductive reasoning skill. For this case, the assistant should treat each side allotting 5 minutes for each session. Review ultrasound treatment guidelines for the upper back, especially larger surface areas, if answered incorrectly.

A130 | Devices, Admin, etc. | Equipment, Modalities

A patient with chronic cervical pain is referred to an outpatient physical therapy clinic. Past medical history reveals appendectomy 12 years ago, chronic heart disease, demand-type pacemaker implanted 8 years ago, and whiplash injury 2 years ago. Presently the patient reports pain and muscle spasm in the cervical region. The modality that is **CONTRAINDICATED** in the case is:

CHOICES:
1. mechanical traction.
2. infrared lamp.
3. hot pack.
4. transcutaneous electrical stimulation.

CORRECT ANSWER: 4

RATIONALE:
All electrical stimulation devices are contraindicated when a patient has a demand-type pacemaker. The electrical signals could interfere with the rhythmic signals of the pacemaker. The other modalities are not contraindicated in this case.

TYPE OF REASONING: DEDUCTIVE
This question requires one to recall the contraindications for treatment modalities with a patient who has a demand-type pacemaker. This necessitates the recall of factual guidelines, which is a deductive reasoning skill. For this situation, the modality that is contraindicated is transcutaneous electrical stimulation, as the signals can interfere with the pacemaker signals. If answered incorrectly, review use of modalities with patients who have demand-type pacemakers.

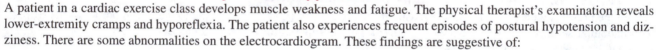

A131 | Cardiovascular/Pulmonary | Clinical Applications

A patient in a cardiac exercise class develops muscle weakness and fatigue. The physical therapist's examination reveals lower-extremity cramps and hyporeflexia. The patient also experiences frequent episodes of postural hypotension and dizziness. There are some abnormalities on the electrocardiogram. These findings are suggestive of:

CHOICES:
1. hyperkalemia.
2. hypocalcemia.
3. hyponatremia.
4. hypokalemia.

CORRECT ANSWER: 4

RATIONALE:
Hypokalemia, decreased potassium in the blood, is characterized by the above signs and symptoms. Other possible symptoms include respiratory distress, irritability, confusion or depression, and gastrointestinal disturbances. Electrocardiogram abnormalities would include flat T wave, prolonged QT interval and depressed ST segment. Hyperkalemia is excess potassium in the blood. Hyponatremia is decreased sodium in the blood, and hypocalcemia is decreased calcium in the blood. These conditions cannot produce this battery of symptoms. Refer to Chapter 7 for signs and symptoms of these and other imbalances.

TYPE OF REASONING: ANALYTICAL
This question provides a group of symptoms and the test taker must analyze the symptoms to make a determination of the likely diagnosis. This requires analytical reasoning skill. For this situation, the symptoms are characteristic of hypokalemia or low blood potassium. If answered incorrectly, review signs and symptoms of hypokalemia.

A132 | Other Systems | Clinical Applications

A patient has a 5 year history of acquired immunodeficiency syndrome (AIDS). The case worker reports that the patient has had a gradual increase in difficulty with walking. The patient rarely goes out anymore. A referral to physical therapy is initiated. The physical therapist assistant has been directed to provide functional training including bed mobility and transfer training. The physical therapist assistant would expect which of the following neuromuscular symptoms with this patient?

CHOICES:
1. paraplegia or tetraplegia.
2. widespread sensory loss resulting in sensory ataxia.
3. motor ataxia and paresis with pronounced gait disturbances.
4. progressive rigidity and akinesia with severe balance disturbances.

CORRECT ANSWER: 3

RATIONALE:

Alterations in memory, confusion and disorientation are characteristic of AIDS dementia complex, a common central nervous system manifestation of HIV infection. Motor deficits may include ataxia, paresis with gait disturbances and loss of fine motor coordination. Patients may also develop peripheral neuropathy with distal pain and sensory loss. Paraparesis (not paraplegia) might be a finding.

TYPE OF REASONING: INFERENTIAL
This question requires the test taker to infer the likely neuromuscular symptoms for a patient with AIDS. This requires inferential reasoning skill, as one must determine what is likely to be true. For this case, the assistant should expect motor ataxia and paresis with pronounced gait disturbances. If answered incorrectly, review neuromuscular symptoms associated with AIDS.

A133 | Musculoskeletal | Data Collection

An assistant is seeing a postal worker who reports numbness and tingling in the right hand after returning to work yesterday. Symptoms are reported on the palm and palmar surface and tips of the first two fingers, and the pad of the thumb. The assistant would report to the therapist that the patient was demonstrating diminished sensation in the distribution of which peripheral nerve?

CHOICES:
1. radial nerve.
2. ulnar nerve.
3. median nerve.
4. accessory nerve.

CORRECT ANSWER: 3

RATIONALE:

The symptoms best typify median nerve distribution. Sensory distribution of the radial nerve covers the dorsum of the thumb and dorsal surface of the thumb and first two fingers. The ulnar nerve covers the thenar eminence, little finger and medial border of the ring finger.

TYPE OF REASONING: DEDUCTIVE
One must recall the symptoms of median nerve dysfunction to arrive at a correct conclusion. This requires the recall of factual symptoms and guidelines, which is a deductive reasoning skill. For this case, the symptoms typify median nerve dysfunction, which should be reviewed if answered incorrectly.

A134 | Other Systems | Clinical Applications

Following a cesarean section, a patient tells the physical therapist assistant that she is anxious to return to her pre-pregnancy level of physical activity (working out at the gym 3 days a week and running 5 miles every other day). The assistant's **BEST** advice is to tell the patient to resume activities with:

CHOICES:

1. pelvic floor exercises and refrain from all other exercise and running for at least 6 to 8 weeks.
2. pelvic floor and gentle abdominal exercises for the first 4 to 6 weeks.
3. abdominal crunches with return to running after 1 month.
4. a walking program progressing to running after 5 weeks.

CORRECT ANSWER: 2

RATIONALE:

Post-cesarean physical therapy can include postoperative TENS, assisted breathing and coughing techniques, and gentle abdominal exercises with incisional support provided by a pillow. Pelvic floor exercises are also important because hours of labor and pushing are typically present before surgery. Vigorous exercise is contraindicated for at least 6 weeks.

TYPE OF REASONING: EVALUATIVE

One must weigh the merits of the courses of action presented and determine which response best addresses the patient's needs and desires. This requires evaluative reasoning skill. For this case, the assistant should tell the patient to complete pelvic floor and gentle abdominal exercises for the first 4 to 6 weeks. If answered incorrectly, review post-cesarean exercises and restrictions.

A135 | Neuromuscular | Clinical Applications

It is reasonable to expect that a young child with Down syndrome will:

CHOICES:

1. learn to walk by age 6 or 7 years.
2. learn to walk by age 2 or 3 years.
3. be unable to walk independently.
4. keep up with typically developing peers in walking skills.

CORRECT ANSWER: 2

RATIONALE:

Research shows that most children with Down syndrome learn to walk by the time they are 2 to 3 years of age. Initially they are delayed in their gross motor skill development compared with their typically developing peers. Children with Down syndrome do achieve their gross motor milestones, but most often these milestones are delayed.

TYPE OF REASONING: INFERENTIAL

This question requires one to determine what may be true for a child with Down syndrome. Questions of this nature often require inferential reasoning skill. For this situation, one can expect a child with Down syndrome to learn to walk by age 2 to 3 years. If answered incorrectly, review developmental milestones and expectations for children with Down syndrome, especially motor skills such as walking.

A136 | Musculoskeletal | Data Collection

During treatment for chronic shoulder pain in a recreational swimmer, the assistant observes excessive medial (internal) rotation of the shoulders and winging of the scapula during overhead motion. The physical therapist diagnosis is chronic shoulder impingement. To restore balance between the anterior chest muscles and posterior trunk muscles the therapist asks the physical therapist assistant to focus on:

CHOICES:
1. strengthening of pectoral muscles and stretching of upper trapezius.
2. strengthening of upper trapezius and stretching of pectoral muscles.
3. strengthening middle and lower trapezius and stretching of pectoral muscles.
4. strengthening of rhomboids and stretching of upper trapezius.

CORRECT ANSWER: 3

RATIONALE:

Abnormal posture that produces excessive medial (internal) rotation of the shoulders may result in chronic shoulder impingement syndrome attributable to a loss of scapular stability with overhead motion. Shoulder pain is likely to continue until a balance between anterior and posterior trunk musculature is achieved. The anterior chest muscles (pectorals) are shortened and need stretching and posterior trunk muscles (middle and lower trapezius) are stretched and need strengthening.

TYPE OF REASONING: INDUCTIVE

This question requires clinical judgment to determine a best course of action for a patient with chronic shoulder impingement. This requires inductive reasoning skill. For this case, the assistant should focus on strengthening middle and lower trapezius and stretching of pectoral muscles. If answered incorrectly, review treatment approaches for chronic shoulder impingement and loss of scapular stability.

A137 | Musculoskeletal | Data Collection

The condition **MOST** consistent with the diagram shown is:

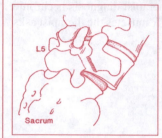

Twomey L, Taylor J (2000) Physical Therapy of the Low Back, 3rd ed. Philadelphia, Churchill Livingstone, Figure 7-1, page 204, with permission.

CHOICES:

1. herniated disc.
2. degenerative joint disease.
3. stenosis.
4. spondylolisthesis.

CORRECT ANSWER: 4

RATIONALE:

The diagram indicates an anterior slippage of one vertebra on the vertebra below, the definition of spondylolisthesis. Stenosis is the narrowing of the vertebral canal, which is not visible in the diagram. Neither degenerative joint disease nor a herniated disc are visible on the diagram.

TYPE OF REASONING: ANALYTICAL

This question requires one to analyze the information presented in a diagram to determine the most likely condition the diagram depicts. Questions that require one to analyze information in the form of pictures, charts and diagrams often necessitate analytical reasoning skill. For this case, the diagram depicts spondylolisthesis. Review signs and symptoms of spondylolisthesis if answered incorrectly.

A138 | Other Systems | Clinical Applications

A physical therapist assistant is working with an office worker, who is a long-term smoker who now has emphysema. The physical therapist diagnosis and treatment plan includes intervention and patient education for thoracic outlet syndrome. The patient reports increased pain and tingling in bilateral hands after sitting at a desk for longer than 1 hour. The assistant should focus treatment on:

CHOICES:
1. stretching the pectoralis major and rhomboid muscles.
2. stretching of the scalenes and pectoralis minor muscles.
3. stretching the wrist and finger flexors.
4. stretching of the biceps brachii and brachialis.

CORRECT ANSWER: 2

RATIONALE:
Patients with emphysema typically present with hypertrophy of the accessory breathing muscles that include the scalenes, which can compress the neurovascular structures of the thoracic outlet; the pectoralis minor can also compress these structures. Stretching of the biceps, brachialis, or wrist and finger flexors will not address the cause of the symptoms.

TYPE OF REASONING: INDUCTIVE
This question requires clinical judgment to determine a best course of action for a patient with emphysema and thoracic outlet syndrome. This requires knowledge of the diagnosis and therapeutic approaches, which is an inductive reasoning skill. For this case, the assistant should focus on stretching of the scalenes and pectoralis minor muscles. If answered incorrectly, review treatment approaches for emphysema and thoracic outlet syndrome.

A139 | Other Systems | Clinical Applications

A physical therapist assistant is working with an individual with a diagnosis of low back pain, degenerative disc disease and gastroesophageal reflux disease. The patient reports that at night upon going to bed the exercises have resulted in upset stomach and inability to sleep very well. The assistant should instruct the patient to:

CHOICES:
1. avoid doing the exercises.
2. drink plenty of water throughout the day.
3. sleep in the supine position.
4. avoid eating large meals.

CORRECT ANSWER: 4

RATIONALE:
Patients who suffer from gastroesophageal reflux disease (GERD) should eat smaller meals; avoiding meals close to bed or exercise time can help as well. Sleeping with the head of their bed elevated can help decrease the symptoms. The supine position should be avoided. Exercising with the upper trunk supported in the elevated position is also recommended. Avoiding exercise will not necessarily help the low back pain. Drinking plenty of water can help decrease the chances of constipation.

TYPE OF REASONING: INDUCTIVE
This question requires one to first determine the cause for the patient's symptoms and then to choose an appropriate course of action. This necessitates clinical judgment, which is an inductive reasoning skill. For this case, the assistant should recommend that the patient avoid eating large meals to alleviate symptoms. Review signs and symptoms of GERD, as well as approaches to alleviating symptoms, if answered incorrectly.

A140 | Other Systems | Interventions

An obese individual who has diabetes is coming to physical therapy to participate in a conditioning program. The assistant should instruct the participant to:

CHOICES:

1. eat a carbohydrate-balanced snack at least 2 hours prior to participating in the conditioning program.
2. avoid eating foods for several hours prior to participating in the conditioning program.
3. inject insulin into the large muscle groups such as the quadriceps prior to participating in the conditioning program.
4. participate in the conditioning program when blood glucose levels are greater than 300 mg/dL.

CORRECT ANSWER: 1

RATIONALE:

Eating a carbohydrate-balanced snack at least 2 hours prior to participating in the conditioning program will ensure regulation of blood sugars. Insulin injections should be given in muscles that are not going to be used heavily during exercises; an abdominal injection is recommended. Participation in exercise programs is contraindicated with fasting blood glucose levels greater than 300 mg/dL, or less than 70 mg/dL.

TYPE OF REASONING: EVALUATIVE

One must weigh the merits of the courses of action presented and then determine the response that will most effectively address the patient's needs. This requires evaluative reasoning skill. For this situation, the assistant should recommend that the patient eat a carbohydrate-balanced snack at least 2 hours prior to participating in the conditioning program. Review guidelines for conditioning programs for patients with diabetes and obesity, as well as regulation of blood sugars with exercise, if answered incorrectly.

A141 | Musculoskeletal | Clinical Applications

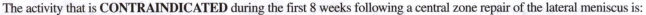

The activity that is **CONTRAINDICATED** during the first 8 weeks following a central zone repair of the lateral meniscus is:

CHOICES:

1. full active knee extension.
2. muscle setting exercises.
3. partial weight-bearing at 25%.
4. knee flexion greater than 60° to 70°.

CORRECT ANSWER: 4

RATIONALE:

Central zone repairs of the meniscus are progressed more conservatively than peripheral zone repairs. Flexion beyond 60° to 70° places posterior translation forces on the repaired meniscus, thus increasing the risk of displacement. Muscle setting and **A-AAROM** exercises begin the day after surgery. Restriction of full active knee extension exercises are part of the protocol following anterior cruciate ligament repair, not following meniscus repair.

TYPE OF REASONING: DEDUCTIVE

One must recall the contraindications for activity after a central zone repair of the lateral meniscus. This requires the recall of factual guidelines, which is a deductive reasoning skill. For this scenario, the patient should avoid knee flexion greater than 60° to 70°. If answered incorrectly, review contraindications and activity limitations for patients with central zone repair of the lateral meniscus.

A142 | Other Systems | Clinical Applications

A physical therapist assistant is providing home care for an older adult patient. Upon arrival, the assistant notices that the patient is confused. The patient's skin color is pale and the turgor is poor. The patient reports an intestinal upset for the past few days with frequent vomiting and diarrhea. The assistant's **BEST** course of action is to:

CHOICES:

1. monitor vital signs; if heart rate is not elevated, get the patient up and walking.
2. notify the family, and insist that the patient not be alone until the illness is over.
3. cancel therapy for today, carefully document the findings and notify the physician.
4. give the patient water and notify the physician and physical therapist immediately.

CORRECT ANSWER: 4

RATIONALE:

The patient is exhibiting signs of dehydration. Confusion is a red flag and requires immediate action: administer fluids and notify the physician and therapist immediately. Getting the patient up and walking or warning the family to stay with the patient will not address the dehydration.

TYPE OF REASONING: EVALUATIVE

One must first analyze the symptoms and then weigh the courses of action to determine the best approach that effectively meets the patient's needs. This requires evaluative reasoning skill. For this case, the patient's symptoms are those of dehydration and the assistant should give the patient water and notify the physician and physical therapist immediately. If answered incorrectly, review signs and symptoms of dehydration as well as first aid approaches for this diagnosis.

A143 | Neuromuscular | Data Collection

To assess a patient's ability to perceive light touch sensations a physical therapist assistant should lightly:

CHOICES:

1. brush a cotton ball across the area being tested.
2. touch the tip of a pin on the area being tested.
3. touch the blunt end of a paper clip on the area being tested.
4. apply pressure through the tip of a double-tipped cotton swab on the area being tested.

CORRECT ANSWER: 1

RATIONALE:

Light touch sensations are tested by brushing the tip of a cotton swab or camel hair brush across the area being tested. The clinician asks the patient to identify by a "yes" or "no" response after the stimulus has been provided. The sharp end of a pin or the tip of a straightened paper clip test the patient's ability to perceive pain, the blunt ends of the pin or paper clip are used to assess dull sensation. Pressure applied through the tip of a cotton swab tests pressure sensation. All of these tests assess superficial-level sensations.

TYPE OF REASONING: DEDUCTIVE

One must recall the procedures for testing light touch to arrive at a correct conclusion. This necessitates the recall of procedures and guidelines, which is a deductive reasoning skill. For this case, the assistant should brush a cotton ball across the area being tested. If answered incorrectly, review light touch testing procedures.

A144 | Musculoskeletal | Interventions

A patient with a traumatic injury to the right hand had a flexor tendon repair to the fingers. Physical therapy interventions following this type of repair would begin:

CHOICES:

1. after the splint is removed 2 to 3 weeks to allow full active range of motion of all affected joints.
2. after the splint is removed 4 to 6 weeks to allow ample healing time for the repaired tendon.
3. within a few days following surgery to preserve tendon gliding.
4. within a few days following surgery to allow for early initiation of strengthening exercises.

CORRECT ANSWER: 3

RATIONALE:

Early passive and active assistive exercises promote collagen remodeling to allow free tendon gliding. When rehabilitation is delayed by several weeks, adhesions form, which restrict free tendon gliding.

TYPE OF REASONING: INFERENTIAL

One must infer or draw a reasonable conclusion about the likely intervention approach for a patient with a flexor tendon repair to the fingers. This requires one to determine what may be true of a situation, which is an inferential reasoning skill. For this situation, one should expect interventions to begin within a few days following surgery to preserve tendon gliding. Review intervention approaches for patients with flexor tendon repair if answered incorrectly.

A145 | Cardiovascular/Pulmonary | Data Collection

A physical therapist assistant is gait training a patient who has obstructive pulmonary disease. When assessing the patient's respiratory status the assistant should find:

CHOICES:

1. the thorax size decreased.
2. decreased rib excursion with respirations.
3. an uneven rise between the two sides of the thorax.
4. a decreased respiratory rate.

CORRECT ANSWER: 2

RATIONALE:

Persons with obstructive lung diseases will typically present with decreased rib excursion during respirations and an enlarged thorax, especially in the advanced stages. This occurs secondary to the loss of elastic recoil of the lung tissues. One would expect an uneven rise in the thorax if a lung or portion of a lung were collapsed, filled with fluid or compromised, not in a person with obstructive lung disease. Persons with chronic obstructive pulmonary disease will present with increased and more shallow respirations.

TYPE OF REASONING: INFERENTIAL

This question requires the test taker to determine what is likely to be true for a patient with obstructive pulmonary disease. This requires inferential reasoning skill. For this scenario, the assistant should find decreased rib excursion with respirations. If answered incorrectly, review signs and symptoms associated with obstructive lung disease.

A146 | Musculoskeletal | Data Collection

A patient is recovering from a left tibial amputation and reports numbness and tingling affecting the dorsal foot and big toe. The patient knows the extremity is gone and cannot understand why this is happening. The physical therapist assistant informs the physical therapist of the patient's newly reported symptom. The therapist suspects the source of discomfort is **MOST LIKELY** pressure from residual limb wrapping and asks the assistant to check to make sure there is **NO** pressure on the peripheral nerve. The assistant knows to check for pressure on the:

CHOICES:
1. sural nerve.
2. medial calcaneal nerve.
3. tibial nerve.
4. common peroneal (fibular) nerve.

CORRECT ANSWER: 4

RATIONALE:

Sensation to the dorsum of the foot and big toe is supplied by the superficial peroneal (fibular) nerve, a branch off the common peroneal (fibular) nerve. The sural nerve is a distal branch of the tibial nerve that supplies the back of the lower extremity and the lateral side of the foot and little toe. The medial calcaneal nerve is also a branch of the tibial nerve that supplies the heel and medial sole of the foot. Phantom limb sensation (sensation of an extremity that is no longer there) usually occurs in the immediate postoperative phase and can be stimulated by external pressure (residual limb wrapping or rigid dressing). It typically dissipates over time though some patients may experience the sensation for the rest of their lives. This is a common finding and should not interfere with prosthetic rehabilitation.

TYPE OF REASONING: ANALYTICAL

This question requires the test taker to analyze the symptoms to determine the likely nerve that is affected. This requires analytical reasoning skill. For this situation, the assistant should test the common peroneal (fibular) nerve for pressure, as symptoms indicate dysfunction of this nerve. If answered incorrectly, review signs and symptoms of dysfunction of the common peroneal nerve.

A147 | Neuromuscular | Interventions

A patient with a complete T10 paraplegia resulting from a spinal cord injury is ready to begin community wheelchair training. The plan of care includes instruction in wheelchair skills to manage curbs. The **BEST** training strategy is to instruct the patient to:

CHOICES:
1. throw their head and trunk backward to rise up on the large wheels.
2. place hand on the top of the handrims to steady the chair while throwing the head and trunk forward.
3. lean backward while moving the hands slowly backward on the rims.
4. grasp the handrims posteriorly and pull them forward abruptly and forcefully.

CORRECT ANSWER: 4

RATIONALE:

A wheelie can be assumed by having the patient place the hands posterior on the handrims and pulling them abruptly and sharply forward. If the patient is unable to lift the casters in this manner, he or she can throw the head back forcefully when pulling the handrims. An alternate technique is to grasp the handrims anteriorly, pull backward, then abruptly and forcefully reverse the direction of pull. The therapist can assist by steadying the chair at the patient's balance point until he or she learns to adjust the position through the use of handrim movements forward and backward.

TYPE OF REASONING: INDUCTIVE

One must recall guidelines for curb management using a wheelchair and then utilize clinical judgment to determine the best course of action for teaching a patient with T10 paraplegia to manage curbs. This requires inductive reasoning skill. For this case, the assistant should instruct the patient to grasp the handrims posteriorly and pull them forward abruptly and forcefully. If answered incorrectly, review curb management techniques with wheelchairs.

A148 | Devices, Admin, etc. | Equipment, Modalities

A patient presents with multiple fractures of both hands and wrists as a result of a mountain bike accident. Now, 5 weeks later, the patient has limited wrist and finger motion, and dry scaly skin over the previously casted areas. The physical agent **MOST** appropriate to aid in increasing range of motion in this case would be:

CHOICES:
1. paraffin.
2. hot packs.
3. functional electrical stimulation.
4. contact ultrasound.

CORRECT ANSWER: 1

RATIONALE:
Paraffin bath will provide circumferential heating of the hands and fingers and will aid in softening the skin. Active exercise, including functional electrical stimulation, would be more effective after the application of paraffin as tissue extensibility and pliability would be increased. Hot packs or ultrasound using direct contact would not completely cover the area to be treated.

TYPE OF REASONING: INDUCTIVE
This question requires clinical judgment to determine a best course of action to address the patient's symptoms. This is an inductive reasoning skill. For this situation, the most appropriate modality choice to increase range of motion is paraffin. If answered incorrectly, review indications for use of paraffin, especially for increasing range of motion.

A149 | Musculoskeletal | Data Collection

A male child who plays catcher on his baseball team complains of bilateral knee pain that is exacerbated with forceful quadriceps contraction. The physical therapist examination noted pain and swelling at the distal attachment of the patellar tendon. The therapist has instructed the physical therapist assistant to begin treatment that addresses the pain and swelling. Early management should focus on:

CHOICES:
1. isometric exercises to decrease inflammation.
2. active range of motion exercises to prevent contracture.
3. decreased loading of the knee by the quadriceps femoris muscle.
4. casting followed by decreased loading of the knee.

CORRECT ANSWER: 3

RATIONALE:
Baseball catchers must make forceful contractions of the quadriceps muscles each time they stand up to throw the ball to the pitcher. This may precipitate Osgood–Schlatter disease in the adolescent boy. Early intervention of this condition focuses on reduction of the loading by the quadriceps but still retaining normal lower-extremity function.

TYPE OF REASONING: INDUCTIVE
This question requires the test taker to determine a best course of action for a child with bilateral knee pain and swelling. This requires clinical judgment, which is an inductive reasoning skill. For this case, the assistant should focus on decreased loading of the knee by the quadriceps femoris muscle. If answered incorrectly, review intervention approaches for knee pain associated with forceful contractions of the quadriceps.

A150 | Other Systems | Clinical Applications

An obese patient who is 70 pounds overweight is recovering from a mild myocardial infarction and needs cardiovascular conditioning. The exercise class will be used in conjunction with a dietary program to promote weight reduction. The **MOST** appropriate protocol for exercise for this patient is:

CHOICES:

1. jogging, for 10 minutes at 4 miles per hour.
2. walking, intensity set at 50% target heart rate.
3. walking, intensity set at 75% of heart rate reserve.
4. swimming, intensity set at 75% age-adjusted heart rate.

CORRECT ANSWER: 2

RATIONALE:

Obese individuals are typically sedentary with lower initial levels of physical conditioning. The initial exercise prescription should focus on a lower intensity exercise progressing to longer durations. Higher intensity exercise (75% or 85% of heart rate maximum) should be avoided initially. Jogging is also too intense and may yield additional orthopedic problems.

TYPE OF REASONING: INDUCTIVE

One must have knowledge of exercise and reconditioning approaches for patients with obesity to arrive at a correct conclusion. This requires inductive reasoning skill, as clinical judgment is paramount to arriving at a correct conclusion. For this situation, the most appropriate protocol for exercise should include walking with the intensity set at 50% target heart rate. Review exercise guidelines for patients with obesity if answered incorrectly.

Examination B

B1 | Musculoskeletal | Interventions

The physical therapist evaluation of a patient's gait identifies the patient as having a positive Trendelenburg sign on the right. The plan of care includes functional activities for strengthening the affected musculature. Which of the following treatments **BEST** addresses the weakness?

CHOICES:

1. bridging.
2. lateral step-ups bilaterally.
3. quadruped leg extension.
4. supine hip abduction.

CORRECT ANSWER: 2

RATIONALE:

A Trendelenburg gait pattern is the result of weak hip abductors, specifically the gluteus medius. Lateral step-ups bilaterally will increase the strength of the gluteus medius muscle; the right gluteus medius is strengthened during weight-bearing while raising the left lower extremity up to the step as the muscle is working against gravity. Supine hip abduction does strengthen the gluteus medius if done correctly; however, it is not as functional as the weight-bearing lateral step-ups as gravity is not a factor. Bridging increases hip extensor strength, as does quadruped leg extension.

TYPE OF REASONING: INDUCTIVE

One must determine the best exercise for a patient, given the diagnosis provided. This is an inductive reasoning skill, where clinical judgment is utilized to draw conclusions. For this patient with a Trendelenburg gait pattern, the best intervention approach to address the weakness is lateral step-ups bilaterally. If answered incorrectly, review signs and symptoms of Trendelenburg gait pattern as well as exercises for this diagnosis.

B2 | Neuromuscular | Clinical Applications

A patient has muscle weakness in elbow flexion; however, pronation and supination strength of the forearm is normal. The muscle that requires strengthening in this case is the:

CHOICES:

1. brachialis.
2. biceps brachii.
3. brachioradialis.
4. coracobrachialis.

CORRECT ANSWER: 1

RATIONALE:

The brachialis is an elbow flexor (only). Pronation and supination are normal; this eliminates biceps brachii, as it is also responsible for supination. Coracobrachialis performs shoulder flexion and adduction, and the brachioradialis also assists with pronation.

TYPE OF REASONING: ANALYTICAL

One must analyze the symptoms presented and then draw a conclusion about what these symptoms represent. This requires analytical reasoning skill, where various pieces of information are analyzed to draw a correct conclusion. In this case, the pattern of weakness indicates that the brachialis muscle is weak and requires strengthening. Review symptoms of brachialis weakness if answered incorrectly.

B3 | Neuromuscular | Interventions

A 5 year-old child with cerebral palsy has persistence of the symmetrical tonic neck reflex. For the child to maintain stability in the quadruped position, the physical therapist assistant should:

CHOICES:

1. turn the head to the nondominant side.
2. tap on the paraspinal musculature.
3. apply approximation to both shoulders.
4. keep the chin elevated.

CORRECT ANSWER: 4

RATIONALE:

If the symmetrical tonic neck reflex persists, elevating the chin will cause the upper extremities to extend and the lower extremities to flex, thus helping to maintain the quadruped position. Turning the head toward the nondominant side will increase awareness of the nondominant side. Tapping on the paraspinal musculature is appropriate if the goal is to increase trunk extension. Applying approximation through the shoulder joint can stimulate increased firing of the shoulder joint musculature, while this may improve shoulder girdle firing it will not assist in hip control.

TYPE OF REASONING: INDUCTIVE

One must determine the position that will maintain stability in the quadruped position in a child with cerebral palsy. This requires inductive reasoning skill, a skill that requires clinical judgment to determine a best course of action. In this case, a child with symmetrical tonic neck reflex in the quadruped position should keep the chin elevated to maintain stability in this position. If answered incorrectly, review symmetrical tonic neck reflex, especially head positioning for quadruped stability.

B4 | Devices, Admin, etc. | Equipment, Modalities

As part of a home program, a patient is using a mechanical cervical traction unit. When the physical therapist assistant arrives, the patient indicates that the cervical condition is improving; however, there is now discomfort in the area of the occiput. The assistant should:

CHOICES:

1. have the patient demonstrate the procedure used, and check to see if the set-up is correct.
2. instruct the patient to place a soft pad between the teeth during traction.
3. have the patient discontinue the traction.
4. have the patient decrease the amount of weight used during traction.

CORRECT ANSWER: 1

RATIONALE:

In this situation the physical therapist assistant should assess whether the patient is setting up the traction machine correctly. The patient should lie supine with the occipital pads lined up with the ears, tighten the occipital pads and then apply the traction force. There should be no traction force applied through the mandible, and soft pads between the teeth are inappropriate in any situation while using cervical traction. The decision to discontinue is inappropriate if set-up has not been assessed. Decreasing the weight may make the traction ineffective and does not address the cause of the discomfort.

TYPE OF REASONING: INDUCTIVE

This question requires one to utilize clinical judgment to determine a best course of action for a patient with discomfort after using mechanical cervical traction. This necessitates inductive reasoning skill. For this case, the assistant should have the patient demonstrate the procedure used and check to see if the set-up is correct. Review guidelines for mechanical cervical traction and set-up if answered incorrectly.

B5 | Musculoskeletal | Interventions

The plan of care calls for manual stretch of a patient's piriformis muscle. To **BEST** accomplish this the patient should be positioned:

CHOICES:

1. supine with the hip flexed to 70° and the knee extended.
2. side-lying with hip extended and medially (internally) rotated.
3. side-lying with the hip abducted and laterally (externally) rotated.
4. supine with the hip flexed and laterally (externally) rotated.

CORRECT ANSWER: 4

RATIONALE:

Because of its attachments, the piriformis is best stretched with the hip in a flexed and laterally (externally) rotated position. The position of hip flexion and knee extension will provide a stretch to the hamstrings, provided the range of motion is limited at the 70° range. Hip extension and medial (internal) rotation or abduction place the piriformis on slack.

TYPE OF REASONING: DEDUCTIVE

One must recall the guidelines for manual stretch of the piriformis muscle to arrive at a correct conclusion. This is factual information, which requires deductive reasoning skill. For this case, the therapist should position the patient in supine with the hip flexed and laterally (externally) rotated. Review hip stretching exercises, especially for the piriformis muscle, if answered incorrectly.

B6 | Cardiovascular/Pulmonary | Clinical Applications

Six weeks after a myocardial infarction, a patient enters an outpatient physical therapy cardiac rehabilitation program. Now that the patient is in phase 2, exercise should predominantly focus on:

CHOICES:
1. low-level weight training using a starting weight at one repetition maximum.
2. circuit training using various upper-extremity resistance devices.
3. continuous aerobic activities using large muscle groups.
4. recreational activities such as jogging and swimming.

CORRECT ANSWER: 3

RATIONALE:
Phase 2 of cardiac rehabilitation functional work capacity should be between 4 and 6 metabolic equivalents (METs). Jogging and swimming are between 6 and 8 METs. Resistive upper-extremity exercises are contraindicated for patients at this stage of cardiac rehabilitation.

TYPE OF REASONING: DEDUCTIVE
One must recall factual guidelines of outpatient cardiac rehabilitation to arrive at a correct conclusion. Recall of factual guidelines requires deductive reasoning skill. For this question, the focus for exercise in phase 2 rehabilitation should be continuous aerobic activities using large muscle groups. If answered incorrectly, review cardiac rehabilitation guidelines, especially for phase 2.

B7 | Devices, Admin, etc. | Safety Roles, Teaching, EBP

A physical therapist assistant has just completed instructing a family member in how to transfer a patient from bed to wheelchair and back to bed. The assistant should document the family member's ability to complete the transfer in which section of the SOAP note?

CHOICES:
1. Subjective.
2. Objective.
3. Assessment.
4. Plan.

CORRECT ANSWER: 3

RATIONALE:
An interpretation or report of the family member's ability level in performing the transfer should be included in the Assessment section of the note. The Objective portion of the note should include a description of the technique taught to the family member. Subjective information is information provided by the patient or the family member. The Plan section should identify if further training of the family member is planned.

TYPE OF REASONING: DEDUCTIVE
This question requires a test taker to recall the factual guidelines for SOAP note documentation. Factual guidelines often necessitate deductive reasoning skill. For this situation, the family member's ability to complete the transfer should be documented in the assessment section of the SOAP note. If answered incorrectly, review SOAP note documentation guidelines, including information to be placed in the assessment section.

B8 | Cardiovascular/Pulmonary | Clinical Applications

A patient who has congestive heart failure (CHF) will likely be on a digitalis medication such as Digoxin. A physical therapist assistant treating this patient in a skilled nursing facility should be alert for digitalis toxicity. Adverse reactions could affect the:

CHOICES:

1. gastrointestinal and central nervous systems.
2. genitourinary and endocrine systems.
3. pulmonary and genitourinary systems.
4. gastrointestinal and integumentary systems.

CORRECT ANSWER: 1

RATIONALE:

Digitalis (cardiac glucosides) is a very common medication used in the treatment of CHF because it increases contractility and decreases heart rate of the cardiac muscle, thus decreasing oxygen demand and increasing coronary blood flow. Digitalis toxicity is a somewhat common and potentially fatal adverse reaction. The central nervous system is often impacted with drowsiness, confusion and visual disturbances. The gastrointestinal system reactions can be in the form of vomiting, diarrhea and nausea. Cardiac arrhythmias can also occur. The genitourinary, integumentary and pulmonary systems are not involved with adverse digitalis reactions. The physical therapist assistant should be alert for early signs of digitalis toxicity.

TYPE OF REASONING: DEDUCTIVE

One must recall the signs of digitalis medication toxicity to arrive at a correct conclusion. This is factual information, which is a deductive reasoning skill. For this scenario, the assistant should monitor the patient for adverse reactions affecting the gastrointestinal and central nervous systems, which are symptoms indicating toxicity. If answered incorrectly, review side effects of taking digitalis medication and signs of toxicity.

B9 | Devices, Admin, etc. | Safety Roles, Teaching, EBP

In an acute care center, a physical therapist assistant is gait training an obese teenager with a long lower-extremity cast when the patient suddenly falls to the floor and is unresponsive. The assistant calls a nurse standing nearby and activates the emergency system in the hospital. The assistant assesses the airway, breathing and circulation and finds a weak, thready pulse and no respirations. The assistant should next begin:

CHOICES:

1. respirations at one breath every 15 seconds.
2. chest compressions at 15 per minute.
3. respirations at one breath every 5 seconds.
4. chest compressions at 60 to 80 per minute.

CORRECT ANSWER: 3

RATIONALE:

The physical therapist assistant should begin respirations at one breath every 5 seconds. Chest compressions are inappropriate as the patient has a pulse, even if it is weak and thready. After the first minute the patient should be reassessed; at that time, if the patient has no pulse and is not breathing, then chest compressions and rescue breathing are initiated; if the patient continues to have a pulse and no breathing, rescue breathing is continued. By this time in a hospital situation, persons from the emergency response team would have already shown up to take over care.

TYPE OF REASONING: DEDUCTIVE

This question requires a test taker to recall the factual guidelines for the administration of cardiopulmonary resuscitation (CPR). Factual guidelines often necessitate deductive reasoning skill. For this situation, after assessing the airway, breathing and circulation, the assistant should begin respirations at one breath every 5 seconds. If answered incorrectly, review CPR guidelines.

B10 | Other Systems | Clinical Applications

The physical therapist has just evaluated and established a plan of care for a patient with rheumatoid arthritis affecting the hands. A physical therapist assistant treating this patient should **MOST LIKELY** expect the patient to present with:

CHOICES:

1. stiffness of the fingers of short duration.
2. osteophytes (bone spurs).
3. radial drift of the metacarpophalangeal joints.
4. bilateral symmetrical deformities.

CORRECT ANSWER: 4

RATIONALE:

Rheumatoid arthritis can result in a variety of deformities of the small joints of the hand, including but not limited to swan neck or boutonniere deformities, ulnar drift of the digits and metacarpophalangeal joints, and morning stiffness that can last until noon. Bilateral symmetrical deformities are a characteristic of rheumatoid arthritis. Short duration stiffness and bone spurs are characteristic of osteoarthritis. Symmetrical deformities can occur with osteoarthritis although this is a variable occurrence.

TYPE OF REASONING: INFERENTIAL

This question provides a diagnosis in which the test taker must determine the most likely symptoms. Questions of this nature often require inferential reasoning skill, which requires one to determine what is most likely to be true of a situation. For this situation, the symptoms most consistent with rheumatoid arthritis of the hands are bilateral symmetrical deformities. If answered incorrectly, review symptoms of rheumatoid arthritis, especially those affecting the hands.

B11 | Cardiovascular/Pulmonary | Clinical Applications

A physical therapist assistant working with a patient who is receiving treatment for a venous thrombosis may note the formation of areas of ecchymosis on the skin secondary to which of the following medications?

CHOICES:

1. heparin.
2. hydrocortisone.
3. Dilantin.
4. digoxin.

CORRECT ANSWER: 1

RATIONALE:

Heparin is a blood thinner used to prevent thrombosis from occurring. It is not unusual for the patient to display ecchymosis (bruising black and blue) under his or her skin. Patients receiving heparin need to be cautious, as they will tend to bleed and bruise more easily if injured. Digoxin is used to increase cardiac muscle contractility and decreases heart rate. Dilantin is used to decrease seizures, especially with epilepsy. Hydrocortisone is used to decrease the effects of psoriasis and other skin disorders.

TYPE OF REASONING: ANALYTICAL

One must analyze the symptoms presented to determine the medication that is secondary to these symptoms. This requires analytical reasoning skill, where pieces of information are analyzed to draw a conclusion. For this case, the symptoms are secondary to the medication heparin. Review side effects of taking blood thinner medication, especially heparin, if answered incorrectly.

B12 | Devices, Admin, etc. | Equipment, Modalities

A child with spastic quadriplegia demonstrates a strong extensor thrust pattern while seated. To help decrease the extensor thrusting response when in a wheelchair the chair should be modified so that:

CHOICES:

1. just the forefoot portion of the feet touch the foot rests.
2. both the seat and seat back are reclined backwards approximately 15°.
3. the leg rests are kept elevated at 80°.
4. the wheelchair is equipped with an electric reclining back.

CORRECT ANSWER: 2

RATIONALE:

When both the seat and the seat back are tilted backward, the patient's center of gravity will be displaced posteriorly. This will assist with combating extensor thrusting response and decrease the likelihood of the patient sliding out of the wheelchair. Elevating the leg rests will not decrease overall tone. Placing the forefoot portion of the foot on the foot rest is likely to place undue stress on the metatarsal heads and may stimulate a clonus response in the gastrocsoleus musculature. Just a reclining back may place the patient at risk for scooting forward in the seat of the wheelchair if the extensor thrusting pattern is initiated; the patient would then be at risk for sliding out the front of the chair.

TYPE OF REASONING: INDUCTIVE

This question requires the test taker to determine the most appropriate position for a patient with a strong extensor thrust while seated in a wheelchair. This requires clinical judgment, which is an inductive reasoning skill. For this case, the wheelchair seat and back should be reclined backwards 15° to reduce the extensor thrust. If answered incorrectly, review wheelchair seating and positioning guidelines for children with spastic quadriplegia.

B13 | Neuromuscular | Interventions

A patient presents with a flexion synergy pattern and spastic hemiparesis on the left. To **BEST** decrease the tone in the upper extremity the physical therapist assistant should:

CHOICES:

1. perform slow passive range-of-motion exercises with the left upper extremity in diagonal patterns.
2. have the patient perform right-extremity active exercise with the left upper extremity placed in a weight-bearing position with the shoulder laterally (externally) rotated and wrist extended.
3. perform functional activities and right upper-extremity exercise with the left upper extremity supported in a hemi sling.
4. apply a slow stretch to the left shoulder extensors, elbow extensors and wrist extensors.

CORRECT ANSWER: 2

RATIONALE:

Performing weight-bearing activities with extremity placed out of the synergy pattern is the best mechanism identified in this question to decrease the flexion synergy pattern identified. Performing slow passive range-of-motion exercises will help decrease triggering a spastic response with that movement; a hemi sling is not functional and does not help promote normal movement patterns or decrease tone; and a slow stretch applied to the agonist muscle groups (flexors) can help decrease tone; however, applied to the antagonists, it is not likely to decrease the tone pattern.

TYPE OF REASONING: INDUCTIVE

One must determine the best approach to decreasing tone in the upper extremity of a patient with flexor synergy pattern and spastic hemiparesis. This is an inductive reasoning skill, where clinical judgment is utilized to draw conclusions. For this patient, it is best to perform right-extremity active exercise with the left upper extremity placed in a weight-bearing position with the shoulder laterally rotated and wrist extended. If answered incorrectly, review exercise guidelines to decrease tone for patients with flexor synergy.

B14 | Neuromuscular | Clinical Applications

A physical therapist assistant is working with a patient who has Parkinson's disease. The assistant should expect the patient to be taking L-dopa or Sinemet, which affect:

CHOICES:

1. alpha motor neuron excitability.
2. transmission of impulses within the spinal cord.
3. synaptic transmission at the neuromuscular synapse.
4. neurochemical imbalances in the basal ganglia.

CORRECT ANSWER: 4

RATIONALE:

Levodopa and Sinemet are both anti-parkinsonism medications. Levodopa replaces L-dopa that is normally produced by the basal ganglia. Patients with Parkinson's disease have a deficiency of this neurotransmitter. Valium (diazepam) is a muscle relaxant that affects alpha motor neuron excitability. Baclofen is an antispasticity drug that affects transmission of impulses within the spinal cord. Botulinum toxin is a muscle relaxant that affects synaptic transmission.

TYPE OF REASONING: DEDUCTIVE

This question requires the test taker to recall the properties of anti-parkinsonism medications to arrive at a correct conclusion. This is factual information, which is a deductive reasoning skill. For this situation, the medications will affect neurochemical imbalances in the basal ganglia. If answered incorrectly, review anti-parkinsonism medication, especially levodopa and Sinemet.

B15 | Devices, Admin, etc. | Safety Roles, Teaching, EBP

A patient with traumatic brain injury has a convulsive seizure during treatment. The patient loses consciousness and presents with tonic–clonic convulsions of all extremities. The physical therapist assistant's **BEST** response is to:

CHOICES:

1. position the patient in side-lying, check to see if airway is open, and immediately call for emergency assistance.
2. initiate cardiopulmonary resuscitation (CPR) immediately and call for help to restrain the patient.
3. position in supine with head supported with a pillow and wait out the seizure.
4. use straps to secure the limbs so the patient cannot be harmed.

CORRECT ANSWER: 1

RATIONALE:

This is an emergency situation. To prevent aspiration, turn the head to the side or position in side-lying. Check to see if the airway is open and wait for tonic–clonic activity to subside before initiating artificial ventilation if needed. A patient who is having a seizure should never be restrained; the area around the patient should be cleared to prevent injury.

TYPE OF REASONING: EVALUATIVE

This question requires the test taker to determine the best response for a patient who is experiencing a convulsive seizure during treatment. Questions that require one to weigh the implications of an action or response often require evaluative reasoning skill. For this situation, the best response is to position the patient in side-lying, then check to see if the airway is open and immediately call for emergency assistance. If answered incorrectly, review emergency first aid and CPR guidelines, especially for patients having seizures.

B16 | Neuromuscular | Clinical Applications

A patient has damage to the lower branches of the femoral nerve. The physical therapist assistant should expect the patient to have the **MOST** difficulty:

CHOICES:

1. ascending stairs.
2. walking on level surfaces.
3. descending stairs.
4. performing bridging exercises.

CORRECT ANSWER: 3

RATIONALE:

An injury to the femoral nerve will affect the quadriceps muscles. Eccentric control of the quadriceps is needed to descend the stairs. The gluteus maximus and hamstrings are the primary muscles involved in bridging exercises. A patient can compensate for weak quadriceps during ambulation on level surfaces by knee or hip hyperextension.

TYPE OF REASONING: INFERENTIAL

Questions that provide a diagnosis and ask the test taker to determine the likely functional difficulties associated with that diagnosis often require inferential reasoning skill. For this question, damage to the lower branches of the femoral nerve will likely produce difficulty with descending stairs. If answered incorrectly, review signs and symptoms of femoral nerve damage, especially engagement in functional activities with damage.

B17 | Devices, Admin, etc. | Safety Roles, Teaching, EBP

A physical therapist assistant with a head cold should have limited contact with patients who:

CHOICES:

1. are in the acute stage of rheumatoid arthritis.
2. are undergoing chemotherapy.
3. have had a recent cerebrovascular accident.
4. have recently had a spinal tap.

CORRECT ANSWER: 2

RATIONALE:

Patients undergoing chemotherapy treatments have a compromised immune system. Precautions should be taken when a person is experiencing a cold or other infection. Patients undergoing chemotherapy are especially susceptible to viral transmissions associated with a head cold. Patients diagnosed with rheumatoid arthritis, cerebrovascular accident or who recently have undergone a spinal tap will not be as susceptible to the effects of exposure to a person with a head cold.

TYPE OF REASONING: INDUCTIVE

This question requires one to utilize clinical judgment to determine a best course of action. For this case, an assistant with a cold should limit contact with patients who are undergoing chemotherapy because of the patients' compromised immune system. If answered incorrectly, review precautions for working with patients who are immunocompromised, especially patients undergoing chemotherapy.

B18 | Other Systems | Clinical Applications

A patient has been discharged to home following a recent ORIF for a pathological fracture of the tibia. The patient also has metastatic carcinoma of the lung. During treatment the patient reports sharp pain in the right hip which frequently causes a loss of sleep. The physical therapist assistant should:

CHOICES:

1. continue with treatment as tolerated and attribute the pain to increased use during treatment.
2. suggest the use of heat and monitor response at the next visit.
3. modify the treatment to avoid walking.
4. recommend that the patient see the physician as soon as possible.

CORRECT ANSWER: 4

RATIONALE:

New night pain is a red flag for possible metastasis to a new site. In addition to suggesting a visit to the physician, the physical therapist assistant should notify the physical therapist and document the findings. The other choices do address minimizing stress to the area; however, they do not address the underlying concern of possible metastasis.

TYPE OF REASONING: EVALUATIVE

For this question, the test taker must determine an appropriate course of action for a patient reporting sharp pain in the right hip. This requires one to weigh the significance of all the information presented to arrive at a correct conclusion, which is an evaluative reasoning skill. For this scenario, the assistant should recommend that the patient sees the physician as soon as possible, especially in light of the patient's history of metastatic cancer. If answered incorrectly, review signs and symptoms of metastatic cancer.

B19 | Cardiovascular/Pulmonary | Clinical Applications

A physical therapist assistant who is providing interventions for a patient following radiation treatments for prostate cancer identifies that the patient is developing edema in the right lower extremity. A secondary effect of the radiation treatment that can cause the edema is:

CHOICES:

1. lymphatic obstruction.
2. disuse atrophy.
3. orthostatic hypotension.
4. the onset of congestive heart failure.

CORRECT ANSWER: 1

RATIONALE:

A patient who has completed radiation treatments for prostate cancer should be a candidate for developing lymphatic disease secondary to damage to the lymphatic system from the radiation. Disuse atrophy will result in tissue wasting, not edema. Increased upright activities will assist in the return of fluid via the muscle pumping action. Although congestive heart failure (CHF) can result in peripheral edema, or is not likely to be unilateral and nothing in the scenario described indicates that the patient is at risk for CHF. Orthostatic hypotension can result from immobility, blood volume depletion, side effects of medication and other causes; however, it is not a secondary effect of radiation therapy or a cause of edema.

TYPE OF REASONING: INFERENTIAL

One must determine the secondary effects of radiation treatment causing edema in the lower extremity. This requires one to infer what may be true, which is an inferential reasoning skill. For this case, the secondary effects of radiation causing lower extremity edema can be attributable to lymphatic obstruction. If answered incorrectly, review radiation treatment guidelines for patients with cancer, especially edema associated with radiation treatment.

B20 | Devices, Admin, etc. | Safety Roles, Teaching, EBP

A physical therapist assistant working in an early intervention program arrives at a home to treat a 2 year-old child. Upon arrival the physical therapist assistant is greeted at the door by the 8 year-old sibling. The sibling tells the assistant to come in as the parent has gone to the store. The assistant determines that the 2 year-old and 8 year-old children are at home alone. The physical therapist assistant should:

CHOICES:

1. call the parent's cell phone.
2. enter the home as invited and treat the child.
3. call the Department of Social Services to report maltreatment.
4. take the children to the local police station.

CORRECT ANSWER: 3

RATIONALE:

A physical therapist assistant working in the home care setting is considered to be a mandatory reporter. Mandatory reporters are required to report cases of suspected child abuse or maltreatment. As PTAs are mandatory reporters, it is inappropriate to attempt to contact the parent on their cell phone since they did find the children at home alone and unattended to.

TYPE OF REASONING: EVALUATIVE

One must determine an appropriate course of action for children who have been left home alone. This requires weighing the choices presented to determine the course of action that best resolves the issue. This is an evaluative reasoning skill. For this case, the assistant should call the Department of Social Services to report the issue. If answered incorrectly, review child abuse and maltreatment guidelines, including mandatory reporting guidelines.

B21 | Devices, Admin, etc. | Safety Roles, Teaching, EBP

A physical therapist and physical therapist assistant team are treating a patient whose plan of care includes: "therapeutic exercise to strengthen core stabilizers." Upon reading the documentation for the previous treatment the physical therapist notes that the assistant has progressed the exercise program to include single knee extension in supine. The physical therapist assistant:

CHOICES:

1. is working within the scope of practice.
2. should have checked with the physical therapist prior to starting the new exercise.
3. should have immediately contacted the physical therapist following the last visit.
4. is working beyond the scope of practice.

CORRECT ANSWER: 1

RATIONALE:

It is within the scope of practice for a physical therapist assistant to progress a patient through an exercise program if it is included in the plan of care. If the plan of care identifies specific exercises, modalities, or therapeutic activities the assistant needs to get verbal or written consent from the physical therapist to modify it.

TYPE OF REASONING: DEDUCTIVE

This question requires one to recall factual guidelines about physical therapy scope of practice. This is a deductive reasoning skill where factual guidelines are often utilized to make decisions. For this situation, the assistant is working within the scope of practice. If answered incorrectly, review physical therapy scope of practice guidelines.

B22 | Other Systems | Interventions

A patient is referred to physical therapy following three weeks of bedrest. The patient has multiple problems including an acute flare-up of rheumatoid arthritis in both hands, a recent surgical repair of an intertrochanteric fracture of the hip, bilateral knee flexion contractures and an abnormal electrocardiogram (EKG). The patient is now permitted to walk with partial weight-bearing on the operated side. The plan of care includes increasing range of motion and improving endurance. The physical therapist assistant could **BEST** meet the plan of care by having the patient:

CHOICES:

1. walk as tolerated with a standard walker and perform passive stretch to bilateral hamstrings.
2. use a recumbent bike and perform contract/relax to bilateral hamstrings.
3. participate in contract/relax exercises to stretch bilateral hamstrings and walk on a treadmill.
4. use an upper-extremity ergometer set at moderate resistance and prone-lying passive stretch of the hamstrings.

CORRECT ANSWER: 2

RATIONALE:

Recumbent bike riding is a safe mechanism to maintain partial weight-bearing on the hip while still increasing endurance, and contract/relax is an effective means of stretching the hamstrings. Because of the recent abnormal EKG, the patient's heart rate and blood pressure should also be closely monitored throughout exercise. The upper-extremity ergometer may not be safe considering the recent abnormal EKG and is not a good choice for a patient with a flare-up of rheumatoid arthritis in the joints of the hands. The treadmill should be avoided as the weight-bearing status would be exceeded. Ambulation as tolerated with the standard walker may increase endurance; however, a passive stretch is not as effective as contract/relax mechanisms to increase range of motion.

TYPE OF REASONING: INDUCTIVE

One must determine the best therapeutic exercise for a patient with a hip fracture, rheumatoid arthritis and an abnormal EKG. Clinical judgment is utilized with questions of this nature, which require inductive reasoning skill. For this situation, the assistant should use a recumbent bike and perform contract/relax to bilateral hamstrings to best meet the plan of care. If answered incorrectly review therapeutic exercises for patients with hip fracture, rheumatoid arthritis and abnormal EKGs.

B23 | Other Systems | Interventions

A patient has rheumatoid arthritis in bilateral elbows and is having difficulty tolerating the long hours required at a desk job. **INITIAL** physical therapy treatment should include:

CHOICES:

1. use of cold and avoidance of active elbow flexion.
2. application of topical analgesics and light resistance strengthening.
3. splinting in 90° of flexion and isometric exercise at 80% effort.
4. use of heat modalities and joint protection.

CORRECT ANSWER: 4

RATIONALE:

Initially the patient should be treated with modalities to decrease tissue irritation. Heat and joint protection may be effective. At this stage strengthening is not appropriate. Splinting should be avoided and is not realistic for this patient. Use of cold with rheumatoid arthritis can be problematic because of cold intolerance, cryoglobulinemia or Raynaud's phenomenon.

TYPE OF REASONING: INDUCTIVE

One must determine the best intervention approach for a patient with rheumatoid arthritis in both elbows. This requires clinical judgment, which is an inductive reasoning skill. For this case, initial intervention should include the use of heat modalities and joint protection to decrease symptoms. If answered incorrectly, review treatment approaches for rheumatoid arthritis.

B24 | Neuromuscular | Clinical Applications

A physical therapist has been asked to consult with a physical education teacher regarding exercises to incorporate with a child who has Down syndrome. Which of the following is a **CONTRAINDICATION** and potentially dangerous?

CHOICES:
1. jumping jacks during strength and conditioning training.
2. batting during softball.
3. long-distance running during track.
4. forward rolls during gymnastics.

CORRECT ANSWER: 4

RATIONALE:

One complication of Down syndrome can be atlanto–axial instability because of ligamentous laxity at the junction between the C1 and C2 vertebrae. If this joint is unstable the pressure exerted through the area with a forward roll could put the patient at risk for spinal cord injury. The other activities are not contraindicated; however, a determination should be made with each individual as to whether that activity is advisable for the patient.

TYPE OF REASONING: EVALUATIVE

One must determine the activity to avoid for a child with Down syndrome. This requires the test taker to weigh the information and its significance to reach a correct conclusion. This is an evaluative reasoning skill. For this situation, the child should not participate in exercise that places stress on the atlanto–axial joint, such as forward rolls. If answered incorrectly, review precautions and contraindications for exercise in children with Down syndrome.

B25 | Devices, Admin, etc. | Safety Roles, Teaching, EBP

While a physical therapist assistant is gait training a patient who has a history of cardiac disease, the patient becomes hypotensive. The physical therapist assistant should:

CHOICES:
1. immediately contact the supervising physical therapist.
2. terminate the activity, sit the patient down and elevate the lower extremities.
3. offer a drink of orange juice.
4. decrease the speed of walking.

CORRECT ANSWER: 2

RATIONALE:

If a cardiac patient experiences hypotension with activity, the activity should be stopped. The patient is not tolerating the activity and the heart cannot keep up with the physical demands of the activity.

TYPE OF REASONING: EVALUATIVE

For this question, the test taker must determine an appropriate response for a patient who has become hypotensive during gait training. This requires one to weigh the courses of action and determine the action that effectively addresses the patient's needs. This is an evaluative reasoning skill. For this situation, the assistant should terminate the activity, sit the patient down and elevate the lower extremities. If answered incorrectly, review guidelines for addressing hypotensive episodes.

B26 | Other Systems | Interventions

The plan of care for a patient immediately following a cesarean delivery should include:

CHOICES:

1. progressive cardiovascular training.
2. partial curl-ups.
3. pelvic floor exercises.
4. practice lifting techniques.

CORRECT ANSWER: 3

RATIONALE:

Following a pregnancy and a cesarean delivery the patient should present with decreased tone in the pelvic floor muscles; pelvic floor exercises will help to rebuild muscle strength and control. Partial curl-ups are contraindicated immediately following cesarean delivery; this exercise will be indicated following appropriate healing time for the abdominal muscles and tissues. Cardiovascular training and lifting techniques do not address the diagnosis identified.

TYPE OF REASONING: INDUCTIVE

One must determine the best exercises to include for a patient post-cesarean delivery. This requires inductive reasoning skill, a skill that requires clinical judgment to determine a best course of action. In this case, the plan of care should include pelvic floor exercises to help rebuild muscle strength and control. If answered incorrectly, review exercises for patients post-cesarean delivery.

B27 | Neuromuscular | Clinical Applications

A physical therapist assistant preparing to treat a patient who was recently admitted to the hospital with a diagnosis of Guillain–Barré syndrome should expect the patient to present with:

CHOICES:

1. symmetrical distribution of extremity weakness with possible involvement of the lower cranial nerves.
2. asymmetrical weakness with hyperreflexia.
3. unilateral facial paralysis; affected eye does not close.
4. sensory loss (stocking and glove distribution) with minor loss of motor function.

CORRECT ANSWER: 1

RATIONALE:

Guillain–Barré syndrome is an acute polyneuritis characterized by rapid development of progressive muscle weakness. The weakness is typically symmetrical and ascends the body (starting first in the lower extremities, progressing to trunk, upper extremities, and, finally, cranial nerves). Stocking and glove sensory loss could be found but not with minor loss of motor function. Unilateral facial paralysis is indicative of Bell's palsy.

TYPE OF REASONING: INFERENTIAL

This question provides a diagnosis and the test taker must determine the likely symptoms of this diagnosis. Questions of this nature often require inferential reasoning skill. For this case, one should expect the patient to present with symmetrical distribution of extremity weakness with possible involvement of the lower cranial nerves. If answered incorrectly, review signs and symptoms of Guillain–Barré syndrome.

B28 | Musculoskeletal | Data Collection

The stationary arm of a goniometer is placed in line with the lateral midline of the trunk, the fulcrum is placed at the greater trochanter, and the movable arm is aligned with lateral femoral condyle. What motion is being measured?

CHOICES:
1. hip abduction.
2. trunk lateral flexion.
3. hip flexion.
4. trunk extension.

CORRECT ANSWER: 3

RATIONALE:

Correct goniometer placement when measuring hip flexion is: stationary arm of the goniometer is aligned with the midline of trunk, the movable arm is placed on the lateral femur aligned with the lateral femoral condyle, and the fulcrum is placed over the greater trochanter at the center of movement for the hip. Hip abduction is measured with the fulcrum over the axis of motion on the anterior hip, the stationary arm is aligned parallel to the anterior superior iliac spines of the ilium, and the movable arm is placed along the anterior thigh aligned with the patella. Trunk range of motion is more accurately measured with an inclinometer and not a goniometer.

TYPE OF REASONING: DEDUCTIVE

This question requires one to recall the procedures for measuring hip flexion with a goniometer. This is factual recall of information, which is a deductive reasoning skill. For this situation, the measurement being taken is that of hip flexion. If answered incorrectly, review goniometry guidelines, including hip measurements.

B29 | Devices, Admin, etc. | Equipment, Modalities

A patient with bilateral short transfemoral amputations will require a wheelchair for functional mobility in the home and community. An appropriate wheelchair modification is:

CHOICES:
1. placement of the drive wheels 2 inches anterior to the vertical back supports.
2. lowering the seat height by 3 inches.
3. increasing the seat depth by 2 inches to accommodate the length of the residual extremity.
4. placement of the drive wheels 2 inches posterior to the vertical back supports.

CORRECT ANSWER: 4

RATIONALE:

Placement of the drive wheels 2 inches posterior to the vertical back supports is an appropriate modification for a patient with bilateral transfemoral amputations. This increases the length of the base of support and provides increased posterior stability. Lowering the seat height by 3 inches is an appropriate modification for a patient with stroke who will use his sound extremity for wheelchair propulsion. Increasing the seat depth is not appropriate.

TYPE OF REASONING: INDUCTIVE

This question requires one to utilize clinical judgment to determine the best wheelchair modification for a patient with bilateral transfemoral amputations. This is an inductive reasoning skill. For this case, an appropriate modification is placement of the drive wheels 2 inches posterior to the vertical back supports to increase posterior stability. If answered incorrectly, review wheelchair modification guidelines, including modifications for patients with bilateral lower-extremity amputations.

B30 | Musculoskeletal | Data Collection

In sitting, a patient is able to flex the hip through 75% of the available range of motion without manual resistance and in side-lying, the patient is able to flex the hip through the full available range of motion. The hip flexor muscle grade is:

CHOICES:
1. fair minus (3-/5).
2. good (4/5).
3. fair (3/5).
4. poor (2/5).

CORRECT ANSWER: 1

RATIONALE:

When a person can move an extremity through the available range of motion against gravity without manual resistance, the muscle grade ascribed should be 3 (fair); a grade of 3- (fair minus)/5 is given when movement against gravity can be achieved through at least half of the available range. A grade of 4 (good)/5 is movement against gravity with moderate manual resistance applied. A grade of 2 (poor)/5 is full range of motion in a gravity-eliminated position.

TYPE OF REASONING: DEDUCTIVE

One must recall the procedures for manual muscle testing to arrive at a correct conclusion. This is factual recall of guidelines, which is a deductive reasoning skill. For this case, the description of the patient's movement should receive a grade of fair minus for the hip flexor muscle. If answered incorrectly, review manual muscle testing guidelines, especially for the hip.

B31 | Neuromuscular | Interventions

A physical therapist assistant is positioning a patient in bed following treatment. The patient has spastic left hemiparesis. The physical therapist assistant should position the upper extremities so that the scapula is:

CHOICES:
1. retracted with the shoulder adducted and medially (internally) rotated.
2. protracted with the shoulder abducted and laterally (externally) rotated.
3. retracted with the shoulder abducted and laterally (externally) rotated.
4. protracted with the shoulder adducted and medially (internally) rotated.

CORRECT ANSWER: 2

RATIONALE:

Positioning is aimed at decreasing the tone-dependent and reflex-dependent postures. The patient should be positioned supine in bed with the scapula positioned in protraction with the shoulder abducted and laterally (externally) rotated.

TYPE OF REASONING: DEDUCTIVE

One must recall the guidelines for positioning a patient with spastic hemiparesis in bed. This is factual information, which necessitates deductive reasoning skill. For this case, the assistant should position the upper extremities so that the scapula is protracted with the shoulder abducted and laterally rotated. If answered incorrectly, review bed positioning for patients with spasticity.

B32 | Integumentary | Interventions

The appropriate position in which to splint a patient with a deep partial thickness burn to the anterior neck is:

CHOICES:

1. chin tucked.
2. chin forward.
3. neck hyperextension.
4. neck flexion.

CORRECT ANSWER: 3

RATIONALE:

When a patient has suffered a deep partial thickness burn to the anterior neck, it is best to position the neck in hyperextension. The scar that forms will shorten because of the contractile or pulling forces of the scar tissue, which will limit range of motion and function.

TYPE OF REASONING: DEDUCTIVE

This question requires the test taker to recall the guidelines for splinting the neck after burns. This is factual information, which is a deductive reasoning skill. For this situation, the neck should be splinted after a deep partial thickness burn to the anterior neck in hyperextension to prevent contractures. If answered incorrectly, review splinting guidelines for patients with burns, especially burns to the neck region.

B33 | Devices, Admin, etc. | Equipment, Modalities

When considering treating a patient using a cryo-cuff, caution must be taken if the patient:

CHOICES:

1. exhibits an acute inflammatory process.
2. presents with very fair complexion.
3. presents with obesity.
4. exhibits Raynaud's disease.

CORRECT ANSWER: 4

RATIONALE:

Extreme caution should be taken when applying cold (cryotherapy) to a patient with Raynaud's disease because of the increased sensitivity to cold. Raynaud's disease is a condition caused by an abnormal degree of spasm of the blood vessels of the extremities in response to cold temperatures. Cryotherapy, in many cases, is contraindicated for someone with Raynaud's disease. Cryotherapy is indicated (in fact, is the first choice of treatment) for an acute inflammatory process. Cryotherapy or thermotherapy (heat) may not be effective on a person who is obese. A patient with a very fair complexion may be at risk if radiant heat were being used rather than cold.

TYPE OF REASONING: DEDUCTIVE

One must recall the contraindications and precautions for the use of cryotherapy to arrive at a correct conclusion. This requires the recall of factual information, necessitating deductive reasoning skill. For this scenario, when one is using a cryo-cuff, caution must be taken with patients who have Raynaud's disease. If answered incorrectly, review symptoms of Raynaud's disease and the use of modalities, especially cryotherapy.

B34 | Neuromuscular | Data Collection

When assessing a child with spina bifida (myelomeningocele), a characteristic the physical therapist assistant should not expect to find is:

CHOICES:

1. increased tone in the lower extremities.
2. inadequate bladder emptying.
3. sensory impairment in the lower extremities.
4. disturbances of bone growth and development.

CORRECT ANSWER: 1

RATIONALE:

Spina bifida usually does not have increased tone in the lower extremities. The child most often exhibits low tone. Spina bifida is a defective closure of the vertebral column. The residual deficits vary according to the severity of the disability. Myelomeningocele most often involves the spinal cord and the lumbosacral nerve roots. Lumbar nerve root involvement results in inadequate bladder emptying and sensory impairments to the lower extremities. Often disturbances in bone growth and development are seen because the paralysis has been present prior to birth during fetal development. The bones have not had the proper alignment or weight-bearing to allow for full development.

TYPE OF REASONING: INFERENTIAL

This question provides a diagnosis and the test taker must determine the symptoms not consistent with this diagnosis. This requires one to determine what is not likely to be true, which is **an** inferential reasoning skill. For this situation, the child with spina bifida is not likely to demonstrate increased tone in the lower extremities. If answered incorrectly, review signs and symptoms of spina bifida.

B35 | Devices, Admin, etc. | Equipment, Modalities

Following a cerebrovascular accident, a patient uses a wheelchair, is independent in stand-pivot transfers and can walk a limited distance. The feature **MOST** important to consider for this patient's wheelchair is:

CHOICES:

1. a swing-away detachable leg rest.
2. a one-arm drive.
3. standard nonremovable desk arms.
4. removable desk arms.

CORRECT ANSWER: 1

RATIONALE:

Because the patient is ambulatory, he or she will most likely walk or take a few steps out of the wheelchair. With safety as the primary concern, it will be important to remove obstacles that may cause the patient to trip; therefore, a swing-away removable leg rest is the most important feature of the wheelchair. Removable desk arms are important for a patient who transfers by using a sliding board or squat pivot technique. A patient who has hemiplegia will require a one-arm drive; however, the swing-away leg rest is the most important feature in this case because hemiplegia was not mentioned.

TYPE OF REASONING: INDUCTIVE

One must utilize clinical judgment to determine the most important feature for a patient's wheelchair. This requires inductive reasoning skill. For this case, the patient with cerebrovascular accident would benefit most from a swing-away detachable leg rest on the wheelchair. If answered incorrectly, review wheelchair prescription guidelines for patients with cerebrovascular accident.

B36 | Devices, Admin, etc. | Safety Roles, Teaching, EBP

If a patient with Alzheimer's disease is becoming frustrated in mastering a skill during treatment, the **BEST** strategy is to:

CHOICES:

1. move the patient to a quiet treatment area to minimize any distractions and enhance concentration.
2. end the treatment session and try the skill later in the day when the patient may be less agitated.
3. redirect the patient to a less challenging skill.
4. increase the time and number of demonstrations of the skill before the patient tries it again.

CORRECT ANSWER: 3

RATIONALE:

When one is treating a patient with Alzheimer's disease, it is best to keep tasks simple and to minimize frustration. Although moving the patient to a quiet treatment area may help, the task may still be too difficult. The physical therapist assistant should not end a session with a negative or frustrating task. If the task is too difficult for the patient's skill level, the patient will not be successful regardless of the amount of repetition or demonstration given.

TYPE OF REASONING: INDUCTIVE

One must determine the best strategy to assist a patient with Alzheimer's disease who is demonstrating frustration during a task. This requires clinical judgment, which is an inductive reasoning skill. For this situation, it is best to redirect the patient to a less challenging skill. If answered incorrectly, review treatment guidelines for patients with Alzheimer's disease.

B37 | Neuromuscular | Data Collection

When one is assessing the development of an 11-month-old child, a normal expectation is that the child can:

CHOICES:

1. run independently.
2. stand alone for several seconds.
3. walk up stairs with assistance.
4. walk up stairs one step at a time without assistance.

CORRECT ANSWER: 2

RATIONALE:

Standing alone for several seconds should be within the ability of an 11-month-old child. All of the other developmental milestones are reached at a much later stage—run independently: 24 months; walk up stairs with assistance: 18 months; and walk up stairs one step at a time without assistance: 24 months.

TYPE OF REASONING: DEDUCTIVE

This question requires the test taker to recall developmental milestones of infants. This is factual information, which is a deductive reasoning skill. For this case, an 11-month-old child can be expected to stand alone for several seconds. Review developmental milestones of infants, especially motor skills of 11-month-old infants, if answered incorrectly.

B38 | Musculoskeletal | Data Collection

During gait assessment the physical therapist assistant notes that the patient's affected hip laterally (externally) rotates during the swing phase of gait. The muscle that if weak will **MOST** likely result in lateral hip rotation is the:

CHOICES:

1. tensor fascia lata.
2. gluteus medius.
3. rectus femoris.
4. iliopsoas.

CORRECT ANSWER: 4

RATIONALE:

The iliopsoas is the strongest hip flexor and is likely weak in this scenario. The tensor fascia latae only assists with hip flexion and increases hip lateral (external) rotation as it is compensating for a weak iliopsoas muscle. The gluteus medius performs hip abduction; weakness of it does not contribute to this gait pattern. The rectus femoris is also an assist for hip flexion, but does not contribute to the lateral (external) rotation during gait.

TYPE OF REASONING: INFERENTIAL

This question requires one to infer or draw a reasonable conclusion about the likely muscle that is weak with a patient who demonstrates lateral rotation of the hip during the swing phase of gait. This requires inferential reasoning skill. For this situation, the iliopsoas muscle is most likely weak causing the lateral rotation. If answered incorrectly, review gait patterns for patients with weak hip musculature.

B39 | Musculoskeletal | Interventions

When using a prosthesis for the **FIRST** time, the safest gait pattern to teach a patient with a transfemoral amputation is:

CHOICES:

1. 2-point gait.
2. swing-through gait.
3. 4-point gait.
4. step-to gait.

CORRECT ANSWER: 3

RATIONALE:

As always, patient safety is the primary concern. When one is first teaching a patient to walk with a prosthesis, the 4-point gait pattern will allow for the most stable and natural gait pattern. With the 4-point gait, the crutches and extremities will always be in contact with the floor except during swing. The 4-point gait also allows for a natural reciprocal gait for good step-through with the prosthesis and facilitates good weight-bearing through the prosthesis. The patient should not perform a swing-through or a step-to gait, as this does not promote a natural gait pattern and can limit weight-bearing through the prosthesis. A 2-point gait, in which the crutches and lower extremities move simultaneously, may be too difficult at this time; however, eventually this will be the gait pattern of choice and should be included in the long-term goals for the patient.

TYPE OF REASONING: INDUCTIVE

One must determine the safest gait pattern to teach a patient with transfemoral amputation to arrive at a correct conclusion. This requires clinical judgment, which is an inductive reasoning skill. For this case, when using a prosthesis for the first time, the patient should be instructed in the use of a 4-point gait pattern. Review gait training guidelines for patients with lower-extremity amputations if answered incorrectly.

B40 | Musculoskeletal | Clinical Applications

A physical therapist assistant is working at bedside with a patient who underwent a rotator cuff repair of a grade 3 tendon injury 2 days ago. It is inappropriate for the physical therapist assistant to incorporate:

CHOICES:

1. pendulum exercises.
2. submaximal isometric exercise.
3. passive range of motion.
4. cryotherapy techniques.

CORRECT ANSWER: 2

RATIONALE:

A grade 3 tendon repair includes suturing of a tear in the tissues, and resistance 2 days following suturing of a tear would put the tissue at risk for tearing of the sutures. Pendulum exercises, passive range of motion and cryotherapy are all indicated to promote healing, safe tissue movement and decreased inflammation.

TYPE OF REASONING: EVALUATIVE

One must weigh all of the potential approaches presented to determine the approach that is inappropriate for a patient with grade 3 rotator cuff tendon injury. This is an evaluative reasoning skill. For this situation, it is inappropriate to incorporate submaximal isometric exercise because of the risk for tearing of the sutures. If answered incorrectly, review intervention approaches for patients with rotator cuff repairs, especially grade 3 tendon injuries.

B41 | Musculoskeletal | Clinical Applications

A patient has just undergone a total knee arthroplasty secondary to severe degenerative joint disease. In the recovery room, a continuous passive movement (CPM) machine has been applied. One purpose of CPM placement after surgery is to:

CHOICES:

1. decrease range of motion.
2. increase edema.
3. increase risk of a deep vein thrombosis.
4. decrease postoperative pain.

CORRECT ANSWER: 4

RATIONALE:

Decreasing postoperative pain is one of the goals and benefits of the continuous passive motion (CPM) machine. Keeping the lower extremity moving prevents the extremity from "stiffening up," thereby decreasing range of motion. The CPM will actually increase range of motion, and may actually decrease edema and decrease the risk for deep vein thrombosis by keeping the joint moving.

TYPE OF REASONING: DEDUCTIVE

This question requires one to recall the purposes of the CPM machine for patients with a status of post–total knee arthroplasty. This is factual information, which necessitates deductive reasoning skill. For this scenario, the purpose of CPM placement after surgery is to decrease postoperative pain. Review indications for CPM machines after joint arthroplasty if answered incorrectly.

B42 I **Neuromuscular** I **Clinical Applications**

The physical therapy plan of care for a patient with spastic diplegia includes gait training and management of flexor hyper-tonicity. This patient's gait pattern will **MOST** likely demonstrate:

CHOICES:

1. excessive hip and knee flexion with decreased stride length.
2. increased double limb support with decreased stride width.
3. pillarlike rigidity on weight bearing with ankle varus.
4. excessive hip flexion with increased stride width.

CORRECT ANSWER: 1

RATIONALE:

The typical position of both lower extremities for a patient with spastic diplegia and flexor hypertonicity is excessive hip and knee flexion, with adduction and medial (internal) rotation of the hips. Having the lower extremities both adducted and medially (internally) rotated will decrease the stride length, not increase stride length. The patient will exhibit pillarlike rigidity with increased extensor tone.

TYPE OF REASONING: INFERENTIAL

One must infer or draw a reasonable conclusion about the likely features of a gait pattern for a patient with spastic diplegia. This requires one to determine what may be true, which is an inferential reasoning skill. For this case, one should expect the patient to most likely demonstrate excessive hip and knee flexion with decreased stride length. Review gait patterns for patients with spastic diplegia if answered incorrectly.

B43 I **Devices, Admin, etc.** I **Equipment, Modalities**

A patient with post-polio syndrome exhibits foot slap at heel strike (initial contact). An ankle–foot orthosis with this patient should include a (an):

CHOICES:

1. medial T strap.
2. lateral T strap.
3. posterior stop.
4. anterior stop.

CORRECT ANSWER: 3

RATIONALE:

Foot slap is a result of weak dorsiflexors. At initial contact, the heel hits the floor and the dorsiflexors eccentrically lower the foot to the floor. When these muscles are weak, foot slap occurs. A posterior stop limits the amount of plantar flexion. An anterior stop should be used if someone were exhibiting increased dorsiflexion. Medial and lateral T straps are used to decrease excessive abduction or adduction of the foot or to decrease excessive supination.

TYPE OF REASONING: INDUCTIVE

One must utilize clinical judgment to determine the appropriate ankle–foot orthosis for a patient with post-polio syndrome and a foot slap. This is an inductive reasoning skill. For this situation, the ankle–foot orthosis should include a posterior stop to address the foot slap. Review orthoses for patients with weak dorsiflexors if answered incorrectly.

B44 | Musculoskeletal | Data Collection

A patient begins to fall forward during static balance testing with a moderate perturbation force displacing the patient anteriorly. What muscle group should the physical therapist assistant expect to contract strongly to re-establish the trunk position over the lower extremities?

CHOICES:

1. hip extensors.
2. hip flexors.
3. trunk extensors.
4. dorsiflexors.

CORRECT ANSWER: 1

RATIONALE:

To preserve the center of gravity the physical therapist assistant should expect to see contraction of the plantar flexors first (with a small disturbance) followed by the hip extensors with a greater disturbance. Activation of the hip extensors will re-establish the trunk position. In standing with the feet fixed, the hip extensors work by reverse action. As the trunk falls forward, the gluteus maximus will contract and return the trunk to upright. The trunk extensors may fire with a large disturbance or in the case of impaired balance responses. One should not expect the dorsiflexors to engage unless a posterior disturbance was applied.

TYPE OF REASONING: INFERENTIAL

One must determine what may be true for a patient with balance deficits whose balance is displaced forward during balance testing to arrive at a correct conclusion. This requires inferential reasoning skill. For this scenario, the muscle group that is likely to contract strongly to re-establish the trunk position is the hip extensors. If answered incorrectly, review standing balance guidelines and the role of muscles in maintaining balance during balance disturbances.

B45 | Musculoskeletal | Clinical Applications

When teaching a group of workers with **NO** history of back injury to lift heavy objects off the floor, the physical therapist assistant should instruct them to:

CHOICES:

1. keep the lumbar spine flexed during the lift.
2. stoop down to the object before trying to lift it.
3. increase the lordotic posture to increase stability when lifting.
4. keep objects as far away from the center of gravity as possible.

CORRECT ANSWER: 2

RATIONALE:

When instructing workers to lift heavy objects you must emphasize proper body mechanics. One of the main principles of body mechanics is to stoop down (squat) to the object before lifting it. This allows the person the ability to then "lift with the legs." The spine should be held in a "neutral position," neither flexed nor in increased lordosis. Increasing the base of support will increase stability when lifting. One should also instruct the workers to keep objects close to the body.

TYPE OF REASONING: DEDUCTIVE

One must recall body mechanics guidelines to arrive at a correct conclusion for this question. This is factual information, which is a deductive reasoning skill. For this scenario, the assistant should instruct the workers to stoop down to the object before trying to lift it. If answered incorrectly, review proper body mechanics for lifting heavy objects from the floor.

B46 | Integumentary | Clinical Applications

A physical therapist assistant has been asked to treat a patient who is 6 months post-injury for deep partial-thickness burns to the posterior distal lower extremity. The patient now has a 20° plantar flexion contracture. Before stretching the ankle joint, the massage technique **MOST** appropriate to help release soft tissue adhesions is:

CHOICES:
1. kneading.
2. effleurage.
3. percussion.
4. friction.

CORRECT ANSWER: 4

RATIONALE:
The patient who has a deep partial-thickness burn may develop hypertrophic scarring. The scars are thick and "stiff." Scarring and shortening of the tissue caused the contracture. To increase range of motion and stretch the area, the scar needs to become more supple. Friction massage is used to "break up" scar tissue, and this should be used prior to stretching the area. Kneading and effleurage are massage techniques used more for relaxation and to treat muscle tightness. Percussion is used as a chest physical therapy technique.

TYPE OF REASONING: INDUCTIVE
This question requires the test taker to use knowledge of massage techniques to arrive at a correct conclusion. This necessitates clinical judgment, which is an inductive reasoning skill. For this case, the most appropriate massage technique for a patient with a plantar flexion contracture after deep partial-thickness burns is friction massage. Review massage techniques for hypertrophic scarring after burns if answered incorrectly.

B47 | Neuromuscular | Clinical Applications

To encourage functional reintegration of the affected side, a patient with hemiplegia should be encouraged to roll and sit up over the edge of the bed from a supine position by:

CHOICES:
1. rotating the upper trunk toward the unaffected side to encourage use of the hemiplegic side when pushing to sitting.
2. first grabbing the bed rail with the unaffected upper extremity to help roll to the hemiplegic side.
3. first flexing and rotating the upper trunk diagonally toward the hemiplegic side to achieve a side-lying on-elbow posture.
4. first flexing the upper trunk by extending both shoulders to achieve a bilateral on-elbows position before rolling onto the unaffected side.

CORRECT ANSWER: 3

RATIONALE:
Having the patient roll onto the affected side facilitates use of his or her affected side by using the upper extremity to push up. This will best help to functionally reintegrate the affected side. A patient with hemiplegia will have great difficulty in rolling toward the unaffected side, because the affected side must initiate the movement.

TYPE OF REASONING: INDUCTIVE
One must utilize clinical judgment to determine the best approach for encouraging bed mobility for a patient with hemiplegia. This is an inductive reasoning skill. For this situation, the patient should be encouraged to roll and sit up over the edge of the bed from a supine position by flexing and rotating the upper trunk diagonally toward the hemiplegic side to achieve a side-lying on-elbow posture. Review bed mobility guidelines for patients with hemiplegia if answered incorrectly.

B48 | Devices, Admin, etc. | Safety Roles, Teaching, EBP

A physical therapist assistant is using ultrasound to assist in the healing and stretching of an injury to the musculotendinous junction that is status post–15 days. The **MOST** effective application should include:

CHOICES:

1. stretching of the tissues followed by continuous ultrasound then resting in a support device for protection.
2. ultrasound at a pulsed setting followed immediately by gentle stretching, then active assistive use of the muscle in the newly acquired range.
3. active exercise of the muscle followed by gentle static stretch to end range with pulsed ultrasound.
4. continuous ultrasound to the tissues followed by active exercise within available range of motion.

CORRECT ANSWER: 2

RATIONALE:

Ultrasound helps promote collagen synthesis, minimize adhesions, and increase protein synthesis to assist with the healing response of tissue. It is particularly effective if applied at the nonthermal setting during the acute phase and thermal ranges during the subacute phases of tissue healing. This injury would be considered still in the acute stage and would best respond to nonthermal (pulsed or low-intensity) ultrasound. Tissue extensibility is the greatest following ultrasound and it has been demonstrated that tissues will best remain at the lengthened state if they are used in that newly gained range of motion. The other choices include splinting the area, stretch to end range (not beyond), and exercise within available range; none of these will address increasing range of motion in a way that is effective.

TYPE OF REASONING: INDUCTIVE

This question requires the test taker to determine the most effective application of ultrasound for a patient with an injury to the musculotendinous junction. This requires knowledge of ultrasound guidelines and clinical judgment, which is an inductive reasoning skill. For this situation, the most effective application of ultrasound should include a pulsed setting followed immediately by gentle stretching and active assistive use of the muscle in the newly acquired range. Review ultrasound guidelines for patients with musculotendinous junction injury if answered incorrectly.

B49 | Musculoskeletal | Data Collection

During observation of the patient's gait in the sagittal view a physical therapist assistant observes the patient fully extend the knee and hip at midstance and hyperextend the trunk in the stance phase. Weakness of which muscle results in knee, hip and trunk extension during stance phase?

CHOICES:

1. rectus femoris.
2. gluteus medius.
3. gluteus maximus.
4. gastrocnemius.

CORRECT ANSWER: 3

RATIONALE:

This gait deviation is termed the gluteus maximus or hip extensor gait deviation. To compensate for a weak gluteus maximus the patient fully extends the knee and hip while extending the trunk to "lock" the kinetic chain and assist with maintaining hip extension during stance.

TYPE OF REASONING: ANALYTICAL

One must assess the patient's gait deviation features to determine the muscle that is likely weak and contributing to the deviation. This requires analytical reasoning skill. For this case, the knee, hip and trunk extension during the stance phase indicates weakness of the gluteus maximus. Review common gait deviations and their cause if answered incorrectly.

B50 | Neuromuscular | Data Collection

A patient with a supracondylar fracture of the humerus also has radial nerve involvement. A physical therapist assistant should expect this patient to demonstrate:

CHOICES:

1. inability to flex the fingers.
2. impaired sensation to the volar surface of the hand.
3. inability to flex the metacarpophalangeal joints.
4. deviation of the wrist to the ulnar side.

CORRECT ANSWER: 4

RATIONALE:

The radial nerve innervates the extensor carpi radialis as well as the abductor pollicis, both of which are responsible for radial deviation. Because of the radial nerve damage, the muscles that are responsible for radial deviation are inactive; the wrist will exhibit ulnar deviation. Inability to flex the fingers is a result of damage to the ulnar and median nerves, as is impaired sensation to the volar aspect. Inability to flex the metacarpophalangeal joints is the result of damage to the ulnar nerve.

TYPE OF REASONING: INFERENTIAL

This question provides a diagnosis and the test taker must determine the likely symptoms, which is an inferential reasoning skill. For this patient with a supracondylar fracture and radial nerve involvement, one should expect to see deviation of the wrist to the ulnar side. If answered incorrectly, review signs and symptoms of radial nerve damage.

B51 | Musculoskeletal | Interventions

The application of large- and small-amplitude oscillation joint mobilization techniques in combination with myofascial techniques is **MOST** appropriate for which condition?

CHOICES:

1. locked facet joints of the lumbar vertebrae.
2. ankylosing spondylitis.
3. osteoporosis of the lumbar spine.
4. scoliosis affecting mobility of the spine.

CORRECT ANSWER: 1

RATIONALE:

Joint mobilization and myofascial techniques are effective and safe to use on locked facet joints of the spine. Ankylosing spondylitis is an inflammatory condition in which the ligaments and soft tissues, discs and potentially the bone itself can be weakened; this makes it inappropriate for large- and small-oscillation joint mobilization. Osteoporosis is a contraindication for the higher grades of mobilization. Scoliosis is the lateral curvature of the spine and is not treated with joint mobilization techniques.

TYPE OF REASONING: INDUCTIVE

One must utilize clinical judgment to determine the most appropriate condition for utilizing large- and small-amplitude oscillation joint mobilization techniques and myofascial techniques. This requires inductive reasoning skill. For this situation, the condition appropriate for these treatment techniques is locked facet joints of the lumbar vertebra. Review indications for joint mobilization techniques, as well as myofascial techniques, if answered incorrectly.

B52 | Other Systems | Clinical Applications

A physical therapist assistant is teaching a water exercise class for participants who are in a phase III cardiac rehabilitation program. One of the participants has an additional diagnosis of spinal stenosis. The assistant should instruct this patient to perform the back stroke during the class in place of:

CHOICES:

1. the crawl.
2. float-assisted jogging.
3. lower-extremity resistance exercises with floats.
4. upper-extremity resisted rows.

CORRECT ANSWER: 1

RATIONALE:

Activities such as the crawl swim stroke places the spine in extension, and positioning patients with spinal stenosis in spinal extension can increase symptoms. All other activities described do not place the patient into a position that maintains an extended spine and will not likely pose a problem for this patient.

TYPE OF REASONING: INDUCTIVE

For this question, the test taker must determine the appropriate water exercise for a patient with spinal stenosis. This requires knowledge of the diagnosis and precautions, which is an inductive reasoning skill. For this case, the assistant should instruct the patient to perform the back stroke in place of the crawl swim to avoid an extended spine during activities. If answered incorrectly, review water-based exercises for patients with spinal stenosis.

B53 | Musculoskeletal | Clinical Applications

A patient presents with neck pain and spasm of the left sternocleidomastoid muscle. To apply myofascial techniques and gentle stretch, what motions should the physical therapist assistant perform with the cervical spine?

CHOICES:

1. lateral flexion to the right.
2. lateral flexion to the right and rotation to the left.
3. lateral flexion and rotation to the right.
4. lateral flexion to the left and rotation to the right.

CORRECT ANSWER: 2

RATIONALE:

The left sternocleidomastoid laterally flexes the neck to the left and rotates the neck to the right. To increase the range of motion, the physical therapist assistant must stretch the muscle in the opposite direction, in this case, lateral flexion to the right and rotation to the left.

TYPE OF REASONING: INDUCTIVE

One must utilize clinical judgment to determine the appropriate cervical motions for a patient with sternocleidomastoid spasm and neck pain. This is an inductive reasoning skill. For this scenario, the assistant should perform lateral neck flexion to the right and rotation to the left to stretch the muscle. If answered incorrectly, review myofascial techniques, especially for the cervical region.

B54 | Musculoskeletal | Clinical Applications

The trigger point for the levator scapula is found:

CHOICES:

1. immediately medial to the superior portion of the acromion process.
2. immediately medial to the inferior angle of the vertebral border of the scapula.
3. just superior to the superior angle of the vertebral border of the scapula.
4. just inferior to the mastoid process.

CORRECT ANSWER: 3

RATIONALE:

The trigger points for the levator scapula are just superior to its attachment on the superior angle of the scapula and immediately inferior to its attachment on the occiput. The trapezius has trigger points just medial to the acromion process on the superior portion, as well as at the midway point of the vertebral border of the scapula. The sternocleidomastoid muscle has a trigger point just inferior to the mastoid process.

TYPE OF REASONING: DEDUCTIVE

This question requires the test taker to recall factual information regarding a trigger point for the levator scapula muscle. This is a deductive reasoning skill, as guidelines are utilized to reach a reasonable conclusion. For this case, the trigger point is located just superior to the superior angle of the vertebral border of the scapula. If answered incorrectly, review trigger points for the cervical muscles.

B55 | Devices, Admin, etc. | Equipment, Modalities

To electrically stimulate a denervated anterior tibialis muscle, a physical therapist assistant should use:

CHOICES:

1. interrupted alternating current (biphasic current).
2. continuous direct current (monophasic current).
3. transcutaneous electrical neural stimulation (monophasic or biphasic current).
4. interrupted direct current (monophasic current).

CORRECT ANSWER: 4

RATIONALE:

Interrupted direct current (monophasic current) is used to stimulate denervated muscles. Studies on animals and clinical studies have indicated that denervated muscle can be stimulated by interrupted monophasic current producing a vermicular contraction. One electrode is always positive and one is always negative during the time of stimulation, producing residual charges in the tissues under the respective electrodes, which will facilitate a muscle contraction.

TYPE OF REASONING: DEDUCTIVE

One must recall the guidelines for use of electrical stimulation to stimulate denervated muscles. This is factual information, which necessitates deductive reasoning skill. For this situation, to stimulate a denervated anterior tibialis muscle, the assistant should use interrupted direct current (monophasic current). If answered incorrectly, review electrical stimulation guidelines for denervated muscles.

B56 | Musculoskeletal | Clinical Applications

A patient who has ankylosis of both subtalar joints will have the **MOST** difficulty walking:

CHOICES:

1. on uneven terrain.
2. up ramps.
3. rapidly.
4. down stairs.

CORRECT ANSWER: 1

RATIONALE:

When the subtalar joints are ankylosed, they have limited motion and may, in fact, be fused. The subtalar joint allows for medial and lateral movements that enable the foot to adjust to uneven surfaces. Therefore, the patient who has ankylosis of both subtalar joints will have difficulty walking on uneven terrain. Ascending and descending stairs require dorsiflexion and plantar flexion motions that occur at the talocrural joint.

TYPE OF REASONING: INFERENTIAL

One must infer or draw a reasonable conclusion about the likely difficulty a patient with ankylosis of both subtalar joints will have while walking. This requires one to determine what may be true, which is an inferential reasoning skill. For this case, the patient will have the most difficulty walking on uneven terrain. Review ankylosis of the subtalar joints if answered incorrectly, especially challenges in walking.

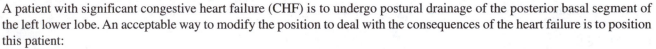

B57 | Cardiovascular/Pulmonary | Interventions

A patient with significant congestive heart failure (CHF) is to undergo postural drainage of the posterior basal segment of the left lower lobe. An acceptable way to modify the position to deal with the consequences of the heart failure is to position this patient:

CHOICES:

1. side-lying on the right with the bed flat.
2. side-lying on the right with the foot of the bed elevated 18 inches.
3. prone with the foot of the bed elevated 18 inches.
4. prone with the bed flat.

CORRECT ANSWER: 4

RATIONALE:

A patient with CHF will not tolerate the Trendelenburg position, (foot of the bed elevated 18 inches); this position will increase dyspnea (shortness of breath). A possible modification of the position for treating the posterior basal segment of the lung will involve placing the patient prone with the bed flat. The prone position will allow gravity to assist in draining the posterior segments of the lung. Although the ideal method to drain the basal segment of the lung is with the foot of the bed elevated, it is contraindicated for a patient with CHF.

TYPE OF REASONING: INDUCTIVE

One must determine the best modified position for postural drainage for a patient with congestive heart failure. This requires clinical judgment and knowledge of the diagnosis to arrive at a correct conclusion, which is an inductive reasoning skill. For this situation, the position should be modified to prone with the bed flat. If answered incorrectly, review postural drainage techniques and positioning for patients with CHF.

B58 | Neuromuscular | Interventions

A patient has a lesion at T10 resulting in paraplegia. The **FIRST** position in the mat activity sequence that allows weight-bearing through the hips and is useful for facilitating initial control of the lower trunk and hips is:

CHOICES:
1. supine on elbows.
2. quadruped.
3. long sitting without using the hands or upper extremities for support.
4. prone on elbows.

CORRECT ANSWER: 2

RATIONALE:
Having the patient in the quadruped position on the mat allows for weight-bearing through the femur into the hip joint. In this position, the lower trunk musculature must work to keep the hips aligned and to prevent lateral sway and/or anterior/posterior sway. The remaining positions do not allow weight-bearing through the hips, nor do they facilitate use of the lower trunk musculature. Long sitting uses more upper-trunk musculature than lower-trunk musculature.

TYPE OF REASONING: ANALYTICAL
One must analyze the activities presented to determine the activity that facilitates weight-bearing to the hips and initial control of the lower trunk and hips. This requires analytical reasoning skill. For this situation, the first position in the mat activity sequence for this patient should be quadruped. Review mat activity for patients with thoracic spinal cord injury, especially lower thoracic injuries, if answered incorrectly.

B59 | Devices, Admin, etc. | Safety Roles, Teaching, EBP

During gait training at home, a patient falls and strikes his head. The physical therapist assistant determines that the patient is unconscious and no longer breathing. The assistant is the only person present. The **FIRST** thing the assistant should do is:

CHOICES:
1. establish an open airway.
2. immediately begin rescue breathing.
3. call the emergency response system before administering care.
4. begin one-person cardiopulmonary resuscitation (CPR) for 1 minute.

CORRECT ANSWER: 3

RATIONALE:
When the physical therapist assistant is alone with a patient and help is not readily available, the assistant should call the emergency response system first to enter the emergency medical services (EMS) system. It is important to take the few seconds to call the emergency response system to send help on the way. This is the first step in participation in the EMS system.

TYPE OF REASONING: EVALUATIVE
This question requires the test taker to weigh the courses of action and determine the action that best addresses the patient's immediate concerns. This is an evaluative reasoning skill. For this scenario, the first thing the assistant should do is call the emergency response system before administering care. If answered incorrectly, review emergency first aid and CPR guidelines.

B60 | Musculoskeletal | Clinical Applications

A patient who has just undergone repair for a chronic anterior shoulder dislocation is participating in an exercise program. Early rehabilitation should avoid glenohumeral:

CHOICES:

1. lateral (external) rotation.
2. abduction.
3. medial (internal) rotation.
4. flexion.

CORRECT ANSWER: 1

RATIONALE:

Lateral (external) rotation will move the humeral head forward and place the repair in a position of stress. Moving the head of the humerus forward into an anterior position should be avoided as this could cause an anterior dislocation. Medial (internal) rotation of the humerus is allowed, because this motion does not cause the head of the humerus to move anteriorly. The remaining movements will cause the humeral head to move anteriorly; however, early in rehabilitation, lateral rotation must be avoided.

TYPE OF REASONING: INDUCTIVE

One must utilize clinical judgment and knowledge of chronic anterior shoulder dislocation to arrive at a correct conclusion. This necessitates inductive reasoning skill. For this situation, early rehabilitation should avoid glenohumeral lateral rotation to avoid anterior dislocation. If answered incorrectly, review chronic anterior shoulder dislocation guidelines and intervention approaches.

B61 | Musculoskeletal | Clinical Applications

The supervising physical therapist has asked the physical therapist assistant to continue providing range-of-motion exercises to a patient with traumatic brain injury (TBI). The patient has hip flexor tightness and decreased knee extension bilaterally. The optimal position in which to place the patient to achieve maximal range of motion is:

CHOICES:

1. sitting.
2. prone.
3. supine.
4. side-lying.

CORRECT ANSWER: 4

RATIONALE:

If the patient is in side-lying, the physical therapist assistant is able to stretch the hips and knees into extension, as side-lying is a supportive position and a relaxed position for a patient who has suffered a TBI. If the patient is placed in prone, the assistant will be able to stretch the patient; however, the patient may exhibit an increase in flexion and flexor tone if the tonic labyrinthine reflex is present. The supine or sitting positions will make it difficult to stretch the patient into extension.

TYPE OF REASONING: INDUCTIVE

This question requires the test taker to use knowledge of muscle-stretching guidelines and TBI to reach a correct conclusion. This requires clinical judgment, which is an inductive reasoning skill. For this case, the optimal position to place the patient in to achieve maximal range of motion is side-lying. If answered incorrectly, review muscle-stretching guidelines for the lower extremity in patients with TBI.

B62 | Other Systems | Clinical Applications

While reviewing the patient's medical record prior to gait training, the physical therapist assistant notes that the patient is experiencing increased shortness of breath and the physician has just written an order for a ventilation perfusion scan. The assistant should:

CHOICES:

1. withhold treatment and contact the supervising therapist.
2. proceed with the treatments as usual because there is no definitive change in the patient's status.
3. hold the breathing exercises and perform gait training only.
4. proceed with the treatments while monitoring the patient's respiration rate and vital signs very carefully.

CORRECT ANSWER: 1

RATIONALE:

The first concern is the patient's safety. A ventilation perfusion scan is performed to identify the presence of a pulmonary embolus (PE). If there is a possibility of a PE, physical therapy is contraindicated. A PE is a serious condition, which, if left untreated, could be life-threatening. If there is any question of a PE, the safest thing to do is to delay the treatment (remember, safety first). The physical therapist assistant should then contact the supervising physical therapist for him/her to investigate and assess whether the patient is appropriate for treatment.

TYPE OF REASONING: EVALUATIVE

One must weigh the value of the approaches provided to determine the approach that is most appropriate for the patient and the potential diagnosis of PE. For this situation, having knowledge of the reasons for a physician ordering a ventilation perfusion scan, the assistant should withhold treatment and contact the supervising therapist. If answered incorrectly, review ventilation perfusion scan information.

B63 | Integumentary | Clinical Applications

A patient who is receiving home physical therapy reports experiencing increased aching in the left lower extremity, which is only alleviated when the lower extremity is elevated. The physical therapist assistant inspects the feet and lower extremities and notes some mild edema, a darker pigmentation to the tissues and a dermatitis-type condition to the tissues on the medial distal lower extremity. The assistant should report to the physical therapist that the patient demonstrates symptoms that seem consistent with:

CHOICES:

1. diabetic ulcers.
2. venous ulcers.
3. arterial ulcers.
4. decubitus ulcers.

CORRECT ANSWER: 2

RATIONALE:

In addition to the description of a venous ulcer that is included, one should note that the pedal arterial pulses are present. Arterial ulcers will more likely present as very painful (pain is relieved with the dependent position), and with trophic changes, and an ischemic and pale appearance. In addition, the ulcers will appear anywhere on the leg or dorsum of the foot or toes and over the bony prominence of the anterior tibia. Diabetic ulcers are typically not painful; paresthesia may be present, and they will have a more round or "punched-out" appearance. One would expect decubitus ulcers to appear over bony landmarks in weight-bearing or pressure areas.

TYPE OF REASONING: ANALYTICAL

This question provides symptoms and the test taker must determine the possible diagnosis of the patient. This requires one to analyze the symptoms presented to draw a conclusion, which is an analytical reasoning skill. For this case, the symptoms seem consistent with venous ulcers. Review signs and symptoms of venous ulcers if answered incorrectly.

B64 | Musculoskeletal | Data Collection

If a physical therapist assistant measures the patient's ankle range of motion to be 25° to −7°, it should be interpreted that the patient has:

CHOICES:

1. −7° of plantar flexion.
2. 25° of dorsiflexion and limited plantar flexion.
3. 25° of plantar flexion and 7° of dorsiflexion.
4. −7° of ankle dorsiflexion.

CORRECT ANSWER: 4

RATIONALE:

Normal range of motion of the ankle is 50° to 0° to 20° indicating 50° of plantar flexion, ability to return to neutral ankle position, and obtaining 20° of dorsiflexion. This patient's range of motion for ankle dorsiflexion would read −7° indicating the inability to achieve the neutral ankle position of zero.

TYPE OF REASONING: ANALYTICAL

One must analyze the range-of-motion numbers presented for the ankle and determine their significance to arrive at a correct conclusion. This requires analytical reasoning skill, as pieces of information are analyzed to determine significance. For this situation, the range-of-motion numbers indicate 7° of ankle dorsiflexion. If answered incorrectly, review range-of-motion measurement guidelines for the ankle.

B65 | Other Systems | Clinical Applications

An adult runner collapses after being brought to the first aid station. Ambient temperature is 92°F (33°C) and body temperature is measured at 101°F (38°C). The runner presents with a rapid pulse, rapid respirations and skin that is warm and dry to touch. When questioned by the assistant helping to monitor the runners, the runner is confused. The assistant reports to a supervising sports physical therapist specialist that the findings seem consistent with:

CHOICES:

1. hypovolemic shock.
2. hypervolemic shock.
3. anaphylactic shock.
4. septic shock.

CORRECT ANSWER: 1

RATIONALE:

This runner is demonstrating signs and symptoms of dehydration (inadequate fluid intake) and hypovolemic shock. Pulse and respirations are increased; blood pressure may decline. Restlessness, anxiety and confusion may all be present as well.

TYPE OF REASONING: ANALYTICAL

This question provides a group of symptoms and the test taker must determine a possible cause. This requires analysis of pieces of information to draw a correct conclusion, which is an analytical reasoning skill. For this scenario, the findings seem consistent with hypovolemic shock. If answered incorrectly, review symptoms of hypovolemic shock.

B66 | Cardiovascular/Pulmonary | Data Collection

A home health physical therapist assistant is treating an older adult patient. On this day the patient is confused and presents with shortness of breath and generalized weakness. Given the patient's history of hypertension and hyperlipidemia, the physical therapist assistant suspects the patient is:

CHOICES:

1. demonstrating mental changes indicative of early Alzheimer's disease.
2. potentially experiencing unstable angina.
3. presenting with early signs of myocardial infarction.
4. forgetting to take prescribed hypertension medication.

CORRECT ANSWER: 3

RATIONALE:

An elderly patient with a cardiac history may present with initial symptoms of mental confusion when experiencing early myocardial infarction, the result of oxygen deprivation to the brain. The shortness of breath and generalized weakness may also be caused by generalized circulatory insufficiencies coexisting with the developing myocardial infarction.

TYPE OF REASONING: ANALYTICAL

This question requires the test taker to determine a cause for the patient's symptoms. Questions that require one to determine a diagnosis based on a group of symptoms often require analytical reasoning skill. For this situation, the assistant could conclude that the patient's symptoms indicate early signs of myocardial infarction. If answered incorrectly, review signs and symptoms of myocardial infarction, especially in older adults.

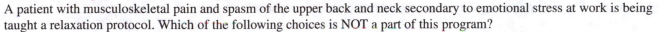

B67 | Other Systems | Clinical Applications

A patient with musculoskeletal pain and spasm of the upper back and neck secondary to emotional stress at work is being taught a relaxation protocol. Which of the following choices is NOT a part of this program?

CHOICES:

1. active strengthening exercises to the affected musculature.
2. progressive tensing, holding and releasing of the affected muscle groups.
3. hot packs to the neck and back for 20 minutes.
4. controlled, diaphragmatic breathing.

CORRECT ANSWER: 1

RATIONALE:

Active strengthening exercises are not considered a relaxation technique. Although hot packs are considered a modality, heat is typically used in conjunction with relaxation techniques.

TYPE OF REASONING: DEDUCTIVE

One must recall the relaxation protocol for patients with pain and spasm to arrive at a correct conclusion. This requires the recall of factual information, which is a deductive reasoning skill. For this case, the only approach that is not part of a relaxation protocol is active strengthening exercises to the affected musculature. If answered incorrectly, review relaxation guidelines for patients with musculoskeletal pain and spasm.

B68 | Other Systems | Interventions

As a result of a traumatic brain injury a patient is demonstrating significant static standing balance deficits. Which of the following is the **BEST** intervention strategy for this patient?

CHOICES:

1. use of a standing equilibrium board.
2. rhythmic stabilization in standing.
3. weight-shifting to pick up objects from the floor.
4. performing reaching tasks outside the base of support.

CORRECT ANSWER: 2

RATIONALE:

Rhythmic stabilization applied in the standing position will help to increase the patient's static standing balance. The remaining activities listed address the patient's dynamic standing balance. In addition, they would be too advanced for a patient unable to maintain static balance.

TYPE OF REASONING: INDUCTIVE

This question requires one to determine the best intervention strategy for a patient with static standing balance deficits. This requires knowledge of the intervention approaches to arrive at a correct conclusion, which is an inductive reasoning skill. For this situation, the best intervention strategy is rhythmic stabilization in standing. Review static standing balance approaches for patients with traumatic brain injury, especially static standing activities, if answered incorrectly.

B69 | Devices, Admin, etc. | Equipment, Modalities

An athlete with no other medical conditions incurred blunt trauma to the right thigh. An ice pack was applied for 40 minutes. The physical therapist assistant should expect the skin to initially exhibit:

CHOICES:

1. erythema followed by blanching at about 30 minutes.
2. blanching followed by decreased blood pressure and increased pulse rate.
3. reflex vasodilation followed by decreased blood pressure and increased pulse rate.
4. blanching followed by erythema at about 10 minutes.

CORRECT ANSWER: 4

RATIONALE:

Blanching, caused by vasoconstriction of the superficial blood vessels, is the initial response to cold. With extended exposure to cold, the body's response is to move relatively warmer blood to the affected area; this is accomplished by vasodilation. Changes in blood pressure or heart rate are not expected responses with application of a local cold application to a healthy individual. If blanching develops, the tissues are demonstrating intolerance for cold and may be frostbitten. Ten to 15 minutes is the recommended treatment time for the application of cold; reapplication an hour or so later is appropriate.

TYPE OF REASONING: INFERENTIAL

One must infer the likely initial response of the skin to blunt trauma and cryotherapy to arrive at a correct conclusion. This requires inferential reasoning skill. For this scenario, the assistant should expect the skin to initially exhibit blanching followed by erythema at about 10 minutes. If answered incorrectly, review skin responses to cryotherapy after injury.

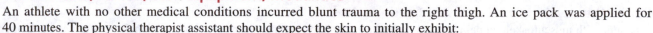

B70 | Devices, Admin, etc. | Safety Roles, Teaching, EBP

When a physical therapist assistant is writing a home program to be administered by family members for a child with cerebral palsy, the primary consideration should be the:

CHOICES:

1. educational level of the family members.
2. gender of the child.
3. religion or beliefs of the family.
4. nationality of the family.

CORRECT ANSWER: 1

RATIONALE:

Educational level is the most important factor to consider when one is administering any program that family members are going to follow. The physical therapist assistant should make sure not to develop a program written higher than the family members' level of understanding. The gender of the child, the religious beliefs of the family or their nationality are not primary considerations of the home program.

TYPE OF REASONING: INDUCTIVE

One must determine the primary consideration when providing a home program for family members. This requires one to determine the outcomes of each of the choices presented to assess the primary benefit of these choices. This is an inductive reasoning skill. For this situation, primary consideration should be the educational level of the family members to ensure understanding of the program and follow-through. If answered incorrectly, review development of home programs for family members.

B71 | Integumentary | Interventions

A physical therapist assistant is performing gait training with a patient who has a venous insufficiency ulcer on the medial side of the left ankle. After gait training the assistant should specifically ensure that:

CHOICES:

1. the lower extremity is elevated and a support garment or elastic bandage is in place.
2. the dressing is changed and an antiseptic ointment is applied to the wound.
3. the patient returns to bed and that the head of the bed is moderately elevated to improve circulation to the lower extremities.
4. there are no signs of deep venous thrombosis.

CORRECT ANSWER: 1

RATIONALE:

A patient with a venous insufficiency ulcer will present with edema, likely minimal pain, and skin changes including hemosiderin staining. In this case the patient's lower extremity should not be left in a dependent position, as this will contribute to the development of further edema. The best treatment is to elevate the lower extremity and to apply a support garment or elastic bandage to the area. Dressing changes are not within the scope of gait training. The patient should be assessed for signs of any deep venous thrombosis prior to, not following, gait training.

TYPE OF REASONING: INDUCTIVE

This question requires one to have knowledge of venous insufficiency ulcers to arrive at a correct conclusion. This requires inductive reasoning skill. For this situation, after gait training, the assistant should ensure that the affected lower extremity is elevated and a support garment or elastic bandage is in place. If answered incorrectly, review treatment guidelines for patients with venous insufficiency ulcers.

B72 | Devices, Admin, etc. | Equipment, Modalities

A patient is receiving iontophoresis using hydrocortisone for chronic overuse tendonitis. The hydrocortisone is used as an:

CHOICES:
1. analgesic.
2. antispasmodic.
3. antiinflammatory agent.
4. antifungal agent.

CORRECT ANSWER: 3

RATIONALE:

Hydrocortisone is used as an antiinflammatory agent. Dexamethasone is another common antiinflammatory medication used with iontophoresis. Lidocaine or xylocaine should be used to decrease pain. Calcium or magnesium should be used to decrease muscle spasm, and copper may be used to treat fungal infections.

TYPE OF REASONING: DEDUCTIVE

One must recall the benefits for using hydrocortisone in iontophoresis. This is factual information and recall of guidelines, which is a deductive reasoning skill. For this scenario, the hydrocortisone is used as an antiinflammatory agent. If answered incorrectly, review iontophoresis guidelines, including indications for the use of hydrocortisone.

B73 | Other Systems | Clinical Applications

The physical therapist assistant is instructed to provide gait training for an older adult patient who has a grade 2 left ankle sprain and fair balance. The patient is to maintain partial weight-bearing during gait. The **MOST** appropriate gait training method in this case should include:

CHOICES:
1. wheeled walker using a reciprocal gait.
2. standard walker, advancing the left lower extremity, then the right.
3. axillary crutches using a 3-point partial-weight-bearing gait.
4. bilateral small-base quad canes using a 3-point gait pattern.

CORRECT ANSWER: 2

RATIONALE:

The standard walker with the involved lower extremity advancing followed by the unaffected lower extremity will allow for partial weight-bearing as indicated. Given that the patient has identified balance difficulty, axillary crutches or quad canes are less safe than the walker. A reciprocal gait pattern with a wheeled walker will not allow for partial weight-bearing.

TYPE OF REASONING: INDUCTIVE

One must determine the most appropriate gait training method for an older adult with grade 2 ankle sprain and fair balance to arrive at a correct conclusion. This requires clinical judgment, which is an inductive reasoning skill. For this case, gait training should include use of a standard walker, advancing the left lower extremity, then the right. Review gait training guidelines for patients with ankle sprain and balance deficits if answered incorrectly.

B74 I Neuromuscular I Interventions

When one is working with a group of patients who have multiple sclerosis, which of the following is the **MOST IMPORTANT** course of action?

CHOICES:
1. use a therapeutic pool.
2. avoid resistance exercises.
3. implement exercise sets with specific repetitions for each.
4. schedule morning treatment sessions.

CORRECT ANSWER: 4

RATIONALE:
Patients who have multiple sclerosis (MS) can fatigue easily and will likely respond best to treatment scheduled in the morning to avoid the afternoon fatigue. A therapeutic pool will likely be kept at a temperature that is too high for a patient with MS and can contribute to fatigue. Group exercise sessions should allow for a variety of abilities, strength and endurance; therefore, a variety of resistance strengths and exercise repetitions would be appropriate and need not be avoided.

TYPE OF REASONING: EVALUATIVE
This question requires the test taker to evaluate the courses of action and determine the one that is most beneficial for a group of patients with MS. This requires evaluative reasoning skill. For this scenario, it is most important to schedule morning treatment sessions to avoid afternoon fatigue. If answered incorrectly, review signs and symptoms of MS and intervention approaches.

B75 I Musculoskeletal I Interventions

To **BEST** stretch the pectoralis major muscle the patient should be positioned:

CHOICES:
1. sitting on heels, forward trunk flexion, with upper extremities in 180° of shoulder flexion.
2. supine with the shoulder abducted to 45° and medially (internally) rotated.
3. supine with the shoulder flexed and abducted to 145°.
4. with hands clasped together behind the low back and extended.

CORRECT ANSWER: 3

RATIONALE:
The pectoral muscles, located on the anterior chest, adduct and medially (internally) rotate the shoulder. To stretch the pectoral muscles, the shoulders must be abducted and laterally (externally) rotated. This is best accomplished in supine with the shoulder flexed and abducted to 145° with the weight of gravity providing a stretching force. The remaining positions do not place the pectoralis on stretch.

TYPE OF REASONING: DEDUCTIVE
One must recall the guidelines for stretching the pectoralis major muscle to arrive at a correct conclusion. This is factual information, which is a deductive reasoning skill. For this case, the pectoralis major muscle should be stretched in supine with the shoulder flexed and abducted 145°. If answered incorrectly, review muscle stretching techniques for the pectoralis major.

B76 | Devices, Admin, etc. | Safety Roles, Teaching, EBP

A physical therapist assistant observes a patient who is walking into the clinic suddenly fall to the ground. When the assistant arrives at the patient's side the patient is unresponsive. The assistant should:

CHOICES:

1. call out for someone to activate a code, open airway and assess breathing.
2. contact physical therapist, determine heart rate and, if absent, begin chest compressions.
3. call for emergency help, take vital signs and begin chest compressions as needed.
4. call code, stay with patient, monitor vital signs and wait for the emergency team.

CORRECT ANSWER: 1

RATIONALE:

This is an emergency situation and immediate action is appropriate. Because the physical therapist assistant is in the clinic, calling out for help is an appropriate first step, followed immediately by opening the airway and assessing the individuals ABCs (airway, breathing, circulation). Initiation of chest compressions is inappropriate until assessment of a lack of pulse is completed and no pulse is detected. Calling the physical therapist or waiting for the emergency team to arrive may cost the individual their life.

TYPE OF REASONING: EVALUATIVE

One must evaluate the courses of action presented and then determine the action that will effectively address the patient's needs. This requires evaluative reasoning skill. For this situation, the assistant should call out for someone to activate a code, open airway and assess breathing. If answered incorrectly, review emergency first aid and CPR guidelines.

B77 | Musculoskeletal | Interventions

A physical therapist suggests that a patient will benefit from isokinetic exercises. The physical therapist assistant should realize that in carrying out this form of exercise the:

CHOICES:

1. speed of exercise should be preset and resistance will vary depending upon the patient's ability.
2. resistance should be preset and the speed of exercise will vary depending upon the patient's ability.
3. resistance should be increased if the patient can achieve a preset 10-repetition maximum.
4. speed of exercise should be increased for the patient to generate more torque.

CORRECT ANSWER: 1

RATIONALE:

In isokinetic exercise the speed is preset and the resistance changes. As the patient "works" harder, the machine responds by increasing the resistance while keeping the speed constant. The machine will resist with as much effort as the patient exerts.

TYPE OF REASONING: INDUCTIVE

This question requires one to recall the benefits of isokinetic exercises to arrive at a correct conclusion. This requires knowledge of isokinetic exercise guidelines, which necessitates inductive reasoning skill. For this case, in carrying out this form of exercise, the speed of exercise should be preset and resistance will vary depending upon the patient's ability. If answered incorrectly, review isokinetic exercise guidelines.

B78 | Devices, Admin, etc. | Safety Roles, Teaching, EBP

A physical therapist assistant is treating a patient who has a diagnosis of AIDS in stage I. Current research demonstrates that exercise:

CHOICES:
1. further suppresses the immune system.
2. will help increase the helper CD4 T cells.
3. training should be performed at 50% to 60% of maximum heart rate.
4. should be avoided.

CORRECT ANSWER: 2

RATIONALE:
Current research demonstrates that exercise is important and effective in enhancing the overall health of the person with AIDS, especially in the earlier stages. Exercise training should be done at 70% to 80% of maximum heart rate to achieve the best results. Vital signs and lab values should be closely monitored, especially in the presence of comorbidities.

TYPE OF REASONING: INFERENTIAL
This question requires one to draw a reasonable conclusion about current research regarding exercise for patients with AIDS. This requires inferential reasoning skill. For this scenario, current research demonstrates that exercise will help increase the helper CD4 T cells, thereby enhancing overall health. If answered incorrectly, review current research regarding benefits of exercise for patients with AIDS.

B79 | Neuromuscular | Clinical Applications

A physical therapist assistant working with a patient who has a lower motor neuron injury should expect the patient to present with:

CHOICES:
1. positive Babinski's sign.
2. clonus.
3. extensor muscle spasms.
4. flaccidity.

CORRECT ANSWER: 4

RATIONALE:
Lower motor neuron lesions include those involving the cranial nerves, anterior horn cell, spinal roots and peripheral nerves. Symptoms of a lower motor neuron injury include decreased reflexes, muscle fasciculations and severe muscle wasting. Upper motor neuron injuries include injuries to the central nervous system, cortex, brain stem, corticospinal tracts and spinal cord. Symptoms of upper motor neuron injury include hypertonicity, hyperreflexia and exaggerated cutaneous and autonomic reflexes, disuse muscle atrophy, and impaired or absent voluntary movement with mass synergy pattern movement.

TYPE OF REASONING: INFERENTIAL
One must infer or draw a reasonable conclusion about the likely presentation of a patient with lower motor neuron injury. This requires one to determine what may be true of a patient, which is an inferential reasoning skill. For this situation, one should expect the patient to present with flaccidity. If answered incorrectly, review signs and symptoms of lower motor neuron injury.

B80 | Musculoskeletal | Clinical Applications

During gait observation the physical therapist assistant notes that the patient has decreased hip extension during stance phase. A likely cause of decreased hip extension will be:

CHOICES:

1. decreased range of motion of the biceps femoris.
2. decreased range of motion of the iliopsoas.
3. weakness of the hip flexors.
4. weakness of the hip extensors.

CORRECT ANSWER: 2

RATIONALE:

Decreased hip extension in stance phase most likely illustrates decreased range of motion of the hip flexors; iliopsoas is the biggest hip flexor muscle. Decreased range of motion of the biceps femoris will likely result in decreased knee extension and will affect stance phase as well as swing phase. Weakness of the hip flexors affects the amount of hip flexion achieved during swing phase. Weakness of the hip extensors will result in lateral or backward bending of the trunk during stance phase to compensate.

TYPE OF REASONING: INFERENTIAL

This question provides a deficit and the test taker must determine the most likely cause for it. This requires one to infer the reason for the deficit, which is an inferential reasoning skill. For this situation, the most likely reason for the deficit is decreased range of motion of the iliopsoas muscle. If answered incorrectly, review gait abnormalities, including decreased hip extension during stance phase.

B81 | Cardiovascular/Pulmonary | Data Collection

While assisting a physical therapist in treating a critically ill patient in the intensive care unit, the therapist asks the physical therapist assistant to quickly find out the most recent PO_2 and PCO_2 results for the patient. These values can be located in the medical record by looking for:

CHOICES:

1. pulmonary function test results.
2. hematocrit.
3. arterial blood gases.
4. vital signs.

CORRECT ANSWER: 3

RATIONALE:

PO_2 and PCO_2 are values obtained by drawing the patient's arterial blood, and indicate the levels of oxygen and carbon dioxide in the blood. This test is called arterial blood gases or ABGs.

TYPE OF REASONING: DEDUCTIVE

This question requires one to recall the abbreviations indicating arterial blood gas values to arrive at a correct conclusion. This is factual information, necessitating deductive reasoning skill. For this situation, PO_2 and PCO_2 can be found in the medical record by looking for arterial blood gas values. If answered incorrectly, review lab values for patients in the intensive care unit, including arterial blood gases.

B82 | Devices, Admin, etc. | Equipment, Modalities

Posting on a lower extremity orthosis will help correct for:

CHOICES:

1. pes planus (flat foot).
2. weak dorsiflexors.
3. a lower-extremity length discrepancy.
4. rearfoot varus.

CORRECT ANSWER: 4

RATIONALE:

Posting is a wedge that is placed on the forefoot or rearfoot portion of an orthosis to correct for a varus or valgus deformity; in the rearfoot it can help control the calcaneus and subtalar joint during gait. A longitudinal arch support will help prevent pes planus and help control the subtalar joint. A lower-extremity length discrepancy will likely be managed with a heel lift. Weak dorsiflexors would best be managed with an ankle–foot orthosis; it may be solid, have a dorsiflexion assist, or have an ankle articulation with a plantar flexion stop.

TYPE OF REASONING: DEDUCTIVE

One must recall the purpose of posting on a lower-extremity orthosis to arrive at a correct conclusion. This is factual recall of guidelines, which is a deductive reasoning skill. For this case, posting on the orthosis will help correct for rearfoot varus. If answered incorrectly, review lower-extremity orthotics, especially orthotics for correction of rearfoot varus.

B83 | Devices, Admin, etc. | Equipment, Modalities

A patient who has rheumatoid arthritis should MOST LIKELY use a/an:

CHOICES:

1. airplane splint.
2. cock-up splint.
3. dynamic wrist extension splint.
4. Milwaukee brace.

CORRECT ANSWER: 2

RATIONALE:

A cock-up or resting splint will likely be used to protect and rest the wrist; the smaller joints of the wrist and hand are often affected when a person has rheumatoid arthritis. An airplane splint is used to position the shoulder at 90° of abduction, and 90° of elbow flexion; it is commonly used following a fracture or surgery when the neutral position is not desirable. A dynamic wrist extension splint will more likely be used by a patient who has weak or no prehension or grasp; it facilitates the tenodesis grasp in a patient with quadriplegia. A Milwaukee brace is a specialized trunk orthosis used to control scoliosis.

TYPE OF REASONING: INFERENTIAL

This question requires one to determine the likely device that would be used by a patient who has rheumatoid arthritis. The test taker must infer the likely conclusion, which is an inferential reasoning skill. For this case, the patient is likely to wear a cock-up splint, as these splints are often worn to protect and rest the wrists. If answered incorrectly, review splinting guidelines for patients with rheumatoid arthritis.

B84 | Integumentary | Clinical Applications

When discussing the care of a patient in the home environment, a physical therapist assistant should explain to the family that the primary cause of decubitus ulcers is:

CHOICES:

1. excessive pressure.
2. the breakdown of skin.
3. lack of moisture on the skin surface.
4. too much moisture (such as urine) in contact with the skin.

CORRECT ANSWER: 1

RATIONALE:

Excess pressure is the primary reason for decubitus ulcers. It is important to teach the family to change the patient's position frequently to avoid excess pressure, especially over bony prominences, which are particularly susceptible to pressure ulcers. Excess moisture on the skin can lead to skin breakdown but is not a primary cause of decubitus ulcers.

TYPE OF REASONING: DEDUCTIVE

One must recall the causes of decubitus ulcers to arrive at a correct conclusion. This necessitates the recall of factual information, which is a deductive reasoning skill. For this situation, the primary cause of decubitus ulcers is excess pressure. If answered incorrectly, review decubitus ulcer guidelines and common causes.

B85 | Devices, Admin, etc. | Equipment, Modalities

An athlete received a contusion to the left thigh nearly a week ago. There is still some local inflammation. It is **MOST** likely that the physical therapist assistant should elect to put a hot pack on that site prior to exercise to:

CHOICES:

1. anesthetize the area.
2. decrease muscle spasm.
3. decrease tissue extensibility.
4. decrease the extensibility of collagen tissue.

CORRECT ANSWER: 2

RATIONALE:

Application of superficial heat for approximately 20 minutes will increase the extensibility of collagen tissue resulting in the reduction of muscle spasms. During the initial 24 to 48 hours, cold should be used to decrease pain and inflammation.

TYPE OF REASONING: INFERENTIAL

One must determine the likely reason for use of a hot pack on a site of contusion prior to exercise to arrive at a correct conclusion. This requires one to determine what may be true of a situation, which is an inferential reasoning skill. For this scenario, it is most likely that the hot pack is being used to decrease muscle spasm prior to exercise. If answered incorrectly, review benefits and indications for use of heat prior to exercise.

B86 | Musculoskeletal | Data Collection

Gait observation reveals a patient ambulating with a steppage gait pattern. The **MOST** likely cause of this compensatory gait pattern is:

CHOICES:
1. weakness of the gastrocnemius and soleus muscles.
2. spasticity of the tibialis anterior muscle.
3. weakness of the extensor digitorum longus and tibialis anterior muscles.
4. extensor spasticity of both the quadriceps and gastrocnemius soleus muscles.

CORRECT ANSWER: 3

RATIONALE:
Weakness of the ankle dorsiflexors, extensor digitorum longus and the tibialis anterior results in a steppage gait pattern (exaggerated hip and knee flexion during swing phase). It also results in foot slap as initial contact rather than heel strike (initial contact). Weakness of the gastrocnemius and soleus muscles will affect knee stability at midstance, and, most significantly, limit push-off into swing phase.

TYPE OF REASONING: INFERENTIAL
One must infer or draw a reasonable conclusion about the most likely cause for a patient ambulating with a steppage gait pattern. This requires inferential reasoning skill. For this case, the most likely cause is weakness of the extensor digitorum longus and tibialis anterior muscles. If answered incorrectly, review gait pattern deviations, including steppage gait pattern.

B87 | Integumentary | Data Collection

Following a deep partial thickness burn the physical therapist assistant should expect the wound bed to appear:

CHOICES:
1. red with slight edema, no blisters and some tenderness.
2. black or charred, and dry; edema is present with little pain.
3. blistered and inflamed with severe pain.
4. reddened or white, with edema and/or blistering, with severe pain.

CORRECT ANSWER: 4

RATIONALE:
A deep partial-thickness burn involves the epidermis and dermis with injury to the nerve endings, hair follicles and sweat glands. Superficial burns involve damage to the epidermis only and appear red, with slight edema and no blistering. A full-thickness burn involves complete destruction of the epidermis, dermis and subcutaneous tissues and may involve the muscle as well. It will appear black or charred, have a dry surface with a scab and present with little pain as the nerve endings have been destroyed.

TYPE OF REASONING: DEDUCTIVE
One must recall the features of a deep partial-thickness burn to arrive at a correct conclusion. This is factual recall of information, which is a deductive reasoning skill. For this situation, one should expect the wound bed to appear reddened or white, with edema and/or blistering, and with severe pain. Review characteristics of deep partial-thickness burns if answered incorrectly.

B88 | Neuromuscular | Clinical Applications

A newborn has a brachial plexus injury that is a result of a breech birth presentation. Nerve roots C8 and T1 have been affected. The infant will **MOST** likely present with:

CHOICES:

1. paralysis of the intrinsic muscles and wrist flexors.
2. a shoulder that is adducted and medially (internally) rotated.
3. the waiter's tip deformity.
4. winging of the scapula.

CORRECT ANSWER: 1

RATIONALE:

A brachial plexus injury results when the nerve and nerve roots are stretched and the nerve is damaged. In this case, the nerve roots of C8 and T1 were affected. The nerve roots of C8 and T1 and the peripheral nerves that come from these roots innervate the muscles of the wrist flexors and the intrinsic muscles of the hand. Damage of these will result in a clawed hand known as Klumpke's paralysis. Waiter's tip deformity and an adducted and medially rotated shoulder are characteristic of Erb's palsy (C5–C6).

TYPE OF REASONING: INFERENTIAL

This question provides a diagnosis and the test taker must determine the most likely symptoms of this diagnosis. This requires inferential reasoning skill. For this case, an incident with C8 and T1 nerve root damage will most likely present with paralysis of the intrinsic muscles and wrist flexors. If answered incorrectly, review brachial plexus injuries in infants, including Klumpke's paralysis.

B89 | Other Systems | Clinical Applications

Following an organ transplant, a patient has been on a long-term regimen of corticosteroids. Possible side effects include:

CHOICES:

1. dyspnea, increased blood pressure and weight loss.
2. osteoporosis, slowness of wound healing and weight gain.
3. low blood sugar levels, increased heart rate and weight gain.
4. osteoporosis, increased healing and weight loss.

CORRECT ANSWER: 2

RATIONALE:

There are many side effects from using steroids, including weight gain, decreased healing and osteoporosis. All of the options listed are a result of steroid use except weight loss, and low blood sugar levels; weight gain and elevated blood sugar levels are associated with corticosteroid use. A patient taking steroids usually has a weight gain because of the side effects of water retention and appetite stimulation.

TYPE OF REASONING: DEDUCTIVE

One must recall the side effects of long-term corticosteroid use to arrive at a correct conclusion. This is factual recall of information, which is a deductive reasoning skill. For this scenario, possible side effects of corticosteroids include osteoporosis, slowness of wound healing and weight gain. If answered incorrectly, review side effects of corticosteroid use.

B90 | Neuromuscular | Clinical Applications

A physical therapist assistant working with a patient who has a C6-level spinal cord injury should expect that the patient:

CHOICES:

1. is dependent for transfers.
2. has active elbow extension control.
3. is able to perform a sliding board transfer on level surfaces.
4. has active finger extension control.

CORRECT ANSWER: 3

RATIONALE:

A patient with C6 motor control should be able to perform sliding board transfers on level surfaces and may need assistance with more difficult transfers. The patient will likely be able to become independent in wheelchair activities with projection or friction surface hand rims; for longer and community distances the patient may need a power chair. Active elbow and finger extension is not intact until the C7 level. It is beneficial to do a thorough review of functional capabilities per injury level for persons with spinal cord lesions.

TYPE OF REASONING: INFERENTIAL

This question requires one to determine what may be true for a patient with C6 spinal cord injury. Questions of this nature often require inferential reasoning skill. For this situation, one should expect that the patient is able to perform a sliding board transfer on level surfaces. If answered incorrectly, review functional abilities for patients with C6 spinal cord injury, especially transfer abilities.

B91 | Devices, Admin, etc. | Safety Roles, Teaching, EBP

An example of an engineering control the hospital should employ to decrease the potential for an exposure of an employee to a bloodborne pathogen is:

CHOICES:

1. color-coded red or labeled containers.
2. gloves.
3. face shield.
4. eye irrigation station.

CORRECT ANSWER: 1

RATIONALE:

The Occupational Safety and Health Administration (OSHA) regulates work environments and has identified methods to control exposure to biohazardous materials. Engineering controls isolate or remove the biohazard from employees; they must be used in conjunction with work practices to be effective. Examples of engineering controls are puncture-resistant and leak-proof containers that are color-coded red or labeled. Engineering controls also provide a process by which reusable contaminated sharps are handled in a way to minimize the potential for exposure. Work practice controls are those mechanisms that have been provided to minimize the splashing, spraying, splattering and generation of droplets. Work practice requirements include hand washing immediately after removing gloves, provision of mechanism for eye irrigation in the event of an exposure and limiting recapping of needles. Personal protective equipment must be used by workers to decrease their chance of exposure. They include gloves, gowns, masks and surgical hoods or caps.

TYPE OF REASONING: DEDUCTIVE

One must recall engineering control guidelines to arrive at a correct conclusion. This is factual information, which is a deductive reasoning skill. For this scenario, an example of an engineering control to reduce the risk of exposure to bloodborne pathogens is color-coded red or labeled containers. If answered incorrectly, review OSHA guidelines for engineering controls to reduce exposure to bloodborne pathogens.

B92 | Musculoskeletal | Clinical Applications

Scar tissue mobilization is safe to initiate during which stage of healing?

CHOICES:

1. first, or inflammatory phase.
2. third, or fibroblastic phase.
3. second, or granulation phase.
4. fourth, or maturation phase.

CORRECT ANSWER: 2

RATIONALE:

The first phase to assist in the reorganization of scar tissue through mobilization is during the fibroblastic phase. During this phase the collagen fibers are laid down with weaker hydrostatic bonds that make tissue elongation easier and safe. Scar mobilization can occur during the fourth phase of healing, or maturation, with increased stress placed on the scar and with less chance of tissue damage. Near or at the end of the maturation phase, tissue remodeling becomes significantly more difficult. During the first and second phases of healing, inflammation is present and granulation tissue is being laid down. Granulation tissue is fragile and care must be taken not to damage it. Less vascular tissues (tendons, ligaments) require longer time frames to progress through the granulation phase.

TYPE OF REASONING: DEDUCTIVE

Knowledge of scar tissue mobilization guidelines is paramount to arriving at a correct conclusion for this question. This requires the recall of factual information, which is a deductive reasoning skill. For this situation, it is safe to initiate scar tissue mobilization during the third or fibroblastic phase of healing. Review scar tissue mobilization guidelines if answered incorrectly.

B93 | Cardiovascular/Pulmonary | Data Collection

Chronic pulmonary changes following a left pneumonectomy should include:

CHOICES:

1. decreased tidal volume.
2. increased tidal volume.
3. decreased breath sounds on the right.
4. decreased residual volume.

CORRECT ANSWER: 4

RATIONALE:

Decreased breath sounds on the side of the pneumonectomy would be likely, not on the opposite side. Residual volume will decrease as there is less air housed in the lung at the end of exhalation as there is only one lung present. Tidal volume (the amount of air inhaled and exhaled during rest) will not change, i.e., it will not increase or decrease.

TYPE OF REASONING: INFERENTIAL

One must infer or draw a reasonable conclusion about the likely chronic pulmonary changes following a pneumonectomy. Questions of this nature require one to determine what may be true, which is an inferential reasoning skill. For this case, chronic pulmonary changes should include decreased residual volume. If answered incorrectly, review pulmonary changes following pneumonectomy.

B94 | Devices, Admin, etc. | Equipment, Modalities

In providing ultrasound treatment for a patient with acute medial epicondylitis, the physical therapist assistant should administer ultrasound at:

CHOICES:

1. 3.0 w/cm^2.
2. 1.0 MHz.
3. 1.0 w/cm^2.
4. 3.0 MHz.

CORRECT ANSWER: 4

RATIONALE:

The superficial tissues over the epicondyle require 3.3 MHz ultrasound, which does not penetrate as deeply into the tissues as does the 1 MHz ultrasound setting. A setting of 3.3 MHz penetrates up to 1 cm, and 1 MHz can penetrate 3 cm to 5 cm deep into the tissues. Watts per centimeter squared (w/cm^2) is a measurement of intensity. An intensity of 3.3 w/cm^2 is too high and could burn the patient; 1.0 w/cm^2 may be an appropriate intensity; however, there is no mention of how long the treatment is delivered which makes the answer inappropriate.

TYPE OF REASONING: DEDUCTIVE

One must recall the guidelines for ultrasound treatment for patients with acute medial epicondylitis. This requires recall of factual guidelines, which is a deductive reasoning skill. For this situation, the assistant should administer ultrasound at 3.0 MHz to treat the superficial tissues over the epicondyle. If answered incorrectly, review ultrasound treatment guidelines for medial epicondylitis.

B95 | Cardiovascular/Pulmonary | Data Collection

A physical therapist assistant determines the resting heart rate of an infant is 115 beats per minute. This should indicate that the infant is demonstrating:

CHOICES:

1. tachycardia.
2. a normal heart rate.
3. tachypnea.
4. bradycardia.

CORRECT ANSWER: 2

RATIONALE:

The normal heart rate of an infant is a range of 100 to 140 beats per minute. A heart rate of 115 is within normal range. Tachycardia (rapid heart rate) and bradycardia (slow heart rate) are not appropriate descriptors. Tachypnea refers to respiratory rate.

TYPE OF REASONING: DEDUCTIVE

One must recall the normal resting heart rate of an infant to arrive at a correct conclusion. This is factual recall of guidelines, which is a deductive reasoning skill. For this case, the resting heart rate of 115 beats per minute indicates a normal heart rate. If answered incorrectly, review resting heart rates of infants.

B96 | Devices, Admin, etc. | Safety Roles, Teaching, EBP

A physical therapist assistant is working with a patient who has been diagnosed with a brain injury. The patient displays agitation while in therapy sessions. The **BEST** way to decrease this behavior is to:

CHOICES:

1. treat the patient in a calm, nonstimulating environment.
2. ignore it as it is expected behavior.
3. reward good behavior if the patient controls the agitation.
4. discontinue treatment when agitation occurs.

CORRECT ANSWER: 1

RATIONALE:

Patients can become overstimulated in a clinic environment. Moving the patient to calm, nonstimulating environment will potentially decrease his or her agitation and help him or her to attend to therapy sessions. The other strategies are not appropriate in managing agitation.

TYPE OF REASONING: INDUCTIVE

This question requires clinical judgment to determine a best course of action for a patient displaying agitation while in therapy. Questions of this nature often require inductive reasoning skill. For this situation, it is best to treat the patient in a calm, nonstimulating, environment. If answered incorrectly, review intervention techniques for patients with brain injury, including behavioral intervention guidelines.

B97 | Musculoskeletal | Clinical Applications

A patient has unilateral weakness of the gastrocnemius/soleus and shortening of the tibialis anterior on the same side. It would be **MOST** difficult for this patient to:

CHOICES:

1. walk up an incline.
2. go up stairs.
3. walk down an incline.
4. go down stairs.

CORRECT ANSWER: 3

RATIONALE:

Shortening of the tibialis anterior will limit plantar flexion. In addition, weakness of the gastrocnemius and soleus muscles will also result in weak plantar flexion. When a person descends an incline, plantar flexion range is necessary for the foot to be flat on surface, and the plantar flexors must act in reverse action to hold back the tibia. The combination of shortened tibialis anterior and weakness of the plantar flexors will result in difficulty descending an incline.

TYPE OF REASONING: INDUCTIVE

One must have knowledge of the impact of weakness of the gastrocnemius/soleus with shortening of the tibialis anterior to arrive at a correct conclusion. This requires clinical judgment, which is an inductive reasoning skill. For this case, it would be most difficult for this patient to walk down an incline because of the limited and weak plantar flexion. If answered incorrectly, review functional limitations from lower-extremity weakness, especially gastrocnemius/soleus weakness and tibialis anterior shortening.

B98 | Devices, Admin, etc. | Equipment, Modalities

A physical therapist assistant is preparing to perform electrical stimulation on a patient for pain management following principles of the Gate Control Theory. The physical therapist assistant should select:

CHOICES:

1. a rate of 1 to 5 pps.
2. a rate of 80 to100 pps.
3. a pulse width of 150 μsec.
4. a treatment duration of 5 minutes.

CORRECT ANSWER: 2

RATIONALE:

Electrical stimulation following the Gate Control Theory incorporates comfortable stimulus that stimulates the nociceptor low-threshold, large-diameter A-beta fibers. It is theorized that stimulation of the nociceptor sensory afferents causes presynaptic inhibition of the T cells and closes the spinal gate to the cerebral cortex to decrease the sensation of pain. A pulse rate between 80 to 100 pulses per second (pps) is in the comfortable range and will produce an analgesic effect. A more noxious effect can be achieved with pulse rates lower than 10 pps, thus according to the endorphin release theory are better used to control chronic pain. A pulse width of 150 μsec is high enough to get a muscle contraction, which is not appropriate in pain reduction. A treatment duration of 20 to 60 minutes is recommended for pain relief following the principles of the Gate Control Theory.

TYPE OF REASONING: DEDUCTIVE

One must recall the guidelines for performing electrical stimulation for pain management following principles of the Gate Control Theory. This is factual recall of guidelines, which is a deductive reasoning skill. For this situation, the assistant should select a rate of 80 to 100 pps. If answered incorrectly, review electrical stimulation guidelines for pain management and the Gate Control Theory.

B99 | Devices, Admin, etc. | Equipment, Modalities

The **BEST** form of cryotherapy that a physical therapist assistant can use to both reduce muscle spasm and facilitate the stretching of a tight muscle group is:

CHOICES:

1. cold pack.
2. ice massage.
3. contrast bath.
4. vapocoolant spray.

CORRECT ANSWER: 4

RATIONALE:

The best form of cryotherapy is the vapocoolant spray because of its multiple effects. Not only will it cool the area, but it also serves as an analgesic to decrease the pain. By interrupting the pain cycle and "blocking" some of the pain the physical therapist assistant will be able to stretch the muscle more effectively. "Numbing" the area and decreasing or eliminating the pain input can disrupt the pain/spasm cycle. The analgesic effects of vapocoolant spray are longer lasting than those with cold packs or ice massage. Contrast baths are better used to stimulate circulation and not appropriate to decrease the pain response to allow tissue stretching.

TYPE OF REASONING: INDUCTIVE

One must have knowledge of cryotherapy techniques for muscle spasm and stretching to arrive at a correct conclusion. This requires clinical judgment, which is an inductive reasoning skill. For this scenario, the best form of cryotherapy to reduce muscle spasm and facilitate stretching of tight muscles is vapocoolant spray. If answered incorrectly, review cryotherapy guidelines, including uses of vapocoolant spray.

B100 | Devices, Admin, etc. | Safety Roles, Teaching, EBP

A physical therapist assistant is assisting the physical therapist in performing a reassessment of a patient prior to the assistant carrying out treatment. The therapist has modified the plan of care to include lateral costal expansion. In the medical record, using the "SOAP" format, this information will be located in the section labeled:

CHOICES:
1. Subjective.
2. Objective.
3. Assessment.
4. Plan.

CORRECT ANSWER: 4

RATIONALE:

This information will be in the "Plan" section of the note. The physical therapist has developed a plan of care for the patient including goals, interventions and the frequency and duration of interventions. "Assessment" is for the professional opinion of what the outcome may be and how the patient may respond to treatment. The "Subjective" section of the note is what the patient says or reports. The "Objective" section is the measurable data obtained through observation tests and measures. The "Plan" section outlines the physical therapy interventions for treatment.

TYPE OF REASONING: DEDUCTIVE

This question requires a test taker to recall the factual guidelines for SOAP note documentation. Factual guidelines often necessitate deductive reasoning skill. For this situation, the plan to include lateral costal expansion should be documented in the Plan section of the SOAP note. If answered incorrectly, review SOAP note documentation guidelines, including information to be placed in the Plan section.

B101 | Musculoskeletal | Interventions

During gait training a patient demonstrates a "hip drop" on the swing limb at midstance. To help correct this gait deviation the physical therapist assistant should provide facilitation to the:

CHOICES:
1. gluteus medius on the swing limb.
2. iliopsoas on the stance limb.
3. quadratus lumborum on the swing limb.
4. hamstrings on the swing limb.

CORRECT ANSWER: 3

RATIONALE:

A "hip drop" on the swing limb can be caused by a weak quadratus lumborum on that side or a weak gluteus medius on the stance limb; facilitation of either will help to decrease the gait deviation. Facilitation of the hamstrings will help to stabilize the knee in stance, assist with knee flexion during swing or control knee "snap" at terminal swing if facilitated at the appropriate time.

TYPE OF REASONING: INDUCTIVE

One must determine the best therapeutic approach for a patient with a hip drop. This requires knowledge of the diagnosis and appropriate courses of action, which is an inductive reasoning skill. For this case, the assistant should provide facilitation to the quadratus lumborum on the swing limb to decrease the gait deviation. If answered incorrectly, review intervention approaches for hip drop.

B102 | Musculoskeletal | Interventions

Graded oscillation techniques that are performed at the limit of available motion are indicated to:

CHOICES:

1. improve free movement of the joint surfaces.
2. improve joint nutrition.
3. decrease pain.
4. decrease accessory motions of the joints.

CORRECT ANSWER: 1

RATIONALE:

Grades III (large-amplitude) and IV (small-amplitude) oscillation techniques are used to improve joint capsule range of motion (accessory motion) and joint motion at the end ranges of motion. Grades I (small-amplitude) and II (large-amplitude) oscillation techniques are used at the beginnings of range of motion of a joint and are used to decrease pain and promote joint nutrition through stimulation of the synovium.

TYPE OF REASONING: DEDUCTIVE

This question requires one to recall the indications for use of graded oscillation techniques performed at the limit of available motion to arrive at a correct conclusion. This is factual recall of information, which is a deductive reasoning skill. For this scenario, grades III and IV oscillation techniques are used to improve free movement of the joint surfaces. Review joint mobilization techniques if answered incorrectly, especially indications for grade III and IV techniques.

B103 | Devices, Admin, etc. | Safety Roles, Teaching, EBP

A physical therapist assistant works in a clinic in which the majority of patients are newly arrived from Asia. It is important for the assistant and other practitioners to **FIRST**:

CHOICES:

1. teach the patients what is to be expected and acceptable regarding healthcare delivery in the United States.
2. find a translator who is not a family member to objectively determine the patient's state of health.
3. try to understand each patient's attitudes and beliefs regarding healthcare.
4. ensure that the plan of care is tailored to meet the needs of the patient.

CORRECT ANSWER: 3

RATIONALE:

The physical therapist assistant will need to first understand the attitudes and beliefs of the patient. Attitudes, expectations and beliefs will greatly affect treatment, outcomes and what interventions will be appropriate for this patient. Although teaching the patient what is expected of the healthcare system in the United States is important, the assistant must first assess whether the patient understands the delivery of healthcare. Finding a translator and objectively determining the patient's state of health is important; however, that is not be the first action to take. Tailoring the plan of care for each individual is appropriate for all patients, and is not specific to this situation.

TYPE OF REASONING: EVALUATIVE

One must evaluate the potential courses of action presented and determine the action that is most effective in addressing the immediate needs of the patients. This requires one to weigh the merits of the actions, which is an evaluative reasoning skill. For this situation, it is important to first try to understand each patient's attitudes and beliefs regarding healthcare. If answered incorrectly, review guidelines for working with culturally diverse patients.

B104 | Musculoskeletal | Data Collection

When one is assessing joint range of motion for ankle dorsiflexion and plantar flexion, the preferred goniometric technique is to align the stationary arm parallel to the midline of the:

CHOICES:

1. fibula and the moving arm parallel to the fifth metatarsal keeping the knee stabilized and fully extended.
2. tibia and the moving arm parallel to the first metatarsal keeping the patient's knee somewhat flexed.
3. tibia and the moving arm parallel to the first metatarsal keeping the knee stabilized and fully extended.
4. fibula and the moving arm parallel to the fifth metatarsal keeping the patient's knee somewhat flexed.

CORRECT ANSWER: 4

RATIONALE:

When one is measuring ankle dorsiflexion and plantar flexion, the goniometer is aligned on the lateral aspect of the lower extremity. The stationary arm is aligned along midline of the fibula and the moving arm is parallel to the fifth metatarsal. The knee should be slightly flexed to put slack on the long head of the gastrocnemius so that ankle dorsiflexion is not limited by this muscle.

TYPE OF REASONING: DEDUCTIVE

This question requires the test taker to recall procedural guidelines for range-of-motion measurement of the ankle. This necessitates the recall of factual information, which is a deductive reasoning skill. For this case, the ankle should be measured by aligning the stationary arm of the goniometer parallel to the midline of the fibula and the movable arm parallel to the fifth metatarsal, keeping the patient's knee somewhat flexed. If answered incorrectly, review range-of-motion measurement procedures, especially for the ankle.

B105 | Neuromuscular | Clinical Applications

Use of rim projections, friction rims or leather gloves for wheelchair mobility is **MOST** appropriate for:

CHOICES:

1. patients whose grip strength is 4-/5.
2. patients whose grip strength is 3-/5.
3. patients with quadriplegia at the C4 neurological level.
4. those who race in wheelchairs at relatively high speeds.

CORRECT ANSWER: 2

RATIONALE:

Rim projections, friction rims and leather gloves will help compensate for weak or decreased grip strength; a patient with a 3-/5 strength is more appropriate than a patient with 4-/5 strength. Patients with quadriplegia at the C4 level have no hand function; therefore, a manually propelled wheelchair is inappropriate. Those who race wheelchairs must use leather gloves to adequately grip the rim and to prevent abrasions or blisters on their hands and fingers; however, they should not need handrim projections.

TYPE OF REASONING: ANALYTICAL

This question requires one to analyze the adaptive devices presented and determine the type of patient who would be most appropriate to utilize such devices. This requires analytical reasoning skill as the evaluation of the devices is utilized to arrive at a correct conclusion. For this situation, the use of rim projections, friction rims or leather gloves for wheelchair mobility is most appropriate for patients whose grip strength is 3-/5. If answered incorrectly, review indications for use of rim projections, friction rims and leather gloves for wheelchair mobility.

B106 | Neuromuscular | Interventions

A patient with a complete spinal cord lesion at the C6 level exhibits signs of orthostatic hypotension. The appropriate course of action is to:

CHOICES:

1. reacclimate the patient to the upright position.
2. walk the patient in the parallel bars using an abdominal binder and elastic wraps on the limbs to prevent venous pooling.
3. immediately check the catheter for blockage.
4. have the patient concentrate on diaphragmatic breathing and lateral costal expansion.

CORRECT ANSWER: 1

RATIONALE:

Orthostatic hypotension is defined as a decrease in blood pressure when a person stands or is placed in an upright position. To prevent this decrease in blood pressure, the physical therapist assistant should gradually bring the patient upright to reacclimate the patient to a standing position. A tilt table is usually utilized to assist by gradually progressing the patient to an upright position. Ambulation is not an option because a patient with a lesion at the C6 level will not be ambulatory. Immediately checking the catheter for blockage is the first course of action if autonomic dysreflexia is suspected. Diaphragmatic breathing and lateral costal expansion will help with aeration of the lungs, but will not help to prevent a drop in blood pressure.

TYPE OF REASONING: EVALUATIVE

This question requires one to determine a best course of action for a patient with orthostatic hypotension. One must weigh the benefits of the courses of action presented to determine the action that will have the most beneficial outcome, which is an evaluative reasoning skill. For this case, the best course of action is to reacclimate the patient to an upright position. Review guidelines for intervention with patients with spinal cord injury who experienced orthostatic hypotension if answered incorrectly.

B107 | Cardiovascular/Pulmonary | Interventions

It is unusual for a physical therapist assistant treating a patient with early stage cystic fibrosis to note in the medical record:

CHOICES:

1. excessive appetite and weight gain.
2. increased pulmonary secretions with airway obstruction.
3. frequent recurrent respiratory infections.
4. salty skin and sweat.

CORRECT ANSWER: 1

RATIONALE:

Cystic fibrosis (CF) is an inherited disorder affecting the exocrine glands of the hepatic, digestive and respiratory systems. The patient with CF is prone to chronic bacterial airway infections and progressive loss of pulmonary function from progressive obstructive lung disease. Early clinical manifestations include an inability to gain weight despite excessive appetite and adequate caloric intake. Excessive weight gain is rarely a finding in a patient with CF. All the other choices are typically present along with persistent coughing, wheezing and reduced exercise tolerance.

TYPE OF REASONING: INFERENTIAL

One must infer or draw a reasonable conclusion about the potential symptoms of a patient with CF to determine the symptoms the assistant would be unlikely to document in the medical record. This requires knowledge of the diagnosis and determining what may be true of a situation, which is an inferential reasoning skill. For this case, it would be unusual to document weight gain for this disease. If answered incorrectly, review signs and symptoms of CF.

B108 | Other Systems | Clinical Applications

A patient with human immunodeficiency virus is hospitalized with a viral infection and has a history of four infectious episodes within the past year. The assistant recognizes that ongoing systemic effects for this patient are likely to include:

CHOICES:

1. low-grade fever, malaise, anemia and fatigue.
2. decreased erythrocyte sedimentation rate.
3. redness, warmth, swelling and pain.
4. fever, tachycardia and hypermetabolic state.

CORRECT ANSWER: 1

RATIONALE:

Repeat infections produce a chronic inflammatory state. Systemic effects include low-grade fever, weight loss, malaise, anemia, fatigue, leukocytosis and lymphocytosis. Inflammatory activity can be detected by an elevated erythrocyte sedimentation rate. Redness, warmth, swelling and pain are signs of the systemic effects of an acute inflammation.

TYPE OF REASONING: INFERENTIAL

One must utilize knowledge of the diagnosis and likely symptoms to arrive at a correct conclusion. This determination of likely symptoms necessitates inferential reasoning skill. For this case, ongoing systemic effects are likely to include low-grade fever, malaise, anemia and fatigue. If answered incorrectly, review signs and symptoms of human immunodeficiency virus, including ongoing systemic effects of the condition.

B109 | Devices, Admin, etc. | Equipment, Modalities

A patient was instructed to apply conventional (high-rate) transcutaneous electrical nerve stimulation (TENS) to the low back to modulate a chronic pain condition. The patient now states that the TENS unit is no longer effective in reducing the pain in spite of increasing the intensity to maximum. The assistant should now:

CHOICES:

1. switch to low-rate TENS.
2. increase the treatment frequency.
3. switch to modulation mode TENS.
4. decrease the pulse duration.

CORRECT ANSWER: 3

RATIONALE:

Because of the long-term continuous use of TENS, the sensory receptors accommodated to the continuous current and no longer responded to the stimuli. Changing to modulation mode (i.e., burst modulation), which periodically interrupts the current flow, does not allow accommodation to occur.

TYPE OF REASONING: INDUCTIVE

This question requires one to utilize clinical judgment to determine a best course of action. This requires knowledge of the application of TENS to arrive at a correct conclusion, which is an inductive reasoning skill. For this scenario, the patient should be switched to modulation mode TENS. If answered incorrectly, review treatment parameters for TENS for patients with chronic pain.

B110 | Musculoskeletal | Interventions

A physical therapist assistant is working with a patient who delivered her first child 2 weeks ago. The physical therapist diagnosis is a 4-cm diastasis recti abdominis. The **BEST INITIAL** intervention that the physical therapist assistant should implement for this patient is to teach:

CHOICES:
1. pelvic tilts and bilateral straight leg raising.
2. pelvic floor exercises and sit-ups.
3. gentle stretching of hamstrings and hip flexors.
4. protection and splinting of the abdominal musculature.

CORRECT ANSWER: 4

RATIONALE:
Diastasis recti abdominis is a condition in which there is lateral separation or split of the rectus abdominis. It is important to teach protection (splinting) of the abdominal musculature. Patients should be instructed to avoid full sit-ups or bilateral straight leg raising. Pelvic floor exercises are done but are not remediation for diastasis recti.

TYPE OF REASONING: INDUCTIVE
One must utilize clinical judgment to determine the best initial intervention for a patient with diastasis recti abdominis. Questions of this nature often require inductive reasoning skill. For this situation, the best initial intervention is teaching protection and splinting of the abdominal musculature. If answered incorrectly, review intervention guidelines for diastasis recti abdominis.

B111 | Neuromuscular | Interventions

To facilitate functional capabilities in children with considerable developmental delay and persistence of the tonic labyrinthine reflex, it is **BEST** to have them practice reaching for objects by positioning them:

CHOICES:
1. supine.
2. prone.
3. long-sitting.
4. side-lying.

CORRECT ANSWER: 4

RATIONALE:
The tonic labyrinthine reflex results in increased flexor tone/flexion of all extremities when the child is placed in the prone position, and increased extensor tone/extension of all the extremities when the child is placed in the supine position. Therefore, to limit the effect of either flexion or extension, the side-lying position will provide the child with the best potential for success in reaching.

TYPE OF REASONING: INDUCTIVE
This question requires the test taker to use clinical judgment to determine a best course of action. This necessitates inductive reasoning skill. For this scenario, the best position for the child with tonic labyrinthine reflex is in side-lying while practicing reaching for objects. If answered incorrectly, review the tonic labyrinthine reflex and the influence of positioning on tone.

B112 | Neuromuscular | Interventions

Following a cerebrovascular accident, a patient with right hemiplegia is beginning ambulation using a large-base quad cane after completing gait training in the parallel bars. The patient is having difficulty advancing the right lower extremity. The **INITIAL** feedback the physical therapist assistant should provide to the patient is:

CHOICES:

1. a verbal cue to shift the weight to the left.
2. to physically assist the patient to shift the weight to the left.
3. to verbally instruct the patient to lift the right lower extremity.
4. to physically assist the patient to advance the right lower extremity.

CORRECT ANSWER: 1

RATIONALE:

The correct feedback is to verbally cue the patient on the technique previously mastered in the parallel bars. To advance the right lower extremity the patient must first shift the weight toward the left—the stance limb. If the patient is unable to complete this with verbal cues, then provide further assistance and physically assist the patient to weight shift. Cueing the patient to lift the right lower extremity should not be performed until a weight shift has occurred.

TYPE OF REASONING: INDUCTIVE

For this question, one must have knowledge of gait training guidelines for patients with stroke to arrive at a correct conclusion. This necessitates clinical judgment, which is an inductive reasoning skill. For this case, the patient with difficulty advancing the right lower extremity during ambulation should be given a verbal cue to shift weight to the left. If answered incorrectly, review gait training guidelines for patients with stroke, especially difficulty advancing a leg during ambulation.

B113 | Devices, Admin, etc. | Equipment, Modalities

The **BEST** choice to control medial ankle joint motion in a patient who has spasticity is a:

CHOICES:

1. floor reaction orthosis.
2. valgus correction strap.
3. solid, molded plastic ankle–foot orthosis (AFO).
4. patellar tendon-bearing brim.

CORRECT ANSWER: 3

RATIONALE:

Using a molded plastic ankle–foot orthosis is the best mechanism to control medial–lateral motion; it is superior to the varus or valgus correction strap. It can be especially effective if thicker plastic is used, if rolled edges are contoured into the brace, and if carbon reinforcements are embedded into the AFO on the appropriate side. A floor reaction orthosis is typically used to resist knee flexion. A patellar tendon-bearing brim is used to decrease weight through the foot.

TYPE OF REASONING: INDUCTIVE

One must determine the best choice to control medial ankle joint motion in a patient with spasticity to arrive at a correct conclusion. This requires knowledge of orthotic devices and therapeutic benefits, which is an inductive reasoning skill. For this situation, the best choice is a solid molded plastic AFO. If answered incorrectly, review orthotic devices to control ankle motion in patients with spasticity.

B114 | Cardiovascular/Pulmonary | Clinical Applications

Which of the following positions is **MOST** effective for a patient with advancing chronic lung disease to catch one's breath?

CHOICES:

1. supine in the recumbent position.
2. sitting and leaning forward on the hands or forearms.
3. side-lying opposite the symptomatic side.
4. prone over a pillow.

CORRECT ANSWER: 2

RATIONALE:

Sitting and leaning forward on the forearms or hands assists the patient with chronic lung disease to increase the effectiveness of using the pectoralis and serratus anterior as accessory motions for ventilation. The other positions will likely increase the amount of energy used to breathe and should be avoided whenever possible.

TYPE OF REASONING: INDUCTIVE

This question requires the test taker to have knowledge of advancing chronic lung disease and strategies for catching one's breath to arrive at a correct conclusion. This requires inductive reasoning skill. For this situation, it is most effective to catch one's breath by assuming a "tripod posture" or sitting and leaning forward on the hands or forearms. If answered incorrectly, review breathing strategies and postures for chronic lung disease.

B115 | Devices, Admin, etc. | Safety Roles, Teaching, EBP

A physical therapist assistant is visiting a patient at home. There is no air conditioning and the day is hot and humid. The patient reports having a headache, being dizzy and experiencing nausea. The patient refuses to take part in therapy. The assistant should:

CHOICES:

1. call the emergency response system, report a case of heat stroke and remain with the patient until help arrives.
2. move the patient to a cool place and administer salt tablets if available.
3. elevate the patient's lower extremities and begin stroking massage to improve circulation.
4. give the patient cold water, and elevate the lower extremities.

CORRECT ANSWER: 4

RATIONALE:

The patient's symptoms indicate the early signs of dehydration. Elevating the lower extremities (to prevent distal edema), giving the patient cold water and attempting to decrease the patient's body temperature are the most appropriate ways to address the situation. The situation described is not a medical emergency and the emergency response system should not be activated. Moving the patient to a cool place is a good option, but administering salt tablets is not advisable. The patient may have another medical condition in which excess sodium is contraindicated. There is not a problem with the patient's circulation; therefore, massage is not indicated.

TYPE OF REASONING: EVALUATIVE

This question requires one to determine the best course of action for a patient with symptoms of dehydration. One must weigh the courses of action and determine the one that best addresses the patient's symptoms, which is an evaluative reasoning skill. For this scenario, the assistant should give the patient cold water and elevate the lower extremities. If answered incorrectly, review first aid approaches for dehydration.

B116 | Cardiovascular/Pulmonary | Interventions

A physical therapist assistant is preparing to perform postural drainage on a patient. A precaution for postural drainage with the patient in the Trendelenburg position (feet elevated) is:

CHOICES:
1. humeral fracture.
2. claustrophobia.
3. rib fractures.
4. congestive heart failure.

CORRECT ANSWER: 4

RATIONALE:

Congestive heart failure is a precaution for postural drainage in the Trendelenburg position. One may be able to perform postural drainage in a modified position. A humeral fracture does not preclude use of the Trendelenburg position—precautions must be taken when using this position; however, side-lying on the side of the fracture is contraindicated. For rib fractures, this position is also allowed with precautions for the fractures. The Trendelenburg position should not bother a person who is claustrophobic.

TYPE OF REASONING: DEDUCTIVE

One must recall the precautions for postural drainage to arrive at a correct conclusion. This necessitates the recall of factual information, which is a deductive reasoning skill. For this situation, a precaution for postural drainage in the Trendelenburg position is congestive heart failure. If answered incorrectly, review precautions for postural drainage techniques, especially the Trendelenburg position.

B117 | Devices, Admin, etc. | Safety Roles, Teaching, EBP

A patient is uncooperative and frequently expresses displeasure about what is being done during treatment sessions. Under these circumstances the physical therapist assistant should **FIRST**:

CHOICES:
1. ask the supervisor to discharge this patient from the assistant's patient load as there is no therapeutic relationship.
2. accept the patient's criticism as a phase of anger related to the disability.
3. tell the patient that the negative attitude could retard rehabilitation.
4. ask the patient to be more specific as to why there is so much dissatisfaction with treatment.

CORRECT ANSWER: 4

RATIONALE:

When a patient frequently expresses displeasure regarding a treatment session, the physical therapist assistant should ask the patient to be more specific about why he or she is dissatisfied to more accurately address the problem(s). The remaining options are not appropriate. Neither switching patients nor accepting the patient's criticism as a phase of anger will address the patient's dissatisfaction. Indicating that a negative attitude could retard rehabilitation will most likely only cause more anger.

TYPE OF REASONING: EVALUATIVE

This question requires the test taker to weigh the merits of the courses of action presented and then determine the response that will most effectively resolve the patient's concerns. This requires evaluative reasoning skill. For this scenario, the assistant should first ask the patient to be more specific about the dissatisfaction with treatment to accurately address the problem. If answered incorrectly, review patient interaction skill guidelines and conflict resolution procedures.

B118 | Devices, Admin, etc. | Equipment, Modalities

A patient is using a portable functional electrical stimulator at home to regain functional wrist extension. The physical therapist assistant should instruct the patient to increase the intensity until the patient:

CHOICES:

1. obtains a maximal wrist extension contraction.
2. feels a very strong stimulus.
3. visualizes a twitch contraction of the wrist extensor muscles.
4. sees the hand begin to rise off the treatment surface.

CORRECT ANSWER: 1

RATIONALE:

The intensity of electrical stimulation for functional strength gains must create a strong, tetanic, muscle contraction; a maximal contraction meets that criteria. A twitch contraction will not create appreciable gains in strength of a muscle for functional use. A contraction to raise the hand off the treatment surface may not be strong enough to increase the strength of the muscle.

TYPE OF REASONING: INDUCTIVE

One must utilize knowledge of functional electrical stimulation to arrive at a correct conclusion for this question. This necessitates clinical judgment, which is an inductive reasoning skill. For this scenario, the assistant should instruct the patient to increase the intensity until the patient obtains a maximal wrist extension contraction. If answered incorrectly, review functional electrical stimulation guidelines.

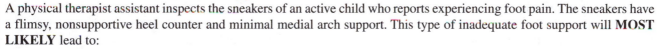

B119 | Musculoskeletal | Clinical Applications

A physical therapist assistant inspects the sneakers of an active child who reports experiencing foot pain. The sneakers have a flimsy, nonsupportive heel counter and minimal medial arch support. This type of inadequate foot support will **MOST LIKELY** lead to:

CHOICES:

1. depressed metatarsal heads.
2. excessive pronation.
3. excessive supination.
4. pes cavus (claw foot).

CORRECT ANSWER: 2

RATIONALE:

Excessive pronation results in the medial aspect of the foot touching the ground during weight-bearing because of the flattening of the medial arch of the foot. This can occur because of inadequate support of the medial arch. A flimsy heel counter also contributes to excessive pronation by allowing the heel to move medially. Depressed metatarsal heads are usually a result of wearing high heels. Excessive supination and pes cavus are caused by anatomical malalignment or neurological deficits rather than inadequate footwear.

TYPE OF REASONING: INFERENTIAL

One must infer the most likely condition that can result from inadequate foot support when a child is wearing nonsupportive shoes. This requires one to determine what may be true of a situation, which is an inferential reasoning skill. For this case, inadequate foot support will most likely lead to excessive pronation. If answered incorrectly, review guidelines for appropriate footwear and support for children.

B120 | Musculoskeletal | Clinical Applications

Following removal of a cast for a fracture of the distal third of the radius, a patient now has limited wrist extension. To increase wrist extension, gentle stretching can be initiated by:

CHOICES:

1. supinating the forearm and extending the wrist and fingers.
2. pronating the forearm and extending the wrist while allowing the fingers to flex.
3. supinating the forearm and extending the wrist while allowing the fingers to flex.
4. pronating the forearm and extending the wrist and fingers.

CORRECT ANSWER: 2

RATIONALE:

Stretching after cast removal should be initiated gently. Limited wrist extension indicates tight wrist flexors. Extending the wrist and allowing the fingers to flex allows the two joint muscles (long finger flexors) to stretch over only one joint. Keeping the forearm pronated allows the wrist and finger flexors to be slack. The remaining positions stretch the muscles over several joints and begin with a position that has the wrist flexors in an already lengthened position.

TYPE OF REASONING: INDUCTIVE

One must determine a best approach for gentle stretching after a distal radius fracture to arrive at a correct conclusion. This requires clinical judgment, which is an inductive reasoning skill. For this situation, gentle stretching can be initiated by pronating the forearm and extending the wrist while allowing the fingers to flex. If answered incorrectly, review stretching guidelines for the upper extremity after cast removal, especially the wrist.

B121 | Other Systems | Data Collection

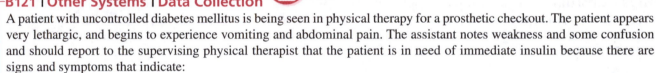

A patient with uncontrolled diabetes mellitus is being seen in physical therapy for a prosthetic checkout. The patient appears very lethargic, and begins to experience vomiting and abdominal pain. The assistant notes weakness and some confusion and should report to the supervising physical therapist that the patient is in need of immediate insulin because there are signs and symptoms that indicate:

CHOICES:

1. ketoacidosis.
2. respiratory acidosis.
3. ketoalkalosis.
4. lactic acidosis.

CORRECT ANSWER: 1

RATIONALE:

An insulin deficiency in a patient with diabetes leads to the release of fatty acids from adipose cells with a production of excess ketones by the liver (diabetic ketoacidosis). Signs and symptoms include alterations in gastrointestinal function (anorexia, nausea and vomiting, abdominal pain), neural function (weakness, lethargy, malaise, confusion, stupor, coma, depression of vital functions), cardiovascular function (peripheral vasodilation, decreased heart rate, cardiac dysrhythmias), and skin (warm, flushed), and increased rate and depth of respiration. The assistant should report these changes immediately; the patient is in need of immediate insulin, fluid and electrolyte replacement solutions.

TYPE OF REASONING: ANALYTICAL

This question provides symptoms from a patient in which the test taker must determine the likely problem that necessitates informing the therapist immediately. This requires analyzing the symptoms to draw a reasonable conclusion, which is an analytical reasoning skill. For this case, the patient's symptoms indicate ketoacidosis. If answered incorrectly, review signs and symptoms of ketoacidosis and procedures to address this condition.

B122 | Other Systems | Clinical Applications

A physical therapist assistant performing conditioning exercises with a patient who has hyperthyroidism should expect to see:

CHOICES:

1. trigger points and bradycardia.
2. rheumatoidlike symptoms and muscle stiffness.
3. muscular and joint edema, and poor peripheral circulation.
4. proximal muscle weakness and potential dysrhythmia.

CORRECT ANSWER: 4

RATIONALE:

A patient with hyperthyroidism will commonly present with muscle weakness and fatigue, muscle atrophy and chronic periarthritis symptoms; as well as increased pulse rate, cardiac output and blood volume. The other symptoms listed all are manifestations of hypothyroidism.

TYPE OF REASONING: INFERENTIAL

This question provides a diagnosis and the test taker must infer the likely symptoms of this diagnosis. This requires one to determine what may be true for a patient's diagnosis, which is an inferential reasoning skill. For this scenario, one should expect to see proximal muscle weakness and potential dysrhythmia. If answered incorrectly, review signs and symptoms of hyperthyroidism.

B123 | Cardiovascular/Pulmonary | Clinical Applications

A patient with the diagnosis of left-sided heart failure, class II, is being seen in physical therapy. With exercise this patient can be expected to demonstrate:

CHOICES:

1. dyspnea with fatigue and muscular weakness.
2. severe, uncomfortable chest pain with shortness of breath.
3. weight gain with dependent edema.
4. anorexia, nausea with abdominal pain and distention.

CORRECT ANSWER: 1

RATIONALE:

Left-sided heart failure is the result of the left ventricle failing to pump enough blood through the arterial system to meet the body's demands. It produces pulmonary edema and disturbed respiratory control mechanisms. Patients can be expected to demonstrate progressive dyspnea (exertional at first, then paroxysmal nocturnal dyspnea), fatigue and muscular weakness, pulmonary edema, cerebral hypoxia and renal changes. Severe chest pain and shortness of breath are symptoms of impending myocardial infarction. The other choices describe symptoms associated with right-sided ventricular failure.

TYPE OF REASONING: INFERENTIAL

One must infer or draw a reasonable conclusion about the likely symptoms of a patient who has left-sided heart failure. This requires inferential reasoning skill, as one must determine what may be true of a diagnosis. For this situation, one can expect the patient to demonstrate dyspnea with fatigue and muscular weakness. If answered incorrectly, review signs and symptoms of left-sided heart failure.

B124 | Neuromuscular | Data Collection

Which test should a physical therapist assistant employ to assess fine motor activity?

CHOICES:

1. bilateral, symmetrical foot tapping.
2. rapid, alternating forearm pronation/supination.
3. bilateral finger-to-thumb opposition.
4. unilateral finger-to-nose activity.

CORRECT ANSWER: 3

RATIONALE:

Finger-to-thumb opposition is fine motor activity. The remaining activities are gross motor activities. Gross motor coordination is movement of larger muscle groups and larger movements. Such activities should include foot tapping, forearm pronation/supination and bringing the finger to the nose.

TYPE OF REASONING: INDUCTIVE

One must utilize clinical judgment to determine the best test to employ to assess fine motor activity. This requires inductive reasoning skill. For this case, the only test that assesses fine motor activity is bilateral finger-to-thumb opposition. If answered incorrectly, review assessment guidelines for fine motor skills.

B125 | Neuromuscular | Interventions

Following surgery, a patient has effusion of the right knee joint and is unable to initiate quadriceps setting exercises. The **BEST** facilitation method is:

CHOICES:

1. transcutaneous nerve stimulation to the thigh.
2. quick icing to the quadriceps muscle.
3. joint approximation at the knee.
4. firm pressure on the patellar tendon.

CORRECT ANSWER: 2

RATIONALE:

Quick icing is the most appropriate method to facilitate the quadriceps activity. Quick icing stimulates the alpha motor neuron that results in muscle contraction. The icing may also have a secondary effect of decreasing the joint effusion. Transcutaneous nerve stimulation will facilitate quadriceps activity; however, it could be quite uncomfortable and is not the easiest or most efficient method for doing so. Joint approximation and pressure on the patellar tendon are contraindicated because both of these activities actually inhibit the quadriceps.

TYPE OF REASONING: INDUCTIVE

This question requires the test taker to utilize knowledge of modalities to facilitate quadriceps activity to arrive at a correct conclusion. This requires clinical judgment, which is an inductive reasoning skill. For this case, the best facilitation method is quick icing to the quadriceps muscle. Review muscle facilitation methods, especially quadriceps facilitation, if answered incorrectly.

B126 | Devices, Admin, etc. | Safety Roles, Teaching, EBP

Researchers examined the benefits of strength training on functional performance in older adults. The data analysis involved a meta-analysis. This refers to:

CHOICES:
1. pooling of data of randomized controlled studies to yield a larger sample.
2. a mechanism to critically evaluate studies.
3. data analysis performed by the Cochrane Collaboration.
4. the retrospective study of individuals with similar conditions.

CORRECT ANSWER: 1

RATIONALE:

Meta-analysis refers to pooling of data of randomized controlled trials (RCTs) to yield a larger sample. Non-RCTs (case studies, case reports) are excluded. The Cochrane Collaboration is one source of meta-analysis reviews. Critically evaluating systematic reviews is a separate process. A retrospective review of a group of individuals with similar conditions is an example of a case–control study.

TYPE OF REASONING: DEDUCTIVE

This question requires one to recall the guidelines for a meta-analysis to arrive at a correct conclusion. This is factual information, necessitating deductive reasoning skill. For this scenario, meta-analysis refers to the pooling of data of randomized controlled studies to yield a larger sample. If answered incorrectly, review meta-analysis study guidelines.

B127 | Devices, Admin, etc. | Equipment, Modalities

A patient has a deep wound on the thigh secondary to the incision from a saphenous vein harvest site failing to heal. There are moderate to large amounts of exudate, tunneling and fragile wound edges. Which of the following dressing categories is the **BEST** selection for this patient?

CHOICES:
1. a hydrocolloid dressing.
2. a transparent film cut 2 inches larger than the wound edges.
3. a rope-shaped alginate covered with a thick gauze pad.
4. hydrophilic foam.

CORRECT ANSWER: 3

RATIONALE:

A rope-shaped alginate is an effective treatment to manage tunneling to help fill up dead space in the wound tunnel. Alginate absorbs significant amounts of wound exudates. A hydrocolloid dressing is best used for shallow wound beds and wounds with less drainage and is not recommended for fragile tissues. A transparent film is nonabsorptive and not recommended for fragile wound edges. Although films can absorb moderate amounts of exudates they do not conform well to wound beds.

TYPE OF REASONING: INDUCTIVE

One must utilize knowledge of wound-dressing techniques to arrive at a correct conclusion for this question. The use of clinical judgment to determine a best course of action often necessitates inductive reasoning skill. For this case, the best dressing selection for this patient is a rope-shaped alginate covered with a thick gauze pad. If answered incorrectly, review wound dressing techniques, especially for wounds with tunneling and significant amounts of exudate.

B128 | Cardiovascular/Pulmonary | Clinical Applications

A patient who has recently and successfully completed a 2-week program of phase III cardiac rehabilitation will **MOST LIKELY** demonstrate a decrease in:

CHOICES:

1. heart rate at a given level of submaximal work.
2. CO_2 elimination in maximal work.
3. cardiac output in maximal work.
4. stroke volume at a given level of submaximal work.

CORRECT ANSWER: 1

RATIONALE:

Successful cardiac rehabilitation will result in decreased heart rate at a given level of submaximal work. Conditioning of the heart musculature will result in more effective pumping with decreased contractions. The other choices are not expectations and would be worrisome if any were true at the end of phase III.

TYPE OF REASONING: INFERENTIAL

One must infer or draw a reasonable conclusion about the most likely characteristics of a patient in a cardiac rehabilitation program. This requires one to determine what may be true, which is an inferential reasoning skill. For this situation, the patient will most likely demonstrate a decrease in heart rate at a given level of submaximal work. If answered incorrectly, review cardiac rehabilitation guidelines, especially patient characteristics, after phase III program completion.

B129 | Neuromuscular | Clinical Applications

The plan of care for a patient recently returned home with right hemiparesis indicates the patient demonstrates good recovery. Spasticity is in decline, there is no indication of synergistic movement and the patient is ambulatory with a small-based quad cane. The **MOST** appropriate activity for a patient at this stage of recovery is:

CHOICES:

1. standing, picking the foot up behind and slowly lowering it.
2. supine, bending the hip and knee up to the chest with some hip abduction.
3. sitting, marching in place (alternate hip flexion movement).
4. standing, small-range knee extension movement to gain quadriceps control.

CORRECT ANSWER: 1

RATIONALE:

This phase of recovery is characterized by some movement combinations that do not follow the paths of either flexion or extension obligatory synergies. Knee flexion in standing is an out-of-synergy movement. All other choices represent synergistic movements: the supine and sitting options are flexion synergy movements and the other standing option focuses on knee extensor movement within an extended position.

TYPE OF REASONING: INDUCTIVE

One must determine the most appropriate activity for a patient with hemiparesis and decline in spasticity. This requires knowledge of rehabilitation guidelines for patients with spasticity to arrive at a correct conclusion. This requires inductive reasoning skill. For this case, the most appropriate activity for a patient is standing, picking the foot up behind and slowly lowering it. If answered incorrectly, review rehabilitation guidelines for patients with spasticity.

B130 | Musculoskeletal | Clinical Applications

Following a deep contusion to the lower back, a patient who is receiving thermotherapy has also been advised to take ibuprofen. The patient asks what the medication does. The **BEST** response is that ibuprofen is:

CHOICES:

1. a corticosteroid that will help to inhibit inflammatory reactions and help heal the wound.
2. a muscle relaxant that relieves serious muscle spasms associated with painful conditions.
3. a nonsteroidal antiinflammatory drug that is useful in treating mild to moderate pain and inflammation.
4. an analgesic generally used to provide symptomatic relief from pain for people.

CORRECT ANSWER: 3

RATIONALE:

Ibuprofen is a nonsteroidal antiinflammatory drug (NSAID). NSAIDs are used to treat mild to moderate inflammation and pain. Some commonly used NSAIDs are Advil, Bayer Select, Motrin and Nuprin Caplets. NSAIDs are contraindicated for persons who are allergic to or who cannot tolerate aspirin.

TYPE OF REASONING: DEDUCTIVE

This question requires the test taker to recall the properties of ibuprofen to arrive at a correct conclusion. This is factual recall of guidelines, which is a deductive reasoning skill. For this case, ibuprofen is a nonsteroidal antiinflammatory drug that is used to treat mild to moderate pain and inflammation. If answered incorrectly, review indications for use of ibuprofen.

B131 | Cardiovascular/Pulmonary | Interventions

When trying to improve the breathing pattern of a patient with a diagnosis of chronic emphysema, a technique the physical therapist assistant should emphasize is:

CHOICES:

1. having the patient supine with a pillow under the knees.
2. pursed-lip expiration.
3. forceful inspiration.
4. maximal use of accessory muscles during the breathing pattern.

CORRECT ANSWER: 2

RATIONALE:

The primary problem for patients with emphysema is air trapping, resulting in overly inflated lungs. Use of accessory muscles will only increase the trapping of the air and continue the overinflation of the lungs. A pursed-lip breathing pattern facilitates the goal of emptying the lungs. A seated rather than supine position is best. Expiration, not inspiration, should be emphasized.

TYPE OF REASONING: DEDUCTIVE

Knowledge of breathing techniques for patients with chronic emphysema is paramount for arriving at a correct conclusion for this question. One must recall breathing technique guidelines, which is a deductive reasoning skill. For this situation, the assistant should emphasize pursed-lip breathing strategies to facilitate emptying the lungs. If answered incorrectly, review breathing strategies and techniques for patients with chronic emphysema.

B132 | Devices, Admin, etc. | Equipment, Modalities

When one is instructing a patient in descending a curb utilizing a cane, the **BEST** procedure is for the patient to hold the cane on the side:

CHOICES:

1. of the weaker extremity, with the weaker extremity and cane leading, when descending followed by the stronger extremity.
2. of the weaker extremity, with the stronger extremity leading, when descending followed by the weaker extremity and cane.
3. opposite the weaker extremity, with the stronger extremity leading, when descending followed by the weaker extremity and cane.
4. opposite the weaker extremity, with the weaker extremity and cane leading when descending, followed by the stronger extremity.

CORRECT ANSWER: 4

RATIONALE:

When one is using a one-handed device, the device is used opposite the weaker lower extremity. Holding the cane on the opposite side is important in reducing forces created by the abductor muscles at the hip. When descending a step, the patient is instructed to lead with the weaker lower extremity for the stronger lower extremity to eccentrically contract the quadriceps muscles to lower the body to the next step. This protects the affected (weaker) lower extremity.

TYPE OF REASONING: DEDUCTIVE

One must recall the proper procedures for descending a curb utilizing a cane to arrive at a correct conclusion. This necessitates the factual recall of guidelines and procedures, which is a deductive reasoning skill. For this case, the patient should hold the cane on the side opposite the weaker extremity, with the weaker extremity and cane leading when descending, followed by the stronger extremity. If answered incorrectly, review gait training guidelines, including procedures for descending a curb with an assistive device.

B133 | Other Systems | Clinical Applications

A patient who is 3 months post–cerebrovascular accident is being treated in physical therapy for adhesive capsulitis of the right shoulder. Today, the patient reports new symptoms including burning pain in the right upper extremity that is increased by the dependent position along with lowered pain threshold and heightened sensitivity to light touch. The right hand is mildly edematous and the skin is dry and warm to touch. The intervention that should be **AVOIDED** by the physical therapist assistant in this case is:

CHOICES:

1. stress-loading activities with weight-bearing on the affected extremity.
2. passive manipulation of the shoulder.
3. positional elevation, compression and gentle massage.
4. active assistive range of motion exercises of the shoulder.

CORRECT ANSWER: 2

RATIONALE:

This patient is demonstrating early signs of complex regional pain syndrome (CRPS), type I (also known as reflex sympathetic dystrophy). Stage I (early) changes include those described in the question and typically begin up to 10 days following injury. Stage II (dystrophic stage) and stage III (atrophic stage) changes typically develop later (3 to 6 months and 6 to 12 months, respectively) and are less responsive to treatment. In stage I CRPS all the treatments listed can be used except passive manipulation, which may aggravate sympathetically maintained pain.

TYPE OF REASONING: ANALYTICAL

This question provides symptoms and the test taker must first determine the likely diagnosis and the intervention approach to be avoided. This requires analytical reasoning skill. For this case, the intervention to be avoided is passive manipulation of the shoulder, as the symptoms indicate complex regional pain syndrome. If answered incorrectly, review intervention guidelines for complex regional pain syndrome.

B134 | Cardiovascular/Pulmonary | Clinical Applications

A physical therapist assistant is working with a patient who had a myocardial infarction 4 weeks ago. Resistive training using weights to improve muscular strength and endurance is appropriate:

CHOICES:
1. if exercise intensities are kept below 85% maximal voluntary contraction.
2. if exercise capacity is greater than 5 METs with no anginal symptoms or ST segment depression.
3. during all phases of rehabilitation if judicious monitoring of heart rate is used.
4. only during post–acute phase III cardiac rehabilitation.

CORRECT ANSWER: 2

RATIONALE:

Resistance training is typically initiated after patients have completed 4 to 6 weeks of supervised cardiorespiratory endurance exercise. Lower intensities are prescribed. Careful monitoring of blood pressure is necessary as blood pressure will be higher and heart rate lower than for aerobic exercise. Contraindications to resistance training include unstable angina, uncontrolled arrhythmias, recent history of congestive heart failure, left ventricular outflow obstruction, severe valvular disease and uncontrolled hypertension. Patients should demonstrate an exercise capacity greater than 5 METs without anginal symptoms or ST segment depression (source: American College of Sports Medicine: *Guidelines for Exercise Testing and Prescription*, ed. 6).

TYPE OF REASONING: INDUCTIVE

One must have knowledge of cardiac rehabilitation guidelines for patients with myocardial infarction to arrive at a correct conclusion. This knowledge is coupled with clinical judgment, which necessitates inductive reasoning skill. For this situation, resistive training using weights to improve muscular strength and endurance is appropriate if the exercise capacity is greater than 5 METs with no anginal symptoms or ST segment depression. If answered incorrectly, review cardiac rehabilitation guidelines and use of resistive training.

B135 | Musculoskeletal | Interventions

To instruct a patient to perform assisted hamstring stretching in the pool a physical therapist assistant should instruct the patient to submerge to the waist, place a buoyant ankle strap around the ankle and have the patient:

CHOICES:
1. walk forward and backward taking very large steps and not allow the foot to raise toward the top of the water.
2. stand facing the wall and allow knee flexion to occur.
3. stand with the back against the pool wall allowing hip flexion to occur.
4. lie supine in the water and perform large, slow flutter kicks.

CORRECT ANSWER: 3

RATIONALE:

Standing with the back against the pool wall and allowing hip flexion to occur will assist with hamstring range of motion as the buoyant ankle weight will create a flexion movement at the hip. Standing and facing the wall while allowing the buoyant ankle strap to raise the foot will work to increase knee flexion. Performing work to overcome the buoyancy of the ankle strap will increase strength of a muscle. Both walking with large steps and performing flutter kicks will increase the work of the lower-extremity musculature and strengthen, not stretch, the muscles.

TYPE OF REASONING: INDUCTIVE

This question requires clinical judgment to determine a best course of action for a patient performing hamstring stretches in a pool. This requires knowledge of therapeutic muscle-stretching guidelines, which is an inductive reasoning skill. For this case, the patient should stand with the back against the pool wall, allowing hip flexion to occur. If answered incorrectly, review water-based stretching exercises, especially hamstring stretches.

B136 | Cardiovascular/Pulmonary | Clinical Applications

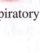

A patient with chronic obstructive pulmonary disease has developed respiratory acidosis. The physical therapist assistant working with the patient should monitor the patient closely for:

CHOICES:

1. disorientation.
2. tingling or numbness of the extremities.
3. dizziness or lightheadedness.
4. hyperreflexia.

CORRECT ANSWER: 1

RATIONALE:

A patient with respiratory acidosis may present with many symptoms of increased carbon dioxide levels in the arterial blood. Significant acidosis may lead to disorientation, stupor or coma. The other choices are signs and symptoms of respiratory alkalosis or a decrease of carbon dioxide in the arterial blood.

TYPE OF REASONING: DEDUCTIVE

This question requires one to recall the common symptoms of respiratory acidosis to arrive at a correct conclusion. This is factual information, which is a deductive reasoning skill. For this case, one should monitor the patient closely for disorientation, a common symptom of respiratory acidosis. If answered incorrectly, review signs and symptoms of respiratory acidosis.

B137 | Devices, Admin, etc. | Safety Roles, Teaching, EBP

A physical therapist assistant is working in a single-story long-term care facility. The emergency call for a tornado warning has been announced over the speaker system. The assistant should respond by:

CHOICES:

1. evacuating residents from the building to the designated gathering location outside the building.
2. removing residents from rooms, closing doors and placing residents in hallways.
3. removing residents from the location of the building most affected and closing safety doors at the entrance to that hallway.
4. immediately discontinuing treatment in the gym area and returning residents to their rooms.

CORRECT ANSWER: 2

RATIONALE:

In a tornado situation the general rule is to remove residents from the exterior of the building near windows, shutting room doors and keeping residents and personnel on the interior of the building away from glass and flying debris. Evacuating residents from a building or removing them from an area and isolating that area is the response in the case of a fire. One should not return residents to their rooms in the case of a natural disaster as it is typical to cluster or protect the residents in some way.

TYPE OF REASONING: EVALUATIVE

One must determine the best course of action by weighing the merits of the actions presented to determine a correct conclusion. This requires evaluative reasoning skill, where one evaluates actions and determines their benefits. For this case, the assistant should remove residents from rooms, closing doors and placing residents in hallways. Review tornado response guidelines in healthcare facilities if answered incorrectly.

B138 | Neuromuscular | Clinical Applications

The **MOST** appropriate positioning strategy for a patient recovering from acute stroke who is in bed and who demonstrates a flaccid upper extremity is:

CHOICES:

1. side-lying on the sound side with the affected shoulder protracted, and arm extended resting on a pillow.
2. supine with the affected arm flexed with hand resting on stomach, pillow placed under knees.
3. supine with the affected elbow extended and arm positioned close to the side of the trunk.
4. side-lying on the sound side with the affected upper extremity flexed overhead.

CORRECT ANSWER: 1

RATIONALE:

Most patients with stroke recover from the flaccid stage and develop spasticity. Positioning for the patient with early stroke stresses (1) protects against ligamentous strain and the development of a painful subluxed shoulder and (2) positions counter to the typical spastic posture of flexion and adduction with pronation. Side-lying with the affected upper extremity supported on a pillow with the shoulder protracted and elbow extended accomplishes both of these goals. The other positions do not.

TYPE OF REASONING: DEDUCTIVE

One must recall the guidelines for positioning patients with stroke and a flaccid upper extremity in bed to arrive at a correct conclusion. This is factual information, necessitating deductive reasoning skill. For this situation, the patient should be positioned side-lying on the sound side with the affected shoulder protracted, and arm extended resting on a pillow. If answered incorrectly, review bed positioning guidelines for patients with stroke.

B139 | Devices, Admin, etc. | Equipment, Modalities

The effect that will not occur by placing a hot pack around the ankle is:

CHOICES:

1. increased subcutaneous tissue temperature.
2. hyperemia.
3. increased sympathetic response.
4. increased collagen tissue extensibility.

CORRECT ANSWER: 3

RATIONALE:

A sympathetic response does not occur when peripheral/superficial heat is applied to an area. Sympathetic responses are the "fight or flight" responses and affect the viscera of the body. It will not occur as a result of application of superficial heat.

TYPE OF REASONING: INFERENTIAL

This question requires one to determine what will not occur when one is using a hot pack. This requires one to infer a potential outcome, which is an inferential reasoning skill. For this case, increased sympathetic response will not occur by placing a hot pack around the ankle. If answered incorrectly, review outcomes of using superficial heat on joints.

B140 | Other Systems | Data Collection

A physical therapist assistant working with a patient who has a blood glucose level that is 68 mg/dL should:

CHOICES:
1. administer a carbohydrate snack and continue to exercise unless further symptoms occur.
2. call for immediate emergency assistance and prepare to initiate life-saving measures.
3. continue to exercise as usual but do not add more activities into the routine.
4. administer a carbohydrate snack and retest in 15 minutes prior to proceeding.

CORRECT ANSWER: 4

RATIONALE:
The ideal range for blood glucose is between 80 mg/dL and 120 mg/dL for individuals. Blood glucose levels below 70 mg/dL and above 120 mg/dL should be closely monitored and a carbohydrate snack should be given to individuals whose levels are 70 mg/dL or lower. Once a carbohydrate snack is administered one must wait 15 minutes and retest the blood glucose level to ensure appropriate levels prior to beginning activity.

TYPE OF REASONING: EVALUATIVE
This question requires one to determine the benefits of the courses of action presented to determine the one that will effectively resolve the patient's issue. This is an evaluative reasoning skill. For this scenario, the assistant should administer a carbohydrate snack and retest in 15 minutes prior to proceeding. If answered incorrectly, review intervention approaches for patients with low blood glucose.

B141 | Musculoskeletal | Data Collection

During gait training the physical therapist assistant observes a patient exhibit an anterior trunk lean from heel strike (initial contact) through midstance. This gait deviation is likely the result of:

CHOICES:
1. weak hip extensors.
2. weak knee extensors.
3. weak hip flexors.
4. tight hip extensors.

CORRECT ANSWER: 2

RATIONALE:
Leaning forward from heel strike (initial contact) through midstance will biomechanically lock the knee. When the foot is in a weight-bearing position, the upper body is in front of the knee, and the center of gravity is behind the knee. Having the center of gravity behind the knee causes the knee to be locked in extension, which compensates for the weakened quadriceps muscles. If the patient did not lean forward the knees might buckle at initial contact.

TYPE OF REASONING: INFERENTIAL
One must determine the likely reason for an anterior trunk lean from heel strike through midstance to arrive at a correct conclusion. This requires one to determine what may be true of a situation, which is an inferential reasoning skill. For this case, the likely reason for this gait deviation is weak knee extensors. If answered incorrectly, review gait deviation patterns, including patterns resulting from week knee extensors.

B142 | Cardiovascular/Pulmonary | Interventions

Three days following a myocardial infarction it is **CONTRAINDICATED** to include:

CHOICES:

1. upper extremity exercise using 5 pound weights.
2. exercise that increases the heart rate 10 to 15 beats per minute over the resting level.
3. exercises in the 2 to 3 MET range.
4. short-duration exercise sessions.

CORRECT ANSWER: 1

RATIONALE:

Upper-body resistive exercise is contraindicated immediately following a myocardial infarction. These exercises are avoided to prevent or minimize the occurrence of the Valsalva maneuver, which occurs when a person holds his or her breath during a strenuous activity. Also, upper-extremity exercises put too much strain on the patient's heart.

TYPE OF REASONING: DEDUCTIVE

This question requires the test taker to recall the contraindications for exercise for patients with myocardial infarction to arrive at a correct conclusion. This is factual recall of guidelines, which is a deductive reasoning skill. For this situation, it is contraindicated to include upper-extremity exercise using 5-pound weights. If answered incorrectly, review cardiac rehabilitation guidelines for patients with myocardial infarction.

B143 | Cardiovascular/Pulmonary | Interventions

When instructing a patient in diaphragmatic breathing, the physical therapist assistant should:

CHOICES:

1. ensure that the upper chest, not the abdomen, rises on inspiration.
2. place the hands at the lateral costal margins for proprioceptive feedback.
3. place the hands on the rectus abdominis just below the anterior costal margin.
4. have the patient shrug the shoulders on inspiration to facilitate diaphragmatic movement.

CORRECT ANSWER: 3

RATIONALE:

Diaphragmatic breathing is taught to increase use of the diaphragm versus accessory muscles during inspiration. The patient should be in a semi-Fowler position as the assistant places the hands over the abdomen and anterior ribs. The upper chest and shoulders should remain quiet. Lateral costal expansion is not desirable when one is emphasizing diaphragmatic breathing.

TYPE OF REASONING: DEDUCTIVE

One must recall the diaphragmatic breathing guidelines to arrive at a correct conclusion. This necessitates the recollection of factual information, which is a deductive reasoning skill. For this case, the assistant should place the hands on the rectus abdominis just below the anterior costal margin. If answered incorrectly, review diaphragmatic breathing guidelines.

B144 | Devices, Admin, etc. | Safety Roles, Teaching, EBP

A researcher expects to find **NO** significant difference between 20- and 30 year-olds after a 12-week exercise training program using exercise heart rates and myocardial oxygen consumption as measures of performance. This is an example of which kind of hypothesis?

CHOICES:
1. experimental hypothesis.
2. research hypothesis.
3. null hypothesis.
4. directional hypothesis.

CORRECT ANSWER: 3

RATIONALE:

The null hypothesis is a statistical hypothesis that states that there is no relationship (or difference) between variables. Any relationship found will be a chance relationship, not a true one. A directional or research (experimental) hypothesis predicts an expected relationship between variables (e.g., 20 year-olds will demonstrate improved measures of performance compared with 30 year-olds).

TYPE OF REASONING: ANALYTICAL

This question provides a research definition and the test taker must determine the term associated with this principle. This requires one to analyze the information provided to determine the appropriate definition, necessitating analytical reasoning skill. For this scenario, the definition is an example of a null hypothesis. If answered incorrectly, review research guidelines, especially hypothesis definitions.

B145 | Devices, Admin, etc. | Equipment, Modalities

Following a dorsal hand burn, an upper-extremity orthosis designed to provide functional positioning should accentuate slight wrist:

CHOICES:
1. extension, MCP extension and IP extension.
2. flexion, MCP flexion and IP flexion.
3. extension, MCP flexion and IP extension.
4. flexion, MCP extension and IP flexion.

CORRECT ANSWER: 3

RATIONALE:

After a burn, it is important to splint the affected area in a functional position. The functional position of the hand is slight wrist extension, metacarpophalangeal (MCP) flexion and interphalangeal (IP) extension. Splinting in this position will prevent wrist and finger flexion contractures.

TYPE OF REASONING: DEDUCTIVE

This question requires one to recall the guidelines for hand splinting after burns. This is factual information, requiring deductive reasoning skill. For this case, the functional hand splinting position includes slight wrist extension, MCP flexion and IP extension. Review splinting guidelines for patients with hand burns if answered incorrectly.

B146 | Devices, Admin, etc. | Safety Roles, Teaching, EBP

The **FIRST** step in a motor relearning program includes observation and analysis of the functional activity. The next step is to:

CHOICES:

1. practice the activity in the realistic environment.
2. practice components of the activity in a controlled environment.
3. practice the activity in a controlled environment.
4. practice the activity in a new environment.

CORRECT ANSWER: 2

RATIONALE:

Motor learning focuses on the patient learning correct movement patterns through observation, explanation and practice. To best accomplish this, components of the functional activity are practiced before the entire activity; components of the activities do not have to be perfected to progress to the next step. As components of tasks are practiced and mastered, then the entire activity itself is incorporated into controlled environments with appropriate feedback. The last step is to transfer the skills to new contexts.

TYPE OF REASONING: DEDUCTIVE

One must recall the steps in a motor relearning program to arrive at a correct conclusion. This necessitates the recall of a therapeutic procedure, which is factual information and a deductive reasoning skill. For this situation, the next step is to practice components of the activity in a controlled environment. If answered incorrectly, review motor relearning program procedures.

B147 | Other Systems | Interventions

A patient with diabetes is exercising. The patient reports feeling weak, dizzy and somewhat nauseous. The assistant notices that the patient is sweating profusely and is unsteady when standing. The assistant's **FIRST** course of action should be to:

CHOICES:

1. administer orange juice for developing hypoglycemia.
2. call emergency services for an insulin reaction.
3. have a nurse administer an insulin injection for developing hyperglycemia.
4. insist that the patient sit down until the orthostatic hypotension resolves.

CORRECT ANSWER: 1

RATIONALE:

Hypoglycemia, abnormally low blood glucose, results from too much insulin (insulin reaction). It requires accurate assessment of symptoms and prompt intervention. Have the patient sit down and give an oral sugar (e.g., orange juice). Once the patient is stabilized, the physician should be notified. Profuse sweating does not usually accompany orthostatic hypotension.

TYPE OF REASONING: EVALUATIVE

For this question, the test taker must determine an appropriate course of action among the choices provided to determine the action that will effectively resolve the patient's symptoms. This requires evaluative reasoning skill. For this case, the assistant's first course of action should be to administer orange juice for developing hypoglycemia. If answered incorrectly, review first aid procedures for patients with hypoglycemia.

B148 | Other Systems | Clinical Applications

A physical therapist assistant is reviewing the plan of care of a patient prior to initiating balance training activities. The initial evaluation revealed that upon admission the patient had a positive fecal blood test. Which lab value is **MOST IMPORTANT** for the assistant to check prior to administering balance retraining activities today?

CHOICES:

1. hematocrit.
2. leukocytes.
3. platelet count.
4. erythrocyte sedimentation rate.

CORRECT ANSWER: 1

RATIONALE:

If the hematocrit (HCT) value is within the normal range for both males and females it indicates that the fecal blood loss is not significant at treatment time and should not affect the patient's ability to tolerate activity. Low HCT levels can be significant as decreased levels can lead to decreased exercise tolerance, decreased endurance and orthostatic intolerance. The leukocytes, platelets and erythrocyte sedimentation rate can be low, but will not impact balance.

TYPE OF REASONING: INDUCTIVE

One must utilize clinical judgment to determine the most important lab value to check prior to administering balance retraining activities for patients with a positive fecal blood test. This is an inductive reasoning skill. For this scenario, it is most important to check the hematocrit prior to administering balance retraining, as it can provide an indication of fecal blood loss. If answered incorrectly, review lab values for patients with blood loss.

B149 | Other Systems | Clinical Applications

Patients with diabetes are at risk for developing plantar ulcers and should be reminded by the physical therapist assistant to avoid:

CHOICES:

1. pressure from footwear and walking barefoot.
2. soaking the feet daily in tepid water.
3. applying mineral oil or lotion to the feet daily.
4. wearing well-fitting jogging shoes instead of leather shoes for use as primary footwear.

CORRECT ANSWER: 1

RATIONALE:

A patient with diabetes often has circulation and sensory impairments. Because of these impairments the patient is at great risk for skin breakdown and open wounds that may go undetected. This can lead to chronic open areas, skin ulcers and/or infections, which could ultimately lead to amputation. The remaining options will assist the patient in maintaining the integrity of the skin on the plantar surface of the foot. The other suggestions are appropriate foot care for patients with diabetes.

TYPE OF REASONING: INDUCTIVE

One must utilize knowledge of diabetic foot care guidelines to arrive at a correct conclusion. This requires inductive reasoning skill, as clinical judgment is paramount to arriving at a correct conclusion. For this case, the patient should be instructed to avoid pressure from footwear and walking barefoot to avoid pressure ulcers. If answered incorrectly, review diabetic foot care guidelines and appropriate footwear.

B150 | Neuromuscular | Data Collection

A physical therapist assistant working with a patient who had an injury to the median nerve following a Colles' fracture should expect to see a strength deficit of which muscle?

CHOICES:

1. pronator teres.
2. extensor indicis.
3. flexor digiti minimi.
4. flexor digitorum superficialis.

CORRECT ANSWER: 4

RATIONALE:

Both the flexor digitorum superficialis (FDS) and the pronator teres are innervated by the median nerve. However, the distal nerve supply to the FDS is more likely to be injured in a Colles' fracture than is the more proximal innervation of the pronator teres muscle. The extensor indicis is innervated by the radial nerve, and the flexor digiti minimi is innervated by the ulnar nerve and neither is likely to be affected with a median nerve injury.

TYPE OF REASONING: INFERENTIAL

One must infer or draw a reasonable conclusion about the likely muscle that will be weakened after a Colles' fracture. This requires the test taker to determine what may be true for a diagnosis, which is an inferential reasoning skill. For this scenario, one should expect to see a strength deficit of the flexor digitorum superficialis. If answered incorrectly, review muscle strength deficits following a Colles' fracture.

Examination C

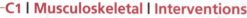

C1 | Musculoskeletal | Interventions

A physical therapist has directed a physical therapist assistant to provide strengthening exercises for a patient with a chronically inflamed biceps brachii muscle that has a painful arc of motion. The **MOST** efficient intervention is:

CHOICES:

1. isometric exercises at the end of range of movement.
2. active concentric contractions through partial range of motion.
3. active eccentric contractions in the pain-free range.
4. isokinetic exercises through the full range of motion.

CORRECT ANSWER: 3

RATIONALE:

Isokinetic, isometric and isotonic exercises do not allow for pain-free muscle contractions and can cause further inflammation of the muscle. For a muscle that is chronically inflamed, focus should be placed on eccentric contractions because there is less effort and stress placed on the contractile units compared with concentric contractions at the same level of work.

TYPE OF REASONING: INDUCTIVE

This question requires one to assess the benefits of each of the intervention approaches presented and then to determine the approach that will minimize pain and improve function. This requires inductive reasoning skill, which is often utilized when one is making judgments about a best therapeutic approach. In this situation, the assistant should choose active eccentric contractions in the pain-free range. If answered incorrectly, review therapeutic exercises for chronically inflamed muscles.

C2 | Devices, Admin, etc. | Safety Roles, Teaching, EBP

A patient who is terminally ill with cancer begins to cry during the physical therapy session. The **BEST** approach should be to:

CHOICES:

1. ask the patient questions while continuing to administer therapy.
2. ignore the tears and focus on therapy in a compassionate manner.
3. take time to allow the patient to express any feelings.
4. encourage denial to enable them to better cope with the challenges that lie ahead.

CORRECT ANSWER: 3

RATIONALE:

It is important to be supportive of a patient who is confronting death. Allow the patient to verbalize feelings and frustrations. The patient will develop a trust level and will engage in therapy.

TYPE OF REASONING: EVALUATIVE

This question requires one to determine the best approach for a patient who is confronting death. Questions of this nature that ask one to evaluate the statements made to others and their effectiveness require evaluative reasoning skill. In this situation, it is best to take time to allow the patient to express any feelings. If answered incorrectly, review strategies for helping patients cope with illness experiences.

C3 | Other Systems | Interventions

A patient with a right transtibial amputation, secondary to complications of diabetes, has just completed ambulating 100 feet with a walker. The patient now reports dizziness, shaking, fatigue and weakness. Upon questioning, the patient also reports not having eaten breakfast because of lack of appetite. The **MOST** appropriate intervention should be to:

CHOICES:

1. have the patient take insulin.
2. give the patient orange juice.
3. give the patient a glass of water.
4. have the patient rest, and then continue therapy.

CORRECT ANSWER: 2

RATIONALE:

The patient is exhibiting signs of hypoglycemia and needs a quick intake of glucose, which orange juice contains. Continuing therapy, water intake and insulin will only decrease the blood sugar level and not be beneficial for the patient.

TYPE OF REASONING: ANALYTIC

This question requires the test taker to analyze the symptoms presented and then determine the cause for these symptoms. Once this determination is made, one must then decide the best course of action. This necessitates analytical reasoning skill. For this case, the patient's symptoms are caused by hypoglycemia and the best course of action is to give the patient orange juice. If answered incorrectly, review symptoms of and remedies for hypoglycemia.

C4 | Cardiovascular/Pulmonary | Data Collection

A physical therapist assistant is working with a patient who has pulmonary disease. The patient's oxygen saturation levels are being monitored continuously with a pulse oximeter attached to the patient's finger. The patient's saturation levels are approximately 90% to 92%. The physical therapist assistant should stop treatment if the oximeter reading initially drops below:

CHOICES:

1. 90%.
2. 82%.
3. 72%.
4. 88%.

CORRECT ANSWER: 4

RATIONALE:

Normal oxygen saturation levels are between 96% and 100%. Systems are being deprived of oxygen if the oxygen saturation point is below 90% to 95%, and become dangerously low if readings fall below 88%. Activity should be stopped and appropriate personnel as well as the supervising physical therapist should be informed.

TYPE OF REASONING: INDUCTIVE

One must determine the pulse oximetry reading that indicates the need to stop treatment. This requires inductive reasoning skill, a skill that requires clinical judgment to determine a best course of action. In this case, when the initial reading drops below 88%, the treatment should stop. If answered incorrectly, review pulse oximetry monitoring guidelines, especially when to stop activity during monitoring.

C5 | Cardiovascular/Pulmonary | Data Collection

A physical therapist assistant checks the vital signs of a patient who has a history of cardiac disease. The heart rate is steady at 60 beats per minute; respiratory rate is eight breaths per minute; blood pressure is 120/70 mmHg and the oral temperature is 98.6°F. The vital sign that presents the **GREATEST** concern at this time is the patient's:

CHOICES:

1. respiratory rate.
2. heart rate.
3. blood pressure.
4. temperature.

CORRECT ANSWER: 1

RATIONALE:

The normal adult respiratory rate should be 12 to 18 breaths per minute. A rate of eight breaths per minute is cause for concern. If it continues, there will be changes in other vital signs and the patient may be in danger. Although the heart rate is on the low end of normal, it is not cause for concern. However, with the decreased respiratory rate, the heart rate may begin to further drop. The blood pressure is well within normal limits for an adult. The temperature is normal for an adult.

TYPE OF REASONING: DEDUCTIVE

One must review all of the vital signs presented and then determine the vital sign that is of greatest concern, based on one's understanding of factual guidelines. This is a deductive reasoning skill, where factual guidelines are utilized to determine normal versus abnormal parameters. In this case, the only vital sign that is not within normal parameters is the patient's respiratory rate. If answered incorrectly, review vital signs guidelines, especially normal respiratory rate.

C6 | Devices, Admin, etc. | Equipment, Modalities

The physical therapist has identified that a patient needs a spiral ankle–foot orthosis. A spiral ankle–foot orthosis is utilized primarily for:

CHOICES:

1. limiting dorsiflexion.
2. limiting plantar flexion.
3. medial or lateral instability of the ankle.
4. increasing plantar flexion.

CORRECT ANSWER: 3

RATIONALE:

A spiral ankle–foot orthosis can correct either medial or lateral ankle instability. This type of orthotic device places pressure on either side of the ankle to aid in stability. A spiral ankle–foot orthosis would not discourage dorsiflexion or plantar flexion, as it does not provide anterior or posterior control.

TYPE OF REASONING: INFERENTIAL

One must infer or draw a reasonable conclusion about the purpose of a spiral ankle–foot orthosis. This necessitates inferential reasoning skill, which often requires one to determine what may be true of a therapeutic process or procedure. In this case, the spiral ankle–foot orthosis is utilized primarily for medial or lateral instability of the ankle. Review lower-extremity orthotics, especially spiral ankle–foot orthoses, if answered incorrectly.

C7 | Integumentary | Data Collection

Prior to beginning prosthetic training with a patient, the physical therapist assistant notices an area of redness and a slight blister on the distal aspect of the residual limb. This is consistent with:

CHOICES:

1. a stage I pressure ulcer.
2. a stage II pressure ulcer.
3. a normal tissue response to weight-bearing in the new prosthesis.
4. the need to decrease the number of sock plies during gait training.

CORRECT ANSWER: 2

RATIONALE:

A stage II pressure ulcer presents clinically as an abrasion, blister or shallow crater; it is partial-thickness and involves the epidermis, dermis or both and is considered superficial. A stage I pressure ulcer presents clinically as nonblanchable erythema of intact skin; it may include changes in skin temperature (warm or cool), tissue consistency (boggy or firm), and/or sensation (pain, itching). Any stage pressure ulcer formation is cause to discontinue gait training with a prosthesis. The physical therapist assistant should inform the supervising physical therapist as well as the nurse in charge of the patient.

TYPE OF REASONING: ANALYTICAL

One must analyze the symptoms presented and then draw a conclusion about what these symptoms represent. This requires analytical reasoning skill, where various pieces of information are analyzed (such as symptoms) to draw a conclusion. In this case, the symptoms indicate a stage II pressure ulcer. Review symptoms and features of pressure ulcers if answered incorrectly.

C8 | Neuromuscular | Clinical Applications

A physical therapist assistant working with a patient 4 weeks following a right-sided cerebrovascular accident (CVA) should expect the patient to exhibit:

CHOICES:

1. poor judgment and decreased safety awareness.
2. negative disposition, self-deprecating comments and depression.
3. slow, cautious behaviors.
4. hesitancy, requiring more feedback and support.

CORRECT ANSWER: 1

RATIONALE:

A patient who has suffered a right-sided CVA will typically demonstrate poor judgment with numerous safety issues. The patient with left-sided CVA will demonstrate cautious, slow behaviors and require more feedback and support.

TYPE OF REASONING: INFERENTIAL

Questions that ask one to determine the likely presentation or deficits of a patient often necessitate inferential reasoning skill. Inferential reasoning skill asks one to determine what is likely to be true in a situation, though one cannot always be absolutely certain. In this case, the patient with a right-sided CVA will most likely exhibit poor judgment and decreased safety awareness. If answered incorrectly, review differences between right- versus left-sided CVA symptomatology, especially symptoms of right-sided CVA.

C9 | Neuromuscular | Clinical Applications

A physical therapist assistant is treating a patient who has a diagnosis of Parkinson's disease. Which of the following should the assistant expect to see during ambulation?

CHOICES:

1. Shuffling gait pattern and weakness on one side.
2. Decreased trunk rotation and decreased arm swing.
3. Decreased step length bilaterally and unilaterally decreased weight-bearing.
4. Forward stooped posture and internally rotated hips bilaterally.

CORRECT ANSWER: 2

RATIONALE:

Gait changes characteristic of Parkinson's disease include those noted, as well as a shuffling gait and festinating cadence. One should expect to see one-sided weakness and potentially leaning toward the affected side during ambulation with a person who had suffered a stroke. A patient may demonstrate decreased step lengths on the surgical side following a hip arthroplasty and should likely also demonstrate decreased weight-bearing on the surgical side. There are different types of cerebral palsy, one of which may include bilateral internally rotated hips; however, cerebral palsy is not associated with forward stooped posture.

TYPE OF REASONING: INFERENTIAL

One must determine the most likely ambulation pattern of a patient who has Parkinson's disease. This requires one to infer the likely features, which is an inferential reasoning skill. For this situation, the assistant should expect to see decreased trunk rotation and decreased arm swing. Review symptoms of Parkinson's disease if answered incorrectly, especially ambulation patterns.

C10 | Musculoskeletal | Clinical Applications

A physical therapist has directed a physical therapist assistant to provide therapeutic exercises to a patient in the early stages of care for a musculoskeletal injury to the shoulder. Which of the following exercises should the assistant implement?

CHOICES:

1. pendulum exercise.
2. active range of motion exercises focused on abduction and lateral (external) rotation.
3. strengthening of the rhomboids and lower trapezius.
4. strengthening of the rotator cuff muscles.

CORRECT ANSWER: 1

RATIONALE:

During the initial phase of rehabilitation the damaged structures should be protected to allow healing. Pendulum exercises are passive exercises; thus, they do not stress the damaged tissues. In addition, they provide movement of the joint surfaces and maintain movement and nutrition within the joint itself. Immediately following a muscular or soft tissue injury the structures are protected and resistance is avoided.

TYPE OF REASONING: INDUCTIVE

One must determine the best exercises to implement for a patient, considering the diagnosis provided. This is an inductive reasoning skill, where clinical judgment is utilized to draw conclusions. For this patient with musculoskeletal injury to the shoulder, it is best to initiate intervention with pendulum exercises. If answered incorrectly, review indications for use of pendulum exercises and interventions for musculoskeletal shoulder injuries.

C11 | Neuromuscular | Data Collection

The physical therapist has directed the physical therapist assistant to monitor a patient's equilibrium reactions during functional activity training. The physical therapist assistant should accomplish this by:

CHOICES:

1. having the patient sit unsupported while reaching forward, and by observing the patient's recovery.
2. having the patient bring his knee to his chest, while the assistant applies manual resistance in the sitting position.
3. having the patient bring his finger from his nose to the assistant's finger.
4. having the patient tap his toe as fast as possible.

CORRECT ANSWER: 1

RATIONALE:

To test a patient's equilibrium reactions a physical therapist assistant can observe whether a patient has adequate recovery when reaching outside the base of support. Appropriate responses would include elongation of the trunk with shortening on the opposite side, or abduction or extension of the upper extremity. Knee to chest is for testing strength of the hip flexors. Toe tapping tests the patient's coordination. Finger to nose tests coordination and would reveal dysmetria if present.

TYPE OF REASONING: INFERENTIAL

This question requires one to determine the best way to assess a patient's equilibrium reactions. This necessitates inferential reasoning skill, where the test taker infers a best course of action. In this scenario, the assistant should perform this test by having the patient sit unsupported while reaching forward and observing the patient's recovery. If answered incorrectly, review equilibrium reaction testing guidelines.

C12 | Neuromuscular | Data Collection

The grasp reflex in an infant develops with:

CHOICES:

1. voluntary release first, then transfers from hand to hand, followed by reflexive grasp, and finally voluntary grasp.
2. voluntary grasp first, then reflexive grasp, followed by voluntary release, and finally transfers from hand to hand.
3. reflexive grasp first, then voluntary release, followed by voluntary grasp, and finally transfers from hand to hand.
4. reflexive grasp first, then voluntary grasp, followed by voluntary release, and finally transfers from hand to hand.

CORRECT ANSWER: 4

RATIONALE:

Grasping skills progress from a reflexive grasp to a voluntary grasp. Only after the child can grasp voluntarily do release skills develop. Transferring skills need both voluntary grasp and release, and develop last.

TYPE OF REASONING: DEDUCTIVE

One must recall factual guidelines of infant motor development to arrive at a correct conclusion. Recall of factual guidelines requires deductive reasoning skill. For this question, the grasp reflex in an infant develops with reflexive grasp first, then voluntary grasp, followed by voluntary release, and transfers from hand to hand. If answered incorrectly, review infant motor development guidelines, especially the grasp reflex.

C13 | Devices, Admin, etc. | Safety Roles, Teaching, EBP

A patient with hepatitis B receives a bleeding skin tear on the right calf during a treatment session. To prevent transmission of the disease while cleaning up, the physical therapist assistant should:

CHOICES:

1. wash both hands before and after cleaning up.
2. wipe up the blood with gauze and dispose in a trash container.
3. wear disposable gloves.
4. wear a mask with a splash guard.

CORRECT ANSWER: 3

RATIONALE:

Hepatitis B is a bloodborne pathogen that causes a viral infection. It is transmitted only via body fluids to noninfected people. Universal (standard) precautions should be followed including wearing gloves, washing after touching the patient and using a disinfectant. Although universal (standard) precautions call for washing hands prior to patient contact for their protection, this does nothing to prevent transmission of the pathogen to the physical therapist assistant. Healthcare workers should always wash hands after contact with body fluids. This situation is unlikely to cause blood or body fluid spray and a mask with a splash guard is not necessary.

TYPE OF REASONING: DEDUCTIVE

One must recall the guidelines for universal (standard) precautions to arrive at a correct conclusion. This is a factual guideline that requires deductive reasoning skill. For this case the therapist should wear disposable gloves to prevent transmission of the hepatitis B virus. Review universal (standard) precautions if answered incorrectly.

C14 | Cardiovascular/Pulmonary | Data Collection

Symptoms of cystic fibrosis include:

CHOICES:

1. rapid respirations with prolonged exhalation phase.
2. persistent cough, shortness of breath, thick greasy stools.
3. persistent cough, thickening of the lining of the bronchial passages.
4. cough, fever, chest pain with deep breathing.

CORRECT ANSWER: 1

RATIONALE:

Cystic fibrosis is a genetic disease that is usually diagnosed within the first year of life. It is an obstructive disorder because of the thickened mucus produced in the lungs and other organs of the body. Other symptoms that can be observed include foul-smelling bowel movements, production of viscous secretions, salty skin secondary to high amounts of salt secreted in perspiration. Chronic bronchitis produces thickening of the lining of the bronchial passages. Chronic bronchitis is often associated with smokers. Emphysema is a pulmonary disease that may develop secondary to prolonged smoking. Symptoms include initial dyspnea with exertion progressing to dyspnea at rest, and rapid respirations with prolonged exhalation phase; cough is uncommon and nonproductive. A cough that may be productive, and is associated with fever and chills, is symptomatic of pneumonia.

TYPE OF REASONING: INFERENTIAL

This question provides a diagnosis and the test taker must determine the symptoms that are associated with cystic fibrosis. Questions of this nature often require inferential reasoning skill, which requires one to infer what is most likely to be true of a situation. For this situation, the symptom most consistent with cystic fibrosis is persistent cough, shortness or breath, and thick greasy stools. If answered incorrectly review symptoms of cystic fibrosis.

C15 | Cardiovascular/Pulmonary | Interventions

A physical therapist assistant is treating a patient on the tilt table secondary to orthostatic hypotension. The patient has been gradually raised from supine to 60° when the patient's blood pressure begins to suddenly decrease. The **MOST** appropriate response is for the assistant to lower the tilt table:

CHOICES:

1. back to 0°, and call the physical therapist for assistance.
2. down in 5° to 10° increments until the blood pressure stabilizes.
3. back to 45° and stay at this level for the remainder of the session.
4. to 0° and call a medical emergency.

CORRECT ANSWER: 2

RATIONALE:

The drop in blood pressure indicates the heart's inability to adapt to the increased demand. The therapeutic outcome of the tilt table is to reacclimate the patient to an upright posture while maintaining appropriate blood pressure responses. Once the patient's blood pressure stabilizes at a certain degree of elevation gradually increase the tilt.

TYPE OF REASONING: INDUCTIVE

This question requires one to utilize clinical judgment to determine a best course of action for a patient with orthostatic hypotension. This necessitates inductive reasoning skill. For this case, the physical therapist assistant should lower the tilt table down in 5° to 10° increments until the blood pressure stabilizes. Review guidelines for the use of a tilt table for orthostatic hypotension if answered incorrectly.

C16 | Musculoskeletal | Clinical Applications

A physical therapist assistant is treating a patient who has a diagnosis of right shoulder adhesive capsulitis with accessory motion dysfunction and noted loss of proper scapulohumeral rhythm. The intervention **MOST** likely to help achieve proper scapulohumeral rhythm of the shoulder complex is:

CHOICES:

1. strengthening exercises for the parascapular muscles and stretching the glenohumeral structures.
2. immobilization to protect joint biomechanics.
3. strengthening exercises for the glenohumeral joint at end range.
4. a manual stretch to achieve normal internal and external rotation at the glenohumeral joint.

CORRECT ANSWER: 1

RATIONALE:

The moving relationship between the scapula and humerus promotes the most effective balance of length and strength for all shoulder girdle muscles; stretching the glenohumeral structures will promote normal joint biomechanics, and strengthening the scapular stabilizers will help maintain the appropriate biomechanical relationship. By definition, the relationships of the scapula and the humerus encourage the fullest amount of functional motion for the shoulder girdle. If the scapulohumeral rhythm is working effectively, the shear and tensile forces should be reduced. Scapulohumeral rhythm has greater impact for flexion and abduction than medial (internal) and lateral (external) rotation.

TYPE OF REASONING: INFERENTIAL

This question requires the test taker to determine an intervention approach that will most likely result in functional improvement. Questions that ask one to determine what may be most beneficial in a therapeutic approach often require inferential reasoning skill. For this scenario, the assistant should initiate strengthening exercises for the parascapular muscles and stretch the glenohumeral structures to achieve the most benefit. If answered incorrectly, review intervention guidelines for adhesive capsulitis.

C17 | Integumentary | Clinical Applications

The physical therapy team members should be **MOST** concerned about the development of keloid scarring with what patient population?

CHOICES:

1. persons of Asian descent.
2. infants and children.
3. the elderly.
4. persons of African American descent.

CORRECT ANSWER: 4

RATIONALE:

The development of keloid scarring is a concern with persons of African, or African American descent, and typically does not develop in persons of Caucasian ancestry. Age is not a factor in the development of keloid scarring. Keloid scarring is characterized as a red and raised scar that extends beyond the boundaries of the original wound.

TYPE OF REASONING: INDUCTIVE

One must utilize clinical judgment to determine the patient population that would present the most concern with the development of keloid scarring. Questions that require clinical judgment often necessitate inductive reasoning skill. For this scenario, team members should be most concerned about keloid scarring in persons of African American descent. If answered incorrectly review information related to keloid scar development.

C18 | Devices, Admin, etc. | Safety Roles, Teaching, EBP

A physical therapist assistant comes upon an unresponsive adult on the floor of the hospital room. After properly position-ing the patient, the physical therapist assistant opens the airway and attempts two slow breaths; the air does not go in. The physical therapist assistant should:

CHOICES:

1. perform the Heimlich maneuver.
2. have someone else perform chest compressions.
3. reposition the head and attempt two more breaths.
4. do nothing, as the person has expired.

CORRECT ANSWER: 3

RATIONALE:

If you have positioned the patient and attempted two breaths but are unsuccessful, you may not have properly positioned the head the first time. The tongue may have fallen into the back of the throat blocking it. You should retilt the head and give two breaths before you assume it is an airway obstruction; you cannot assume an airway obstruction until you retilt the head and try again. Having someone else perform the process will not solve the problem unless the first person is un-trained. You cannot determine whether a person has expired just because you cannot get air into the lungs. After the retilt of the head and an attempt to get air into the lungs is unsuccessful, the Heimlich maneuver must be performed. If there is no pulse once the airway has been opened, cardiac compressions must be started. Only the medical professionals at a hos-pital can pronounce a patient as expired.

TYPE OF REASONING: DEDUCTIVE

This question requires a test taker to recall the factual guidelines for the administration of cardiopulmonary resuscitation (CPR). Factual guidelines often necessitate deductive reasoning skill. For this situation, after one has tried to administer two slow breaths and the air does not go in, the head should be repositioned and two more breaths should be attempted. If answered incorrectly, review CPR guidelines.

C19 | Integumentary | Data Collection

A physical therapist assistant providing intervention to the lower extremity for a patient with a diagnosis of venous insufficiency would expect:

CHOICES:

1. abnormal nail growth, hair loss, dry skin and increased pain.
2. hemosiderin staining, wounds at the proximal medial malleolus and increased tissue temperatures.
3. tissues that appear whitish in color and are very painful.
4. mild pain, edema in one extremity, numbness and tingling.

CORRECT ANSWER: 2

RATIONALE:

Additional signs and symptoms of venous insufficiency include swelling of bilateral lower extremities; there is likely minimal pain, wet tissue in and around the wound, and granulation tissue in the wound bed. Arterial insufficiency presents more closely with wounds located on the lateral malleoli and dorsum of the feet, however can occur proximal to the medial malleolus as well. Arterial insufficiency can also produce trophic changes such as abnormal nail growth, hair loss, and dry skin, much pain, and a necrotic pale wound base. Raynaud's disease typically does not generate wounds, is usually very painful, and is triggered by exposure to cold temperatures. Lymphedema presents as edema of the affected extremity(ies), resultant numbness and tingling, discomfort that ranges from mild to intense, and possibly pitting edema. Review texts for further information on wounds, appearance and treatments.

TYPE OF REASONING: INFERENTIAL

One must infer or draw a reasonable conclusion about the likely signs and symptoms of venous insufficiency. Determining what may be true of a situation often requires inferential reasoning skill. For this situation, one would expect hemosiderin staining, wounds at the proximal medial malleolus and increased tissue temperatures. If answered incorrectly, review signs and symptoms of venous insufficiency.

C20 | Cardiovascular/Pulmonary | Interventions

A physical therapist assistant is working in an outpatient clinic and has been assigned to conduct a group exercise program with patients in phase III of their cardiac rehabilitation program. For this phase of rehabilitation the **MOST** appropriate therapeutic exercise is:

CHOICES:

1. resistance exercises using less than 15 pounds, in sitting position.
2. slowly performing active range of motion activities of the upper and lower extremities.
3. walking on a treadmill at 2 mph.
4. running on a treadmill at 5 mph.

CORRECT ANSWER: 1

RATIONALE:

Patients in phase III of a cardiac rehabilitation program should have returned to their previous functional levels and should be able to safely perform resistance exercises, in sitting position, using less than 15 pounds. Slowly performing active range-of-motion activities will not increase the heart rate enough for cardiac rehabilitation in phase III. Walking on a treadmill at 2 mph is included in phase II of the cardiac rehabilitation program; this slow speed would not require enough endurance for any of the patients to increase function. Running on a treadmill at 5 mph exceeds the MET level appropriate for many of the patients in this age group and may be unsafe.

TYPE OF REASONING: INDUCTIVE

One must determine the most appropriate therapeutic exercise for patients in phase III of a cardiac rehabilitation program. This requires clinical judgment, which is an inductive reasoning skill. For this case the most appropriate therapeutic exercise is resistance exercises using less than 15 pounds, in sitting position. If answered incorrectly, review cardiac rehabilitation guidelines, especially phase III cardiac rehabilitation and exercises.

C21 | Other Systems | Clinical Applications

The plan of care for a patient in the third trimester of pregnancy includes strengthening exercises for the abdominal muscles. Which exercise represents the **MOST** conservative modification for abdominal exercise during pregnancy?

CHOICES:

1. supine "short-arch bicycle" exercises.
2. supine single heel sliding.
3. curl-ups and curl-downs with hands placed across the abdomen to approximate the rectus muscle.
4. head lift with pelvic tilt while hands approximate the rectus muscle.

CORRECT ANSWER: 2

RATIONALE:

Strengthening of the abdominal muscles should be performed with caution to avoid causing or progressing the separation of the fibers of the rectus abdominis muscle. All exercises listed are appropriate modifications to protect the rectus muscle during pregnancy. The supine single heel slide exercise does not require the woman to overcome gravity to perform the exercise whereas the others do, thus making it the most conservative and least strenuous for the woman to perform.

TYPE OF REASONING: INDUCTIVE

This question requires the test taker to determine the most conservative modification for abdominal exercise during pregnancy. Clinical judgment is utilized to arrive at a correct conclusion, which necessitates inductive reasoning skill. For this situation, the most conservative modification for abdominal exercise during pregnancy is supine single heel sliding. Review abdominal exercises during pregnancy if answered incorrectly.

C22 | Cardiovascular/Pulmonary | Interventions

After reading a patient's medical history, the physical therapist assistant notes that the patient has arterial insufficiency. Participation in therapy may be limited by:

CHOICES:

1. signs of intermittent claudication.
2. increased pedal pulses.
3. peripheral neuropathy.
4. cool skin.

CORRECT ANSWER: 1

RATIONALE:

Arterial insufficiency results in ischemia to the exercising muscle causing intermittent claudication which is a precaution for therapy. The patient experiences cramping in the calf area with increased use such as walking. Relief of pain is accomplished by resting the extremity. Walking programs can help improve collateral circulation and should be done as frequently as possible for short durations to control the pain level. Caution in daily living activities is needed for peripheral neuropathy and cool skin. Pedal pulses actually diminish with arterial insufficiency.

TYPE OF REASONING: INFERENTIAL

One must infer or draw a reasonable conclusion about the likely limitations for participation in therapy by a patient who has arterial insufficiency. Inferential reasoning is utilized whenever one must determine what may be true in a therapeutic circumstance. For this case, participation in therapy is likely to be limited by intermittent claudication. If answered incorrectly, review arterial insufficiency signs and symptoms as well as intermittent claudication.

C23 | Musculoskeletal | Clinical Applications

To decrease the progression of a scoliosis curvature a child has been fitted with a wheelchair seating system with three-point support. The three points of support stabilize:

CHOICES:

1. both sides of the pelvis and the upper trunk on the convex side of the curve.
2. the pelvis and the upper ribcage on the concave side of the curve, and the apex of the curve on the convex side.
3. the head, pelvis and ribcage.
4. the shoulder, pelvis and knee, all on the convex side of the curve.

CORRECT ANSWER: 2

RATIONALE:

To minimize the progression of a spinal curve, the apex of the curve needs to be supported as well as the stabilizing counterpoints on the pelvis and upper ribcage on the opposite side of the body. The head, shoulder and knee do not stabilize the spine as well as the pelvis and ribcage itself.

TYPE OF REASONING: DEDUCTIVE

One must recall the features of a wheelchair seating system with three-point support. This is factual information, which requires deductive reasoning skill. For this situation, a three-point support system stabilizes the pelvis and the upper rib cage on the concave side and the apex of the curve on the convex side. If answered incorrectly, review wheelchair seating systems, especially three-point supports.

C24 | Musculoskeletal | Clinical Applications

Passive stretching exercises are not recommended for a child with:

CHOICES:

1. cerebral palsy.
2. osteogenesis imperfecta.
3. Duchenne's muscular dystrophy.
4. spina bifida.

CORRECT ANSWER: 2

RATIONALE:

Children with osteogenesis imperfecta have very fragile bones and hypermobile joints. Passive stretching is not recommended. It can cause fractures in the long bones. Passive stretching is recommended for children with cerebral palsy, Duchenne's muscular dystrophy and spina bifida.

TYPE OF REASONING: INDUCTIVE

This question requires one to use clinical judgment to determine the diagnosis that is inappropriate for passive stretching. Questions requiring reasoning through clinical situations often necessitate inductive reasoning skill. For this scenario, passive stretching is not recommended for a child with osteogenesis imperfecta. If answered incorrectly, review exercises for children with osteogenesis imperfecta as well as contraindicated exercises.

C25 | Devices, Admin, etc. | Equipment, Modalities

A patient returns for therapy two days after receiving cervical traction for the first time. The patient reports increased pain. The established plan of care calls for traction, therapeutic exercise, education regarding proper body mechanics and modalities to decrease pain. Following consultation with the supervising physical therapist the therapy session should focus on:

CHOICES:

1. modalities to decrease the pain.
2. cervical traction, but with decreased tension or pull.
3. therapeutic exercises to strengthen the cervical musculature.
4. educating the patient about correct body mechanics with all activities of daily living.

CORRECT ANSWER: 1

RATIONALE:

The patient has increased pain after the initial traction treatment. Do not perform the traction again as it appears to have aggravated the cervical condition. The best intervention at this time is to decrease the patient's pain. Consultation with the physical therapist is warranted as the plan of care may need modification.

TYPE OF REASONING: INDUCTIVE

One must determine a best course of action for a patient with increased pain after traction. This requires clinical judgment, which is an inductive reasoning skill. For this case, the therapy session should focus on modalities to decrease the pain. If answered incorrectly, review cervical traction guidelines, especially interventions for pain after traction.

C26 | Devices, Admin, etc. | Equipment, Modalities

A physical therapist has directed a physical therapist assistant to measure a patient for a manual wheelchair. The patient's measurements are 22 inches from hip to hip and 16 inches from buttocks to the back of the knees. The **MOST** appropriate size wheelchair is:

CHOICES:

1. standard adult.
2. narrow adult.
3. extra-wide adult.
4. standard child.

CORRECT ANSWER: 3

RATIONALE:

A standard adult chair measures 18 inches in width and 16 inches in depth. The procedure for measuring a patient for a wheelchair is to add 2 inches to the hip width and subtract 2 inches from the measurement from the buttocks to the popliteal space behind the knee. In this case, the patient's measurements should be 22 inches for width and 16 inches for depth. The patient should require an extra-wide wheelchair.

TYPE OF REASONING: DEDUCTIVE

One must recall the factual guidelines for wheelchair measurement to arrive at a correct conclusion. The recall of facts often requires deductive reasoning skill. For this case, the patient's measurements indicate that an extra-wide adult wheelchair is most appropriate. If answered incorrectly review wheelchair prescription guidelines, especially wheelchair measurements.

C27 | Musculoskeletal | Interventions

A patient is attending outpatient physical therapy for a right rotator cuff strain that occurred 2 weeks ago. The plan of care indicates to begin with isometric exercises for the rotator cuff muscles. The advantage of isometric exercises in this case is:

CHOICES:

1. limiting the joint position of the exercise.
2. facilitation of greater work by the rotator cuff muscles.
3. increased muscle action to increase swelling and decrease circulation.
4. a low risk of joint irritation.

CORRECT ANSWER: 4

RATIONALE:

The fixed range of motion of isometric exercises promotes a low risk of joint irritation. Strengthening may occur but it is not considered an advantage. There is no movement with isometric exercises so no work is performed. Physical work is defined as force times distance. Muscle pump action as related to isometrics decreases swelling and increases circulation, not vice versa as stated.

TYPE OF REASONING: INFERENTIAL

One must determine the advantages of isometric exercises to arrive at a correct conclusion. This requires one to infer the benefits of such an approach, which is an inferential reasoning skill. For this situation the advantage of isometric exercises is a low risk of joint irritation. Review benefits of isometric exercise guidelines if answered incorrectly.

C28 | Devices, Admin, etc. | Equipment, Modalities

The physical therapy plan of care for a patient with a diagnosis of acute biceps tendonitis includes modalities to decrease inflammation. The **MOST** appropriate modality for this patient is:

CHOICES:

1. iontophoresis using lidocaine at 40 mAmp minutes.
2. iontophoresis using dexamethasone at 40 mAmp minutes.
3. phonophoresis delivered at 1.5 w/cm² × 5 minutes.
4. phonophoresis delivered at 1.0 w/cm² × 8 minutes.

CORRECT ANSWER: 2

RATIONALE:

Both iontophoresis and phonophoresis are used to deliver medications into the tissues. This patient's diagnosis calls for modalities to decrease inflammation; dexamethasone is appropriately used to decrease inflammation, whereas lidocaine is used to decrease pain. Phonophoresis used with a nonpulsed ultrasound beam will introduce heat into the area; this can increase inflammation. An appropriate modality is pulsed ultrasound with the antiinflammatory ointment.

TYPE OF REASONING: INDUCTIVE

This question requires the test taker to determine the most appropriate modality for a patient with acute biceps tendonitis. This requires clinical judgment, which is an inductive reasoning skill. In this case, the therapy plan of care should include iontophoresis using dexamethasone at 40 mAmp minutes. If answered incorrectly, review treatment modalities for acute biceps tendonitis, especially iontophoresis.

C29 | Cardiovascular/Pulmonary | Data Collection

The physical therapist assistant is working with a patient who has lymphedema of the lower extremity following radiation treatment for cancer of the prostate. The physical therapist assistant should measure the girth of the limb from the inferior angle of the lateral malleolus in:

CHOICES:

1. centimeters, every 10 cm proximally from the metatarsal heads to the groin.
2. inches, at 5-inch increments proximally to the groin.
3. centimeters, at 3-centimeter increments proximally to the superior patellar angle.
4. inches, at 1-inch increments proximally to an area just proximal to the area of edema.

CORRECT ANSWER: 1

RATIONALE:

Circumference is best measured in centimeters as it is more sensitive than inches. Measurements along the length of the limb should be based from bony landmarks and at increments sufficient (about every 1 to 2 inches) to identify the extent of the edema. Because the condition affects the entire lower extremity the entire lower extremity should be measured.

TYPE OF REASONING: DEDUCTIVE

This question requires one to recall the guidelines for lower-extremity measurement of lymphedema. Deductive reasoning skills are utilized whenever one must recall factual guidelines or protocols. For this scenario, the limb should be measured in centimeters, every 10 cm proximally from the metatarsal heads to the groin. If answered incorrectly, review lymphedema measurement guidelines of the lower extremity.

C30 | Integumentary | Interventions

A patient is recovering from a full-thickness burn to the shoulder, anterior chest and axillary area. Range-of-motion activities should focus on shoulder:

CHOICES:

1. abduction, medial (internal) rotation and flexion.
2. extension, lateral (external) and medial (internal) rotation.
3. flexion, abduction and lateral (external) rotation.
4. adduction, extension and medial (internal) rotation.

CORRECT ANSWER: 3

RATIONALE:

The common deformity for burns of the shoulder and axillary area is into adduction and medial (internal) rotation; range of motion then should focus on reversing that—flexion, abduction and lateral (external) rotation. The other shoulder motions are important; however, they do not include the specific area of concern for deformity.

TYPE OF REASONING: INDUCTIVE

This question requires the use of clinical judgment to determine a best course of action. Questions requiring clinical judgment often necessitate inductive reasoning skill. For this question, one must recall the common deformity for burns to the shoulder and axillary area to determine the best range-of-motion activities. In this case, range-of-motion activities should focus on shoulder flexion, abduction and lateral rotation. If answered incorrectly, review range-of-motion exercises for patients with burns to the upper body.

C31 | Musculoskeletal | Clinical Applications

A physical therapist is monitoring a patient who is participating in a work conditioning program. When the patient squats to lift a box the physical therapist assistant observes that the client lifts with a posteriorly rounded lower back. The assistant's instructions to the patient regarding proper lifting technique should include:

CHOICES:
1. performing a slight anterior pelvic tilt.
2. keeping the back in a neutral position.
3. exaggerating the posterior rounded low back.
4. maintaining knees in extension and hyperextension of the shoulders.

CORRECT ANSWER: 2

RATIONALE:
The back should be maintained in the patient's neutral position, with the hips and knees in a flexed position. Increased flexion or extension (anterior pelvic tilt) puts the spine in a position of weakness and the patient at greater risk of injury during the lift.

TYPE OF REASONING: DEDUCTIVE
One must recall the guidelines for proper lifting techniques to arrive at a correct conclusion. This is factual information, which is a deductive reasoning skill. For this case, the assistant's instructions should include keeping the back in a neutral position. If answered incorrectly, review proper lifting techniques, especially biomechanical alignment.

C32 | Neuromuscular | Clinical Applications

A child with cerebral palsy has a strong asymmetrical tonic neck reflex (ATNR) when the head is turned to the right side. Because of the ATNR influence, the activity that the child will have the **MOST** difficulty with is:

CHOICES:
1. brushing teeth while sitting in a wheelchair.
2. bringing a spoon to the mouth with the right hand when the head is facing forward.
3. activating a head switch placed on the right side of the wheelchair head support, which requires neck rotation and extension.
4. extending both arms into a T-shirt that is being held to the right side.

CORRECT ANSWER: 4

RATIONALE:
The stimulus for the ATNR is turning the head to the side. The response is flexion of the extremities on the scalp side, and extension of the extremities on the face side. Extending both arms while the head is turned to the side is impossible for the child because of this reflex. Brushing teeth and bringing a spoon to the mouth are accomplished by keeping the head facing forward and not activating the reflex. Activating a switch by the head would likely be a reproducible movement, especially using a combination of extension and rotation to perform the task.

TYPE OF REASONING: INFERENTIAL
This question requires the test taker to infer the most challenging activity to complete with the presence of the ATNR reflex. Questions that require one to determine what may be true of this situation often require inferential reasoning skill. For this case, the child will have the most difficulty with extending both arms into a T-shirt that is being held to the right side. Review ATNR reflex, especially functional activities with the presence of this reflex, if answered incorrectly.

C33 | Other Systems | Clinical Applications

A physical therapist assistant providing cardiac rehabilitation to a patient who has Graves' disease should be cautious to avoid:

CHOICES:
1. bradycardia.
2. cool exercise environment.
3. overheating the patient.
4. decreased blood pressure.

CORRECT ANSWER: 3

RATIONALE:
Persons with hyperthyroid diseases (e.g., Graves' disease) are more susceptible to heat intolerance, and precautions must be taken during exercise to avoid overheating. Other clinical manifestations of hyperthyroidism include increased pulse rate, increased cardiac output and increased blood volume.

TYPE OF REASONING: DEDUCTIVE
This question requires the recall of precautions and contraindications when one is working with a patient who has Graves' disease. This is factual recall of information, which is a deductive reasoning skill. For this scenario, the assistant should be cautious to avoid overheating the patient because of the susceptibility of heat intolerance associated with the disease. If answered incorrectly, review Graves' disease, especially precautions for rehabilitation.

C34 | Neuromuscular | Data Collection

During observation of a young patient attempting bed mobility activities the physical therapist assistant notes that the child exhibits increased extension of the extremities while supine, and increased flexion of the extremities and neck while prone. The physical therapist assistant should report to the physical therapist that the child displays the following during bed mobility activities:

CHOICES:
1. asymmetrical tonic neck reflex.
2. symmetrical tonic neck reflex.
3. righting response.
4. tonic labyrinthine reflex.

CORRECT ANSWER: 4

RATIONALE:
The tonic labyrinthine reflex, when present, is influenced by position. If the patient is supine, both the upper and lower extremities will go into extension. If the patient is prone both the upper and lower extremities will flex. To assist the patient with bed mobility activities it is helpful to place the patient in side-lying position to neutralize the increase in tone.

TYPE OF REASONING: ANALYTICAL
One must analyze the information presented to determine the most likely reflex present during this functional activity. Whenever pieces of information are analyzed to determine a diagnosis or deficit, analytical reasoning skills are utilized. For this case, the description is consistent with tonic labyrinthine reflex. If answered incorrectly, review childhood reflexes, especially tonic labyrinthine reflex.

C35 | Neuromuscular | Clinical Applications

A patient has been diagnosed with Guillain–Barré. The physical therapist assistant preparing to treat this patient in the early rehabilitation phase should expect the patient to present with:

CHOICES:

1. asymmetrical weakness of the upper extremities with hyperreflexia.
2. symmetrical distribution of weakness, progressing from lower extremities to upper extremities.
3. decreased muscle tone of one side of the face, with drooping mouth and an exaggerated open eye.
4. asymmetrical distribution of weakness and tingling, progressing from the upper extremities to the lower extremities.

CORRECT ANSWER: 2

RATIONALE:

Guillain–Barré syndrome is an acute polyneuritis classically characterized by rapid development of progressive muscle weakness. Weakness is typically symmetrical and begins at the distal lower extremities and progresses to the upper extremities. Sensory loss could also be found. The diagnosis of Bell's palsy results in the decreased muscle tone of the facial muscles, which typically presents on one side.

TYPE OF REASONING: INFERENTIAL

One must determine the likely presentation of symptoms of a patient with Guillain–Barré syndrome. This necessitates inferential reasoning skill, which is often utilized when one is determining the likely symptoms or deficits of the patient. In this case, one should expect the patient to present with symmetrical distribution of weakness, progressing from the lower extremities to the upper extremities. If answered incorrectly, review signs and symptoms of Guillain–Barré syndrome.

C36 | Neuromuscular | Clinical Applications

A child is diagnosed with myelomeningocele (spina bifida) with a L3–4 lesion. The child's clinical presentation would include:

CHOICES:

1. intact lower extremity sensation.
2. intact bowel and bladder control.
3. active hip flexion.
4. complete inability to hip hike.

CORRECT ANSWER: 3

RATIONALE:

Children with myelomeningocele at the L3–4 level will be able to perform active hip flexion. Children with an L3–4 lesion have no sensation in the lower extremities and feet, and no bowel and bladder control. Hip hikers (quadratus lumborum) innervated from T12–L3 are mostly intact and functional.

TYPE OF REASONING: INFERENTIAL

This question requires the test taker to infer the likely symptoms of a child with spina bifida, which requires inferential reasoning skill. For this particular situation, a child with spina bifida at the L3–4 level would most likely demonstrate active hip flexion. If answered incorrectly review signs and symptoms of different types of spina bifida especially effects on the lumbar region.

C37 | Other Systems | Clinical Applications

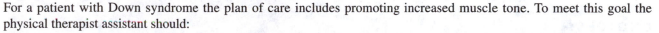

A elderly patient is being treated for depression following the death of her spouse. The patient is currently taking antidepressant medication (tricyclic). The physical therapist assistant should monitor the patient for which of the following based upon the patient's medication usage?

CHOICES:

1. hyperalertness.
2. cardiac arrhythmias.
3. dyspnea.
4. postural hypotension.

CORRECT ANSWER: 4

RATIONALE:

Fall risk is significantly increased with certain medications. Tricyclic antidepressants (e.g., Elavil) can be effective in relieving depression but may cause postural hypotension, fainting or confusion, thus increasing fall risk. The elderly are particularly susceptible to adverse drug effects because of a multitude of factors.

TYPE OF REASONING: DEDUCTIVE

One must recall the common side effects of taking tricyclic antidepressants to arrive at a correct conclusion. This is factual information, which is a deductive reasoning skill. For this scenario, the assistant should monitor the patient for signs of postural hypotension, a common side effect of taking this medication. If answered incorrectly, review side effects of tricyclic antidepressants.

C38 | Neuromuscular | Interventions

For a patient with Down syndrome the plan of care includes promoting increased muscle tone. To meet this goal the physical therapist assistant should:

CHOICES:

1. perform slow, rhythmic movements.
2. lightly bounce the child on her lap.
3. assist the child to perform facilitated somersaults.
4. perform gentle passive range of motion.

CORRECT ANSWER: 2

RATIONALE:

Most children with Down syndrome have low tone. Bouncing and vigorous movement helps stimulate muscle activity and therefore increases tone, whereas slow rhythmic or passive movements tend to relax a child. Somersaults are never appropriate with a child with Down syndrome because of the risk of atlanto–axial dislocation and resultant spinal cord injury.

TYPE OF REASONING: INDUCTIVE

One must determine the best therapeutic activity for a child with Down syndrome. Clinical judgment is utilized with questions of this nature, which require inductive reasoning skill. For this situation, the child should be lightly bounced on the assistant's lap to stimulate muscle activity and increased tone. If answered incorrectly review therapeutic activities for Down syndrome, especially activities to stimulate muscle activity and improve hypotonicity.

C39 | Neuromuscular | Data Collection

Protective extension backwards will most likely be exhibited by an infant that is:

CHOICES:

1. 9 to 10 months old.
2. 3 to 4 months old.
3. 5 to 6 months old.
4. 7 to 8 months old.

CORRECT ANSWER: 1

RATIONALE:

Protective extension backwards usually develops by 9 to 10 months of age. Children 4 to 6 months of age may be able to protect themselves from falling forward, and children aged 6 to 8 months can protect themselves from falling laterally.

TYPE OF REASONING: DEDUCTIVE

One must recall the guidelines for the development of the protective extension reflex to arrive at a correct conclusion. This is factual recall of information, which necessitates deductive reasoning skill. In this case, protective extension backwards usually develops by 9 to 10 months of age. If answered incorrectly, review the protective extension and similar protective reflexes and age of development.

C40 | Musculoskeletal | Interventions

A physical therapist assistant is working with a young, active patient who had a transtibial amputation 2 weeks ago. The patient's condition is complicated by a wound at the incision site. The patient is anxious to begin weight bearing and would like to be measured and fit for a prosthesis immediately. The **MOST** appropriate response by the assistant is to explain:

CHOICES:

1. that patients are not measured or fit for prostheses until 3 months after any amputation.
2. that the patient's arms are not strong enough to assist the patient to stand this soon after the surgery.
3. that the wound on the residual limb needs to heal and swelling needs to minimize before the prosthesis can be measured.
4. that the physician will address that concern and the patient can ask the physician at the next visit.

CORRECT ANSWER: 3

RATIONALE:

It is within the physical therapist assistant's scope to address the patient's concerns. The answer is an appropriate medical explanation as to why this fit is not appropriate at this time. It is also appropriate to inform the supervising physical therapist about the patient's request to supply the patient with a little more information about when he could expect a fitting and begin use of the prosthesis. The patient is young and strong and could certainly bear weight on crutches to support his weight. Asking the patient to wait until he sees the physician does not show respect for the patient's concerns or needs and is not necessary.

TYPE OF REASONING: EVALUATIVE

This question requires the test taker to determine the best response for a patient who is requesting to be fit for a prosthesis and who has a wound at the incision site. Questions that require one to weigh the implications of an action or response often require evaluative reasoning skill. For this situation, the most appropriate response is to explain that the wound on the residual limb needs to heal and swelling needs to minimize before fitting for a prosthesis. If answered incorrectly, review prosthetic fitting guidelines, especially for wounds on the residual limb.

C41 | Neuromuscular | Clinical Applications

A patient has been diagnosed with a stroke of the middle cerebral artery. Which of the following would the physical therapist assistant expect to see?

CHOICES:

1. contralateral sensory loss and hemiparesis with the leg more involved than the arm.
2. unilateral neglect, memory and behavioral impairments, aphasia.
3. contralateral sensory loss, thalamic sensory syndrome, cortical blindness.
4. decreased level of consciousness, dysarthria, tetraplegia, diplopia.

CORRECT ANSWER: 2

RATIONALE:

Symptoms describing a middle cerebral artery occlusion include unilateral neglect, memory and behavioral impairments and aphasia; in addition, apraxia and agraphia may also be present. Occlusion of the anterior cerebral artery results in contralateral sensory loss and hemiparesis with the leg more involved than the arm. A posterior cerebral artery occlusion usually results in contralateral sensory loss, thalamic sensory syndrome, cortical blindness, prosopagnosia (inability to recognize faces, even one's own) and visual agnosia. Signs and symptoms of basilar artery occlusion can include: decreased level of consciousness, dysarthria, pupillary abnormalities, bulbar symptoms, diplopia, bilateral cerebellar lesions, and tetraplegia.

TYPE OF REASONING: INFERENTIAL

Questions that provide a diagnosis and ask the test taker to determine the likely symptoms of that diagnosis often require inferential reasoning skill. For this question, a stroke of the middle cerebral artery will likely produce unilateral neglect, memory and behavioral impairments and aphasia. If answered incorrectly, review signs and symptoms of stroke, especially of the middle cerebral artery.

C42 | Devices, Admin, etc. | Safety Roles, Teaching, EBP

An adolescent is in a high-school class for those with severe disabilities. The physical therapist evaluated the student's physical therapy needs and set up a positioning, standing and strengthening program that the teacher and classroom staff are to carry out. The Individualized Education Plan states that the student is to get consult services from physical therapy. A physical therapist assistant has been assigned to provide follow-up care. The appropriate role for the physical therapist assistant is to:

CHOICES:

1. reassess the student's strength and functional skills on a weekly basis.
2. be available to the teacher and classroom aides to help implement appropriate activities.
3. recommend discharge from physical therapy as the student has no needs.
4. provide therapy as the physical therapist has indicated in the plan of care.

CORRECT ANSWER: 2

RATIONALE:

Adolescents with severe disabilities are not likely to change quickly in their skills or their needs unless an unforeseen or traumatic event occurs such as a fall or surgery. Therefore, being available to consult with the physical therapist assistant regularly should meet this child's needs for physical therapy until the next physical therapy evaluation. The physical therapist is obligated to see the child every few months to support and supervise the assistant, as well as to communicate with the assistant regularly. She or he can update the child's programs as needed at that time. Services for a school-based program should include being available to the teachers and staff to consult on issues that may arise. Direct patient care does not need to occur to meet the child's needs. Once the physical therapist assistant knows the child's physical therapy goals, he or she can work with the classroom staff to ensure that they are following through appropriately.

TYPE OF REASONING: INDUCTIVE

This question requires one to determine the appropriate role for the physical therapist assistant in a high-school setting providing consult services. This requires clinical judgment and knowledge of school-based therapy guidelines, which necessitates inductive reasoning skill. For this situation, the assistant should be available to the teacher and classroom aides to help implement appropriate activities, which best provides consultation services. If answered incorrectly review school-based consult services for physical therapy.

C43 | Integumentary | Clinical Applications

A physical therapist assistant is assigned to perform a whirlpool treatment for a patient with thick, scaly plaques on the skin. This chronic condition results from stress and a lack of medication. The skin disorder characterized by this description is:

CHOICES:

1. polymyositis.
2. scleroderma.
3. eczema.
4. psoriasis.

CORRECT ANSWER: 4

RATIONALE:

Psoriasis is an immune skin disorder that presents with scaly skin caused by rapid skin cell reproduction. Whirlpool baths with oil will help to remove the scaly plaques and improve range of motion. Polymyositis, scleroderma and eczema will not resolve with this intervention. All three require more intense medical management than whirlpool treatments. The clinical presentation of polymyositis, scleroderma and eczema is not thick, scaly plaques on the skin.

TYPE OF REASONING: ANALYTICAL

This question provides a group of symptoms and the test taker must determine the most likely diagnosis. Questions of this nature require analytical reasoning skill as pieces of information are evaluated to determine a diagnosis. For this case, the symptoms are indicative of psoriasis. If answered incorrectly, review signs and symptoms of psoriasis.

C44 | Neuromuscular | Interventions

A physical therapist assistant is working with a patient whose status is posttraumatic brain injury. The patient has developed a flexion synergy pattern in the right upper extremity. To inhibit this pattern during functional activities the physical therapist assistant should position the right:

CHOICES:

1. scapula into retraction, shoulder into abduction and elbow into extension.
2. scapula into protraction, shoulder into lateral (external) rotation and elbow into flexion.
3. shoulder into medial (internal) rotation, elbow into extension and forearm into pronation.
4. elbow into extension, forearm into supination and wrist into flexion.

CORRECT ANSWER: 3

RATIONALE:

To inhibit a synergy pattern during functional activities, the extremity should be positioned out of the pattern of influence. The flexor synergy pattern for the upper extremity includes scapular retraction/elevation, shoulder abduction/lateral (external) rotation, elbow flexion, forearm supination and wrist/finger flexion.

TYPE OF REASONING: INDUCTIVE

One must utilize clinical judgment to determine the best position to inhibit a flexor synergy pattern. Inductive reasoning skills are utilized whenever one must determine a best therapeutic technique for optimal outcomes. For this situation, the assistant should position the right shoulder into internal rotation, elbow extension and forearm pronation. If answered incorrectly review flexor synergy patterns of the upper extremity, especially after traumatic brain injury.

C45 | Devices, Admin, etc. | Safety Roles, Teaching, EBP

A physical therapist assistant finishing gait training with a patient that is on contact precautions secondary to a MRSA infection is preparing to leave the patient's private room. The physical therapist assistant should, in this order:

CHOICES:

1. store the gait belt in the patient's room, remove gloves and protective gown, and wash hands before leaving the patient's room.
2. remove protective gown and gloves, place the gait belt in the lab coat pocket, and wash hands before leaving the patient's room.
3. place the gait belt in a biohazard laundry bag and transport to designated laundry area down the hall, wash hands immediately after disposing of contaminated laundry.
4. remove the mask and dispose in biohazard trash, store the gait belt in patient's room, remove protective gown and gloves, wash hands, place gown in biohazard laundry bag and transport to contaminated laundry area.

CORRECT ANSWER: 1

RATIONALE:

Contact precautions call for a private room with dedicated patient care equipment; gloves and gown must be worn when in contact with the patient, and hands must be washed with antiseptic soap immediately upon leaving the room. It is inappropriate to use the gait belt with other patients or to remove it from the room. It is also inappropriate to remove the biohazard bag without washing hands after disposing of it.

TYPE OF REASONING: DEDUCTIVE

This question requires a test taker to recall the sequential procedures for contact precautions. This is a factual guideline, which necessitates deductive reasoning skill. For this scenario, the assistant should first store the gait belt in the patient room, then remove gloves and protective gown, and finally wash hands before leaving the patient's room. If answered incorrectly, review contact precautions procedures, especially for MRSA.

C46 | Neuromuscular | Clinical Applications

A patient presents with limited shoulder abduction secondary to adhesive capsulitis. The supervising physical therapist determines that grade 2 and 3 joint mobilization techniques will assist in promoting the return of normal joint accessory motion and shoulder abduction. Taking into consideration the articular surfaces of the glenohumeral joint, the correct direction for mobilization is:

CHOICES:

1. superior glide of the humerus on the scapula.
2. inferior glide of the humerus on the scapula.
3. anterior glide of the scapula on the humerus.
4. posterior glide of the humerus on the scapula.

CORRECT ANSWER: 2

RATIONALE:

The convex humerus moves on the concave glenoid fossa. To improve abduction, the head of the humerus needs to be mobilized inferiorly or the opposite direction of the swing of the bone. Superior glides of the glenohumeral joint often result in impingement and should be used judiciously. Anterior glides typically are used to increase lateral (external) rotation of the glenohumeral joint. Posterior glides assist with flexion and medial (internal) rotation of the glenohumeral joint.

TYPE OF REASONING: DEDUCTIVE

This question requires the test taker to recall the proper procedures for joint mobilization techniques. This is a factual procedure, which requires recall of facts and knowledge and necessitates deductive reasoning skill. For this case, when performing joint mobilization techniques of the glenohumeral joint, the assistant should perform an inferior glide of the humerus on the scapula. If answered incorrectly, review joint mobilization procedures of the upper extremity, especially of the glenohumeral joint.

C47 | Devices, Admin, etc. | Equipment, Modalities

The physical therapist plan of care for a patient with acute low back pain identifies the use of interferential current. The best electrode configuration to choose is two channels with the four electrodes placed:

CHOICES:

1. immediately adjacent and parallel to the spinal column with one channel on each side.
2. perpendicular to the spinal column, one channel over the upper lumbar area, and the other channel over lower lumbar area.
3. diagonally to the spinal column so the channels cross near the area of most pain.
4. parallel to the spinal column, one channel from the mid-thoracic spine paravertebrals to the lower lumbar area on the right side, the other mirroring it on the left side.

CORRECT ANSWER: 3

RATIONALE:

The crisscrossed electrode configuration over the lower back focuses treatment on the muscles involved, as well as allows the current interference. The other options do not allow for the currents from both channels to interfere with each other and create the interferential current pattern.

TYPE OF REASONING: INDUCTIVE

The use of clinical judgment in determining the best electrode placement is paramount to arriving at a correct conclusion for this question. This requires inductive reasoning skill. For this case the patient with low back pain should have the electrode configuration placement diagonally to the spinal column so the channels cross near the area of most pain. Review electrode placement for interferential current with low back pain if answered incorrectly.

C48 | Musculoskeletal | Data Collection

A patient who is substituting with the sartorius muscle during manual muscle testing of the iliopsoas muscle would demonstrate which of the following deviations for a muscle that has fair (3/5) strength.

CHOICES:

1. lateral (external) rotation and abduction of the hip.
2. medial (internal) rotation and abduction of the hip.
3. flexion of the hip and extension of the knee.
4. extension of the hip and knee.

CORRECT ANSWER: 1

RATIONALE:

The iliopsoas is the prime flexor of the hip; it originates from T12 to L5 vertebral bodies, the iliac fossa and crest and sacrum, and inserts on the lesser trochanter of the femur. Substitution of the sartorius muscle for a weak iliopsoas will result in lateral (external) rotation and abduction of hip and substitution of the tensor fasciae latae muscle will result in medial (internal) rotation and abduction of the hip (because of its anterior–lateral proximal attachment).

TYPE OF REASONING: INFERENTIAL

This question requires one to infer or draw a reasonable conclusion about the likely substitution pattern for a weak iliopsoas muscle. Questions that require one to determine what may be true of a situation often require inferential reasoning. In this situation, a patient with a weak iliopsoas muscle will likely demonstrate lateral rotation and abduction of the hip. If answered incorrectly, review typical substitution patterns for weak muscles, especially of the lower extremity.

C49 | Neuromuscular | Clinical Applications

An infant with developmental dysplasia of the hip was just referred to physical therapy. This patient is likely to come to therapy in a:

CHOICES:

1. hip flexion and adduction splint.
2. hip extension and adduction splint.
3. hip extension and abduction splint.
4. hip flexion and abduction splint.

CORRECT ANSWER: 4

RATIONALE:

To allow the acetabulum and the head of the femur to form correctly, the hip must be placed in a position of least stress and most congruence of the joint. This position is hip flexion and abduction. Usually the child is placed in a Pavlik harness, which positions both lower extremities in flexion and abduction of the hip.

TYPE OF REASONING: INFERENTIAL

One must infer or draw a reasonable conclusion about what is likely to be true for an infant with developmental dysplasia of the hip. This requires inferential reasoning skill. For this situation, the patient is likely to come to therapy in a hip flexion and abduction splint, also known as a Pavlik harness. If answered incorrectly, review signs and symptoms of developmental dysplasia of the hip and splinting procedures.

C50 | Musculoskeletal | Data Collection

Manual muscle testing strength of the lower trapezius muscle (for scapular depression and adduction) for muscles with good (4/5) to normal (5/5) strength should be conducted with the patient prone and shoulder positioned in:

CHOICES:

1. 180° of abduction and fully externally rotated.
2. 145° of abduction, the forearm in neutral with the thumb pointing at the ceiling.
3. 90° of abduction, elbow flexed to 90° and the forearm in neutral with the thumb pointing inward.
4. neutral position at the side and the shoulder and forearm internally rotated with the thumb pointing inward.

CORRECT ANSWER: 2

RATIONALE:

To get the full effects of gravity for the lower trapezius muscle the patient is positioned prone with the shoulder in 145° of abduction; this aligns the arm with the fiber direction of the lower trapezius muscle. The patient is asked to lift his arm off the table. For a grade of normal (5/5) the patient has to lift his arm so that it is level with the ear and take maximal resistance for that muscle. A position of 18° is inappropriate as it is the end range of motion; muscles are rarely tested at the end range where the muscle is physiologically weaker. At 90° of abduction in the prone position with the elbow flexed the examiner is testing the rhomboids. The lower trapezius muscle cannot be tested with the shoulder in the neutral position at the side.

TYPE OF REASONING: DEDUCTIVE

This question requires the recall of the procedures for manual muscle testing of the lower trapezius muscle. This is factual recall of information, which is a deductive reasoning skill. For this case, the muscle should be tested with the shoulder positioned in 145° of abduction and the forearm neutral with the thumb pointing at the ceiling. If answered incorrectly, review manual muscle testing procedures, especially testing of the lower trapezius muscle.

C51 | Musculoskeletal | Interventions

To relieve pressure on the patient's calcaneus while the patient is in the supine position, the assistant should position a 2-inch towel roll:

CHOICES:

1. under the posterior tibia/fibula just distal to the fossa of the knee.
2. laterally at the proximal femur, running along the length of the femur.
3. under the distal posterior tibia at the area of the Achilles tendon.
4. medially at the medial condyle of the femur, running distally along the length of the tibia.

CORRECT ANSWER: 3

RATIONALE:

A towel roll elevating the calcaneus off the mattress or supporting surface will relieve pressure on the posterior calcaneus, a common place for tissue breakdown. Something placed on the posterior surface and distal to the knee will have the potential to increase extension pressure on the knee joint itself. Towel rolls placed along the length of the femur are used to control medial (internal) and lateral (external) rotation of the hip and to protect the medial or lateral malleolus (as well as bony landmarks on the medial and lateral side of the lower extremities) but not the calcaneus.

TYPE OF REASONING: INDUCTIVE

This question requires one to utilize clinical judgment to determine the best place to place a towel roll to relieve pressure on the patient's calcaneus. This requires inductive reasoning skill. For this case the assistant should place the towel roll under the distal posterior tibia at the area of the Achilles tendon. If answered incorrectly, review pressure relief techniques, including use of towel rolls for pressure relief.

C52 | Other Systems | Clinical Applications

A physical therapist assistant is working in the intensive care unit of the hospital with a patient who was admitted for a flare up of inflammatory bowel disease and dehydration. The physical therapy plan of care calls for ambulation activities for endurance and lower extremity strengthening exercise. It is **MOST** important for the physical therapist assistant to:

CHOICES:

1. limit lower-extremity exercise to active exercise and avoid resisted exercises.
2. frequently offer water throughout treatment.
3. exercise in a semi-Fowler's (head elevated) position.
4. closely monitor heart rate and blood pressure with upright activities.

CORRECT ANSWER: 4

RATIONALE:

A patient with hypovolemia (dehydration) is subject to problems with blood pressure and heart rate management secondary to the condition. A patient with hypovolemia may also present with irritable muscles (muscle fatigue, twitching and cramping), a lower tolerance for exercise and a higher resting heart rate. Older patients' systems will be less able to compensate for hypovolemia by increasing the heart rate, especially if they are on a cardiac medication such as a beta blocker or digoxin.

TYPE OF REASONING: INFERENTIAL

One must determine the most important activity to complete with a patient in an intensive care unit who has inflammatory bowel disease and dehydration. This requires knowledge of both intensive care unit guidelines and the diagnosis of the patient, plus determination of the best course of action, which is an inferential reasoning skill. For this case, the assistant should closely monitor heart rate and blood pressure with upright activities because of the patient's propensity for problems with blood pressure and heart rate management. Review activities for patients with inflammatory bowel disease and hypovolemia if answered incorrectly, especially activities for patients in intensive care.

C53 | Neuromuscular | Interventions

A physical therapist assistant is working with a patient who has a complete spinal cord injury at the level of C6. The plan of care includes instructing the family in exercises to maintain passive range of motion. The physical therapist assistant should instruct the family to focus on:

CHOICES:

1. providing range of motion to individual muscles according to specific functional needs.
2. keeping all muscles fully ranged through normal range of motion.
3. keeping muscles fully ranged, with hyperflexibility in the low back extensors and hamstrings.
4. limiting range of motion in the shoulders to promote stability.

CORRECT ANSWER: 1

RATIONALE:

Selective stretching techniques are indicated for the patient with spinal cord injury. Overstretching the long finger flexors will result in loss of tenodesis grasp. Overstretching the back extensors will result in loss of sitting stability.

TYPE OF REASONING: INDUCTIVE

This question requires one to utilize clinical judgment to determine a best course of action for a patient with cervical spinal cord injury. Questions that require knowledge of therapeutic techniques and approaches often necessitate inductive reasoning skill. For this case, the assistant should instruct the family to provide range-of-motion to individual muscles according to specific functional needs. If answered incorrectly, review family training guidelines for patients with spinal cord injury, especially range-of-motion techniques.

C54 | Neuromuscular | Data Collection

Children with spastic diplegia often have a crouched gait pattern. The common crouched gait pattern associated with spastic diplegia includes:

CHOICES:

1. hip flexion, abduction, lateral (external) rotation and knee flexion.
2. hip flexion, adduction, medial (internal) rotation and knee flexion.
3. hip flexion, adduction, lateral (external) rotation and knee extension.
4. hip extension, abduction, medial (internal) rotation and knee extension.

CORRECT ANSWER: 2

RATIONALE:

Children with spastic diplegia often have spasticity in their hip adductors, internal rotators, medial hamstrings and ankle plantar flexors and significant weakness in their hip extensors, abductors, knee extensors and ankle plantar flexors. They stabilize themselves by adducting and medially (internally) rotating their hips to compensate for their weakness.

TYPE OF REASONING: INFERENTIAL

One must determine the likely gait pattern for a child with spastic diplegia to arrive at a correct conclusion. This requires knowledge of the diagnosis and mobility patterns, which is an inferential reasoning skill. For this situation, one should anticipate hip flexion, abduction, internal rotation and knee flexion. Review gait patterns for children with spastic diplegia if answered incorrectly.

C55 | Musculoskeletal | Clinical Applications

An appropriate modification to accommodate a plantar flexion contracture during gait training is:

CHOICES:

1. use of a heel lift.
2. the addition of a metatarsal pad.
3. use of a dorsiflexion assist ankle–foot orthosis.
4. electrical stimulation of the tibialis anterior.

CORRECT ANSWER: 1

RATIONALE:

A heel lift will accommodate a plantar flexion contracture and attempt to approximate a heel strike on the side with the contracture. A dorsiflexion assist ankle–foot orthosis is used to assist a patient with a weak tibialis anterior. Use of an ankle–foot orthosis with a muscle contracture may result in tissue breakdown. A metatarsal pad may assist to decrease abnormal tone in a lower extremity. Electrical stimulation of the tibialis anterior is appropriate if the muscle is weak.

TYPE OF REASONING: INDUCTIVE

One must determine the most appropriate modification to accommodate a plantar flexion contracture to arrive at a correct conclusion. This requires clinical judgment, which is an inductive reasoning skill. For this scenario, the use of a heel lift is most appropriate as it will accommodate the contracture and approximate a heel strike on the side with the contracture. If answered incorrectly, review ankle contractures, especially plantar flexion contractures and appropriate orthotic devices.

C56 | Cardiovascular/Pulmonary | Clinical Applications

While reviewing a patient's medical record prior to treatment, the physical therapist assistant notes that the patient has a diagnosis of congestive heart failure with right ventricular involvement. The physical therapist assistant should expect the patient to **MOST** likely present with:

CHOICES:

1. pulmonary edema.
2. progressive dyspnea.
3. dependent edema.
4. renal changes increasing blood volume.

CORRECT ANSWER: 3

RATIONALE:

Right ventricular failure is failure of the ventricle to adequately pump blood into the lungs, which results in peripheral edema and venous congestion. The accumulation of fluids in the venous system results in peripheral edema, a back-up of fluids into both lungs. Jugular venous distention and accumulation of fluid in the liver can also develop. The other symptoms noted are those most closely associated with left-sided ventricular failure. Renal changes resulting in increasing blood volumes are associated with failure on both sides of the heart; however, they are more evident with left-sided failure.

TYPE OF REASONING: INFERENTIAL

This question requires the test taker to infer the most likely symptoms for a patient with congestive heart failure with right ventricular involvement. This requires knowledge of the diagnosis to correctly determine symptoms, which is an inferential reasoning skill. For this case, one should expect the patient to have dependent edema. If answered incorrectly, review symptoms of congestive heart failure, especially right ventricular failure.

C57 | Devices, Admin, etc. | Equipment, Modalities

An active child with left hemiplegia, mild knee hyperextension and foot drop has a prescription to obtain an orthosis to correct the lower extremity problems. An appropriate device to decrease the mild knee hyperextension and foot drop is:

CHOICES:

1. a knee–ankle–foot orthosis.
2. a posterior leaf spring orthosis.
3. an ankle–foot orthosis.
4. a hip–knee–ankle–foot orthosis.

CORRECT ANSWER: 3

RATIONALE:

An ankle–foot orthosis, which is set in neutral ankle dorsiflexion or a few degrees of dorsiflexion, will prevent mild knee hyperextension, maintain neutral ankle position and assist with heel strike (initial contact). A knee–ankle–foot orthosis provides knee and ankle control but is bulky and is best for individuals who have decreased hip control and poor to absent knee and ankle control. A posterior leaf spring orthosis provides control for excessive knee flexion with weight-bearing. A hip–knee–ankle–foot orthosis provides support at the hips, knees and ankles and this provides too much support for a child with mild lower extremity weakness.

TYPE OF REASONING: ANALYTICAL

One must analyze the deficits of the child and then determine the most appropriate orthotic device to correct the lower extremity problems. This requires analytical reasoning skill. For this situation, the best device to correct the problems is an ankle–foot orthosis or AFO. If answered incorrectly, review lower-extremity orthotic devices, especially orthoses to correct knee hyperextension and foot drop.

C58 | Devices, Admin, etc. | Equipment, Modalities

A physical therapist assistant is working with an active young child who is ready for a new orthosis. The patient has good ankle dorsiflexion and plantar flexion strength and excessive pronation. The patient will require an orthosis to maintain the foot in neutral alignment and provide medial/lateral stability at the ankle while allowing free ankle dorsiflexion and plantar flexion. The **MOST** effective device is a:

CHOICES:

1. hip–knee–ankle–foot orthosis.
2. hinged ankle–foot orthosis.
3. knee–ankle–foot orthosis.
4. supramalleolar orthosis.

CORRECT ANSWER: 4

RATIONALE:

A supramalleolar orthosis provides positioning at the foot and medial/lateral support at the ankle, but does not block ankle dorsiflexion or plantar flexion nor does it offer knee support. The hip–knee–ankle–foot orthosis, hinged ankle–foot orthosis and knee–ankle–foot orthosis all offer too much support and limit both knee and ankle movement.

TYPE OF REASONING: ANALYTICAL

One must determine the most effective orthosis that will provide medial/lateral stability at the ankle and neutral alignment of the foot. This requires knowledge of orthotic devices and analysis of their features, which is an analytical reasoning skill. For this situation, the most effective device is a supramalleolar orthosis. If answered incorrectly, review lower-extremity orthotic devices, especially supramalleolar orthoses.

C59 | Neuromuscular | Interventions

A physical therapist has directed a physical therapist assistant to provide interventions to address the patient's loss of range of motion caused by hypertonicity. The patient is in a coma following a severe traumatic brain injury. The MOST effective intervention for this patient is:

CHOICES:

1. serial casting and positioning to maintain flexibility.
2. PNF to promote strengthening.
3. therapeutic exercise for sitting balance and coordination.
4. weight-bearing activities.

CORRECT ANSWER: 1

RATIONALE:

Because the patient is in a coma he will most likely not be able to actively participate in strengthening, therapeutic exercise for balance and coordination or weight-bearing activities. The priority at this time is to maintain joint range of motion and muscle flexibility and facilitate upright positioning in a safe device such as a wheelchair, adapted seat or tilt table. Serial casting and positioning will assist with maintaining flexibility.

TYPE OF REASONING: INDUCTIVE

This question requires one to utilize knowledge of therapy processes that will be most effective for a patient who has severe traumatic brain injury. This is an inductive reasoning skill. For this case, the most effective intervention for this patient to address the loss of range of motion is serial casting and positioning to maintain flexibility. If answered incorrectly, review approaches to improve range of motion in patients who are comatose.

C60 | Devices, Admin, etc. | Safety Roles, Teaching, EBP

A physical therapist assistant has been providing physical therapy to a patient following a transtibial amputation of the right lower extremity. The patient's adult children would like to look at the patient's medical record. The physical therapist assistant should:

CHOICES:

1. give the son or daughter the chart as a family member has a right to view the information.
2. deny access to the chart unless written permission is granted from the patient, and then refer the son or daughter to the physical therapist.
3. not let the son or daughter view the chart under any circumstances, because they may misinterpret the information.
4. let the son or daughter look at the chart, but only with the physical therapist present.

CORRECT ANSWER: 2

RATIONALE:

The issue is patient confidentiality. Family members do not have access to medical information unless they have consent either from the patient or from a health care proxy if the patient is deemed incompetent. In accordance with the American Physical Therapy Association's Guide for Professional Conduct Principle 1: Physical therapist assistants respect the rights and dignity of all individuals. After the family member has received written permission, inform the physical therapist in order to review the chart with the family member(s).

TYPE OF REASONING: EVALUATIVE

This question requires one to use both knowledge of guidelines as well as ethical reasoning to determine a best course of action. Questions of this nature often require evaluative reasoning skill to weigh the merits of each approach and determine the one that best addresses the issue at hand. For this situation, the assistant should deny access to the chart unless written permission is granted from the patient and then refer the son or daughter to the physical therapist. Ultimately, the physician in charge is the only one qualified to comment on the medical record if permission has been granted.

C61 | Cardiovascular/Pulmonary | Clinical Applications

Which of the following contraindications to joint mobilization is common for patients with chronic pulmonary disease?

CHOICES:

1. reflex muscle guarding.
2. long-term corticosteroid therapy.
3. concurrent inhalation therapy.
4. functional chest wall immobility.

CORRECT ANSWER: 2

RATIONALE:

Very often patients with chronic pulmonary disease have been managed with corticosteroid therapy. Long-term steroid use affects ligamentous integrity, which often produces joint hypermobility.

TYPE OF REASONING: DEDUCTIVE

This question requires one to recall the contraindications to joint mobilization to arrive at a correct conclusion. This is factual recall of information, which is a deductive reasoning skill. For this case, the typical contraindication to joint mobilization for patients with chronic pulmonary disease is long-term corticosteroid therapy. Review joint mobilization guidelines and contraindications, especially for patients with chronic pulmonary disease, if answered incorrectly.

C62 | Musculoskeletal | Interventions

A patient presents with lateral elbow pain that has persisted for several months as a result of repetitive use of power tools. The patient reports aching in the forearm and transient sharp pain when gripping an object tightly. The supervising physical therapist completed the examination and recommended a treatment program addressing chronic lateral epicondylitis. The **MOST** appropriate intervention strategies for this patient are:

CHOICES:

1. cryotherapy, cross-friction massage followed by electrical stimulation, then flexibility.
2. cryotherapy prior to activities, practice using power tools with review of proper ergonomic positioning and body mechanics, and heat therapy after activities.
3. heat therapy prior to activities, practice using power tools with review of proper ergonomic positioning and body mechanics, and cryotherapy after activities.
4. heat therapy, then ultrasound followed by strengthening activities.

CORRECT ANSWER: 3

RATIONALE:

Heat therapy will assist with relaxing muscles and will warm tissues, followed by protected activity, and cryotherapy will assist with controlling pain after activities. Reviewing proper ergonomic technique and body mechanics is essential to prevent further injury and irritation to the affected area. Massage, electrical stimulation and ultrasound may be correct passive interventions; however, because it has been several months, a more active approach needs to be taken to return to normal function.

TYPE OF REASONING: INDUCTIVE

Knowledge of treatment guidelines for chronic lateral epicondylitis is paramount for arriving at a correct conclusion. Utilizing knowledge of treatment approaches and processes often requires inductive reasoning skill. For this situation, the most appropriate intervention strategies should include heat prior to activities, ergonomic training while using power tools and cryotherapy after activities. Review guidelines for treatment of chronic lateral epicondylitis if answered incorrectly.

C63 | Neuromuscular | Interventions

Typical physical therapy management for a child with myelomeningocele (spina bifida) at the T4–5 level should focus on:

CHOICES:

1. gait training with a knee–ankle–foot orthosis and crutches.
2. strengthening of the hip extensors and quadriceps muscles.
3. standing balance activities with a hip–knee–ankle–foot orthosis.
4. wheelchair mobility training.

CORRECT ANSWER: 4

RATIONALE:

Wheelchair mobility training is the most appropriate and functional intervention for this level. Children with a high thoracic lesion will have innervation to the neck, upper extremity and some trunk muscles. Because there is no innervation distal to T5, the patient will not be able to gain strength in his or her hip extensors or quadriceps muscles. Standing may be included for some children for physiological benefits; however, to do so, a parapodium or standing frame should be used. The child will need extensive wheelchair training as this will be the child's primary mode of mobility.

TYPE OF REASONING: INDUCTIVE

One must utilize knowledge of therapeutic processes for children with thoracic spina bifida to arrive at a correct conclusion, which is an inductive reasoning skill. For this case, children with thoracic spina bifida should receive wheelchair mobility training as this will be the child's primary mode of mobility. If answered incorrectly, review therapeutic activities for children with spina bifida, especially thoracic-level involvement.

C64 | Cardiovascular/Pulmonary | Interventions

A patient who is recovering from surgery is receiving postural drainage as part of the physical therapy plan of care. The physical therapist assistant should discuss decreasing the frequency of sessions per day with the physical therapist if the:

CHOICES:
1. consistency of the sputum changes.
2. patient becomes febrile.
3. amount of productive secretions decreases.
4. patient experiences decreased postoperative pain.

CORRECT ANSWER: 3

RATIONALE:

The purpose of postural drainage is to help remove secretions. If the amount of drainage diminishes, the treatment is likely successful and the frequency can be decreased. Development of increased postoperative pain, a fever or a change in the consistency of the sputum does not indicate readiness to decrease frequency of postural drainage.

TYPE OF REASONING: INFERENTIAL

One must determine the situation that would warrant decreasing the frequency of treatment sessions for a patient receiving postural drainage. This requires one to infer or draw a reasonable conclusion about what is likely to be true. For this situation, the frequency of sessions should be decreased if the patient demonstrates a decreased amount of productive secretions. If answered incorrectly review treatment guidelines for patients requiring postural drainage techniques and frequency of treatment sessions.

C65 | Devices, Admin, etc. | Safety Roles, Teaching, EBP

A patient sustained a left rectus femoris strain while playing volleyball 2 weeks ago. The supervising physical therapist has directed the physical therapist assistant to begin a stretching program to promote a functional gain in range of motion. The patient has complained of pain and discomfort with knee flexion greater than 80°. The **MOST** appropriate treatment program for this patient should include moist heat for 20 minutes followed by:

CHOICES:
1. immediate static stretching at end range with a 10- to 20-second stretch.
2. immediate static, progressive stretching just beyond tissue resistance with a 30- to 60-second stretch.
3. immediate ballistic stretching with 10 passive stretches to end range; repeat two sets.
4. three repetitions of hold–relax with a 30-second hold and 10-second relax with stretch at end range.

CORRECT ANSWER: 2

RATIONALE:

Static stretching at end range with a 30- to 60-second hold just beyond tissue resistance has been reported to increase the length of soft tissues (joint capsule, muscle and tendon). Ballistic stretching is not appropriate when pain and discomfort are present, as well as a muscle strain. In addition, ballistic stretching has been proven to be effective on younger, healthy subjects. Static stretching with a 10- to 20-second hold has not been shown to be as effective as a 30- to 60-second hold. Hold–relax techniques can increase tissue length; however, up to a 10-second hold followed by a 30- to 60-second static progressive hold is effective whereas a 30-second hold and 10-second stretch is not.

TYPE OF REASONING: INDUCTIVE

This question requires knowledge of treatment guidelines for a patient with rectus femoris strain to arrive at a correct conclusion. Knowledge of treatment guidelines often necessitates inductive reasoning skill. For this case, the most appropriate treatment program for this patient should include moist heat followed by immediate static, progressive stretching just beyond tissue resistance. If answered incorrectly, review treatment activities for muscle strain, especially rectus femoris strain.

C66 I Neuromuscular I Interventions

The physical therapy interventions **MOST** effective in decreasing tone in a patient with hypertonia is:

CHOICES:

1. a warm whirlpool to relax muscles and increase range of motion.
2. use of a weighted vest or belts to increase proprioceptive feedback.
3. passive range of motion activities and avoiding strength training.
4. active weight-bearing with aligned limbs and trunk.

CORRECT ANSWER: 4

RATIONALE:

Persons with hypertonia generally have poor motor control and poor muscle strength. Using the principles of biomechanics, positioning limbs and trunk with muscles in a mid position, not overlengthened or in a shortened position, helps to facilitate active control. Even though the patient has hypertonia, strengthening can be emphasized. Concerns of increasing spasticity are not warranted as it has been proven that strengthening a muscle with increased tone does not increase that tone or spasticity. Although passive range of motion will be an important part of treatment, it should be incorporated with active interventions. Whirlpools may assist with relaxing the muscles temporarily but there is no lasting effect and it would be difficult to work on stretching and strengthening in a whirlpool. Weighted vests may be helpful for children with sensory dysfunction or movement disorder such as ataxia.

TYPE OF REASONING: INDUCTIVE

One must have knowledge of the therapeutic approaches that are most effective in decreasing hypertonia to arrive at a correct conclusion. Clinical judgment is utilized in this situation, which is an inductive reasoning skill. For this case, the most effective way to reduce hypertonia is to have the patient perform active weight-bearing with aligned limbs and trunk. Review therapeutic approaches for decreasing hypertonia if answered incorrectly.

C67 I Devices, Admin, etc. I Equipment, Modalities

A physical therapist assistant has observed a child with cerebral palsy to present with severe extensor posturing of the lower extremities. For proper wheelchair positioning, the physical therapist assistant should identify that the wheelchair seat:

CHOICES:

1. positions the hip and knee to create flexion less than 90°.
2. positions the hip and knee to create flexion greater than 90°.
3. be in an anterior tilt with the back of the wheelchair.
4. includes a hip adductor wedge.

CORRECT ANSWER: 2

RATIONALE:

Hip and knee flexion greater than 90° facilitates flexion and would assist in keeping the lower extremities in a flexed posture. Hip flexion less than 90° will facilitate hip extension, which would cause the child's pelvis to slide forward and out of the wheelchair. The same will occur if the chair is in an anterior tilt. If the chair is tilted, it should be in a posterior direction to assist in keeping the pelvis back in the chair. Extensor posturing is often accompanied by adductor spasticity. You do not want to position the child in more adduction as you would if you used an adductor wedge. You would want to minimize adduction and would in fact use an abductor wedge to prevent the lower extremities from adducting and crossing over each other.

TYPE OF REASONING: INFERENTIAL

Knowledge of wheelchair positioning for children with cerebral palsy is paramount to arriving at a correct conclusion for this question. For this scenario, the wheelchair seat should position the hip and knee to create flexion greater than 90° in a child with severe extensor posturing of the lower extremities. If answered incorrectly, review wheelchair positioning guidelines, especially for children with cerebral palsy.

C68 | Musculoskeletal | Interventions

A patient presents with a grade 2 lateral ankle sprain incurred during a volleyball game the previous night. Today, the patient ambulates into the clinic non–weight-bearing using bilateral axillary crutches and has a compression wrap on the involved ankle. During early maximum-protection phase of rehabilitation an appropriate treatment intervention should be to:

CHOICES:

1. encourage full-range-of-motion exercises.
2. incorporate muscle-setting exercises.
3. perform isotonic exercise at 60% maximum strength.
4. use plyometric activities.

CORRECT ANSWER: 2

RATIONALE:

An early goal is to protect the joint from further injury. Thus, muscle setting without motion is appropriate. Although the ultimate goal is for full weight-bearing, typically, partial weight-bearing, as tolerated, is encouraged until pain is lessened or disappears. Plyometric activities are a late intervention to prepare the athlete for return to sports.

TYPE OF REASONING: INDUCTIVE

This question requires the test taker to determine most appropriate treatment intervention for a patient with grade 2 lateral ankle sprain. This requires clinical judgment, which is an inductive reasoning skill. For this case, the assistant should incorporate muscle-setting exercises during the early maximum protection phase. Review exercises for ankle sprains, especially during the early phase of rehabilitation.

C69 | Devices, Admin, etc. | Equipment, Modalities

A young child with cerebral palsy presents with severe spastic quadriplegia, poor head and trunk control, no functional use of upper extremities and extensor posturing. The appropriate piece of equipment for standing activities is a:

CHOICES:

1. posterior rolling walker.
2. parapodium.
3. supine stander.
4. dynamic stander.

CORRECT ANSWER: 3

RATIONALE:

A supine stander provides posterior support, which is helpful for children with poor head and trunk control. A posterior rolling walker or a parapodium does not provide enough support for this child nor does the child have enough upper-extremity control to use these. A dynamic stander is not helpful at this time, secondary to this child's limited upper-extremity control.

TYPE OF REASONING: INDUCTIVE

One must determine the most appropriate piece of equipment for a child with cerebral palsy and severe spastic quadriplegia. This requires the test taker to understand the effects of cerebral palsy and then assess which equipment piece will provide the most benefit. This requires inductive reasoning skill. For this case, a supine stander will provide the most benefit for the child's diagnosis and symptoms. Review therapeutic equipment for children with cerebral palsy if answered incorrectly.

C70 | Neuromuscular | Interventions

The best way to get a 4 year-old child with pervasive developmental disorder (PDD) to participate in strengthening activities is to include:

CHOICES:

1. progressive resistive exercises using cuff weights and resistive band.
2. daily activities such as climbing stairs, running on the playground, and ball activities.
3. imaginative games and role playing of the patient's favorite characters.
4. PNF patterns using timing for emphasis at the end range of motion.

CORRECT ANSWER: 2

RATIONALE:

Using familiar activities and functional activities is most appropriate for this child. Children with PDD do best with familiar and routine activities. They often have impaired receptive and expressive language skills and have difficulty with lots of verbal instructions so it would be difficult to instruct them in an exercise program or PNF techniques. Children with PDD also often have impairments in imagination, thereby making it difficult for the child to participate in imaginative games.

TYPE OF REASONING: INDUCTIVE

This question requires one to utilize clinical judgment to determine a best course of action for a child with PDD. This is an inductive reasoning skill. For this scenario, children with PDD often respond positively to strengthening activities such as climbing stairs, running on the playground and ball activities, as these are familiar activities. If answered incorrectly, review therapeutic activities for children with PDD, especially strengthening activities.

C71 | Neuromuscular | Interventions

A patient recovering from traumatic brain injury is unable to bring her right foot up on the stair during stair-climbing training. The **MOST** functional method to develop this skill is to:

CHOICES:

1. have the patient practice marching in place.
2. passively place the foot on the next step.
3. practice stair climbing inside the parallel bars using a 3-inch step.
4. strengthen the patient's hip flexors by using an isokinetic training device before attempting stair climbing.

CORRECT ANSWER: 3

RATIONALE:

The most appropriate functional activity to promote the skill of stair climbing is practice by using a 3-inch step in the parallel bars. Passive movements do not promote active learning. Marching in place and isokinetic training may improve the strength of the hip flexors but do not promote the same synergistic patterns of muscle activity as the desired skill.

TYPE OF REASONING: INDUCTIVE

One must utilize clinical judgment and reasoning to determine the most functional method to develop stair-climbing skill. Questions of this nature, where determining the most therapeutic course of action is paramount to arriving at a correct conclusion, require inductive reasoning skill. For this scenario, the most functional method to develop this skill is to practice stair climbing inside the parallel bars by using a 3-inch step. Review stair-climbing training guidelines if answered incorrectly.

C72 | Cardiovascular/Pulmonary | Clinical Applications

The primary physical therapy intervention for a young child with cystic fibrosis is:

CHOICES:

1. postural drainage.
2. pursed-lip breathing.
3. assisted cough.
4. diaphragmatic breathing.

CORRECT ANSWER: 1

RATIONALE:

Chest physical therapy, including percussion, vibration and postural drainage, is a primary physical therapy intervention for children with cystic fibrosis to maintain clear airways because of the excessive mucus production caused by cystic fibrosis. To clear these secretions and allow for good aeration, aggressive techniques must be used. Pursed-lip breathing is used with patients with chronic obstructive pulmonary disease for them to exhale fully. Diaphragmatic breathing and assisted cough are techniques used with patients with spinal cord injuries to assist weak muscles.

TYPE OF REASONING: INFERENTIAL

One must infer the symptoms and therapeutic processes for children with cystic fibrosis to arrive at a correct conclusion. This requires inferential reasoning skill. For this situation, young children with cystic fibrosis primarily require postural drainage techniques to maintain clear airways because of excessive mucus production. If answered incorrectly, review the symptoms of cystic fibrosis and treatment interventions for this diagnosis.

C73 | Neuromuscular | Clinical Applications

A patient is being seen in physical therapy with a status of post–tibial plateau fracture. As a result of inappropriate casting the peroneal nerve received a compression injury. The physical therapist assistant should expect to see altered motor and sensory responses in what dermatome?

CHOICES:

1. L5.
2. L4.
3. L3.
4. S1.

CORRECT ANSWER: 1

RATIONALE:

The L5 dermatome covers the anterolateral lower extremity, medial dorsal foot and plantar aspect of the great toe; to think of the L5 dermatome covering the toes (one has five toes) may be a helpful study tool. The L3 dermatome covers the distal anteromedial thigh and knee. L4 covers the anteromedial lower extremity. S1 covers the lateral dorsal foot and most of the plantar foot.

TYPE OF REASONING: INFERENTIAL

This question requires the test taker to infer the symptoms of a patient with a status of post–tibial plateau fracture with compression injury to the peroneal nerve. One must infer the likely dermatome that is affected with this type of injury, which requires inferential reasoning skill. In this case, the L5 dermatome is likely to be damaged. If answered incorrectly, review compression injury to the peroneal nerve and dermatome involvement for the L5 distribution.

C74 | Devices, Admin, etc. | Safety Roles, Teaching, EBP

A physical therapist assistant is working with a patient who has middle-stage Alzheimer's disease and a recent total hip arthroplasty. The patient is having difficulty following directions for ambulation activities with a walker. To best facilitate ambulation with the walker the physical therapist assistant should:

CHOICES:

1. use single-step verbal directions.
2. physically assist the patient to perform the activities.
3. perform ambulation activities on the treadmill.
4. first demonstrate the activity, and then provide physical guidance.

CORRECT ANSWER: 4

RATIONALE:

In earlier stages of Alzheimer's disease, patients may be able to follow single-step verbal direction; however, as the disease progresses, this approach is no longer effective. Patients will likely do better if they receive some visual and tactile cueing to accomplish activities. Manually performing the tasks with the patient may result in involuntary muscle resistance to movement. A patient with Alzheimer's disease will likely be unable to handle the speed of a treadmill.

TYPE OF REASONING: INDUCTIVE

One must determine the best therapeutic approach to assist a patient with Alzheimer's disease to use a walker for ambulation activities. This requires clinical judgment, which is an inductive reasoning skill. For this scenario, the assistant should first demonstrate the activity and then provide physical guidance, as patients with this condition in the middle stages respond positively to visual and tactile cueing. If answered incorrectly, review therapeutic approaches for patients with Alzheimer's disease, especially ambulation activities.

C75 | Musculoskeletal | Clinical Applications

Vertebral instability at the atlanto–axial joint is most often seen in children diagnosed with:

CHOICES:

1. cerebral palsy.
2. Down syndrome.
3. spina bifida.
4. Duchenne's muscular dystrophy.

CORRECT ANSWER: 2

RATIONALE:

Children with Down syndrome have an increased incidence of atlanto–axial instability. This is an important consideration when one is implementing treatment with this patient population; care must be used to avoid extremes of range of motion in the cervical spine. This is not the case for children with cerebral palsy, spina bifida or Duchenne's muscular dystrophy.

TYPE OF REASONING: DEDUCTIVE

This question requires factual recall of information about Down syndrome and common deficits, which is a deductive reasoning skill. For this case, children with Down syndrome commonly have issues with vertebral instability at the atlanto–axial joint. If answered incorrectly, review signs and symptoms of Down syndrome, especially atlanto–axial instability.

C76 | Neuromuscular | Data Collection

A common deviation observed in boys with Duchenne's muscular dystrophy when standing from the floor is:

CHOICES:

1. a forward bent position because of weak back extensors.
2. a protruding abdomen secondary to weak abdominals.
3. use of the upper extremities to push on the knees and "walk" hands up the legs.
4. use of a nearby object for upper-extremity support because of spastic motor recruitment patterns.

CORRECT ANSWER: 3

RATIONALE:

A boy with Duchenne's muscular dystrophy has lower-extremity weakness. To stand up from the floor, the boy must have adequate hip and knee extensor strength. To compensate for this weakness, a boy will likely use the upper extremities to push on the lower extremities and "walk the arms up the legs" to stand; this may be referred to as the Gowers' sign. Although the boy may present with weakness of the back extensors, abdominals, and hip flexors and abductors, these weaknesses are not compensated by using the technique known as the "positive Gowers' sign." The other answers do not correlate with weakness typically observed with Duchenne's muscular dystrophy. Duchenne's muscular dystrophy is sex-linked and only affects males.

TYPE OF REASONING: INFERENTIAL

One must infer or draw a reasonable conclusion about the common deviation observed with boys with Duchenne's muscular dystrophy when standing from the floor. This requires inferential reasoning skill. For this scenario, the common deviation is the use of the upper extremities to push on his knees and walk his hands up the legs because of insufficient lower-extremity strength to stand from the floor. If answered incorrectly review functional abilities of boys with Duchenne's muscular dystrophy, especially mobility patterns.

C77 | Other Systems | Interventions

A patient is receiving physical therapy following a Colles' fracture and the subsequent diagnosis of osteoporosis. The fracture is now well healed and the plan of care includes the development of a home exercise program. At a minimum, the exercise program should include:

CHOICES:

1. wall push-ups and upper-extremity resistive band exercises.
2. aerobic activity and exercises that use eccentric muscle contractions.
3. active upper-extremity diagonals and core stability exercises.
4. submaximal upper-extremity active exercise and bike riding.

CORRECT ANSWER: 1

RATIONALE:

For exercises to promote an increase in bone density they must be performed in a weight-bearing or loading capacity; wall push-ups and resistance exercises will meet those criteria. Exercising muscles eccentrically, aerobic activities, sub-max, or active upper extremity will not stimulate bone growth. Bike riding will likely increase upper-extremity weight-bearing; however, submaximal exercises will not be beneficial for this patient.

TYPE OF REASONING: INDUCTIVE

One must utilize clinical judgment to determine the best exercise program for a patient with a healed Colles' fracture. Questions that require one to determine the best therapeutic approach often require inductive reasoning skill. For this scenario, the exercise program should include wall push-ups and upper-extremity resistive band exercises. Review exercise guidelines for patients with Colles' fracture if answered incorrectly.

C78 | Musculoskeletal | Data Collection

Following a hip fracture that is now healed, a patient presents with weak hip flexors with a muscle grade of poor (2/5). All other muscles are within functional limits. During gait, the assistant expects that the patient may walk with:

CHOICES:
1. forward trunk lean.
2. a circumducted gait.
3. excessive hip flexion.
4. backward trunk lean.

CORRECT ANSWER: 2

RATIONALE:
Circumduction is a compensation for weak hip flexors or an inability to shorten the lower extremity (weak knee flexors and ankle dorsiflexors). Hip hiking can also compensate for an abnormally long lower extremity (lack of knee flexion and dorsiflexion). Excessive hip flexion is a compensation for foot drop. Forward trunk lean and backward trunk lean are stance phase deviations that compensate for quadriceps weakness and gluteus maximus weakness, respectively.

TYPE OF REASONING: INFERENTIAL
This question requires one to infer or draw a reasonable conclusion about what is likely to be true for a patient with weak hip flexors. This requires inferential reasoning skill. For this case, one should expect that the patient will walk with a circumducted gait. If answered incorrectly, review gait patterns for patients with lower-extremity weakness, especially weak hip flexors.

C79 | Musculoskeletal | Interventions

Two weeks after surgical repair of an avulsion injury to the brachial plexus that occurred during delivery, physical therapy intervention for a 2-month-old infant should include:

CHOICES:
1. gentle range-of-motion exercises.
2. developmental activities such as prone on elbows.
3. introduction of assistive devices to promote functional skills.
4. active strengthening exercises.

CORRECT ANSWER: 1

RATIONALE:
Following surgical repair of an avulsion injury, the infant's arm is usually positioned across the chest in adduction and medial (internal) rotation for approximately 1 to 2 weeks to promote healing. Gentle range-of-motion exercises to prevent contractures is recommended for the next few weeks followed by more aggressive exercises including weight-bearing and reaching activities. Because the child is only 2 months old, developmental activities such as prone on elbows are too developmentally advanced. It is also too early at this stage for use of assistive devices, which should not be addressed until the child is older and only if there is a need.

TYPE OF REASONING: INDUCTIVE
One must utilize clinical judgment to determine the best intervention for an infant with brachial plexus injury. Inductive reasoning skills are utilized whenever one must determine a best therapeutic process. For this situation, intervention should include gentle range-of-motion exercises. If answered incorrectly, review intervention approaches for brachial plexus injuries in infants.

C80 | Musculoskeletal | Clinical Applications

A physical therapist assistant is treating a patient who has Paget's disease. The medical management for this patient includes a medication to improve bone strength. A possible side effect of medications for building bone strength the assistant should be aware of is:

CHOICES:

1. impaired blood-clotting times.
2. hypotension.
3. dizziness and lightheadedness.
4. swelling of the feet or abdomen.

CORRECT ANSWER: 1

RATIONALE:

One medication used to treat disorders of the bone is raloxifene (Evista); this medication can impair blood-clotting times. Physical therapist assistants working with patients who are taking this medication should be sure to observe the patient for bruising and encourage the patient to get regular blood tests of blood clotting times. A patient taking ACE inhibitors may be at risk for swelling of the feet or abdomen. Multiple different medications can cause hypotension (e.g., calcium channel blockers, fish oil). Diuretics can cause symptoms of lightheadedness or dizziness. See the medication table in Chapter 4 for further details.

TYPE OF REASONING: DEDUCTIVE

One must recall the side effects of medications that build bone strength to arrive at a correct conclusion. This is factual information, which is a deductive reasoning skill. In this situation, the possible side effect of such medications is impaired blood-clotting times. If answered incorrectly review side effects of medications for patients with Paget's disease, especially bone-building medication.

C81 | Integumentary | Clinical Applications

When discussing the benefits of wheelchair cushions, the physical therapist assistant should explain to a patient with paraplegia that the primary cause of decubitus ulcers is:

CHOICES:

1. friction.
2. excess moisture.
3. soap cleansers.
4. excess pressure.

CORRECT ANSWER: 4

RATIONALE:

A decubitus ulcer is formed from the pressure of prolonged sitting. Friction requires the rubbing of two surfaces. Moisture softens the skin and soap cleansers may contain toxic chemicals, contributing to skin breakdown.

TYPE OF REASONING: DEDUCTIVE

One must recall the causes of decubitus ulcers to arrive at a correct conclusion. This is factual recall of information, which is a deductive reasoning skill. In this case, the primary cause of decubitus ulcers is excess pressure, most commonly attributable to prolonged sitting. If answered incorrectly review decubitus ulcer guidelines, especially causes of decubitus ulcers.

C82 | Other Systems | Data Collection

A patient who has had diabetes since childhood is now receiving hemodialysis. An indication that the hemodialysis is not optimally effective is:

CHOICES:
1. persistent cough.
2. increased peripheral edema.
3. jaundiced coloring.
4. hyperreflexia.

CORRECT ANSWER: 2

RATIONALE:

Patients with type 1 diabetes suffer kidney failure; therefore, they need hemodialysis to replace the kidney's function. The kidney's function is to clear waste products, toxins and excess fluid from the blood. If this is not done satisfactorily there will be an excessive peripheral edema caused by the increased fluid and toxins in the blood and tissues. This manifests itself as edema in the periphery. Persistent cough, jaundiced coloring or hyperreflexia is not caused by increased fluid in the peripheral tissues.

TYPE OF REASONING: INFERENTIAL

One must infer the symptom that would indicate that hemodialysis is not optimally effective. Questions that require the test taker to determine what may be true of a situation often require inferential reasoning skill. In this case, a person with increased peripheral edema demonstrates that hemodialysis is not optimally effective. If answered incorrectly, review hemodialysis guidelines and symptoms indicating ineffective dialysis.

C83 | Musculoskeletal | Clinical Applications

A basketball player is undergoing rehabilitation with a status of post–left knee anterior cruciate ligament reconstruction. The orthopedic surgeon utilized a bone–patellar tendon–bone graft and has ordered that an accelerated rehabilitation protocol be utilized to restore function to the athlete's lower extremities. The best description regarding the positive impact of utilizing closed-chain kinetic exercises as part of an accelerated rehabilitation protocol is that it:

CHOICES:
1. facilitates long axis distraction of the joint.
2. enhances functional movement in the transverse plane.
3. promotes the functional recruitment of motor units.
4. creates shear forces at the articular level.

CORRECT ANSWER: 3

RATIONALE:

Closed-chain exercises encourage functional recruitment of motor units, specifically co-contraction of the flexor and extensor groups. Closed joint compression versus joint distraction occurs as a part of closed-chain exercise. The primary motion of the knee occurs in the sagittal plane, with flexion and extension; the screw home mechanism occurs in the transverse plane; however, it is an accessory movement, thus, one that is not selectively exercised. Closed-chain exercises actually reduce shear forces, not promote forces at a joint.

TYPE OF REASONING: INDUCTIVE

This question requires one to determine the positive impact of utilizing closed-chain kinetic exercises as part of an accelerated rehabilitation protocol. This necessitates clinical judgment, which is an inductive reasoning skill. For this case, closed chain kinetic exercises promote the functional recruitment of motor units. If answered incorrectly, review the benefits of closed-chain kinetic exercises, especially after athletic injuries and anterior cruciate ligament reconstruction.

C84 | Cardiovascular/Pulmonary | Data Collection

A physical therapist assistant is instructed to begin treating a distance runner who has been referred to physical therapy for ankle pain. Prior to beginning treatment the patient's blood pressure is 122/68 mmHg and the resting heart rate is 48 bpm. The assistant should conclude:

CHOICES:

1. that the patient is poorly hydrated and provide water prior to treatment.
2. that the patient has hypoglycemia and provide the patient with sugar immediately.
3. that the patient has hypotension and exercise the patient at a greater than planned on intensity.
4. that endurance training has resulted in a lower heart rate and that the patient will tolerate exercise.

CORRECT ANSWER: 4

RATIONALE:

A benefit of endurance training is that it can result in a decreased resting heart rate and lower resting blood pressure with improved functional capacity. The blood pressure is within normal ranges and should not lead the physical therapist assistant to become concerned. There are no signs and symptoms observed that would lead the physical therapist assistant to suspect dehydration, hypotension or low blood sugar level.

TYPE OF REASONING: INDUCTIVE

One must utilize clinical judgment to determine the meaning of a patient with a resting heart rate of 48 bpm and a blood pressure of 122/68 mmHg. Given that the patient is a distance runner, one should conclude that endurance training has resulted in a lower heart rate and that the patient will tolerate exercise. The patient's blood pressure is unremarkable. If answered incorrectly review vital sign guidelines in athletes, especially distance runners.

C85 | Musculoskeletal | Interventions

Boys with Duchenne's muscular dystrophy often progressively lose their ability to ambulate. Wheelchair mobility will typically become necessary at age:

CHOICES:

1. 3 to 8 years.
2. 15 to 17 years.
3. 9 to 14 years.
4. 18 years to adulthood.

CORRECT ANSWER: 3

RATIONALE:

Boys with Duchenne's muscular dystrophy often lose their ambulation skills between the ages of 9 and 14 years. Between 3 and 8 years of age, children show signs of weakness with gait deviations, decreased endurance and tripping; however, they are still able to ambulate. Adolescents between 15 and 17 years of age often use powered mobility and may need ventilator assistance because of respiratory complications. Individuals aged 18 years and older demonstrate increased dependence and respiratory compromise.

TYPE OF REASONING: DEDUCTIVE

One must recall the typical age range that a child with Duchenne's muscular dystrophy will progressively lose the ability to ambulate to the point of needing a wheelchair for mobility. This is factual information, which is a deductive reasoning skill. For this situation, a boy with Duchenne's muscular dystrophy will typically decline in strength and need to use a wheelchair for mobility between 9 and 14 years of age. If answered incorrectly, review symptoms of Duchenne's muscular dystrophy and mobility patterns as the disease progresses.

C86 | Devices, Admin, etc. | Safety Roles, Teaching, EBP

A physical therapist assistant is working with a patient who is exhibiting signs and symptoms of autonomic dysreflexia. The assistant should:

CHOICES:

1. sit the patient down and monitor blood pressure and pulse rate.
2. administer chest compressions.
3. allow the patient to rest then resume exercise activities at a lighter pace.
4. activate emergency protocols and check for and eliminate irritants to the patient's system.

CORRECT ANSWER: 4

RATIONALE:

Autonomic dysreflexia is an emergency situation encountered by patients with spinal cord lesions, generally at the T7 and above level. It is a dangerous condition in which hypertension will persist if it is not treated immediately. It is generally triggered by noxious stimuli, which initiate an autonomic response that the autonomic system cannot control and correct normally. The most common irritant to the system is bladder distension; other irritants can include rectal distension, pressure sores, bladder infections and noxious cutaneous stimuli (e.g., tight clothing).

TYPE OF REASONING: DEDUCTIVE

This question requires the test taker to recall factual guidelines regarding how to intervene when a patient exhibits signs and symptoms of autonomic dysreflexia. Using factual information to determine a correct course of action often necessitates deductive reasoning skill. For this situation, the assistant should activate emergency protocols and check for and eliminate irritants to the patient's system. If answered incorrectly, review guidelines for intervening during episodes of autonomic dysreflexia.

C87 | Neuromuscular | Interventions

A physical therapist assistant is gait training a patient with a status of post–cerebrovascular accident who demonstrates an upper-extremity flexor synergy pattern. To facilitate a decrease in the upper-extremity synergy pattern during gait training activities, the physical therapist assistant should position the elbow, forearm and wrist in:

CHOICES:

1. flexion, pronation and radial deviation with extension, respectively.
2. extension, pronation and ulnar deviation with extension, respectively.
3. extension, supination and radial deviation with flexion, respectively.
4. flexion, supination and ulnar deviation with flexion, respectively.

CORRECT ANSWER: 2

RATIONALE:

To decrease spasticity, the extremity is positioned out of the synergy pattern. The upper-extremity flexor synergy pattern consists of elbow flexion with forearm supination, and wrist and finger flexion. Positioning the elbow into extension, forearm in pronation, and the wrist and fingers into extension will inhibit the flexor tone.

TYPE OF REASONING: DEDUCTIVE

One must recall the out-of-synergy pattern for a patient with a status of post–cerebrovascular accident to arrive at a correct conclusion. This is factual information, which is a deductive reasoning skill. For this situation, the out-of-synergy pattern consists of elbow, forearm and wrist extension, pronation, and ulnar deviation with extension. If answered incorrectly, review synergy patterns with cerebrovascular accidents, especially out-of-synergy patterns.

C88 | Musculoskeletal | Clinical Applications

A patient presents for outpatient physical therapy services with the diagnosis of hypermobility of the shoulder. The physical therapist directs the physical therapist assistant to provide therapeutic exercise to address the hypermobility. The **MOST** appropriate therapeutic exercise is:

CHOICES:

1. taping and stabilization exercises.
2. grade 2 and 3 manual peripheral joint mobilization.
3. rotator cuff stretching exercises.
4. overhead strengthening exercises.

CORRECT ANSWER: 1

RATIONALE:

For a hypermobile joint, the proper intervention is to stabilize the joint functionally through corrective exercises or taping. If a joint is hypermobile, no joint mobilization is warranted. Because the joint has such hypermobility, the assistant should not do strengthening exercises at the end range in the overhead position; instead, strengthening should be done in the beginning to midrange. Stretching exercises are not indicated for a hypermobile joint.

TYPE OF REASONING: INDUCTIVE

One must utilize clinical judgment to determine the most appropriate therapeutic exercise for shoulder hypermobility. Questions that require one to determine an appropriate therapeutic approach often necessitate inductive reasoning skill. For this situation, the most appropriate therapeutic exercise is taping and stabilization exercises. If answered incorrectly review therapeutic exercises for joint hypermobility, especially shoulder hypermobility.

C89 | Devices, Admin, etc. | Safety Roles, Teaching, EBP

While walking through the parking lot to work, a physical therapist assistant comes upon an individual who is calling for help. The individual is on the ground and reports that he or she fell on the ice. Upon visual inspection the assistant notes a swollen ankle that is resting at an extreme range of inversion. The appropriate first aid intervention is to call for help and/or call the emergency response system, then:

CHOICES:

1. encourage the patient, with verbal cueing only, to come into a sitting position and assess the individual's heart rate.
2. cover the patient for warmth and discourage active movement or weight-bearing until help arrives.
3. straighten the ankle and fabricate and apply a splint from available material.
4. attempt to transfer the patient from the ground into an available vehicle and apply ice to the ankle until help arrives.

CORRECT ANSWER: 2

RATIONALE:

The safest intervention for this patient is to initiate steps to get emergency response and comfort the patient until help arrives. Because the ankle is disfigured and swollen, there is a potential for fracture and/or sprain. Attempting to move a patient in this situation could result in further injury to the ankle or lower extremity, including further damage to bone, nerve or other soft tissue. Attempting to transfer the patient into a car could result in further injury to the patient or cause injury to yourself. Keeping the patient warm with a jacket or blanket will prevent them from going into shock.

TYPE OF REASONING: DEDUCTIVE

This question requires one to recall first aid guidelines to arrive at a correct conclusion. The recall of factual guidelines necessitates deductive reasoning skill. For this scenario, the assistant should cover the patient for warmth and discourage active weight-bearing or movement until help arrives. If answered incorrectly review first aid guidelines and care for injured joints.

C90 | Musculoskeletal | Interventions

Following a complex fracture of the tibia at midshaft, a patient's tibia is immobilized with an external fixation device. While the external fixator is in place, a rehabilitation program for the affected limb should include:

CHOICES:

1. isometric exercises of the distal limb and resisted exercise of the hip and knee musculature.
2. increasing cardiovascular fitness through aerobic exercises.
3. maintaining or increasing muscle strength of the affected limb by using cuff weights at the ankle.
4. increasing muscle strength by using closed-chain activities.

CORRECT ANSWER: 1

RATIONALE:

It is a goal to prevent or minimize muscle atrophy of the entire limb, yet care needs to be taken not to disturb the integrity of the healing site. This is best accomplished by isometric exercises of the distal limb, and resisted exercise of hip and knee (resistance can be as little as gravity itself); active movement is likely not contraindicated at the hip and knee. Increasing cardiovascular fitness will not be contraindicated; however, this will not address the goal of maintaining or increasing strength of the affected limb. Increasing strength through closed-chain activities should be a goal of treatment once the fixator is removed. Cuff weights placed at the ankle should be distal to the fracture and create increased stress at the fracture site; at the same time a cuff weight applied proximal to the fracture will not be contraindicated.

TYPE OF REASONING: INDUCTIVE

Knowledge of rehabilitation guidelines after lower-extremity fractures is paramount to arriving at a correct conclusion for this question. This requires clinical judgment, which is an inductive reasoning skill. For this case, the patient's fracture of the tibia at midshaft warrants isometric exercises of the distal limb and resisted exercise of the hip and knee musculature. If answered incorrectly, review exercises for the lower extremity after fracture, especially tibial fractures.

C91 | Other Systems | Clinical Applications

A patient is recovering from a mild stroke and demonstrates trunk extensor weakness and postural instability. The patient also suffers from severe heartburn and says that previous physical therapy treatments have made it worse. Prior exercises have included holding in side-lying, bridging and prone on elbows. The **BEST** choice to maximize recovery while minimizing heartburn is to:

CHOICES:

1. perform trunk stabilization exercises with the patient in a semi-Fowler's position.
2. reduce the number of repetitions of bridging and focus on dynamic reversals, not holding.
3. perform rhythmic stabilization with the patient sitting.
4. assure the patient that the heartburn is not aggravated by exercise and suggest taking antacids before physical therapy.

CORRECT ANSWER: 3

RATIONALE:

Heartburn is a common symptom of gastrointestinal disorders and can be aggravated by supine and prone positioning. Modifying the patient's position to upright can alleviate the symptoms and demonstrate to the patient the assistant's concern. Recommending medications is outside the scope of the physical therapy assistant.

TYPE OF REASONING: INDUCTIVE

One must utilize clinical judgment to determine the best exercise to perform with a patient who experiences severe heartburn during exercise. Questions that require one to determine a best therapeutic approach often necessitate inductive reasoning skill. For this situation, exercise in an upright position is best; therefore, performing rhythmic stabilization with the patient sitting is best. If answered incorrectly, review exercise approaches for patients with heartburn.

C92 | Musculoskeletal | Clinical Applications

A patient has been admitted to a skilled nursing facility following an open reduction internal fixation to the right hip for a femoral neck fracture. The physical therapy plan of care includes strengthening the lower extremities, gait training, transfer training and patient education. Which of the following complications is **LEAST** likely to be an issue with this patient?

CHOICES:

1. avascular necrosis.
2. deep vein thrombosis.
3. dislocation of the hip joint.
4. respiratory compromise.

CORRECT ANSWER: 3

RATIONALE:

Hip dislocation is more often associated with a total hip arthroplasty than with an open reduction internal fixation. Avascular necrosis, deep vein thrombosis and respiratory compromise are all possible complications of surgery. Avascular necrosis is possible because the blood supply to the head of the femur is often compromised after a femoral neck fracture. The patient will initially have mobility problems. A decrease in mobility can cause a compromise in the peripheral circulation, which can then lead to a deep vein thrombosis. Respiratory compromise is also possible because of decreased mobility as well as a potential side effect from anesthesia during the surgery.

TYPE OF REASONING: INFERENTIAL

One must draw a reasonable conclusion about the least likely complications for a patient with a status of post–open reduction internal fixation of the hip. This requires the test taker to determine what may be true of a patient, which requires inferential reasoning skill. For this scenario, dislocation of the hip joint is the least likely complication after open reduction internal fixation as this is more characteristic of a total hip replacement. If answered incorrectly, review complications after hip open reduction internal fixation.

C93 | Musculoskeletal | Clinical Applications

A patient is receiving physical therapy because of lower back pain. The supervising physical therapist is concerned that the patient may have a pars interarticularis defect (spondylolisthesis) that is responsible for the symptoms. Until the patient's condition can be verified through radiographic imaging the patient should avoid exercises that include:

CHOICES:

1. isometric strengthening of the abdominals.
2. stretching of the hamstrings.
3. isometric strengthening of the back extensors.
4. isotonic strengthening of the back extensors.

CORRECT ANSWER: 4

RATIONALE:

Spondylolisthesis is the definition of a defect with forward slippage of one vertebra on the one below it. Excessive motion especially with extension of the spine can exacerbate symptoms or potentially cause more damage. Activities that include extension of the spine in the area of the spondylolisthesis should be avoided. When one is performing isotonic strengthening exercises there is movement about the joint that needs to be avoided. Isometric strengthening is permissible because there is not movement about the joint. Often there is hamstring tightness associated with spondylolisthesis and to decrease the stress on the spinal segments the hamstrings should be at their optimal length; therefore, hamstring stretching should be encouraged.

TYPE OF REASONING: INDUCTIVE

One must utilize clinical judgment to determine a best course of action for this question. Questions that require knowledge of therapeutic approaches often require inductive reasoning skill. For this situation, a patient with suspected spondylolisthesis should avoid performing isotonic strengthening exercises of the back extensors. Review signs and symptoms of spondylolisthesis and contraindications for exercises if answered incorrectly.

C94 | Musculoskeletal | Interventions

A physical therapist assistant is treating a patient with a transtibial amputation in the outpatient setting. The patient received a prosthesis 2 months ago and is wearing it 8 hours a day. The physical therapy plan is now focused on gait training to minimize gait deviations. During therapy, the physical therapist assistant notes that the patient has developed a small non-blanchable red area on the distal–lateral aspect of the residual limb. The physical therapist assistant should instruct the patient to:

CHOICES:

1. discontinue use of the prosthesis and contact the physical therapist immediately.
2. continue using the prosthesis and make arrangements for the prosthetist to be present at the next treatment session.
3. discontinue use of the prosthesis and make arrangements for the prosthetist to be present at the next treatment session.
4. continue using the prosthesis and tell the physical therapist about the ulcer at the next treatment session.

CORRECT ANSWER: 1

RATIONALE:

With an ulcer already forming, the patient must stop using the prosthesis immediately to prevent further skin breakdown. Because there is a change of patient status (presentation of a skin ulcer) the physical therapist must complete a reexamination of the patient. There will need to be a change in the plan of care because of the patient's status change and that change in the plan of care needs to be determined by the physical therapist. A visit to the prosthetist may be indicated; however, before this occurs, the therapist needs to determine whether there are other factors affecting the patient's change in status.

TYPE OF REASONING: EVALUATIVE

This question requires the test taker to weigh the merits of the potential courses of action and determine the one that best resolves the patient's issue. This requires evaluative reasoning skill. For this scenario, it would be best to instruct the patient to discontinue use of the prosthesis and contact the physical therapist immediately.

C95 | Musculoskeletal | Data Collection
The clinician in the photograph is testing the strength of which muscle?

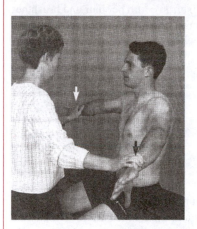

Magee D (2002). Orthopedic Physical Assessment, 4th ed. Philadelphia, W. B. Saunders, Figure 5-94, page 278, with permission.

CHOICES:

1. supraspinatus.
2. anterior deltoid
3. middle deltoid.
4. upper trapezius.

CORRECT ANSWER: 1

RATIONALE:

The muscle being tested is the supraspinatus. The empty-can position puts the supraspinatus muscle in its most effective position for contraction. Weakness may be the result of inflammation, neuropathy of the suprascapular nerve or a tendon tear.

TYPE OF REASONING: ANALYTICAL

This question requires one to evaluate the information presented in the photo to determine which muscle is being tested. Information that is evaluated through pictures and graphs often requires analytical reasoning skill. For this situation, the photo depicts strength testing of the supraspinatus. If answered incorrectly, review muscle testing of the shoulder, especially photos of muscle-testing procedures.

C96 | Musculoskeletal | Interventions

A patient with rheumatoid arthritis is being treated in physical therapy during an acute flare-up. The patient presents with bilateral ulnar drift and swan neck deformities that affect the patient's ability to button her shirts, comb her hair and brush her teeth. During this acute flare-up the intervention that focuses on preventing further deformity and loss of function should be:

CHOICES:

1. paraffin baths.
2. stretching the intrinsic hand muscles and long finger flexors.
3. fabrication of custom resting splints.
4. strengthening the intrinsic hand muscles and long finger flexors.

CORRECT ANSWER: 3

RATIONALE:

Splints to help limit the effects of the deformity are appropriate first steps in preventing further loss of function and deformity. The patient is in an acute flare-up; therefore, any intervention needs to be carefully administered. Paraffin baths are a heating agent and are contraindicated for a patient who is in an acute flare-up; avoid any modality that could potentially increase the swelling of the joint. Strengthening and stretching to the intrinsic hand muscles and finger flexors is appropriate, but not during active flare-ups of rheumatoid arthritis. It is best to prevent further deformity and attempt to relieve some of the discomfort by fabrication and donning of splints.

TYPE OF REASONING: INDUCTIVE

One must determine the best course of action for a patient with an acute rheumatoid arthritis flare-up. This necessitates clinical judgment, which is an inductive reasoning skill. For this patient, intervention should focus on the fabrication of custom resting splints to address the ulnar drift and swan neck deformity of both hands. If answered incorrectly, review therapeutic approaches for rheumatoid arthritis, especially splinting of the hands.

C97 | Musculoskeletal | Interventions

A patient presents in an outpatient rehabilitation clinic with a recent history of pain in the right shoulder that increases when the patient is reaching overhead. The pain has intensified and is growing more consistent; however, there are times when the patient is asymptomatic. The supervising physical therapist's diagnosis is shoulder impingement syndrome and the physical therapist has directed the physical therapist assistant to provide superficial thermal modalities and joint mobilization grades 1 and 2. Joint mobilization is being utilized to:

CHOICES:

1. increase joint nutrition and diminish pain.
2. maintain joint mobility and increase strength.
3. increase joint mobility and reeducate the neuromuscular proprioceptors.
4. increase capsular mobility and decrease pain.

CORRECT ANSWER: 1

RATIONALE:

The effects of grade 1 and 2 joint mobilization are to maintain joint nutrition and decrease pain responses. Only grades 3 and 4 maintain or increase capsular mobility. Joint mobilization techniques do not directly affect strength; however, they may improve biomechanics within a joint and indirectly improve strength or function of a joint. Joint mobilization does not reeducate joint proprioceptors.

TYPE OF REASONING: INFERENTIAL

One must determine the purpose of joint mobilization for a patient with shoulder impingement syndrome. This requires the test taker to determine what may be true of a therapeutic approach, which is an inferential reasoning skill. For this case, the purpose of joint mobilization for this patient is to increase joint nutrition and diminish pain. If answered incorrectly, review purposes and categories of joint mobilization and use of joint mobilization for shoulder impingement syndrome.

C98 | Cardiovascular/Pulmonary | Data Collection

A patient has developed congestive heart failure after a myocardial infarction. The pulmonary signs and symptoms a clinician should expect to find include:

CHOICES:
1. inspiratory wheezing and shortness of breath.
2. crackles and cough.
3. cough productive of thick yellow secretions.
4. crackles and barrel chest.

CORRECT ANSWER: 2

RATIONALE:
Patients who present with a myocardial infarction and congestive heart failure have changes to their pulmonary exam, the most common being crackles and dry cough. Inspiratory wheezing occurs with extreme airway narrowing, which is a hallmark of an obstructive disease process and not of congestive heart failure. The cough associated with congestive heart failure is most likely nonproductive. Crackles or adventitious sounds as well as a barrel-shaped chest are all symptoms of emphysema.

TYPE OF REASONING: INFERENTIAL
This question requires the test taker to infer or draw a reasonable conclusion about the likely pulmonary signs and symptoms of a patient with congestive heart failure. This requires inferential reasoning skill as one must determine what may be true of a diagnosis. For this situation, one should anticipate pulmonary signs of crackles and cough. If answered incorrectly, review signs and symptoms of congestive heart failure, especially pulmonary signs and symptoms.

C99 | Devices, Admin, etc. | Safety Roles, Teaching, EBP

A patient fell out of a wheelchair while in physical therapy. The incident report of this event should include:

CHOICES:
1. the cause of the incident, the name of the injured and the date of the incident.
2. the cause of the incident, the corrective actions taken and names of those involved.
3. the names of those involved, witnesses, what occurred and where it occurred—only in event of an injury.
4. the name of those involved, witnesses, what occurred, time of incident and where it occurred.

CORRECT ANSWER: 4

RATIONALE:
An incident report should avoid interpretive information such as cause of the occurrence or corrective actions that were taken. The typical information included on an incident report is the name of those involved inclusive of witnesses, what occurred, when it occurred and where it occurred. There is no presumption that someone was injured. It is sometimes called an "occurrence" report.

TYPE OF REASONING: DEDUCTIVE
One must recall the factual guidelines for the completion of an incident report. Deductive reasoning skills are often utilized when one is recalling factual guidelines and procedures. For this scenario, an incident report should include the names of those involved, witnesses, what occurred, time of incidents and where it occurred. If answered incorrectly, look over incident report guidelines and procedures.

C100 | Devices, Admin, etc. | Safety Roles, Teaching, EBP

When working with a patient who is coughing and exhibiting signs and symptoms of influenza the physical therapist assistant should:

CHOICES:

1. wear a moisture barrier gown while providing care.
2. ensure that the patient wears gloves prior to touching equipment that is being used by other patients.
3. provide the patient with a trash can to dispose of used tissues.
4. ensure that the patient wears a mask while exercising in the common gym area.

CORRECT ANSWER: 4

RATIONALE:

Standard precautions are based on the principle that all blood and body fluids, secretions and excretions, except sweat, are infections and may contain transmissible infectious agents. By ensuring that the patient wears a mask when out of her room, the assistant ensures that the public and other patients will be shielded from any potential pathogens. This situation does appear to provide a threat to the physical therapist assistant that requires the use of a gown. In addition to the assistant providing a container to dispose of the used tissues, the patient should be offered alcohol-based hand rub or the ability to wash her hands after coughing, sneezing or blowing her nose. Any equipment used by the patient should be disinfected according to procedure.

TYPE OF REASONING: EVALUATIVE

This question requires the test taker to weigh the benefits and merits of each of the potential courses of action and then determine the action that best resolves the issue at hand. Questions of this nature often require evaluative reasoning skill. For this situation, a patient who is coughing and demonstrates symptoms of influenza should wear a mask while exercising in the common gym area. If answered incorrectly, go over standard precautions for patients with viral illness, including influenza.

C101 | Other Systems | Clinical Applications

A physical therapist assistant is reading a plan of care for a patient with the diagnosis of long-standing rheumatoid arthritis. Which of the following clinical presentations is consistent with this diagnosis? Reports of:

CHOICES:

1. morning stiffness, Herberden's nodules, joints of the hand, knee and hip involved.
2. morning stiffness, nodules over bony prominences, joints of the cervical spine, hand, and elbow involved.
3. pain with weight-bearing, ulnar drift and subluxation of the wrist joint, joints of the wrist, hand, elbow and cervical spine involved.
4. stiffness following periods of rest, deformities of interphalangeal joints, joints of the lumbar spine, hips and knees involved.

CORRECT ANSWER: 2

RATIONALE:

Rheumatoid arthritis is an autoimmune-type disorder in which the synovial joints become affected, typically the smaller joints of the body. The associated signs and symptoms include morning stiffness and bilateral involvement of smaller joints such as the joints of the hand, wrists, elbow, shoulders and the cervical spine. Inflammatory signs within the joint are common. Common joint deviations associated with rheumatoid arthritis include ulnar drift, swan neck deformity, boutonniere deformity, hallux valgus, splayfoot and hammer toes. Osteoarthritis is a pathological condition in which the articular cartilage of the joints is destroyed and bony overgrowth occurs within the joint. The larger, weight-bearing joints of the body are more typically affected. Osteoarthritis tends to affect individual joints, unlike the bilateral involvement in rheumatoid arthritis. Joints typically involved include, but are not limited to the lumbar spine, hip, knee and first metatarsal phalangeal joint; the upper-extremity joints can include the carpal metacarpals, distal interphalangeals and proximal interphalangeals.

TYPE OF REASONING: INFERENTIAL

This question requires one to infer or draw a reasonable conclusion about the likely symptoms for a patient with rheumatoid arthritis. This requires inferential reasoning skill. For this case, the most likely symptoms include morning stiffness, nodules over bony prominences, and involvement of the cervical spine, hand and elbow joints. If answered incorrectly, review signs and symptoms of rheumatoid arthritis.

C102 | Cardiovascular/Pulmonary | Clinical Applications

A patient with congestive heart failure is on a regimen of diuretics and calcium channel blockers. The potential side effects of these medications that the physical therapist assistant should be alert for include:

CHOICES:

1. orthostatic hypotension and dizziness.
2. reflex tachycardia and unstable blood pressure.
3. gastrointestinal upset and extreme fatigue.
4. decreased electrolytes and electrical instability evidenced by increased arrhythmias.

CORRECT ANSWER: 1

RATIONALE:

The adverse side effects that diuretics or calcium channel blockers have in common are orthostatic hypotension and dizziness. These represent a safety risk during functional training and gait.

TYPE OF REASONING: DEDUCTIVE

One must recall the potential side effects of both diuretics and calcium channel blockers. This is factual recall of information, which is a deductive reasoning skill. For this case, the likely side effects are orthostatic hypotension and dizziness. If answered incorrectly, review side effects of congestive heart failure medication, especially diuretics and calcium channel blockers.

C103 | Devices, Admin, etc. | Equipment, Modalities

The therapeutic guidelines for using intermittent traction to alleviate symptoms of a lumbar herniated disc protrusion are to:

CHOICES:
1. utilize 75% of the patient's actual body weight.
2. utilize the highest force tolerable by the patient to alleviate symptoms.
3. utilize the lowest force possible to alleviate symptoms.
4. utilize a fixed force, between 80 and 180 pounds.

CORRECT ANSWER: 3

RATIONALE:

The correct answer is to use the lowest force that alleviates the symptoms of pain and discomfort associated with disc herniation and protrusion. A fixed percentage of the patient's actual body weight, usually one half of the patient's body weight, is typically utilized as a starting point for the amount of force to use, not 75%. When one is utilizing a traction table that is not friction free, one half of the patient's body weight is needed just to overcome the effects of gravity. Utilizing the highest force possible to alleviate symptoms can increase joint hypermobility and possibly cause collateral damage.

TYPE OF REASONING: DEDUCTIVE

This question requires the recall of therapeutic guidelines for use of intermittent traction to treat lumbar herniated disc protrusion. This requires the recall of factual guidelines, which is a deductive reasoning skill. For this situation the guidelines for intermittent traction are to utilize the lowest force possible to alleviate symptoms. If answered incorrectly, review intermittent traction guidelines and use of traction for lumbar herniated discs.

C104 | Devices, Admin, etc. | Safety Roles, Teaching, EBP

A physical therapist assistant is preparing to perform cardiopulmonary resuscitation (CPR) on a 14 year-old who has just collapsed in the therapy gym. The physical therapist assistant should place his hands such that the heel of one hand is placed:

CHOICES:
1. on the distal one third and parallel to the length of the sternum, with the heel of the other hand directly over it.
2. on the patient's forehead to stabilize the neck; the other hand is placed with the second and third finger tips over the sternum just below the nipple line.
3. on the middle portion of and parallel to the length of the sternum; the heel of the other hand is placed directly over the top of it.
4. two finger widths proximal to the xiphoid process on the length of the sternum; the other hand is placed just proximal to that hand on the length of the sternum.

CORRECT ANSWER: 1

RATIONALE:

The correct hand placement is on the distal one third of the sternum, parallel to it and two finger widths proximal to the xiphoid process. The heel of both hands on the sternum or hands placed in the middle portion of the sternum would not deliver effective compression forces to the heart and may put the patient at greater risk for fracture of the ribs or puncture of organs lying below the ribs. One hand placed on the forehead and finger tips placed on the sternum to deliver compressions is correct for performing CPR on an infant; a 14 year-old is considered an adult and the physical therapist assistant should use the same placement as that for an adult.

TYPE OF REASONING: DEDUCTIVE

One must recall the guidelines for performing CPR to arrive at a correct conclusion. This is factual information, which is a deductive reasoning skill. For this scenario, the assistant should place the heel of one hand on the distal one third and parallel to the length of the sternum with the heel of the other hand directly over it. If answered incorrectly, review CPR guidelines, especially adult CPR guidelines.

C105 | Integumentary | Interventions

A patient is being seen as an outpatient in the wound care center at the local hospital. The patient presents with a wound that is draining copious amounts of serous fluid. The physical therapist plan of care calls for cleaning and a dressing change. The **MOST** appropriate dressing for this wound is:

CHOICES:

1. a transparent dressing.
2. an autolytic débrider covered with a gauze wrap.
3. an alginate covered with a cushioned dressing.
4. an absorbent dressing.

CORRECT ANSWER: 4

RATIONALE:

An absorbent dressing is best to absorb serous drainage from this wound. A transparent dressing would cover the wound but would likely not be able to contain the amount of drainage from this wound; copious means a large amount of drainage. Autolytic agents or alginates are most often used to débride eschar and slough, respectively.

TYPE OF REASONING: INDUCTIVE

This question requires clinical judgment to determine the most appropriate course of action. Questions of this nature, which require knowledge of therapeutic processes, often require inductive reasoning skill. For this case, the most appropriate dressing for the wound is an absorbent dressing. Review wound care guidelines, especially use of absorbent dressings for wound drainage, if answered incorrectly.

C106 | Musculoskeletal | Data Collection

A patient presented with reports of persistent wrist pain after painting a house 3 weeks ago. The physical therapist plan of care includes soft tissue management for de Quervain's tenosynovitis. The physical therapist assistant should perform soft tissue massage:

CHOICES:

1. on the abductor pollicis longus and extensor pollicis brevis tendons.
2. over the transverse ligament at the distal radius and ulna.
3. on the flexor pollicis longus and opponens pollicis tendons.
4. on the adductor pollicis tendon.

CORRECT ANSWER: 1

RATIONALE:

De Quervain's tenosynovitis is an inflammation of the abductor pollicis longus and extensor pollicis brevis tendons; placing a stretch on those muscles will cause discomfort. Soft tissue massage over the transverse ligament is not an appropriate treatment. The adductor pollicis, flexor pollicis longus or opponens pollicis tendons are not associated with de Quervain's tenosynovitis.

TYPE OF REASONING: INDUCTIVE

This question requires knowledge of treatment procedures for de Quervain's tenosynovitis to arrive at a correct conclusion. Knowledge of therapeutic processes often requires inductive reasoning skill. For this situation, the assistant should perform soft tissue massage on the abductor pollicis longus and extensor pollicis brevis tendons. If answered incorrectly, review treatment techniques for de Quervain's tenosynovitis, especially soft tissue massage techniques.

C107 | Musculoskeletal | Interventions

A physical therapist assistant is seeing a patient in the outpatient setting 4 days after an open repair of the rotator cuff of the right shoulder. The short-term goals include maintenance of range of motion and pain and inflammation control. The physical therapist has directed the assistant to provide therapeutic exercise and modalities to address the goals. The **BEST** choice of interventions at this time is:

CHOICES:
1. passive range-of-motion activity.
2. active range-of-motion activity within pain-free range.
3. isometric exercise in the midrange position at 50% effort.
4. cold pack and interferential current.

CORRECT ANSWER: 1

RATIONALE:

Passive range-of-motion activity will be the most effective method to prevent loss of motion and at the same time protect the musculoskeletal repairs at 4 days post-op. Active range-of-motion activity will help prevent a loss of motion, but may also disrupt the healing process. Isometric muscle contractions, especially at 50% effort, would clearly cause potential harm to the surgically repaired tissue; isometrics do not protect against loss of motion. Cold pack and interferential current do address the short-term goal of pain and inflammation control; however, they do not address maintenance of range of motion.

TYPE OF REASONING: INDUCTIVE

One must determine the best choice for intervention for a patient with open repair of the rotator cuff. This requires clinical judgment, which is an inductive reasoning skill. For this case, the best choice of intervention for a patient who is 4 days post-op is passive range-of-motion activity. If answered incorrectly, review intervention activities for patients with acute rotator cuff repair, including range-of-motion activities.

C108 | Devices, Admin, etc. | Safety Roles, Teaching, EBP

To best implement the concepts of motor learning into a treatment session with a patient who is recovering from a cerebrovascular accident, the physical therapist assistant should demonstrate the functional activity being done correctly, then:

CHOICES:
1. ask the patient to verbally repeat the steps just observed.
2. allow the patient to perform the task in whatever manner is needed to accomplish it, even with errors.
3. assist the patient to perform the task.
4. insist that the patient only perform the task if it can be accomplished without error.

CORRECT ANSWER: 3

RATIONALE:

The principles of motor learning emphasize the patient observing and performing functional activities and tasks to improve performance. Early in the learning the patient learns by observation and guided practice; there is allowance for some trial-and-error learning to occur. Having the patient verbally repeat what has been done will not involve the motor system and will limit learning through movement. Guidance is provided to allow the patient to accomplish a task relatively well, versus learning and reinforcing poor movement patterns.

TYPE OF REASONING: INDUCTIVE

One must utilize clinical judgment to determine the best functional activity for a patient with a cerebrovascular accident. This requires knowledge of motor learning principles, which is an inductive reasoning skill. For this scenario, the assistant should demonstrate the functional activity and then assist the patient to perform the task, which coincides with the principles of motor learning theory. If answered incorrectly, review motor learning principles and engagement in functional activity.

C109 | Other Systems | Clinical Applications

A patient with a 10 year history of diabetes reports cramping, pain and fatigue of the right buttock after walking 400 feet or climbing stairs. When the patient stops exercising, the pain goes away immediately. The skin of the involved lower extremity is cool and pale. The assistant checks the record and finds no mention of this problem. The assistant reports to the therapist that the patient is displaying:

CHOICES:

1. radiating pain.
2. muscle cramps.
3. intermittent claudication.
4. delayed onset of muscle soreness.

CORRECT ANSWER: 3

RATIONALE:

Intermittent claudication, often the earliest indication of peripheral arterial disease, is manifested by cramping, pain or fatigue in the muscles during exercise that is typically relieved by rest. Peripheral arterial disease is a common result of long-standing diabetes. The calf muscle is most commonly affected, but discomfort may also occur in the thigh, hip or buttock. Cessation of pain immediately upon stopping the exercise is characteristic of intermittent claudication, not other spinal problems. With severe disease, however, pain may be present even at rest. The findings cannot explain the incorrect choices.

TYPE OF REASONING: ANALYTICAL

This question requires the test taker to analyze the symptoms presented and then determine the most likely diagnosis. This requires analytical reasoning skill. For this situation, the symptoms are most consistent with intermittent claudication. If answered incorrectly, review signs and symptoms of peripheral arterial disease, including intermittent claudication.

C110 | Cardiovascular/Pulmonary | Clinical Applications

A patient in chronic renal failure is being seen in physical therapy for deconditioning and decreased gait endurance. The assistant needs to schedule the patient's sessions around dialysis, which is received three mornings a week. The patient is also hypertensive and requires careful monitoring. The assistant's **BEST** approach is to take blood pressure:

CHOICES:

1. before and after activities, using the nonshunted arm.
2. in the seated position, when activity has ceased.
3. in the supine position, using the shunted arm.
4. every minute during activity, using the shunted arm.

CORRECT ANSWER: 1

RATIONALE:

A dialysis shunt interferes with taking blood pressure. Use the nonshunted arm. Pre- and postexercise measurements are appropriate; taking blood pressure during walking would result in inaccurate measurements.

TYPE OF REASONING: INDUCTIVE

This question requires clinical judgment to determine a best course of action for a patient with chronic renal failure requiring blood pressure monitoring. This necessitates inductive reasoning skill. For this case, blood pressure should be taken before and after activities, using the nonshunted arm. If answered incorrectly, look over blood pressure techniques, including taking blood pressure for patients on dialysis with shunt access on the upper extremity.

C111 | Devices, Admin, etc. | Equipment, Modalities

A patient presents with partial- and full-thickness burns on the chest and neck region. The assistant plans to apply transcutaneous electrical nerve stimulation (TENS) prior to débridement to modulate pain. Which TENS mode should provide the **BEST** relief?

CHOICES:

1. conventional (high-rate) TENS.
2. acupuncture-like (low-rate) TENS.
3. modulated TENS.
4. brief intense TENS.

CORRECT ANSWER: 4

RATIONALE:

Brief intense TENS is used to provide rapid-onset but short-term relief during painful procedures. The pulse rate and pulse duration are similar to that with conventional TENS; however, the current intensity is increased to the patient's tolerance.

TYPE OF REASONING: INDUCTIVE

One must determine the appropriate TENS mode that will best provide pain relief for a patient with partial- and full-thickness burns. This requires knowledge of therapeutic processes, which is an inductive reasoning skill. For this case, brief intense TENS is best to provide rapid-onset, short-term relief during painful procedures such as débridement. If answered incorrectly, review TENS guidelines, including use of TENS for débridement.

C112 | Musculoskeletal | Clinical Applications

A patient who had a transtibial amputation 3 months ago is receiving physical therapy services. During the therapy session today the patient reports a knifelike pain and electrical shocks in the missing limb. The physical therapist assistant should document this in the medical record as:

CHOICES:

1. local pain.
2. phantom pain.
3. phantom sensation.
4. referred pain.

CORRECT ANSWER: 2

RATIONALE:

Following amputation, it is common for the majority of individuals to experience a phantom limb sensation. For most patients these feelings usually recede. Phantom sensation is usually not painful and is the sensation the patient feels that part or the entire limb is present. Some may experience painful sensations called phantom pain. Phantom pain may be local or diffuse, and may be continuous or intermittent. Local pain refers to pain that is specific to an injured area such as a bruise, cut nerve endings at that specific spot or pressure from a prosthesis. Referred pain is usually involved in problems related to areas where pain is referred from the original nerve root down its pathway. One example is in the back where pain can be referred down the lower extremity because of compression of a nerve root as it exits the spine.

TYPE OF REASONING: ANALYTICAL

One must analyze the symptoms presented and then determine the likely cause of the pain to enter into the medical record. Questions that require the test taker to analyze information to draw conclusions often require analytical reasoning skill. For this situation, the symptoms are indicative of phantom pain. If answered incorrectly, review phantom sensations and pain after amputation.

C113 | Devices, Admin, etc. | Equipment, Modalities

The initial evaluation identifies that a patient has weakness of the knee muscles, grade poor (2/5) resulting from an anterior cruciate ligament injury, moderate pain (5/10) and excessive translation of the tibia during active knee extension. The plan of care includes functional electrical stimulation (FES). The protocol for strengthening the quadriceps and improving stability of the knee should consist of stimulation of the:

CHOICES:

1. quadriceps but not the hamstrings.
2. hamstring immediately before the quadriceps to produce co-contraction.
3. hamstrings but not the quadriceps.
4. quadriceps immediately before the hamstrings to produce co-contraction.

CORRECT ANSWER: 2

RATIONALE:

Stimulating the hamstrings just prior to stimulating the quadriceps will stabilize the tibia and prevent anterior tibial translation during knee extension and during co-contraction of both muscles. This prevents the moving tibia from placing tension on the injured anterior cruciate ligament.

TYPE OF REASONING: DEDUCTIVE

One must recall the guidelines for use of FES with patients demonstrating lower-extremity weakness to arrive at a correct conclusion. The recall of factual information is a deductive reasoning skill. For this case, FES should consist of stimulation of the hamstrings immediately before the quadriceps to produce co-contraction. Review applications of FES for lower-extremity weakness if answered incorrectly.

C114 | Musculoskeletal | Interventions

A patient with diabetes who had a transtibial amputation 3 months ago has recently been fitted with a prosthesis. During ambulation the patient reports pain in the distal and posterior portion of the residual limb. Upon inspection, the physical therapist assistant notes a reddened area developing on the distal tibia. Which of the following should be the physical therapist assistant's response?

CHOICES:

1. Initiate strengthening exercises for the quadriceps muscles.
2. Instruct the patient to avoid excessive lateral thrust of the residual limb during midstance.
3. Adjust the sock layers and continue with gait training, closely monitoring the patient's response.
4. Contact the prosthetist to make modifications to the prosthesis.

CORRECT ANSWER: 3

RATIONALE:

Patients with new amputations fluctuate in volume and use various layers of socks within their temporary prosthesis to maintain proper fit. If a patient uses too few layers of socks it will allow them to "bottom out" in the prosthesis, or fit too far down into it and bear weight on the distal end of the residual limb versus the weight-bearing areas of the socket. Weak quadriceps strength can lead to a gait deviation of excessive knee flexion in the early stance phase. Excessive lateral thrust is likely because of the prosthetic foot being inset too far. If this caused tissue irritation it would likely be on the lateral tibia. Insufficient plantar flexion built into the prosthesis will likely lead to a gait deviation of early knee flexion during stance phase, but would not likely lead to the development of reddened areas in this pattern.

TYPE OF REASONING: EVALUATIVE

One must assess the benefits of the courses of action presented and then determine a course of action that effectively resolves the patient's issue. Weighing information to determine its merits often requires evaluative reasoning skill. For this situation, the assistant should respond by adjusting the sock layers and continue with gait training, closely monitoring the patient's response. If answered incorrectly, review prosthetic training guidelines and appropriate responses for reddened areas on the residual limb after ambulation.

C115 | Neuromuscular | Clinical Applications

A physical therapist assistant is providing physical therapy interventions for a 9 year-old with myelomeningocele (spina bifida) lesion at L4–5. The plan of care indicates continuation of mobility training. The physical therapist assistant should expect this patient's current mobility status to be:

CHOICES:

1. community mobility with a power wheelchair.
2. household ambulation with crutches and knee–ankle–foot orthoses.
3. household ambulation with reciprocating gait orthoses and walker, and wheelchair for community mobility.
4. community ambulation with crutches and ankle–foot orthoses.

CORRECT ANSWER: 4

RATIONALE:

Children with L4–5 lesions generally have good strength in their hip flexors, adductors, knee flexors and extensors and ankle dorsiflexors. They also have some muscle control in their hip extensors and abductors and ankle plantar flexors. Therefore, they usually can ambulate community distances with ankle–foot orthoses and crutches. They do not need reciprocating gait orthoses, knee–ankle–foot orthoses or power wheelchairs because they have functional hip and knee strength.

TYPE OF REASONING: INFERENTIAL

One must infer or draw a reasonable conclusion about the likely mobility status of a child with spina bifida at L4–5. This requires knowledge of the diagnosis and typical mobility patterns, which is an inferential reasoning skill. For this case, one should expect the patient's mobility status to include community ambulation with crutches and use of ankle–foot orthoses. If answered incorrectly, review mobility patterns for children with spina bifida affecting the lumbar region.

C116 | Musculoskeletal | Clinical Applications

When instructing a patient's caregiver to perform sliding board transfers with the patient, the physical therapist assistant should instruct the caregiver to achieve a lower center of gravity by:

CHOICES:

1. using a wide base of support.
2. using a narrow base of support.
3. maintaining an upright posture in the back.
4. flexing at the hips and extending at the knees.

CORRECT ANSWER: 1

RATIONALE:

A wide base of support increases balance as well as lowers the center of gravity; in contrast, a narrow base of support decreases balance and raises the center of gravity, which will decrease the biomechanical advantage of the caregiver. Maintaining the back in an upright posture is correct body mechanics; however, it does nothing to affect the base of support. Correct body mechanics call for flexing both the hips and knees; this also lowers the center of gravity.

TYPE OF REASONING: DEDUCTIVE

One must recall the guidelines for how to achieve a lower center of gravity during sliding board transfers. This is factual information, which is a deductive reasoning skill. For this scenario, using a wide base of support will achieve a lower center of gravity. If answered incorrectly, review biomechanical guidelines for transfer techniques, including sliding board transfers.

C117 | Other Systems | Clinical Applications

A physical therapist assistant is treating a 2 year-old child with Down syndrome who frequently uses a "W" sitting position. The main reason to discourage "W" sitting in this child is that it may cause:

CHOICES:

1. abnormally low tone because of reflex activity.
2. femoral torsion and medial knee stress.
3. developmental delay of normal sitting.
4. hip subluxation and lateral knee stress.

CORRECT ANSWER: 2

RATIONALE:

"W" sitting is a stable and functional position, but may cause later orthopedic problems of femoral torsion and knee stress. Children with Down syndrome typically exhibit low tone and hyperextensibility. "W" sitting is not likely to affect low tone or reflex activity. Hip subluxation is unlikely.

TYPE OF REASONING: INDUCTIVE

This question requires the test taker to utilize clinical judgment to determine the main reason to discourage "W" sitting for a child with Down syndrome. This requires inductive reasoning skill. For this situation, the main reason to discourage "W" sitting is that it may cause femoral torsion and medial knee stress. If answered incorrectly, review sitting posture in children with Down syndrome, including "W" sitting.

C118 | Devices, Admin, etc. | Equipment, Modalities

The supervising physical therapist has instructed a physical therapist assistant to order a wheelchair for an elderly patient whose status is post–total hip arthroplasty surgery. It is critical for the assistant to order:

CHOICES:

1. antitip attachments.
2. elevating adjustable leg rests.
3. adjustable arm rests.
4. a solid seat.

CORRECT ANSWER: 4

RATIONALE:

The solid seat helps maintain the hips in a neutral position. The sling seat promotes the medially (internally) rotated hip position, which is contraindicated following hip arthroplasty surgery. The elevating leg rests might be nice to have, and could potentially help with any edema, but are not critical. Adjustable arm rests and antitip attachments again are nice options but do not seem to be indicated for this individual.

TYPE OF REASONING: INDUCTIVE

One must determine the most appropriate wheelchair feature for a patient whose status is post–hip arthroplasty. This requires clinical judgment, which is an inductive reasoning skill. For this situation, the assistant should order a wheelchair with a solid seat to maintain the hips in a neutral position. If answered incorrectly, review wheelchair prescription guidelines, especially for patients with a status of post–total hip arthroplasty.

C119 | Devices, Admin, etc. | Safety Roles, Teaching, EBP

An elderly and frail resident of a nursing home has developed a stage III pressure ulcer. The wound is open with necrosis of the subcutaneous tissue down to the fascia. This elderly patient, when compared with a younger patient with the same type of ulcer, can be expected to demonstrate:

CHOICES:

1. decreased vascular and immune responses resulting in impaired healing.
2. increased scarring with healing.
3. increased elasticity and eccrine sweating.
4. increased vascular responses with significant erythema.

CORRECT ANSWER: 1

RATIONALE:

Age-associated changes in the integumentary system include decreased vascular and immune responses that result in impaired healing. Rate of healing is considerably slower. In the elderly, scarring is typically less than in a younger individual. Both elasticity and eccrine sweating are decreased in the elderly.

TYPE OF REASONING: INFERENTIAL

One must determine the likely characteristics of wound healing for an elderly patient versus a younger patient. This requires one to determine what may be true of the situation, which is an inferential reasoning skill. For this case, the elderly patient can be expected to demonstrate decreased vascular and immune responses resulting in impaired healing compared with a younger patient with the same type of ulcer. If answered incorrectly, review wound healing guidelines, especially in the elderly.

C120 | Cardiovascular/Pulmonary | Interventions

A physical therapist assistant is following the plan of care for treatment of a patient on the coronary care unit 2 days after a coronary artery bypass surgery. An appropriate exercise regimen at this stage of the patient's recovery should include:

CHOICES:

1. ankle pumps and heel slides to increase the heart rate 1 to 5 beats over the resting level.
2. shoulder flexion and abduction, and elbow flexion with a 3-pound weight at an intensity to increase the heart rate 15 to 25 beats per minute.
3. exercises that increase the heart rate 30 beats over the resting level, such as upper-extremity exercises using a 1 pound weight, or marching in place while seated.
4. ankle pumps and marching in place while seated, at an intensity to increase the heart rate 10 to 15 beats over the resting level.

CORRECT ANSWER: 4

RATIONALE:

For a patient in phase I of a cardiac program, it is important to increase circulation in the lower extremities to decrease the chances of a deep vein thrombosis. Exercises should be in the 1 to 3 MET range and the heart rate should not exceed 20 bpm above the resting heart rate. The systolic blood pressure should not raise more than 20 mmHg or fall more than 10 to 15 mmHg from normal range. The 3 to 4 MET range is too high and might put the patient at risk for increased cardiac problems. Exercising that increases the heart rate only 1 to 5 beats over the resting level is not enough to build up endurance. Upper-extremity exercises will increase the heart rate more quickly than lower-extremity exercises; in addition, they do not achieve the added benefit of promoting blood flow in the lower extremities.

TYPE OF REASONING: INDUCTIVE

One must determine the best therapeutic approach for a patient on the coronary care unit after coronary artery bypass surgery. This requires clinical judgment, which is an inductive reasoning skill. For this situation, a patient who has had a recent coronary artery bypass graft should perform ankle pumps and marching in place, while seated, at an intensity to increase the heart rate 10 to 15 beats over the resting level. If answered incorrectly, review cardiac rehabilitation guidelines, especially for patients in the initial phases of rehabilitation.

C121 | Devices, Admin, etc. | Equipment, Modalities

A physical therapist assistant is reviewing the physical therapist plan of care in preparation to treat a client in an outpatient setting. The client was involved in a severe car accident 21 days ago and suffered a cervical fracture with incomplete spinal cord damage. The plan of care identifies a strengthening, balance and endurance program. What type of stabilization device should the assistant anticipate that the patient will likely be utilizing at this stage of recovery?

CHOICES:

1. a halo with vest attachment.
2. cervical tongs.
3. a Philadelphia collar.
4. a body jacket.

CORRECT ANSWER: 1

RATIONALE:

The halo device will limit motion of the cervical spine, which protects the incomplete spinal cord lesion. Cervical tongs are used with a patient who is immobilized in the supine position in bed, and are typically only temporary. A Philadelphia collar is often used following the initial period of immobilization in the halo device. A body jacket will protect the thoracic or lumbar spine; however, it will offer no protection for the cervical spine.

TYPE OF REASONING: INFERENTIAL

This question requires the test taker to infer the likely stabilization device that will be utilized with a patient who has sustained a cervical fracture. This requires inferential reasoning skill. For this case, one should anticipate that the patient will wear a halo with vest attachment. If answered incorrectly, review stabilization devices for spinal cord injury, including cervical injuries.

C122 | Devices, Admin, etc. | Equipment, Modalities

To appropriately guard a patient who is descending stairs for the first time using crutches and who is non–weight-bearing on the right side, the physical therapist assistant should stand:

CHOICES:

1. behind and slightly to the right side.
2. in front and slightly to the right side.
3. in front and slightly to the left side.
4. behind and slightly to the right side.

CORRECT ANSWER: 2

RATIONALE:

The correct guarding position is to stand in front and slightly to the involved side of the patient (the right side in this case). During ascent, the therapist should stand behind and slightly to the involved side.

TYPE OF REASONING: INDUCTIVE

One must utilize clinical judgment to determine the best guarding position for a client who is descending stairs using crutches and who is non–weight-bearing on the right side. Questions of this nature often require inductive reasoning skill as knowledge of therapeutic guidelines is paramount to arriving at a correct conclusion. For this situation, the assistant should stand in front and slightly to the right side. If answered incorrectly, review stair negotiation guidelines including use of crutches while negotiating stairs.

C123 | Devices, Admin, etc. | Safety Roles, Teaching, EBP

Using a quick or ballistic stretching technique can prove to be dangerous to the integrity of the muscle and the musculo-tendinous unit. The therapeutic disadvantage of ballistic stretching is that it:

CHOICES:

1. is likely to elicit a stretch reflex, which will prohibit a full stretch.
2. will promote plastic elongation of the muscle and tendons.
3. will not facilitate safer shortening of the muscle and tendons.
4. is likely to inhibit the stretch reflex that will allow for a full stretch.

CORRECT ANSWER: 1

RATIONALE:

Quick or ballistic stretching activates the stretch reflex and triggers shortening of the muscle by stimulating the muscle and musculotendinous proprioceptors, not elongation of the muscle. Eliciting the stretch reflex makes stretching the muscle more difficult. A slow stretch will avoid activation of the proprioceptors and make it easier to stretch a muscle that is relaxed.

TYPE OF REASONING: INDUCTIVE

One must determine the therapeutic disadvantage of ballistic stretching to arrive at a correct conclusion. This requires clinical judgment, which is an inductive reasoning skill. For this case, the therapeutic disadvantage of ballistic stretching is that it is likely to elicit a stretch reflex, which will trigger shortening of the muscle, and prohibit a full stretch. If answered incorrectly, review stretching technique guidelines, especially ballistic stretching techniques.

C124 | Neuromuscular | Clinical Applications

A child with autism encounters a change in routine at school. The child is likely to react by:

CHOICES:

1. demonstrating increased excitement and the inability to sit still, disturbing classmates by talking and distracting them.
2. directing others to participate in the new routine to make coping easier.
3. refusing to participate, disagreeing verbally with direction or withdrawing by going to sleep.
4. having a temper tantrum, screaming, displaying stereotypical behaviors such as hand flapping, or social withdrawal.

CORRECT ANSWER: 4

RATIONALE:

Autism is a neurobehavioral disability that includes differences in behavior, speech, socialization and interaction with the environment. Stereotypical behaviors such as hand flapping, as well as difficulty with changes in routine leading to temper tantrums, characterize autism. Poor social skills and poor expressive language skills are also characteristic. Because changes in routine are difficult for children with autism to handle, it is unlikely that this child would demonstrate excitement, verbal interactions or appropriate social skills such as directing his peers.

TYPE OF REASONING: DEDUCTIVE

One must recall the common behaviors of children with autism to arrive at a correct conclusion. This necessitates the recall of factual information, which is a deductive reasoning skill. For this scenario one should anticipate the child reacting by having a temper tantrum, screaming, displaying stereotypical behaviors such as hand flapping or social withdrawal. If answered incorrectly review signs and symptoms of autism and autistic behaviors.

C125 | Neuromuscular | Data Collection

The physical therapist has finished an evaluation on a patient who suffered a traumatic brain injury in a motor vehicle accident 2 weeks ago. The patient is able to respond to simple commands and requires a structured environment. The patient's memory is severely impaired; however, past memory is better than recent memory. Communication is difficult, as the patient tends to confabulate. Which of the following indicate an improvement in the patient's cognitive functioning? The patient:

CHOICES:

1. may follow simple commands in inconsistent or delayed manner; reacts inconsistently to stimuli.
2. shows carry-over for relearned tasks and little carry-over for new tasks, and demonstrates goal-oriented behavior with instruction.
3. appears in a deep sleep, completely unresponsive to any stimuli.
4. shows heightened activity levels with bizarre and nonpurposeful behavior that is not relative to the immediate environment.

CORRECT ANSWER: 2

RATIONALE:

The patient in the question is functioning at Rancho Level V, confused–inappropriate. By demonstrating goal-oriented behavior and carry-over of relearned tasks the patient is functioning at a Rancho Level VI, which is an improvement in cognitive functioning. A patient who is unresponsive to stimuli and appears to be in a deep sleep is functioning at Level 1 and is not showing an indication of improvement. A patient who is functioning at Level IV will demonstrate heightened activity levels and demonstrate bizarre and nonpurposeful behaviors that are unrelated to the immediate environment.

TYPE OF REASONING: ANALYTICAL

This question requires the test taker to analyze the patient's current status and deficits to determine the symptoms that indicate an improvement in cognitive functioning. This requires analytical reasoning skill. For this case, the patient is showing carry-over for relearned tasks and little carry-over for new tasks with goal-oriented behavior, which would indicate an improvement in cognitive functioning. If answered incorrectly, review traumatic brain injury signs and symptoms, including the Rancho Levels of Cognitive Functioning Scale.

C126 | Neuromuscular | Interventions

A physical therapist assistant is working with a patient who has Parkinson's disease. The patient demonstrates a pattern of slow movements, resting tremors and decreased postural reflexes. To meet the identified goal of improved ambulation activities, intervention should include:

CHOICES:

1. sitting "pelvic clock" exercises on a physio-ball.
2. assisted segmental rolling activities.
3. standing marching and foot-placing activities.
4. Frenkel's lower-extremity coordination exercises.

CORRECT ANSWER: 3

RATIONALE:

Standing marching and foot-placing activities will help improve a patient's ability to weight shift and advance the foot for ambulation. Physio-ball activities and segmental rolling will assist with trunk mobility. Frenkel's exercises will help with lower-extremity control but may not transfer into improved gait activities.

TYPE OF REASONING: INDUCTIVE

This question requires one to use clinical judgment to determine the best intervention activities for a patient with Parkinson's disease. This requires inductive reasoning skill. For this case, the best intervention activities should include standing marching and foot-placing activities. If answered incorrectly, review intervention activities for patients with Parkinson's disease, including ambulation activities.

C127 | Devices, Admin, etc. | Safety Roles, Teaching, EBP

A federal law mandates that individualized educational services in the least restrictive environment be provided, free of charge, for qualifying children with disabilities. This includes children from birth to 21 years of age. This mandate is referred to as:

CHOICES:

1. Section 504 of the Rehabilitation Act.
2. the Individuals with Disabilities Education Act (IDEA).
3. the Americans with Disabilities Act.
4. the Technology Assistance Act.

CORRECT ANSWER: 2

RATIONALE:

Both Section 504 of the Rehabilitation Act and the Americans with Disabilities Act are civil rights legislation. These acts legislate access for children to go to school, but do not mandate their education. The Technology Assistance Act provides for technology information and supports for individuals with disabilities, but does not mandate educational services for young children. Only IDEA mandates educational and related services for children with disabilities.

TYPE OF REASONING: DEDUCTIVE

This question requires one to recall factual information about federal laws, which is a deductive reasoning skill. For this situation, the federal mandate described is that of the Individuals with Disabilities Education Act or IDEA. Review information regarding federal mandates for individuals with disabilities, especially IDEA.

C128 | Neuromuscular | Clinical Applications

A physical therapist assistant is treating a patient with Duchenne's muscular dystrophy. A common pattern of characteristics of this disorder includes:

CHOICES:

1. progressive muscular weakness from proximal to distal musculature.
2. hypersensitivity in the tissues of the lower extremity, typically associated with an insult to the central nervous system or a systemic disease process.
3. general weakness of the facial nerves of one side of the face, affecting expression and eyelid control.
4. bilateral lower extremities affected; gait pattern is dominated by a scissoring gait.

CORRECT ANSWER: 1

RATIONALE:

Duchenne's muscular dystrophy is a genetic disorder characterized by progressive weakness in the proximal musculature, progressing to the distal musculature. The child progressively loses mobility and self-care skills by the preteen years, and survives until the late teens or 20s and then most commonly succumbs to respiratory or cardiac problems. Reflex sympathetic dystrophy is a sympathetically mediated response, often following some type of central nervous system lesion or systemic disease process, and leads to severe hypersensitivity of the affected extremity or trunk portion. Bell's palsy affects the facial nerve and leads to weakness or paralysis of the facial muscles. A patient with spastic cerebral palsy will often demonstrate a scissoring gait pattern.

TYPE OF REASONING: INFERENTIAL

This question provides a diagnosis, and the test taker is to determine the likely symptoms associated with this disorder. This requires inferring the symptoms, which is an inferential reasoning skill. For this situation, the expected characteristics of the disorder include progressive muscular weakness from proximal to distal musculature. If answered incorrectly, review signs and symptoms of Duchenne's muscular dystrophy.

C129 | Devices, Admin, etc. | Equipment, Modalities

A physical therapist assistant is working with a patient who has just received a new plastic, solid ankle–foot orthosis. As a part of the adjustment and breaking-in period, the areas that will be closely monitored for proper relief and tissue breakdown include the:

CHOICES:

1. calf band, fibular head, popliteal fossa, malleoli and styloid process of the 5th metatarsal.
2. tibial condyles, tibial tuberosity, anterodistal tibia and metatarsal heads.
3. pelvic band, quadriceps tendon, popliteal space, tibial tuberosity and navicular.
4. popliteal space, posterior calf musculature, malleoli, Achilles tendon and base of the metatarsals.

CORRECT ANSWER: 1

RATIONALE:

When a patient receives a new ankle–foot orthosis it is important to implement patient education regarding wearing and tissue breakdown areas. Physical therapists and physical therapist assistants should carefully monitor the tissues of the limb to avoid skin breakdown caused by improper fit, as well as teach these to the patient and family members. Common areas for tissue breakdown are over bony prominences. Common bony prominences in the lower extremity that would be involved include, but are not limited to, calf band, fibular head, popliteal fossa, malleoli and styloid process of the 5th metatarsal. The tibial condyles and tibial tuberosity are often areas of potential breakdown with a transtibial prosthesis. An ankle–foot orthosis does not come into contact with the pelvis or thigh so it is unnecessary to inspect this area on this patient.

TYPE OF REASONING: INFERENTIAL

One must infer or draw a reasonable conclusion about the likely areas to be closely monitored for tissue breakdown in a patient with a new ankle–foot orthosis. This requires inferential reasoning skill. For this case, the likely areas that will be monitored include the calf band, fibular head, popliteal fossa, malleoli and styloid process of the 5th metatarsal. If answered incorrectly, review prosthetic fitting guidelines, including monitoring for proper fit.

C130 | Neuromuscular | Clinical Applications

A physical therapist assistant is preparing to treat a patient with an injury to the posterior knee that crushed the tibial nerve. The physical therapy evaluation identifies both motor and sensory involvement. The physical therapist assistant should expect the patient to present with:

CHOICES:

1. decreased muscle tone of the knee flexors, as well as paresthesia of the posterior thigh and knee.
2. increased muscle tone and spasticity of the knee flexors, as well as absent sensation over the posterior thigh area.
3. decreased muscle tone of the plantar flexors and invertors of the ankle, as well as paresthesia of the posterior calf and plantar surface of the foot.
4. increased muscle tone and spasticity of the plantar flexors and invertors of the ankle, as well as absent sensation over the posterior calf and plantar surface of the foot.

CORRECT ANSWER: 3

RATIONALE:

Lesions in the upper motor neuron area cause motor spasticity and hyperreflexive muscle responses. A lesion to the nerve at the posterior thigh involves a peripheral nerve, or lower motor neuron. This will result in decreased muscle tone and reflexes. The sciatic nerve splits just proximal to the knee to form the tibial, and common and deep peroneal (fibular) nerves. The common peroneal nerve serves motor and sensory function to the antero-lateral distal limb. The tibial nerve supplies the posterior calf area. It innervates the gastrocnemius, soleus, plantaris, tibialis posterior, flexor digitorum longus and flexor hallucis longus.

TYPE OF REASONING: INFERENTIAL

One must determine the likely symptoms for a patient who has a crushed tibial nerve. This requires the test taker to infer the symptoms, which is an inferential reasoning skill. For this case, one should expect the patient to present with decreased muscle tone of the plantar flexors and inverters of the ankle, with paresthesia of the posterior calf and plantar surface of the foot. If answered incorrectly, review signs and symptoms of lower-extremity nerve injury, especially tibial nerve damage.

C131 | Cardiovascular/Pulmonary | Clinical Applications

A phase 2 outpatient cardiac rehabilitation program uses circuit training with different exercise stations for the 50-minute program. One station uses upper-extremity ergometry. When comparing upper-extremity exercise to lower-extremity exercise, at a given workload, the assistant can expect that:

CHOICES:

1. the principal changes are higher systolic and diastolic BP.
2. exercise capacity is reduced owing to higher stroke volumes.
3. both heart rate (HR) and systolic and diastolic blood pressure (BP) will be higher.
4. HR will be higher while systolic BP will be lower.

CORRECT ANSWER: 3

RATIONALE:

Upper-extremity ergometry uses a smaller muscle mass than leg ergometry, resulting in a lower maximal oxygen uptake. In upper-extremity exercise, both HR and BP will be higher than for the same level of work in the lower extremities.

TYPE OF REASONING: ANALYTICAL

One must analyze the different types of exercises presented to determine their effects on HR and BP. This requires analytical reasoning skill. For this case, one should expect both HR and systolic and diastolic BP to be higher when comparing upper-extremity exercise to lower-extremity exercise. If answered incorrectly, review cardiac rehabilitation guidelines, especially effects of exercise on HR and BP.

C132 | Devices, Admin, etc. | Safety Roles, Teaching, EBP

To find out if a physical therapist assistant is legally permitted to supervise a physical therapy aide in a specific state one should reference the:

CHOICES:
1. appropriate practice act.
2. American Physical Therapy Association's Guide for Conduct of the Physical Therapist Assistant.
3. departmental policy and procedure manual.
4. American Physical Therapy Association's Standards of Practice.

CORRECT ANSWER: 1

RATIONALE:

Each state will set its own supervision requirements for personnel. These can typically be referenced in the state's practice act or in the state's rules and regulations for practice. The American Physical Therapy Association sets acceptable standards for physical therapy and physical therapy personnel; individual states can choose to use those or other requirements. A department's policy and procedure manual is not a reference for legal supervisory requirements.

TYPE OF REASONING: DEDUCTIVE

This question requires the test taker to determine the appropriate resource to refer to find whether an assistant is able to supervise a physical therapy aide. This is factual information, which requires deductive reasoning skill. For this situation, the best resource to refer to is the appropriate practice act for the state in which the physical therapist assistant resides. If answered incorrectly, review supervision of personnel guidelines.

C133 | Neuromuscular | Interventions

A physical therapist assistant is working with a patient who has right hemiparesis and is demonstrating good recovery. Both involved limbs demonstrate some ability to move in patterns that are out of synergy. The patient is ambulatory with a small-base quad cane. The activity that is **MOST** appropriate for a patient at this stage of recovery is:

CHOICES:
1. supine, bending the hip and knee up to the chest and slowly lowering the foot back to the mat.
2. standing with the hip extended while flexing the knee and slowly lowering the foot back to the floor.
3. sitting, marching in place and incorporating elbow flexion with the marching pattern.
4. supine, performing active assistive diagonal flexion patterns with the lower extremities.

CORRECT ANSWER: 2

RATIONALE:

This stage of recovery is characterized by some movement combinations that do not follow the paths of either flexion or extension synergies. Knee flexion in standing is a movement that is an out-of-synergy movement pattern. All other choices represent synergistic movements.

TYPE OF REASONING: INDUCTIVE

This question requires clinical judgment about an appropriate therapeutic activity for a patient with a cerebrovascular accident. Questions of this nature where one must determine a most appropriate therapeutic activity often require inductive reasoning skill. For this case, a most appropriate activity is standing with the hip extended while flexing the knee and slowly lowering the foot back to the floor. If answered incorrectly, review therapeutic exercises for patients with cerebrovascular accident, especially stages of recovery.

C134 | Musculoskeletal | Data Collection

A physical therapist assistant is helping to plan a scoliosis screening for a local school. The assistant should plan it for girls who are between what years of age?

CHOICES:
1. 6–8.
2. 9–11.
3. 12–14.
4. 15–17.

CORRECT ANSWER: 2

RATIONALE:

The most effective age to screen girls for scoliosis is just before the pubescent growth spurt, between ages 9 and 11 years, when the scoliotic curve can increase dramatically. Boys should be screened between 11 and 13 years of age because of differences in the age of puberty onset between girls and boys.

TYPE OF REASONING: DEDUCTIVE

One must recall the guidelines for the assessment of scoliosis in young females to arrive at a correct conclusion. This is factual information, which necessitates deductive reasoning skill. For this situation, the assistant should plan to assess girls between the ages of 9 and 11 years. If answered incorrectly, review scoliosis screening guidelines, especially in females.

C135 | Neuromuscular | Clinical Applications

A physical therapist assistant is working with a patient who is recovering from a complete spinal cord injury at the C6 neurological level. The physical therapist has directed the assistant to strengthen the available musculature. Which of the following muscles would the therapist focus on?

CHOICES:
1. shoulder flexion, extension and all elbow motions.
2. scapular elevation and respiration.
3. shoulder lateral (external) rotation and abduction.
4. all shoulder motions as well as all elbow motions.

CORRECT ANSWER: 1

RATIONALE:

A patient with an intact spinal cord to the C6 level will have intact shoulder flexion, extension and medial (internal) rotation; elbow flexion and extension; pronation; and wrist extension. A patient with an intact spinal cord to the C5 level will have intact shoulder lateral (external) rotation and abduction, elbow flexion, and supination. A patient with an intact spinal cord to the C7 level will have intact all shoulder motions, elbow flexion and extension, wrist flexion and extension, and finger extension. A patient with an intact spinal cord to the C4 level will have intact scapular elevation and respiration.

TYPE OF REASONING: INFERENTIAL

This question requires one to draw a reasonable conclusion about the likely muscles that will be focused on for a patient with C6 spinal cord injury. Questions that require one to determine what may be true of a situation often necessitate inferential reasoning skill. For this case, the assistant is likely to focus on shoulder flexion and extension, and all elbow motions. Review intact musculature for cervical spinal cord injury, including C6 injury, if answered incorrectly.

C136 | Neuromuscular | Data Collection

A physical therapist assistant is working with an infant with Down syndrome. The assistant should expect the infant's tone to be:

CHOICES:

1. hypertonic.
2. hypotonic.
3. fluctuating.
4. absent.

CORRECT ANSWER: 2

RATIONALE:

Most young children with Down syndrome present with low or hypotonic muscle tone. If the tone was fluctuating or absent the patient would not be able to maintain sitting at all.

TYPE OF REASONING: INFERENTIAL

This question requires one to infer the likely tone that is present for a child with Down syndrome. Determining what may be true of a situation often necessitates inferential reasoning skill. For this case, one should expect the infant's tone to be hypotonic. If answered incorrectly, review signs and symptoms of Down syndrome.

C137 | Musculoskeletal | Data Collection

To correctly perform a manual muscle test for grade good (4/5) muscle strength of the sternal head of the pectoralis major, the physical therapist assistant should position the patient supine and the shoulder in abduction to:

CHOICES:

1. 120°.
2. 90°.
3. 60°.
4. 160°.

CORRECT ANSWER: 1

RATIONALE:

The whole muscle is tested in 90° of abduction, the sternal head requires 120° of abduction and the clavicular head is tested in 60° of abduction. Grade poor (2/5) or lower is tested with the upper extremity supported or with the patient sitting with the upper extremity supported on a horizontal surface at the level of the axilla.

TYPE OF REASONING: DEDUCTIVE

This question requires the test taker to recall the procedure for manual muscle testing of the sternal head of the pectoralis major. This is factual information, which is a deductive reasoning skill. For this scenario, the correct testing position is with the patient supine and the shoulder in 120° of abduction. If answered incorrectly, review manual muscle testing procedures, including testing the pectoralis major.

C138 | Cardiovascular/Pulmonary | Clinical Applications

A patient recovering from surgery for triple coronary artery bypass grafts is scheduled to begin a phase III cardiac rehabilitation program. During the resistance training portion of the circuit training program, the assistant instructs the patient to **AVOID** the Valsalva maneuver because:

CHOICES:

1. heart rate and blood pressure are likely to be elevated.
2. slowing of pulse and increased venous pressure are possible.
3. a cholinergic or vagal response can occur.
4. the decreased return of blood to the heart can lead to pitting edema.

CORRECT ANSWER: 2

RATIONALE:

The Valsalva maneuver results from forcible exhalation with the glottis, nose and mouth closed. It increases intrathoracic pressure and causes slowing of the pulse, decreased return of blood to the heart and increased venous pressure. A cholinergic or vagal response is the result of parasympathetic nervous system stimulation.

TYPE OF REASONING: INDUCTIVE

One must determine the reasons to avoid the Valsalva maneuver with a patient who has a status of post–coronary artery bypass grafting. This requires clinical judgment, which is an inductive reasoning skill. For this situation, the reasons to avoid the Valsalva maneuver are the possibility of slowing of the pulse and increased venous pressure. If answered incorrectly, be aware of precautions and contraindications for patients in cardiac rehabilitation.

C139 | Devices, Admin, etc. | Safety Roles, Teaching, EBP

A patient is having difficulty learning how to transfer from mat to wheelchair. The patient cannot seem to get the idea of how to coordinate the movement even after numerous attempts. In this case, the **MOST** effective use of feedback during early motor learning should incorporate:

CHOICES:

1. increased verbal feedback as the patient fatigues.
2. verbal feedback for the correct technique and proprioceptive feedback for incorrect technique.
3. tactile and visual feedback for correct technique.
4. visual feedback rather than other forms of feedback.

CORRECT ANSWER: 3

RATIONALE:

During the early stage of motor learning, learners benefit from seeing the whole task performed correctly as dependence on visual input is high. Tactile feedback for correct technique also provides appropriate feedback into the system. Developing a reference of correctness and success (knowledge of results) is critical to ensure early skill acquisition. Proprioceptive feedback for incorrect techniques is inappropriate.

TYPE OF REASONING: INDUCTIVE

This question requires the test taker to determine the most effective feedback approach to facilitate motor learning during transfer training. This requires knowledge of therapeutic approaches for transfer training, which necessitates inductive reasoning skill. For this case, one should incorporate tactile and visual feedback for correct technique. Review transfer training guidelines using motor learning approaches if answered incorrectly.

C140 | Cardiovascular/Pulmonary | Interventions

A patient who is using an incentive spirometer reports feeling lightheaded. The physical therapist assistant should instruct the patient to:

CHOICES:
1. take a rest period and only use the device 10 times per hour.
2. take a deeper breath on the following attempt.
3. lie down while using the spirometer.
4. try to use the spirometer more frequently to get used to it.

CORRECT ANSWER: 1

RATIONALE:
If a patient feels lightheaded with an incentive spirometer, it may be because of blowing off too much CO_2 by hyperventilating. An incentive spirometer should always be used in the most upright position possible to attain the highest values possible.

TYPE OF REASONING: EVALUATIVE
One must weigh the benefits of the courses of action presented to determine the approach that will most effectively resolve the patient's issue. This requires evaluative reasoning skill. For this situation, the assistant should instruct the patient who is using an incentive spirometer to take a rest period and only use the device 10 times per hour. If answered incorrectly, review guidelines for use of incentive spirometers.

C141 | Neuromuscular | Interventions

Isokinetic training can be used in the rehabilitation of patients following a cerebrovascular accident (CVA) during the late stages of recovery to improve:

CHOICES:
1. strength of synergistic muscle groups.
2. initiation of movements.
3. control of movements at slower speeds.
4. control of movements at faster speeds.

CORRECT ANSWER: 4

RATIONALE:
Patients during later stages of recovery from stroke frequently exhibit problems with control of faster movements. They are able to move at slow speeds, but as speed of movement increases, control decreases. An isokinetic device can be an effective training modality to remediate this problem.

TYPE OF REASONING: INDUCTIVE
One must utilize clinical judgment to determine the benefits of using isokinetic training for patients with CVA. This requires inductive reasoning skill. For this case, the benefits of isokinetic training include improving control of movements at faster speeds. If answered incorrectly, review isokinetic training guidelines, especially for patients with a status of post–CVA.

C142 | Neuromuscular | Clinical Applications

A patient with a traumatic brain injury is inconsistently oriented to time and place. The patient is unable to remember recent events and shows little or no carry-over for new learning. The primary focus of rehabilitation at this stage of recovery is to:

CHOICES:

1. develop an environment and daily structure in which the patient is best able to process stimuli cognitively.
2. promote independence in problem-solving skills and provide as little verbal or tactile input as possible.
3. increase functional independence in bed mobility and transfers.
4. promote increased arousal and attention through the use of sensory stimulation techniques.

CORRECT ANSWER: 1

RATIONALE:

This patient demonstrates recovery consistent with a confused state (Rancho Los Amigos Levels V/VI). The main focus should be on providing environmental and daily structure to reduce distractions and help the patient process stimuli.

TYPE OF REASONING: INDUCTIVE

This question requires the test taker to determine the primary focus for rehabilitation of a patient with traumatic brain injury. This requires clinical judgment, which is an inductive reasoning skill. For this situation, a patient at this stage of recovery would benefit from developing an environment and daily structure where the patient is best able to process stimuli cognitively. If answered incorrectly, review the Rancho Los Amigos Levels of recovery and therapeutic approaches for patients with traumatic brain injury, especially patients at Levels V and VI of recovery.

C143 | Cardiovascular/Pulmonary | Data Collection

The medical record identifies that a patient is walking with a transtibial prosthesis and demonstrates terminal swing impact. The assistant should expect to see the patient perform:

CHOICES:

1. hip external (lateral) rotation at midswing.
2. decreased hip flexion at heel strike.
3. knee hyperextension at heel strike.
4. hip abduction at swing.

CORRECT ANSWER: 3

RATIONALE:

Terminal swing impact refers to the sudden stopping of the prosthesis as the knee extends during late swing. Possible causes can include insufficient knee friction or too much tension in the extension aid; the assistant should note knee hyperextension at heel strike. Additionally, if the patient with an amputation fears the knee will buckle at heel strike (initial contact), the patient can use forceful hip flexion to extend the knee.

TYPE OF REASONING: INFERENTIAL

One must infer or draw a reasonable conclusion about the likely gait pattern of a patient who is using a below-knee prosthesis. Questions that ask one to determine what may be true of a patient often necessitate inferential reasoning skill. For this case, the patient with a terminal swing impact is likely to perform the hyperextension at heel strike. If answered incorrectly, review gait patterns for patients who are using lower-extremity prostheses, especially terminal swing impact.

C144 | Devices, Admin, etc. | Equipment, Modalities

The physical therapist has just finished the evaluation of a patient with the diagnosis of L4–5 paraplegia. The physical therapist has met with the orthotist and discussed the **MOST** appropriate orthotic device to use in the continued care of this patient. This patient is able to perform all transfers independently, perform independent skin inspections, can stand and ambulate with forearm crutches and is independent in all activities of daily living. The **MOST** appropriate orthosis to facilitate improved gait is:

CHOICES:

1. bilateral solid ankle–foot orthoses.
2. bilateral knee–ankle–foot orthoses.
3. a hip–knee–ankle–foot orthosis.
4. a thoracic–lumbar–sacral orthosis.

CORRECT ANSWER: 2

RATIONALE:

A Craig–Scott knee–ankle–foot orthosis is the most common orthosis used for persons with a spinal cord injury at the L4–5 level. It has a shoe attachment and ankle and knee joints with controls and shells for the thigh and calf. A patient at an L4–5 spinal injury level does not have enough support with an ankle–foot orthosis because of poor knee stability. A thoracic–lumbar–sacral orthosis could limit mobility too much and would not provide the support needed at the hips and knees for standing. A hip–knee–ankle–foot orthosis is very bulky and would likely limit the patient's ability to efficiently perform activities of daily living.

TYPE OF REASONING: INDUCTIVE

This question requires one to determine the most appropriate orthosis for a patient with an L4–5 spinal cord injury. This requires knowledge of the diagnosis and orthotic devices to arrive at a correct conclusion, which is an inductive reasoning skill. For this case, the most appropriate orthotic device is a bilateral knee–ankle–foot orthosis. If answered incorrectly, review lower-extremity orthotics for patients with spinal cord injury.

C145 | Other Systems | Clinical Applications

A young woman who is 12 weeks pregnant asks a physical therapist assistant if it is safe to continue with her aerobic exercise. Currently she jogs 3 miles, three times a week and has done so for the past 10 years. After discussion with the therapist, the assistant's **BEST** reply to the woman is:

CHOICES:

1. jogging is safe as long as the target heart rate does not exceed 140 beats per minute.
2. jogging is safe at mild to moderate intensities whereas vigorous exercise is contraindicated.
3. continue jogging only until the 5th month of pregnancy.
4. swimming is preferred over walking or jogging for all phases of pregnancy.

CORRECT ANSWER: 2

RATIONALE:

According to the American College of Sports Medicine, women can continue to exercise regularly (three times a week) at mild to moderate intensities throughout pregnancy if no additional risk factors are present. After the first trimester, women should avoid exercise in the supine position because this position is associated with decreased cardiac output. Prolonged standing with no motion should also be avoided. Non–weight-bearing exercise (swimming) is an appropriate alternative to walking or jogging, depending on the patient's skill and interests.

TYPE OF REASONING: EVALUATIVE

This question requires one to determine a best course of action and to evaluate the benefits of such an action with a patient who is pregnant and who wishes to continue aerobic exercise. This requires evaluative reasoning skill. For this situation, the best reply to the patient is that jogging is safe at mild to moderate intensities whereas vigorous exercise is contraindicated. If answered incorrectly, review exercise guidelines for patients who are pregnant.

C146 | Devices, Admin, etc. | Equipment, Modalities

Evaluation findings for a 10 year-old include pain and limited range of motion following a surgical repair of the medial collateral ligament and the anterior cruciate ligament. The plan of care includes use of physical agents for pain control and tissue healing. The physical therapist assistant should avoid use of:

CHOICES:

1. pulsed shortwave diathermy.
2. pulsed ultrasound.
3. transcutaneous electrical stimulation.
4. interferential current.

CORRECT ANSWER: 2

RATIONALE:

Ultrasound is contraindicated for patients whose epiphyseal areas are still active. The epiphyseal plates close at the end of puberty. All the other physical agents can be used without adverse physiological effects and would contribute to pain control.

TYPE OF REASONING: DEDUCTIVE

One must recall the contraindications for use of specific physical agent modalities to arrive at a correct conclusion. This is recall of factual guidelines, which is a deductive reasoning skill. For this situation, the assistant should avoid use of pulsed ultrasound, as the patient's epiphyseal areas are still active. If answered incorrectly, review contraindications for use of physical agent modalities, especially ultrasound, in children.

C147 | Integumentary | Interventions

Treatment for an infected and draining stage IV pressure ulcer should most likely include the application of a/an:

CHOICES:

1. transparent film.
2. hydrogel covered with a lightly absorbent wrap.
3. hydrocolloid dressing.
4. alginate covered with absorbent dressings.

CORRECT ANSWER: 4

RATIONALE:

A stage IV pressure ulcer will include disruption of the deep tissues such as fascia, muscle and joint structures. It will likely present with necrotic tissue and have exudate. This type of wound needs intervention to clean up the necrotic tissue, such as an alginate to rid the wound of necrotic tissue and dressings to absorb the drainage or exudate. Clean stage I and stage II wounds can be better managed with the transparent film or hydrocolloid; these are designed to provide protection to the wound. A hydrogel dressing is BEST used on stage II and III wounds to maintain a moist wound bed.

TYPE OF REASONING: INFERENTIAL

One must infer the likely treatment approach for an infected and draining stage IV pressure ulcer. Ultimately, such ulcers are managed surgically after infection clears. This requires one to determine what may be true, which is an inferential reasoning skill. For this case, one would most likely include the application of an alginate covered with absorbent dressings. If answered incorrectly, review treatment guidelines for pressure ulcers, especially stage IV.

C148 | Other Systems | Clinical Applications

A physical therapist assistant is providing treatment in a long-term care center for a patient who has decreased core strength with an additional diagnosis of gastroesophageal reflux disease. The patient reports being unable to tolerate lying on his back to perform exercises. The physical therapist assistant should modify the intervention approach by:

CHOICES:

1. performing exercise with the patient prior to eating.
2. modify exercise to fast-paced walking and avoid lying down.
3. modify the supine position to right side-lying.
4. encourage the patient to increase the calories in the food consumed prior to exercise.

CORRECT ANSWER: 1

RATIONALE:

Patients with gastroesophageal reflux disease will tolerate exercise better if there is less body agitation (such as in running or aerobics), if it is performed prior to eating, and if it is not performed in strenuous bouts. Fatty foods or high-calorie foods prior to eating can trigger the reflux response. Reflux symptoms may be decreased in the left side-lying position.

TYPE OF REASONING: INDUCTIVE

This question requires one to determine a best course of action for a patient with gastroesophageal reflux disease. This requires knowledge of the diagnosis and therapeutic courses of action to arrive at a correct conclusion, which is an inductive reasoning skill. For this situation, the assistant should modify the intervention approach by performing exercise with the patient prior to the patient eating to reduce the likelihood of symptoms. If answered incorrectly, review signs and symptoms of gastroesophageal reflux disease and guidelines for exercise.

C149 | Neuromuscular | Data Collection

As a result of a drug overdose, a patient suffered permanent damage to the basal ganglia. It is **MOST** likely that the patient will demonstrate:

CHOICES:
1. hypotonia.
2. ataxia.
3. poor motor planning.
4. dysdiadochokinesia.

CORRECT ANSWER: 3

RATIONALE:

The basal ganglia functions to convert general motor activity into specific, goal-oriented action plans. Dysfunction results in problems with motor planning and scaling of movements and postures. Dysdiadochokinesia is the inability to quickly substitute antagonistic motor impulses to produce antagonistic muscular movements. Hypotonia is decreased muscle tone. Parkinson's disease is an example of a disorder that also affects the basal ganglia; however, the patient presents with difficulty initiating movements.

TYPE OF REASONING: INFERENTIAL

One must infer the likely symptoms of a patient who has damage to the basal ganglia. This requires the test taker to determine what may be true of this patient, which is an inferential reasoning skill. For this case, the patient would most likely demonstrate poor motor planning with damage to the basal ganglia. If answered incorrectly, review signs and symptoms of patients with basal ganglia damage.

C150 | Cardiovascular/Pulmonary | Interventions

A physical therapist assistant should teach a patient segmental breathing by placing:

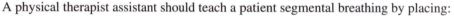

CHOICES:
1. a hand over the area of hypoventilation and applying firm pressure just prior to inspiration, then asking the patient to breathe in against the resistance of the hand.
2. both hands gently over the lower ribs and applying gentle pressure throughout exhalation and increasing pressure at the end of exhalation by asking the patient to inhale against the resistance.
3. a hand over the lower abdomen and applying pressure at or near the end of exhalation.
4. the incentive spirometer in the patient's mouth and encouraging the patient to breathe in as deeply as possible.

CORRECT ANSWER: 1

RATIONALE:

To assist with segmental breathing the clinician places a hand over the area of hypoventilation and applies firm pressure just prior to inspiration and asks the patient to breathe in against the resistance of the hand. In diaphragmatic breathing, the clinician places both hands gently over the lower ribs and applies gentle pressure throughout exhalation and increases pressure at the end of exhalation and asks the patient to inhale against the resistance. During pursed-lip breathing, the exhalation phase can be prolonged by the clinician gently applying pressure through the abdomen near the end of expiration. An incentive spirometer assists with overall inhalation, not inhalation of a specific segment.

TYPE OF REASONING: INDUCTIVE

For this question, the test taker must utilize knowledge of segmental breathing techniques to arrive at a correct conclusion. This requires inductive reasoning skill. For this case, the assistant should teach the patient segmental breathing by placing a hand over the area of hypoventilation and applying firm pressure just prior to inspiration followed by asking the patient to breathe in against the resistance of the hand. If answered incorrectly, review segmental breathing techniques.

References

Adler S, Beckers D, Buck M (2008). PNF in Practice, 3rd ed. New York, Springer.

Andrews J, Wilk K, Harrelson G (2004). Physical Rehabilitation of the Injured Athlete, 3rd ed. Philadelphia, Elsevier Saunders.

American College of Sports Medicine (2002). ACSM's Resources for Clinical Exercise Physiology. Philadelphia, Lippincott Williams & Wilkins.

American College of Sports Medicine (2006). ACSM's Guidelines for Exercise Testing and Prescription, 7th ed. Philadelphia, Lippincott Williams & Wilkins.

American Physical Therapy Association (2001). Guide to Physical Therapist Practice, 2nd ed. Alexandria, VA, APTA.

Baranoski S, Ayello E (2007). Wound Care Essentials: Practice & Principles, 2nd ed. Philadelphia, Lippincott Williams & Wilkins.

Batavia M. (2000). Clinical Research for Health Professionals: A User-Friendly Guide. Boston, Butterworth-Heinemann.

Batavia M. (2006). Contraindications in Physical Rehabilitation—Doing No Harm. St Louis, Elsevier Saunders.

Bear M, Connors B, Paradiso M (2007). Neuroscience—Exploring the Brain, 3rd ed. Philadelphia, Lippincott Williams & Wilkins.

Behrens B, Michlovitz S (2005). Physical Agents: Theory & Practice, 2nd ed. Philadelphia, FA Davis.

Belanger AY (2002). Evidence-Based Guide to Therapeutic Physical Agents. Philadelphia, Lippincott Williams & Wilkins.

Bonham P, Flemister B (2002). Guideline For Management of Wounds in Patients with Lower-Extremity Arterial Disease #1, Glenview.

Bowden BS, Bowden JM. (2005). An Illustrated Atlas of the Skeletal Muscles, 2nd ed. Englewood, CO, Morton Publishing.

Brotzman S (2007). Handbook of Orthopaedic Rehabilitation, 2nd ed. St Louis, Elsevier Mosby.

Brown S, Miller W, Eason J (2005). Exercise Physiology Basis of Human Movement in Health and Disease. Philadelphia, Lippincott Williams & Wilkins.

Cameron M (2008). Physical Agents in Rehabilitation, 3rd ed. St Louis, Elsevier Saunders.

Campbell S (2006). Physical Therapy for Children, 3rd ed. St Louis, Elsevier Saunders.

Ciccone C (2007). Pharmacology in Rehabilitation, 4th ed. Philadelphia, FA Davis.

Clarkson HM (2000). Musculoskeletal Assessment: Joint Range of Motion and Manual Muscle Strength, 2nd ed. Philadelphia, Lippincott Williams & Wilkins

Cook C (2006). Orthopedic Manual Therapy: An Evidence-Based Approach. Upper Saddle River, NJ, Pearson Education.

Craik R, Oatis C (1995). Gait Analysis: Theory and Application. St Louis, Mosby–Year Book.

Crawford, P, Fields-Varnado, M (2004). Guideline For Management of Wounds in Patients with Lower-Extremity Neuropathic Disease, #3, Glenview.

Davies P (2000). Steps to Follow, 3rd ed. New York, Springer.

Davis C (2006). Patient Practitioner Interaction, 4th ed. Thorofare, NJ, Slack.

DeDomenico G (2008). Beard's Massage, 5th ed. St Louis, Elsevier.

Deglin J, Vallerand A (2009). FA Davis's Drug Guide for Nurses, 11th ed. Philadelphia, FA Davis.

Denegar C, Saliba E, Saliba S (2006) Therapeutic Modalities for Musculoskeletal Injuries, 2nd ed. Champaign, IL, Human Kinetics.

DeTurk W, Cahalin L (2004). Cardiovascular and Pulmonary Physical Therapy. New York, McGraw-Hill.

Dohm G Lynis, Fushiki T (2002). Exercise Treatment for Obesity. Endotext.org, Http://www.endotext.org/obesity/obesity19/obesity19.htm. Web Jun.2009.

Domholdt E (2005). Rehabilitation Research: Principles and Applications, 3rd ed. St Louis, Elsevier Saunders.

Donatelli R (2007) Sports-Specific Rehabilitation. St Louis, Elsevier.

Donatelli R, Wooden M (2009). Orthopedic Physical Therapy, 4th ed. New York, Churchill Livingstone.

Drake R, et al (2008) Gray's Atlas of Anatomy. Maryland Heights, MO, Elsevier.

Drench M, Noonan A, Sharby N, Ventura S (2003). Psychosocial Aspects of Health Care. Upper Saddle River, NJ, Prentice Hall.

Durstine J, Moore, G, Durstine (2002). ACSM's Exercise Management for Persons with Chronic Diseases and Disabilities. Champaign, IL, Human Kinetics.

Dutton M (2004). Orthopaedic Examination, Evaluation, and Intervention. New York, McGraw-Hill.

Erickson M, McKnight R, Utzman R (2008). Physical Therapy Documentation: From Examination to Outcome. Thorofare, NJ, Slack.

Effgen S (2005). Meeting the Physical Therapy Needs of Children. Philadelphia, FA Davis.

Field-Fote E (2009). Spinal Cord Injury Rehabilitation. Philadelphia, F A Davis.

Finch E, Brooks D, Stratford P, et al. (2002). Physical Rehabilitation Outcome Measures: A Guide to Enhanced Clinical Decision Making, 2nd ed. Toronto, Canadian Physiotherapy Association.

Frontera W, Slovik D, Dawson D (eds) (2006). Exercise in Rehabilitation Medicine, 2nd ed. Champaign, IL, Human Kinetics.

Frownfelter D, Dean E (2006). Cardiovascular and Pulmonary Physical Therapy: Evidence and Practice, 4th ed. St Louis, Elsevier Mosby.

Gabard D, Martin M (2003). Physical Therapy Ethics. Philadelphia, FA Davis.

Goodman C, Fuller K (2009). Pathology: Implications for the Physical Therapist, 3rd ed. St Louis, Elsevier Saunders.

Goodman C, Snyder T (2007). Differential Diagnosis in Physical Therapy: Screening for Referral, 4th ed. St Louis, Elsevier Saunders.

Griffin L (2005). Essentials of Musculoskeletal Care, 3rd ed. Rosemont, IL, American Academy of Orthopaedic Surgeons.

Gutman S (2008). Quick Reference Neuroscience for Rehabilitation Professionals: The Essential Neurological Principles

Underlying Rehabilitation Professionals, 2nd ed. Thorofare, NJ, Slack.

Guyton A, Hall J (2006). Textbook of Medical Physiology, 10th ed. St Louis, Elsevier Saunders.

Hall C, Brody L (2004). Therapeutic Exercise: Moving Toward Function, 2nd ed. Philadelphia, Lippincott Williams & Wilkins.

Hertling D, Kessler R (2006). Management of Common Musculoskeletal Disorders: Physical Therapy Principles and Methods, 4th ed. Philadelphia, Lippincott Williams & Wilkins.

Hillegass E, Sadowsky H (2001). Essentials of Cardiopulmonary Physical Therapy, 2nd ed. St Louis, Elsevier Saunders.

Hislop H, Montgomery J (2007). Daniels and Worthingham's Muscle Testing: Techniques of Manual Examination, 8th ed. St Louis, Elsevier Saunders.

Hoppenfeld S (1982). Physical Evaluation of the Spine and Extremities. New York, Appleton-Century-Crofts.

Howle J (2002). Neuro-Developmental Treatment Approach: Theoretical Foundations and Principles of Clinical Practice. Laguna Beach, CA, Neuro-Developmental Treatment Association.

Huber F, Wells C (2006). Therapeutic Exercise—Treatment Planning for Progression. St Louis, Elsevier Saunders.

Irion G (2002). Comprehensive Wound Management. Thorofare, NJ, Slack.

Irwin S, Tecklin J (2004). Cardiopulmonary Physical Therapy, 4th ed. St Louis, Elsevier Mosby.

Jenkins D (2009). Hollinshead's Functional Anatomy of the Limbs and Back, 9th ed. Maryland Heights, MO, Elsevier.

Jewell D (2008). Guide to Evidence-Based Physical Therapy Practice. Sudbury, MA, Jones & Bartlett.

Johnson J, Paustian C (2005). Guideline For Management of Wounds in Patients with Lower-Extremity Venous Disease, #4, Glenview.

Kaltenborn F (2007). Manual Mobilization of the Joints. Vol 1. The Extremities, 6th ed. Oslo, Olaf Norlis Bokhandel.

Kanel E, Schwartz J, Jessell T, et al. (2000). Principles of Neural Science, 4th ed. New York, McGraw-Hill.

Kauffman T, Barr J, Moran M (2007). Geriatric Rehabilitation Manual, 2nd ed. St Louis, Elsevier Health Sciences.

Kendall F, McCreary E, Provance P, et al (2005). Muscle Testing and Function, 5th ed. Philadelphia, Lippincott Williams & Wilkins.

Kiernan J (2006). Barr's The Human Nervous System: An Anatomical Viewpoint, 8th ed. Philadelphia, Lippincott Williams & Wilkins.

Kisner C, Colby L (2007). Therapeutic Exercise Foundations and Techniques, 5th ed. Philadelphia, FA Davis.

Kitchen S (2002). Electrotherapy: Evidenced-Based Practice, 2nd ed. St Louis, Elsevier Mosby.

Kizior R, Hodgson B (2009). Saunders Drug Handbook for Health Professionals. St Louis, Elsevier Saunders.

Kloth L, McCulloch J (2002). Wound Healing: Alternatives in Management, 3rd ed. Philadelphia, FA Davis.

Kolt G, Snyder-Mackler L (2007). Physical Therapies in Sport and Exercise, 2nd ed. St Louis, Elsevier Churchill Livingstone.

Lacy C, Amstrong L, Goldman M, et al (2009). Drug Information Handbook, 15th ed. Hudson, OH, Lexi-Comp.

Law M, MacDermid J (2007). Evidence-Based Rehabilitation: A Guide to Practice, 2nd ed. Thorofare, NJ, Slack.

Leavitt R, ed. (1999). Cross-cultural Rehabilitation: An International Perspective. St Louis, Elsevier Saunders.

Levangie P, Norkin C (2005). Joint Structure and Function: A Comprehensive Analysis, 4th ed. Philadelphia, FA Davis.

Lewis C, Bottomley J, (2007). Geriatric Rehabilitation—A Clinical Approach, 3rd ed. Upper Saddle River, NJ, Pearson Education.

Lippert LS (2006). Clinical Kinesiology and Anatomy, 4th ed. Philadelphia, F A Davis.

Long T, Toscano K (2001). Handbook of Pediatric Physical Therapy, 2nd ed. Baltimore, Lippincott Williams & Wilkins.

Lundy-Ekman L (2007). Neuroscience Fundamentals for Rehabilitation, 3rd ed. St Louis, Elsevier Saunders.

Lusardi MM, Nielsen CC (eds) (2006). Orthotics and Prosthetics in Rehabilitation, 2nd ed. St Louis, Elsevier Butterworth-Heinemann.

Magee D (2008). Orthopedic Physical Assessment, 5th ed. St Louis, Elsevier Saunders.

Magee D, Zachazewski J, Quillen W (2007). Scientific Foundations and Principles of Practice in Musculoskeletal Rehabilitation. St Louis, Elsevier Saunders.

Magee D, Zachazewski J, Quillen W (2009). Pathology and Intervention in Musculoskeletal Rehabilitation. St Louis, Elsevier Saunders.

Malone D (2006). Physical Therapy in Acute Care: A Clinician's Guide. Thorofare, NJ, Slack.

Martin S, Kessler M (2006). Neurologic Interventions for Physical Therapy, 2nd ed. St Louis, Elsevier Saunders.

McArdle W, Katch F, Katch V (2006). Exercise Physiology: Energy, Nutrition and Human Performance, 5th ed. Philadelphia, Lippincott Williams & Wilkins.

McKinnis L (2005). Fundamentals of Musculoskeletal Imaging, 2nd ed. Philadelphia, FA Davis.

Michlovitz S (2005). Modalities for Therapeutic Intervention, 4th ed. Philadelphia, FA Davis.

Milne C, Corbett L, Dubuc, D (2003). Wound, Ostomy and Continence Secrets, Philadelphia, Hanley & Belfus.

Minor SM, Minor MS (2005). Patient Care Skills, 5th ed. Upper Saddle River, NJ, Prentice Hall Health.

Moore K (2006). Clinically Oriented Anatomy, 5th ed. Baltimore, Lippincott Williams & Wilkins.

Myers B (2004). Wound Management: Principles and Practice. Upper Saddle River, NJ, Prentice Hall.

Neumann DA (2009). Kinesiology of the Musculoskeletal System: Foundations for Physical Rehabilitation, 2nd ed. St Louis, Elsevier Mosby.

Norkin C, White J (2009). Measurement of Joint Motion: A Guide to Goniometry, 4th ed. Philadelphia, FA Davis.

Nosse L, Friberg D (2004). Managerial and Supervisory Principles for Physical Therapists, 2nd ed. Philadelphia, Lippincott Willliams & Wilkins.

Nyland J (2006). Clinical Decisions in Therapeutic Exercise—Planning and Implementation. Upper Saddle River NJ, Pearson Prentice Hall.

Oatis C (2008). Kinesiology: The Mechanics & Pathomechanics of Human Movement. Philadelphia, Lippincott Williams & Wilkins.

O'Sullivan S, Schmitz T (2007). Physical Rehabilitation, 5th ed. Philadelphia, F A Davis.

O'Sullivan S, Schmitz T (2010) Improving Functional Outcomes in Physical Rehabilitation. Philadelphia, FA Davis.

Pagliarulo M (2007). Introduction to Physical Therapy, 3rd ed. St Louis, Elsevier Mosby.

Paz J, West M (2002). Acute Care Handbook for Physical Therapists, 3rd ed. St Louis, Elsevier Butterworth-Heinneman.

Pierson F, Fairchild S (2008). Principles and Techniques of Patient Care, 4th ed. St Louis, Elsevier Saunders.

Porth C (2005). Pathophysiology, 7th ed. Philadelphia, Lippincott Williams & Wilkins.

Portney L, Watkins M (2008). Foundations of Clinical Research, 3rd ed. Upper Saddle River, NJ, Prentice Hall Health.

Prentice Q (2005). Therapeutic Modalities for Allied Health Professionals. New York, McGraw-Hill Medical.

Prentice WE, Voight MI (2001). Techniques in Musculoskeletal Rehabilitation. New York, McGraw-Hill.

Purtilo R (2005). Ethical Dimensions in the Health Professions, 4th ed. St Louis, Elsevier.

Purtilo R, Haddad A (2002). Health Professional and Patient Interaction, 6th ed. St Louis, Elsevier Saunders.

Quinn L, Gordon J (2009). Documentation for Rehabilitation: A Framework for Clinical Decision-Making, 2nd ed. Maryland Heights, MO, Elsevier.

Ratliff C, Bryant D (2003). Guideline For Prevention and Management of Pressure Ulcers, #2, Glenview.

Reese N (2005). Muscle and Sensory Testing, 2nd ed. St Louis, Elsevier Saunders.

Reese NB, Bandy WD (2002). Joint Range of Motion and Muscle Length. St Louis, Elsevier Saunders.

Robertson V, Ward A, Law J, Reed A (2006). Electrotherapy Explained: Principles and Practice, 3rd ed. Philadelphia, Butterworth-Heinemann.

Rothstein J, Roy S, Wolf S (2005). The Rehabilitation Specialist's Handbook, 3rd ed. Philadelphia, FA Davis.

Rubin M, Safdieh J (2007). Netter's Concise Neuroanatomy. St Louis, Elsevier Health Sciences.

Sackett D, et al. (2000). Evidence-Based Medicine. Philadelphia, Churchill Livingstone.

Sahrmann S (2002). Diagnosis and Treatment of Movement Impairment Syndromes. St Louis, Elsevier Mosby.

Saidoff D, McDonough A (2002). Critical Pathways in Therapeutic Intervention—Extremities and Spine. St Louis, Elsevier Mosby.

Salter R (1999). Textbook of Disorders and Injuries of the Musculoskeletal System, 3rd ed. Baltimore, Williams & Wilkins.

Saunders H, Saunders R (eds) (2004). Evaluation, Treatment and Prevention of Musculoskeletal Disorders & Spine, 4th ed. Chaska, MN, Saunders Group.

Schmidt R, Lee T (2005). Motor Control and Learning, 4th ed. Champaign, IL, Human Kinetics.

Scifers J (2008). Special Tests for Neurologic Examination. Thorofare, NJ, Slack.

Scott R (1998). Professional Ethics: A Guide for Rehabilitation Professionals. St. Louis, Elsevier Mosby.

Scott R (2006). Legal Aspects of Documenting Patient Care for Rehabilitation Professionals, 3rd ed. Boston, Jones & Bartlett.

Scott R, Petrosinol L (2008). Physical Therapy Management. St Louis, Elsevier Mosby.

Scuderi G, McCann P, Bruno P (eds) (2005). Sports Medicine, 2nd ed. St. Louis, Elsevier Mosby.

Seymour R (2002). Prosthetics and Orthotics: Lower Limb and Spinal. Philadelphia, Lippincott Williams & Wilkins.

Shepard K, Jensen G (2002). Handbook of Teaching for Physical Therapists, 2nd ed. St Louis, Elsevier Butterworth-Heinemann.

Shumway-Cook A, Woollacott M (2007). Motor Control—Theory and Practical Applications, 3rd ed. Philadelphia, Lippincott Williams & Wilkins.

Shurr D, Michael J (2001). Prosthetics and Orthotics, 2nd ed. Upper Saddle River, NJ, Prentice Hall.

Snell R (2005). Clinical Neuroanatomy for Medical Students, 6th ed. Philadelphia, Lippincott Williams & Wilkins.

Somers M (2001). Spinal Cord Injury Rehabilitation, 2nd ed. Upper Saddle River, NJ, Prentice Hall.

Standring S (2008). Gray's Anatomy: The Anatomical Basis of Clinical Practice. St Louis, Elsevier Churchill Livingstone.

Starkey C and Johnson G (2005). Athletic Training and Sports Medicine. American Academy of Orthopaedic Medicine. Sudbury MA, Jones & Bartlett.

Starkey C, Ryan J (2002). Evaluation of Orthopedic and Athletic Injuries, 2nd ed. Philadelphia, FA Davis.

Stephenson R, O'Connor L (2000) Obstetric and Gynecologic Care in Physical Therapy, 2nd ed. Thorofare, NJ, Slack.

Sussman C, Bates-Jenson B (2006). Wound Care: A Collaborative Practice Manual for Physical Therapists and Nurses, 3rd ed. Philadelphia, Lippincott Williams & Wilkins.

Swain J, Bush K, Brosing J (2009). Diagnostic Imaging for Physical Therapists. St Louis, Elsevier.

Tecklin J (2007). Pediatric Physical Therapy, 4th ed. Philadelphia, Lippincott Williams & Wilkins.

Thompson JC (2001). Netter's Concise Atlas of Orthopedic Anatomy. St Louis, Elsevier.

Umphred D (ed) (2007). Neurological Rehabilitation, 5th ed. St Louis, Elsevier Mosby.

Watchie J (2009). Cardiovascular and Pulmonary Physical Therapy: A Clinical Manual, 2nd ed. Maryland Heights, MO, Elsevier.

Waxman S (1999). Correlative Neuroanatomy, 25th ed. New York, McGraw-Hill.

Whittle M (2007). Gait Analysis, 4th ed. St Louis, Elsevier.

Wilmore J, Costill D, Kenney W (2007). Physiology of Sport and Exercise, 4th ed. Champaign, IL, Human Kinetics.

Young P, Young P, Tolbert D (2007). Basic Clinical Neuroscience. Philadelphia, Lippincott Williams & Wilkins.

Web Articles

Pino H. "Patient Management: The Exercise Prescription for the Obese Patient." *Bariatric Times* 2.2 (2005: 1044-7946. *Http://bariatrictimes.com/displayArticle.cfm?articleID=article65*. Web 12 Sep 2009.

Gallagher S. "Patient Transferring Challenges." *Bariatric Times*, article archive. (2009). *Http://bariatrictimes.com/2009/08/17/patient-transferring-challenges/*. Web 25 Aug 2009.

United States Government Websites

http://www.osha.gov/pls/oshaweb/searchresults.category?p_text=personal%20protection%20equipment%20in%20healthcare&p_title=&p_status=CURRENT.

http://www.osha.gov/SLTC/emergencypreparedness/index.html.

http://www.osha.gov/SLTC/etools/hospital/clinical/pt/pt.html#equipmenthazards.

http://www.eeoc.gov/types/sexual_harassment.html.

http://www.ed.gov/policy/speced/guid/edpicks.jhtml.

http://www.ada.gov/.

http://www.nlm.nih.gov/medlineplus/patientrights.html#cat1.

Websites

Occupational Health Clinics for Ontario Workers, Inc. *http://www.ohcow.on.ca/resourceshandbooks/patient_handling/patient_handling.htm*. Oct 2009.

Texas Medical Association. http://www.texmed.org/Template.aspx?id=4557. Oct 2009.

Academic Resources, Dean of Students Office Iowa State University, Academic Success Center. *http://www.dso.iastate.edu/asc/academic/test.html*. 27 Jun 2009.

Notetaking Systems, Academic Skill Center, Student Academic Services, California Polytechnic State University San Luis Obispo. *http://sas.calpoly.edu/asc/ssl/notetaking.systems.html*. 27 Jun 2009.

Index

Note: Page numbers followed by *f* and *t* figures and tables, respectively. Boxed material is indicated by *b*